Advanced Porous Biomaterials for Drug Delivery Applications

Advanced Porous Biomaterials for Drug Delivery Applications probes cutting-edge progress in the application of advanced porous biomaterials in drug delivery fields. These biomaterials offer promise in improving upon the design, cost, and creation of potent novel drug delivery systems. The book focuses on two categories: nature engineered and synthetic advanced porous biomaterials, with a wide range of low-cost porous biomaterial-based systems that have been used for the delivery of diverse drugs through in vitro/in vivo approaches.

- Details how advanced porous biomaterial-assisted systems improve essential properties in drug delivery applications
- Explains how advanced porous biomaterials systems are being used and explored to improve overall performances of drug delivery systems in mitigating a variety of diseases
- Emphasizes major applications in drug delivery such as controlled release, cancer therapy, and targeted delivery, and with focus on oral, topical, and transdermal applications
- Focuses on both naturally available and synthetic low-cost advanced porous biomaterials and their role in enhancing important parameters in drug delivery applications
- Accessible to readers with bio and non-bio backgrounds

This book is an ideal reference for academics, researchers, and industry professionals in the interdisciplinary fields of biomedicine and biomedical engineering, pharmaceuticals, materials science, and chemistry.

Emerging Materials and Technologies

Series Editor:
Boris I. Kharissov

Hybrid Polymeric Nanocomposites from Agricultural Waste
Sefiu Adekunle Bello

Photoelectrochemical Generation of Fuels
Edited by Anirban Das, Gyandshwar Kumar Rao, and Kasinath Ojha

Emergent Micro- and Nanomaterials for Optical, Infrared, and Terahertz Applications
Edited by Song Sun, Wei Tan, and Su-Huai Wei

Gas Sensors
Manufacturing, Materials, and Technologies
Edited by Ankur Gupta, Mahesh Kumar, Rajeev Kumar Singh, and Shantanu Bhattacharya

Environmental Biotechnology
Fundamentals to Modern Techniques
Sibi G

Emerging Two Dimensional Materials and Applications
Edited by Arun Kumar Singh, Ram Sevak Singh, and Anar Singh

Advanced Porous Biomaterials for Drug Delivery Applications
Edited by Mahaveer Kurkuri, Dusan Losic, U.T. Uthappa, and Ho-Young Jung

Thermal Transport Characteristics of Nanofluids and Phase Change Materials
S. Harikrishnan and A.D. Dhass

Multidimensional Lithium-Ion Battery Status Monitoring
Shunli Wang, Kailong Liu, Yujie Wang, Daniel-Ioan Stroe, Carlos Fernandez, and Josep M. Guerrero

For more information about this series, please visit: www.routledge.com/Emerging-Materials-and-Technologies/book-series/CRCEMT

Advanced Porous Biomaterials for Drug Delivery Applications

Edited by
Mahaveer Kurkuri, Dusan Losic,
U.T. Uthappa, and Ho-Young Jung

CRC Press
Taylor & Francis Group
Boca Raton London New York

CRC Press is an imprint of the
Taylor & Francis Group, an **informa** business

First edition published 2023
by CRC Press
6000 Broken Sound Parkway NW, Suite 300, Boca Raton, FL 33487-2742

and by CRC Press
4 Park Square, Milton Park, Abingdon, Oxon, OX14 4RN

CRC Press is an imprint of Taylor & Francis Group, LLC

Library of Congress Cataloging-in-Publication Data
Names: Kurkuri, Mahaveer, editor. | Losic, Dusan, editor. | Uthappa, U. T., editor. | Jung, Ho-Young, editor.
Title: Advanced porous biomaterials for drug delivery applications / edited by Mahaveer Kurkuri, Dusan Losic, U.T. Uthappa and Ho-Young Jung.
Description: First edition. | Boca Raton, FL : CRC Press, 2023. | Includes bibliographical references and index.
Identifiers: LCCN 2022023520 | ISBN 9781032107981 (hardback) | ISBN 9781032108025 (paperback) | ISBN 9781003217114 (ebook)
Subjects: MESH: Drug Delivery Systems—methods | Biocompatible Materials—therapeutic use | Porosity | Aluminum Silicates—therapeutic use | Metal-Organic Frameworks—therapeutic use
Classification: LCC RS199.5 | NLM QV 785 | DDC 615/.6—dc23/eng/20220906
LC record available at https://lccn.loc.gov/2022023520

ISBN: 978-1-032-10798-1 (hbk)
ISBN: 978-1-032-10802-5 (pbk)
ISBN: 978-1-003-21711-4 (ebk)

DOI: 10.1201/9781003217114

Typeset in Sabon
by codeMantra

We reverently bow our heads and dedicate this book to God Almighty for giving us the perseverance to complete this work. We also dedicate this contribution to our beloved family members for their unconditional support and blessings throughout our lives.

Prof. Mahaveer Kurkuri

Prof. Dusan Losic

A/Prof. U. T. Uthappa

Prof. Ho-Young Jung

Contents

Foreword by Dr. Chenraj Roychand

It is my great pleasure to introduce this book to the scientific community. I am very proud and honored to introduce this important compilation of advanced porous biomaterials for drug delivery applications. It is increasingly clear that advanced porous biomaterials with cutting-edge properties will play a significant role in meeting the world's future needs, specifically in the field of nanomedicine/pharmaceutics. Most recently, the research community working on advanced porous biomaterials has initiated to tackle the challenges associated with the field of drug delivery applications. The editors of this book are having an outstanding research track record and are capable of compiling and advocating the current trends in advanced porous biomaterials in the drug delivery research domain. Prof. Mahaveer Kurkuri is serving as the Associate Director at the Centre for Research in Functional Materials (CRFM), Jain (Deemed-to-be University); Dr U. T. Uthappa, who is a talented young researcher and Alma Mater of Jain (Deemed-to-be University), is currently serving as an Assistant International Research Professor at Yeungnam University, Republic of Korea.

The other two editors of this book Prof. Dusan Losic, Adelaide University, Australia, and Prof. Ho-Young Jung, Chonnam National University, South Korea, are very well-known scientists of international repute who have joined their hands in bringing up this book. Undoubtedly, all the authors of this book have brought in their best efforts as editors, and the book will set a benchmark in porous materials specifically for drug delivery applications. I extend my appreciation to CRC Press (T&F Group), which has once again proved its commitment to publishing vital, enriching, and research-centric books that are critical to the research and development cycle. The book starts with an introduction to advanced natural and synthetic porous biomaterials for drug delivery applications and covers the significance of all such advanced porous biomaterials. Comprising substantial compilations of advanced research findings, this book would serve as a comprehensive survey of the state of the field. These compilations will be of significant interest to academicians, scientists, researchers, upper-level undergraduates,

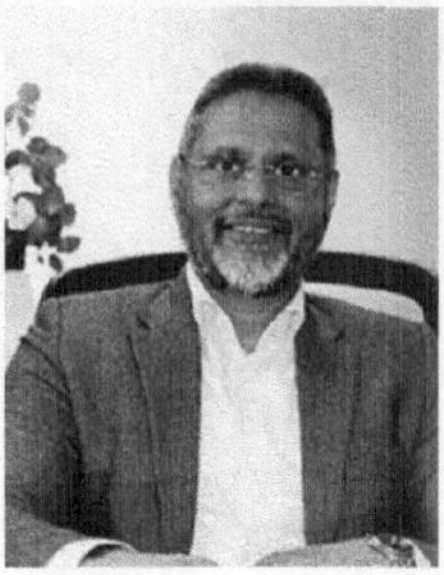

graduates, and engineers as well as technologists working in the field of biomaterials or related areas.

Dr. Chenraj Roychand
Chancellor of Jain (Deemed-to-be University), Bengaluru, Karnataka, India

Preface

This book, written by an excellent group of professionals, is a new and interesting compilation of the latest achievements and developments in one of the most popular fields of interest known as advanced porous biomaterials. Biomaterials developed by engineers, chemists, physicists, biologists, and clinicians with a cooperative effort are being used for more than 60 years in innovative drug delivery systems. These diverse biomaterials have enriched the pharmacokinetic and pharmacodynamics properties of several pharmaceutical drugs/compounds. Many of these biomaterials are intended to release therapeutic materials for prolonged/controlled periods (hours/days/weeks/months). Further, they can be transformed to reach particular target sites/locations within the body. Consequently, they achieve the desired therapeutic effects by decreasing the amount of medication and thereby reducing the associated risks to the patient. Because of all these facts, and in contrast to the existing biomaterials, the exploration of "advanced porous biomaterials" with unique properties, displaying unprecedented advantages over existing biomaterials, is always of high general interest and demand.

Additionally, the surface properties of advanced porous biomaterial systems can be improved in a more advanced manner compared to the existing biomaterials used in the current drug delivery fields. Likewise, such modifications help in the design and development of advanced drug delivery systems. Moreover, as these systems are cost effective, the advanced porous biomaterial systems can be extensively used in the biomedicinal field. The goal of this book is to highlight the recent advances in advanced porous biomaterials research, which includes both natural and synthetic porous biomaterials. Consequently, the book delivers a particular emphasis on understanding its characteristics, preparation/fabrication methods, various surface modifications/functionalization strategies, and their respective drug delivery applications (in vitro/in vivo). The book contains 14 chapters that deal with the most advanced porous biomaterials and their applications in drug delivery systems. We believe that this book will deliver significant contributions to the rapidly evolving field of drug delivery.

Therefore, this book is an ideal source of reference for several readerships in biomedical fields, pharmaceuticals, and nanotechnology-related companies; academicians, researchers, and professionals; industrialists from chemistry, material science, and technological backgrounds; and interested general public/audience as well. Additionally, the book is an ideal source for all those who wish to broaden their knowledge in the field of drug delivery field.

Prof. Mahaveer Kurkuri
Prof. Dusan Losic
A/Prof. U. T. Uthappa
Prof. Ho-Young Jung

Acknowledgments

This book has been reserved on a path through the accomplishment, support, and encouragement of several people, together with our knowledgeable authors, who have contributed their vast scientific knowledge to strengthen this book. The CRC Press team and Allison Shatkin, who guided us throughout the publication process; our parent institutions, Jain (Deemed-to-be University), Bengaluru, Karnataka, India, the University of Adelaide, South Australia, Chonnam National University and Yeungnam University, Republic of Korea. Also, we would like to acknowledge Aimee Wragg, Editorial Assistant, CRC Press team for her kind assistance in every stage, which made us to accomplish this book project in a successful manner. Prof. Kurkuri would like to acknowledge the continuous support being given by Mr. M. S. Parswanath, Director, Projects and Facilities, Jain (Deemed-to-be University), India. This book contribution would never have been possible without their unconditional support.

Prof. Mahaveer Kurkuri
Prof. Dusan Losic
A/Prof. U. T. Uthappa
Prof. Ho-Young Jung

Editors

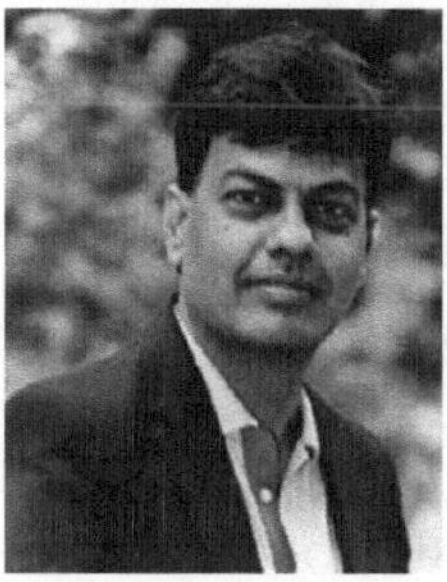

Prof. Mahaveer Kurkuri

Mahaveer Kurkuri is currently working as a Professor and Associate Director at the Centre for Research in Functional Materials (CRFM), Jain (Deemed-to-be University), India. He has received his PhD degree in Polymer Chemistry from Karnataka University, Dharwad, India in 2003. He worked in various well-known reputed universities as Post-Doctoral Fellow at KAIST, South Korea (2004–2006); Research Associate, Flinders University, Australia (2006–2008); and Research Fellow at the University of Adelaide, Australia (2008–2014). Since 2014, he is associated with Jain (Deemed-to-be University), India. He has published more than 70 papers in peer-reviewed journals with more than 2630 citations and h-index: 31. His current research interests are drug delivery, water treatment, energy, microfluidics, supramolecular chemistry, biosensors, ion detection, molecular logic gates, and surface chemistry in general to mimic the nature, particularly utilizing the understandings in nano and bio areas.

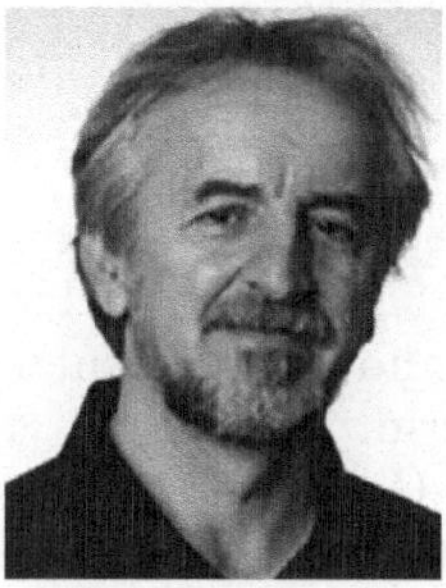

Prof. Dusan Losic

Dusan Losic is a Professor and Graphene Hub Director at the School of Chemical Engineering and Advanced Materials, University of Adelaide, and the leader of Nano Research Group with 20 researchers. He completed his PhD (2003) in Nanoscience and Nanotechnology (Flinders University, Australia), which is one of the first PhDs in Australia in this field. After 3 years of post-doctoral work at Flinders University, in 2007 he received ARC Research Fellowship (5 years) starting his independent research at the University of South Australia (Ian Wark Research Institute). In 2012, he received ARC Future Fellowship and joined the University of Adelaide with his research group. His multidisciplinary research involves fundamental, engineering, and applied aspects across disciplines of nanotechnology, chemistry, materials science, engineering, medicine, and agriculture with focus on engineering of new nanomaterials, new properties, and their applications to address concerning problems in health, environment, agriculture, and energy. He has published more than 470 publications in leading journals and conferences, including 3 edited books, 20 book chapters, 300 journal papers, 80 conference papers, 120 conference abstracts, and 9 patents, attracting ca. 20,500 citations, h-index: 78 and 14 journal covers. He has also presented 5 plenary, 10 key, and 20 invited conference lectures, and 100 invited talks and seminars at universities worldwide. He has received approximately $20 M in research funding in the last 10 years completing 40 research projects, half involving industry with an outstanding track record in research translation (5 licensing technologies).

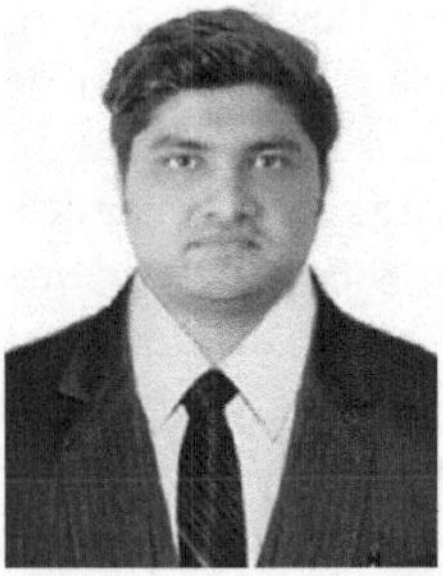

Dr. U. T. Uthappa
Dr. U. T. Uthappa is currently working as an Assistant International Research Professor at the School of Chemical Engineering, Yeungnam University, Republic of Korea. He has received his PhD degree in Chemistry from Jain (Deemed-to-be University), India in 2020. Prior to joining Yeungnam University, he worked as Post-Doctoral Fellow at Chonnam National University, South Korea (2021–2022). His core research interest lies in the design of novel biomaterials for drug delivery (controlled release and targeted drug delivery) and water treatment applications. He has published more than 24 papers in peer-reviewed journals with more than 600 citations and h-index: 14. Dr. Uthappa has published his research works in high-impact journals such as *Journal of Controlled Release*, *Applied Surface Science*, *Trends in Analytical Chemistry*, *Chemosphere*, *Advances in Colloid and Interface Science*, and *ACS Biomaterials Science & Engineering*.

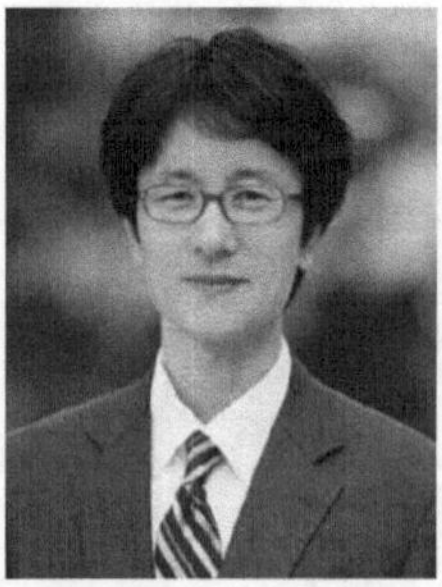

Prof. Ho-Young Jung
Ho-Young Jung serves as full-time Professor for Environment and Energy Engineering Department at Chonnam National University, South Korea. He obtained his PhD in Chemical and Biomolecular Engineering at KAIST in 2007. Prior to joining as Professor at Chonnam National University, South Korea, he worked in various well-known reputed universities as Post-Doctoral Fellow at KAIST (2007–2008), Research Associate at USC (2008–2009), Assistant Professor at Kangwon National University (2009–2012), and Associate

Professor at Chonnam National University, South Korea. His research interests include energy storage devices, batteries, membranes, drug delivery, and water treatments. He has published more than 90 research papers in internationally recognized peer-reviewed journals and has more than 25 patents to his credit.

Contributors

Mahesh P. Bhat
Agricultural Automation Research Center
Chonnam National University
Yeosu, Republic of Korea

Varsha P. Brahmkhatri
Nanomaterials for Drug Delivery and Therapeutics (NDT-Lab), Centre for Nano and Material Science
Jain (Deemed-to-be University)
Bengaluru, India

Tafadzwa Justin Chiome
Division of Nanoscience & Technology, School of Life Sciences
Centre of Excellence in Molecular Biology & Regenerative Medicine
JSS Academy of Higher Education & Research
Mysuru, India

Sharon George
Centre for Nano and Material Sciences
Jain (Deemed-to-be University)
Bengaluru, India

Karan Gulati
School of Dentistry
The University of Queensland
Herston, Australia

M. Hadden
School of Biomedical Engineering
University of Sydney
Sydney, Australia

Heon-Ho Jeong
Department of Chemical and Biomolecular Engineering
Chonnam National University
Yeosu, Republic of Korea

K. Kant
Departamento de Química Física
University of Vigo
Vigo, Spain

Manika Khanuja
Centre of Nanoscience and Nanotechnology
Jamia Millia Islamia
New Delhi, India

Madhuprasad Kigga
Centre for Research in Functional Materials
Jain (Deemed-to-be University)
Bengaluru, India

Ganesh Kokil
School of Materials Science and Engineering
and
Australian Centre for Nanomedicine
University of New South Wales
Sydney, Australia

Tushar Kumeria
School of Materials Science and Engineering
and
Australian Centre for Nanomedicine
University of New South Wales
Sydney, Australia

Mahaveer Kurkuri
Centre for Research in Functional Materials
Jain (Deemed-to-be University)
Bengaluru, India

Kyeong-Hwan Lee
Agricultural Automation Research Center
Chonnam National University
Yeosu, Republic of Korea

Dusan Losic
School of Chemical Engineering and Advanced Materials
The University of Adelaide
Adelaide, Australia

Shaheer Maher
School of Chemical Engineering and Advanced Materials
The University of Adelaide
Adelaide, Australia
and
Faculty of Pharmacy
Assiut University
Assiut, Egypt

Remya Pakkukalayil Narayanan
Global Academy of Technology
Bengaluru, India

Shajesh Palantavida
Centre for Nano and Material Sciences
Jain (Deemed-to-be University)
Kanakapura, India

Arvind Raj
Centre for Research in Functional Materials
Jain (Deemed-to-be University)
Bengaluru, India

Yogambha Ramaswamy
School of Biomedical Engineering
and
Sydney Nano Institute
The University of Sydney
Sydney, Australia

Pranita Rananaware
Nanomaterials for Drug Delivery and Therapeutics (NDT-Lab), Centre for Nano and Material Science
Jain (Deemed-to-be University)
Bengaluru, India

Richelle M. Rego
Centre for Research in Functional Materials
Jain (Deemed-to-be University)
Bengaluru, India

Ayad Saeed
School of Materials Science and Engineering
University of New South Wales
Sydney, Australia

Astha Sharma
School of Materials Science and Engineering
University of New South Wales
Sydney, Australia

Gurvinder Singh
School of Biomedical Engineering
and
Sydney Nano Institute
University of Sydney
Sydney, Australia

Manoj Kumar Singh
Department of Physics
School of Engineering and Technology (SOET)
Central University of Haryana
Jant-Pali, India

Pratap Singh
Department of Physics
Central University of Haryana
Jant-Pali, India

Asha Srinivasan
Division of Nanoscience & Technology, School of Life Sciences
Centre of Excellence in Molecular Biology & Regenerative Medicine
JSS Academy of Higher Education & Research
Mysore, India

R. Tiwari
Department of Chemistry
Kali Charan Nigam Institute of Technology (KCNIT)
Banda, India

Nahid Tyagi
Department of Physics
Central University of Haryana
Jant-Pali, India
and
Jamia Millia Islamia
New Delhi, India

U. T. Uthappa
School of Chemical Engineering
Yeungnam University
Gyeongsan, Republic of Korea

Baiju Kizhakekilikoodail Vijayan
Department of Chemistry/Nanoscience
Kannur University
Payyannur, India

C. Viray
School of Biomedical Engineering
University of Sydney
Sydney, Australia

Zhenxu Yang
School of Biomedical Engineering
The University of Sydney
Sydney, Australia

Part A

Overview of Drug Delivery and Porous Materials

Chapter 1

A Brief Overview of Drug Delivery Systems and Significance of Advanced Porous Biomaterials in the Drug Delivery Field

U.T. Uthappa
Yeungnam University

Heon-Ho Jeong
Chonnam National University

Mahaveer Kurkuri
Jain (Deemed-to-be University)

CONTENTS

1.1 INTRODUCTION

The advent of innovative porous biomaterials designed from advanced nanoengineered techniques in the drug delivery (DD) field has made significant development in the past decade. The ideal drug delivery system (DDS)

DOI: 10.1201/9781003217114-2

delivers an adequate amount of therapeutic agent to definite sites for action in a safe and efficient manner, with improved dosage, required time, and drug release profile, to attain the desired therapeutic effects without causing harm to surrounding cells and tissues in the human body (Mainardes and Silva 2004). In the DD field, one of the key aspects is to find the most efficient, cost-effective, and time-efficient strategy to deliver drugs/therapeutics/biomolecules to specified areas in the shortest feasible period with the least extent of harm and complications. Traditional DDSs fall short of these requirements since they typically deliver rapid drug release into the bloodstream over a short period (Drews 2000). Although frequent dosage might eliminate hazardous peaks and subtherapeutic troughs, it leads to poor patient compliance. Traditional DD via tablets or intravenous injections with toxic drugs can have negative side effects which cause damage to healthy cells/organs, whereas less intrusive measures are ineffective in toxic manifestation when treating diseases that can spread to other parts of the body, despite posing fewer risks (Hoffman 2008).

The global pharmaceutical drug delivery market is projected to reach USD 2,206.5 billion by 2026 from USD 1,656.9 billion in 2021, at a CAGR of 5.9% (https://www.marketsandmarkets.com/Market-Reports/drug-delivery-technologies market-1085.html). It has been observed that current research on porous micro/nano biomaterials is rapidly gaining prominence in the human health care sectors (Santos 2012). Microparticles are substances that range in size from one micron to a few millimeters. They are used in DDSs because when a specific active species, such as a drug, is encapsulated or administered into a carrier or matrices, the drug is protected from the environment, sensitive drugs are prevented, bioavailability is improved, and the toxicity and side effects of the drug are reduced (Kumar et al. 2011). As a result, porous materials have the potential to increase physiochemical capabilities as well as drug dissolving properties in the oral/targeted drug delivery region. Surface modification or functionalization of porous materials can thus be used to increase the adsorption capacity and release rate of specific drug molecules (Solano Umaña and Vega Baudrit 2015). Hierarchical porous materials are well known for having a wide range of structural properties, including a large surface area, a porous network, and small pore sizes. Because of their distinct chemical, physical, and surface morphological qualities, porous materials have crucial characteristics (De Stefano et al. 2011). The overall schematic overview and some specific advantages of porous carriers toward DD applications are shown in Figure 1.1.

1.2 DIFFERENT TYPES OF DRUG DELIVERY SYSTEMS (DDSs)

The main objectives of DDSs are listed below.

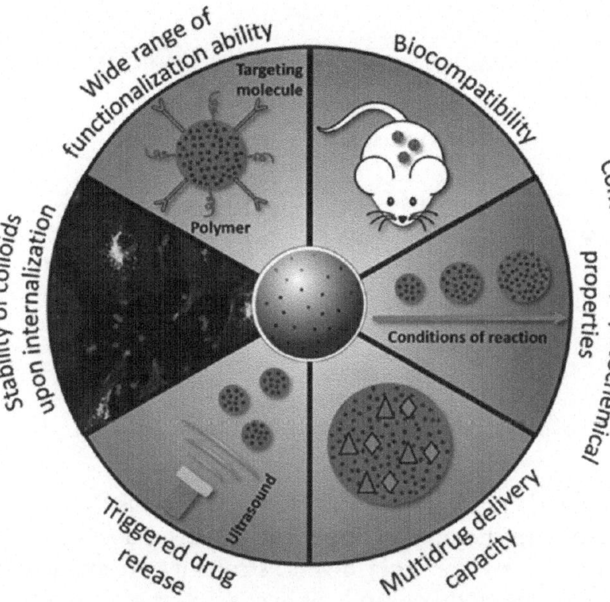

Figure 1.1 Schematic overview and importance of porous carriers for DD applications (Trofimov et al. 2018). (Open access, the Authors under Creative Commons Attribution 4.0 International license (http://creativecommons.org/licenses/by/4.0/), published by MDPI.)

1.2.1 Controlled DDSs

The use of controlled release technologies to deliver drugs was instigated in the 1970s and has extended to grow very rapidly (Li et al. 2004). The word "controlled release" has a connotation that refers to the selection of a long-acting drug release mechanism. Controlled drug delivery systems (CDDSs) aid in the transfer of a uniform concentration of drug to the adsorption site and allow for the maintenance of therapeutic plasma drug concentrations. It also reduces the number of negative effects and drug administrations (Deepu, Mathew, and Shamna 2014). The graph for the plasma drug concentration is shown in Figure 1.2.

1.2.2 Targeted DDSs

The phrase "targeted drug delivery" refers to a smart DDS that enables the therapeutic agent to be carried and delivered to a specific place or site within the body for an extended period. This type of system allows the body to maintain desired plasma and tissue drug levels while avoiding harm to healthy tissues. Targeted drug delivery systems not only deliver therapeutic agents to the exact places or locations where they are needed, but also

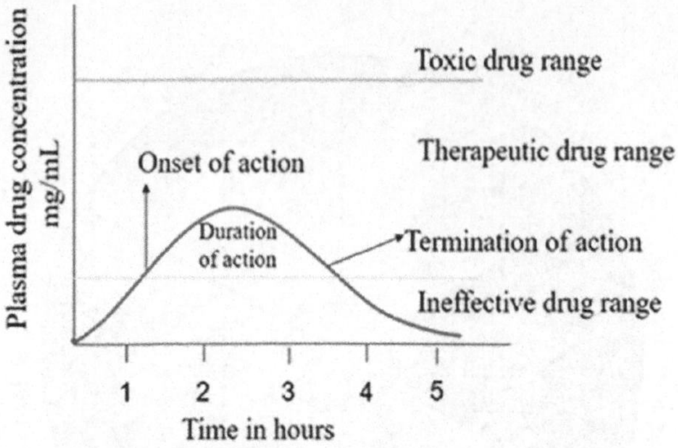

Figure 1.2 Graph explaining plasma drug concentration.

help improve the therapeutic efficiency of medications by lowering the toxicity associated with them, allowing for lower drug doses to be utilized for therapy. As a result, two primary diverse strategies are extensively explored and employed to satisfy these kinds of needs.

1.2.2.1 Passive Targeting

The accumulation of drug/drug carrier system at a necessary definite location or place, where the anti-cancer drug could be ascribed due to the disease's physicochemical or pharmacological features, is known as passive targeting. To avert uptake by the reticuloendothelial system (RES) and increase circulation time for potential targeting ability, the size and surface features of created DDSs must be managed and optimized in cancer treatment. Normally, passive targeting relies on a straightforward medication delivery strategy via blood circulation. The drug release or activities are restricted to certain areas of the body, such as tumors, in this case.

1.2.2.2 Active Targeting

It's a specialized ligand-receptor interface for intracellular localization that can merely happen after blood circulation and extravasations. This type of active targeting is divided into three categories:

1. Limited distribution of drug carrier systems to the capillary bed of a predetermined target site, such as organs or tissues, is denoted as first-level targeting.
2. Second-level targeting denotes the precise delivery of medications to certain cell types, such as tumor cells rather than normal cells.
3. Targeting drug delivery to the intracellular place of targeted cells is referred to as the third level, which is based on the endocytosis-assisted

delivery of a drug complex into a cell using a receptor-based ligand (Rani and Paliwal 2014).

1.3 IMPORTANCE OF POROUS MATERIALS IN DRUG DELIVERY

Porous materials have void regions encased in their bulk structures, providing a large surface area for interaction with drug/guest molecules. This provides additional inherent benefits in applications like drug adsorptions/interactions (Hu and Srinivasan 1999, 2001). Porous materials have acquired tremendous interest as controlled drug delivery matrices due to their outstanding features such as stable identical porous structure, high surface area, controllable pore sizes with a narrow distribution, and tunable surface properties (Sher et al. 2007, Shivanand and Sprockel 1998). Porous carriers are being used in pharmaceuticals for the development of novel, floating, targeted, controlled, sustained DDSs and to improve the solubility of poorly soluble drugs due to their extensive range of useful features (Sharma et al. 2005, Streubel, Siepmann, and Bodmeier 2003, Yuasa, Takashima, and Kanaya 1996, Streubel, Siepmann, and Bodmeier 2002, Salis et al. 2003, Byrne and Deasy 2002). These porous systems have a large number of nanopores, which allow therapeutics to be included in a well-defined manner (Wang et al. 2006). These characteristics enable them to absorb and release various forms of drugs in a more consistent and predictable mode.

1.4 CLASSIFICATION OF POROUS MATERIALS

Drug delivery via mesoporous, microporous, and nonporous carriers is a burgeoning field of study (Song, Hidajat, and Kawi 2005, Andersson et al. 2004). Porous materials, whether formed naturally or artificially, offer wide prospects specifically in the DD field. Their pore structure is usually generated naturally or during the synthetic conditions or crystallization process or after further processing such as calcination or solvent extraction. The synthetic process results in the development of interconnecting mesopores that can be identical or dissimilar in size and shape (Sing 1985). The general class of porous materials/carriers employed in the DD field is represented in Table 1.1 (Ahuja and Pathak 2009). Additionally, the classification of porous materials according to pore size and build-up framework is shown in Figure 1.3.

1. Pore size: A porous material's pore size is essential because it influences drug entrapment and can be used as a DD strategy. The soaking/impregnation using a highly concentrated drug solution is a popular method of drug trapping within the pores (nearly saturated solution).

Table 1.1 The Importance of Textural Properties on Adsorption/Entrapment of Drug Molecules on or into the Porous Materials Is Discussed Below

Types of Pores	*Pore Dimensions*	*Pore Formation*
Microporous	Width less than 2 nm	Created as a result of the defective filling of constituent molecules
Mesoporous	Width between 2 and 50 nm	Effect of key defects in the structure
Macroporous	Width greater than 50 nm	Produced chief lattice structure defects such as racks, fissures, and etching networks

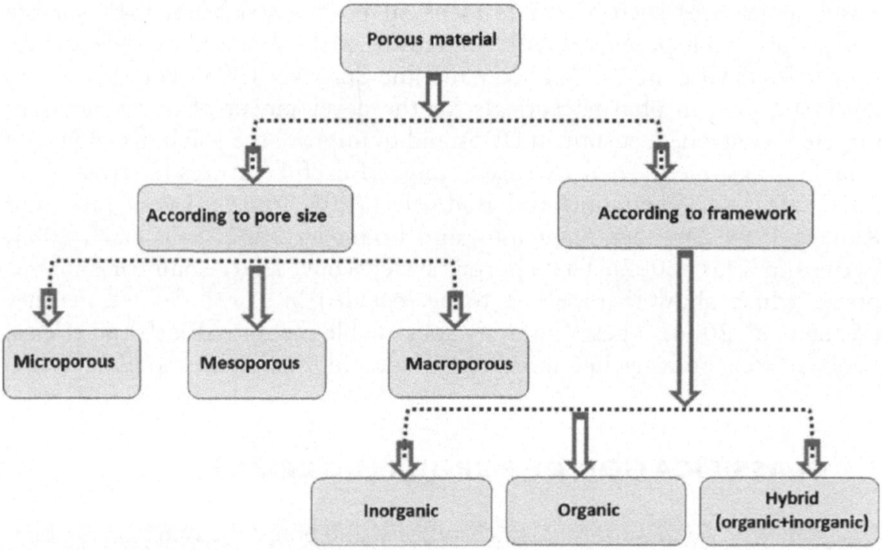

Figure 1.3 General classification of porous materials according to pore size and build-up framework.

Several other parameters must be addressed during the drug loading process, such as solvent, concentration, pH, temperature, speed of mixing, and duration of agitation (Kresge et al. 1992, Fan et al. 2003).

2. Surface area: The adsorptive capabilities of porous material are largely responsible for the drug loading process. The porous material's surface property is a crucial factor for drug adsorption and loading. The material's surface area speeds up the contact time among the host and guest molecules. Various parameters such as size, morphology, texture, and porosity are the functions of surface area (Brunauer, Emmett, and Teller 1938).

3. Pore volume: Encapsulation/loading of drug molecules with an improved payload is potential due to the substantial surface area, and high pore volume is one of the critical points to be considered (Hartmann 2005). In addition, continuous, repeated, and consecutive impregnations result in the total pore volume filling that can attain a superior payload of drug molecules. The constant impregnation enhances the amount of drug loading and assists with intermolecular drug-drug interactions (Charnay et al. 2004).

1.5 NATURAL POROUS MATERIALS

Porous materials, either natural or synthetic, attained more interest due to their exceptional characteristic features. From nature, an extensive range of porous biomaterials can be obtained by employing biological evolution that might be low cost, might have low impact on the environment, and might be abundant in nature. Some of the very important advanced nature designed/naturally available and synthetic porous materials, their evolution, significant properties, and utilization in DD applications are briefly outlined below. However, detailed insights regarding properties, synthesis process, and their application focused on DD domains will be presented in chapters of Parts B and C. The schematic representation with various external and internal triggering mechanisms involved for porous materials for drug delivery applications is shown in Figure 1.4.

a. Silk fibroins: The Food and Drug Administration (FDA) has officially acknowledged silk fibroins (SF) as a biocompatible material for the creation of a variety of nanotechnological tools (Melke et al. 2016). In comparison to other commonly used degradable biological polymers in the pharmaceutical sector, such as polylactide, poly(lactic-co-glycolic acid), and collagen, the majority of studies have indicated that SF has superior biocompatibility and a lesser immunogenic response (Hawe et al. 2012, Numata et al. 2010, Meinel et al. 2004). Among various SF species, mulberry silk generated mostly by the silkworm *Bombyx mori* accounts for 90% of the silk supply (Kaplan et al. 1993). Silk is a natural polymeric biomaterial with unique structural features such as low cost, self-assembling ability, mechanical strength, processing flexibility, biodegradability, and biocompatibility to meet DD requirements (Numata and Kaplan 2010).
b. Diatoms: In 2010, diatoms were explored for the first time as a drug carrier by Losic et al. (2010). Diatoms are well known as photosynthetic algae composed of SiO_2 covered with frustules (Uthappa, Kurkuri, and Kigga 2019). Diatoms offer several unique properties, including nontoxicity, biocompatibility, chemical stability, and low

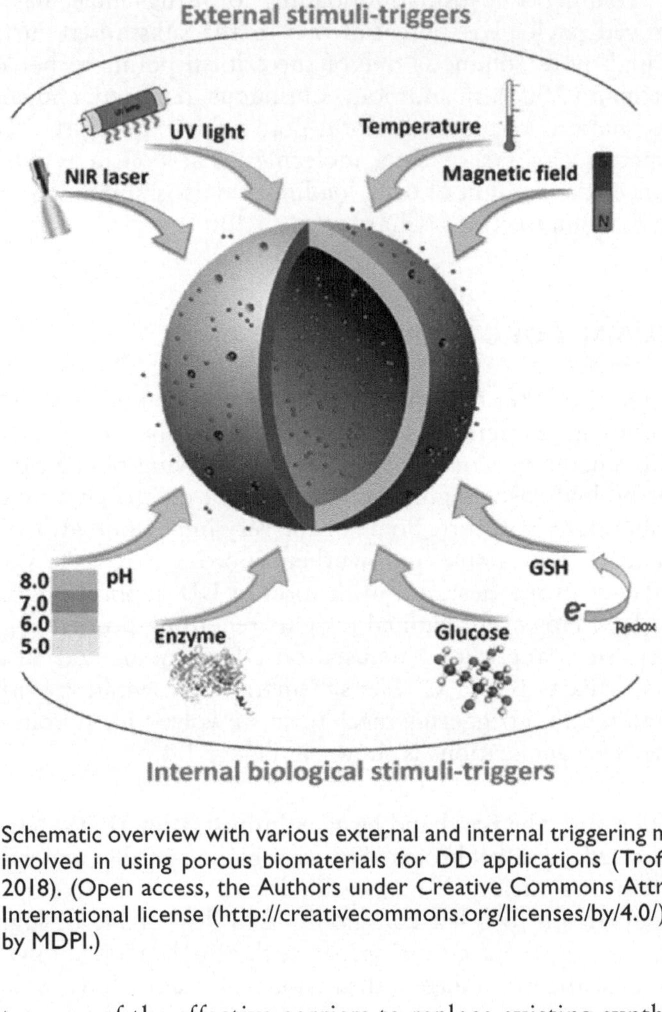

Figure 1.4 Schematic overview with various external and internal triggering mechanisms involved in using porous biomaterials for DD applications (Trofimov et al. 2018). (Open access, the Authors under Creative Commons Attribution 4.0 International license (http://creativecommons.org/licenses/by/4.0/), published by MDPI.)

cost as one of the effective carriers to replace existing synthetic silica (Bariana, Aw, and Losic 2013, Bariana et al. 2013, Uthappa et al. 2018, 2019).

c. Nanoclay: There are around 30 different varieties of nanoclays based on their mineralogical composition, which are employed in various applications depending on their qualities. The arrangement of these layers distinguishes the clay minerals into different classes such as kaolinite, hectorite, halloysite, and montmorillonite. Nanoclays are made up of layers of stacked tetrahedral/octahedral sheets. These nanoclays have some excellent properties such as high porosities with better surface features, low density, exceptional biocompatible, diffusion-controlled release mechanisms, and thermal and chemical stability (Williams and Haydel 2010, Carretero 2002, Khurana et al. 2015).

d. Zeolites: Because of the regular and uniform geometry of their pores and ion exchange capacities, zeolites have been a focus of contemporary drug release system research for the regulated administration of pharmaceuticals (Krajišnik et al. 2019). Some of the extensive scientific studies have leveraged that the enormous pore sizes available in some zeolite architectures help to release loaded drug molecules in a free manner from the porous zeolite architectures (Bacakova et al. 2018).
e. Calcium carbonate ($CaCO_3$) and calcium phosphate ($CaPO_4$):, This nanoparticles have been employed since the early 1990s, and there is no report on their hazardous effects (Biradar et al. 2012). These inorganic nanoparticles have been employed to limit the release of various kinds of drugs in numerous forms due to their extended biodegradation timescales. Indeed, because of the slow degradation of $CaCO_3$ matrices, most of the drugs can be preserved for a long time after administration. These porous inorganic nanoparticles behave as a good drug delivery carrier because of their natural abundance, low cost, safety, biocompatibility, pH sensitivity, osteoconductivity, and slow biodegradability properties (Yang, Sheldon, and Webster 2010, Zhou et al. 2015).

1.6 SYNTHETIC POROUS MATERIALS

a. Metal-organic frameworks (MOFs): In comparison to traditional porous materials like zeolites and activated carbons, MOFs, also known as porous coordination polymers (PCPs), are made up of organic linkers and metal ions or clusters and have emerged as a new type of crystalline material with large surface area (1,000–10,000 m^2/g), high porosity, tunable structural features, and flexible tailorability (Li et al. 2016, Allendorf and Stavila 2015, Furukawa et al. 2013, Uthappa et al. 2020). Porous MOFs for the first time were explored in 2006 by Horcajada et al. for DD application (Horcajada et al. 2006). The main disadvantage of MOFs is their limited stability, which can lead to toxicity issues and poor therapeutic response, limiting their biological applications (Yao, Liu, and Li 2021).
b. Covalent-organic frameworks (COFs): COFs are crystalline porous organic polymeric frameworks that are mostly made up of light elements (H, B, C, N, and O) arranged in a periodic pattern. They are more stable than MOFs because they are made up of molecular building blocks joined by covalent connections. COFs possess excellent properties such as high-specific surface area, precisely tailored pores with geometry, active sites, flexible molecular structures, low density, exclusive electrical, magnetic, and optical properties (Yao, Liu, and Li 2021). As an alternative to MOFs, several series of COFs have

been designed and constructed to overcome such limitations. The first COF was synthesized by Yaghi et al. in 2005 (Cote et al. 2005) and emerged as an innovative drug carrier in 2015 (Fang et al. 2015).

c. Nanoporous anodic alumina (NAA): NAA is produced using an electrochemical anodization process, an inorganic framework of non-erodible porous substrates through distinct morphologies (Jani, Losic, and Voelcker 2013). These are the intrinsic features "bio-inertness, chemical/mechanical/thermal stability, high-specific surface area, tunable pore diameters, and high porosities facilitates to control of the release of drugs" (Santos et al. 2014, Jani, Losic, and Voelcker 2013). NAA has been extensively investigated in a variety of in vitro and in vivo studies to solve a variety of crucial issues in drug delivery fields (Santos et al. 2014, Losic and Simovic 2009).
d. Porous titanium (Ti): Due to its large specific surface area, ordered structure, customizable pore size, excellent biocompatibility, and easily modifiable surface, TiO_2 has gained a lot of attention. Porous TiO_2 with various morphologies, pore diameters, and structures has been widely investigated to date in DD applications (Cui et al. 2021).
e. Porous silicon (Si): Leigh Canham proved the biocompatibility of porous Si in the mid-1990s for its usage in vivo. Insulin administration through monolayers of Caco-2 cells was the first report of drug delivery from porous Si across a cellular barrier (Anglin et al. 2008). Because of its amazing features such as high surface area (up to $800\,m^2/g$), biocompatibility, and biodegradability, while keeping drug bioactivity, porous Si (pSi) is an appealing material for DD applications. Furthermore, nanostructured pSi has demonstrated unique optical and luminescent features (Zhang et al. 2019).
f. Graphene oxides (GO): Graphene has extraordinary physiochemical properties with improved structural geometries, high Young's modulus, better fracture strength, outstanding electrical and thermal conductivity, quick charge carrier mobility, high-specific surface area, and biocompatibility (Geim 2009, Kakran and Li 2012, Kumeria et al. 2013). In 2008, the pioneer work of Dai's team showed PEG-functionalized graphene oxide to load anti-cancer drugs via non-covalent physisorption and has in vitro cellular absorptions (Liu et al. 2008, Sun et al. 2008).
g. Fullerenes: Fullerene, a carbon allotrope, is a nanoscale carbon material with distinctive photochemical, electrochemical, and physical properties. The low systemic toxicity makes it a promising candidate for target-specific drug administration in the body. Fullerenes for drug delivery are still in the initial stages of improvement due to their intrinsic hydrophobicity, which limits their usage in biology (Montellano et al. 2011, Shi et al. 2014).
h. Carbon nanotubes (CNTs): CNTs are carbon graphitic nanomaterials that are hollow and organized, with a wide range of features including

high surface area, high aspect ratio, ultralightweight, facile modifications, and acceptable biocompatibility (Sahoo et al. 2011, Kaur, Gill, and Jeet 2019). Despite their remarkable characteristics, there are technical challenges faced while using CNTs such as lack of solubility, dispersibility, and poor processability issues. Functionalization and solubilization of CNTs have recently attained considerable attention to overcome this problem of poor processability and to fully use the features of CNTs. This greatly broadens their application possibilities specifically in the DD field (Dubey et al. 2021)

1.7 CONCLUSION AND FUTURE PERSPECTIVES

Although, some of the above-mentioned advanced porous biomaterials have been extensively explored and studied for decades. Even at this early stage of progress, these intriguing porous materials exhibited several advantages and prospects for translation into DD applications. Despite several in vitro/in vivo studies that revealed positive efforts in DD applications, many fundamental concerns remain unresolved in some circumstances, such as cell source selection, production of tissue-specific models, and construction of complex organs. However, most of the porous materials have persuaded many of the preliminary conditions and have become viable candidates when it comes to DD applications. Some of the porous materials may be limited by the use of a small number of animals and the short time of implantation. As a follow-up study, it could be worthwhile to investigate in vitro biocompatibility in response to different cell types. Furthermore, more intensive in vitro/in vivo/ex vivo/preclinical/clinical/human trials for all such natural and synthetic advanced porous biomaterials in the field of drug delivery must be carefully reviewed. Even though some of the porous materials are bio-inert and non-toxic, more biocompatibility tests are needed before they can be applied in clinical and human trials.

To summarize, we believe that some of the initial success of all these advanced porous biomaterials, specifically in the DD field, to make them feasible for real-life clinical applications will necessitate a multidisciplinary research attempt in the future. This requires successful collaboration among scientists, engineers, and technologists from various fields. As a result, there may be many more fascinating stories and commercialization of all such natural and synthetic advanced porous biomaterials in the near future.

ACKNOWLEDGMENTS

Dr. Uthappa would like to acknowledge Chonnam National University and Yeungnam University, South Korea. Prof. Kurkuri greatly expresses thanks to DST, India (DST/BDTD/EAG/2019), DST, India (DST/TDT/DDP-31/2021), and provision delivered by CRFM-JAIN (Deemed-to-be University), India. This work was also supported by the National Research Foundation of Korea (NRF) grant funded by the Korean Government (MSIT) (No. NRF-2020R1C1C1005505).

REFERENCES

Ahuja, Gaurav, and Kamla Pathak. 2009. "Porous carriers for controlled/modulated drug delivery." *Indian Journal of Pharmaceutical Sciences* no. 71 (6):599.

Allendorf, Mark D., and Vitalie Stavila. 2015. "Crystal engineering, structure–function relationships, and the future of metal–organic frameworks." *CrystEngComm* no. 17 (2):229–246.

Andersson, Jenny, Jessica Rosenholm, Sami Areva, and Mika Lindén. 2004. "Influences of material characteristics on ibuprofen drug loading and release profiles from ordered micro-and mesoporous silica matrices." *Chemistry of Materials* no. 16 (21):4160–4167.

Anglin, Emily J., Lingyun Cheng, William R. Freeman, and Michael J. Sailor. 2008. "Porous silicon in drug delivery devices and materials." *Advanced Drug Delivery Reviews* no. 60 (11):1266–1277.

Bacakova, Lucie, Marta Vandrovcova, Ivana Kopova, and Ivan Jirka. 2018. "Applications of zeolites in biotechnology and medicine–a review." *Biomaterials Science* no. 6 (5):974–989.

Bariana, Manpreet, Moom Sinn Aw, Mahaveer Kurkuri, and Dusan Losic. 2013. "Tuning drug loading and release properties of diatom silica microparticles by surface modifications." *International Journal of Pharmaceutics* no. 443 (1–2):230–241.

Bariana, Manpreet, Moom Sinn Aw, and Dusan Losic. 2013. "Tailoring morphological and interfacial properties of diatom silica microparticles for drug delivery applications." *Advanced Powder Technology* no. 24 (4):757–763.

Biradar, Santoshkumar, Virupaxi Goornavar, Adaikkappan Periyakaruppan, Jessica Koehne, Robert Jeffers, Joseph C. Hall, Vani Ramesh, M. Meyyappan, and Govindarajan T. Ramesh. 2012. "Optimization of process parameters of polymer solution mediated growth of calcium carbonate nanoparticles." *Nanotechnology* no. 23 (37):375601.

Brunauer, Stephen, Paul Hugh Emmett, and Edward Teller. 1938. "Adsorption of gases in multimolecular layers." *Journal of the American Chemical Society* no. 60 (2):309–319.

Byrne, R.S., and P.B. Deasy. 2002. "Use of commercial porous ceramic particles for sustained drug delivery." *International Journal of Pharmaceutics* no. 246 (1–2):61–73.

Carretero, M. Isabel. 2002. "Clay minerals and their beneficial effects upon human health. A review." *Applied Clay Science* no. 21 (3–4):155–163.

Charnay, Clarence, Sylvie Bégu, Corine Tourné-Péteilh, Lionel Nicole, D.A. Lerner, and Jean-Marie Devoisselle. 2004. "Inclusion of ibuprofen in mesoporous templated silica: Drug loading and release property." *European Journal of Pharmaceutics and Biopharmaceutics* no. 57 (3):533–540.

Cote, Adrien P., Annabelle I. Benin, Nathan W. Ockwig, Michael O'Keeffe, Adam J. Matzger, and Omar M. Yaghi. 2005. "Porous, crystalline, covalent organic frameworks." *Science* no. 310 (5751):1166–1170.

Cui, Xin-gang, Hua Chen, Qing-bang Ye, Xin-yu Cui, Xiao-jing Cui, Hong-jing Cui, Guang-zhi Shen, Miao-jing Li, Jian-tao Lin, and Ya-xin Sun. 2021. "Porous titanium dioxide spheres for drug delivery and sustained release." *Frontiers in Materials* no. 8:204.

De Stefano, Luca, Mario De Stefano, Edoardo De Tommasi, Ilaria Rea, and Ivo Rendina. 2011. "A natural source of porous biosilica for nanotech applications: The diatoms microalgae." *Physica Status Solidi C* no. 8 (6):1820–1825.

Deepu, S., Molly Mathew, and M.S. Shamna. 2014. "Controlled drug delivery system." *IJPCS* no. 3 (3):636–641.

Drews, Jürgen. 2000. "Drug discovery: A historical perspective." *Science* no. 287 (5460):1960–1964.

Dubey, Rama, Dhiraj Dutta, Arpan Sarkar, and Pronobesh Chattopadhyay. 2021. "Functionalized carbon nanotubes: Synthesis, properties and applications in water purification, drug delivery, and material and biomedical sciences." *Nanoscale Advances* no. 3 (20):5722–5744.

Fan, Jie, Chengzhong Yu, Feng Gao, Jie Lei, Bozhi Tian, Limin Wang, Qian Luo, Bo Tu, Wuzong Zhou, and Dongyuan Zhao. 2003. "Cubic mesoporous silica with large controllable entrance sizes and advanced adsorption properties." *Angewandte Chemie International Edition* no. 42 (27):3146–3150.

Fang, Qianrong, Junhua Wang, Shuang Gu, Robert B Kaspar, Zhongbin Zhuang, Jie Zheng, Hongxia Guo, Shilun Qiu, and Yushan Yan. 2015. "3D porous crystalline polyimide covalent organic frameworks for drug delivery." *Journal of the American Chemical Society* no. 137 (26):8352–8355.

Furukawa, Hiroyasu, Kyle E. Cordova, Michael O'Keeffe, and Omar M. Yaghi. 2013. "The chemistry and applications of metal-organic frameworks." *Science* no. 341 (6149):1230444.

Geim, Andre Konstantin. 2009. "Graphene: Status and prospects." *Science* no. 324 (5934):1530–1534.

Hartmann, Martin. 2005. "Ordered mesoporous materials for bioadsorption and biocatalysis." *Chemistry of Materials* no. 17 (18):4577–4593.

Hawe, Andrea, Michael Wiggenhorn, Marco van de Weert, Joerg H.O. Garbe, Hanns-Christian Mahler, and Wim Jiskoot. 2012. "Forced degradation of therapeutic proteins." *Journal of Pharmaceutical Sciences* no. 101 (3):895–913.

Hoffman, Allan S. 2008. "The origins and evolution of "controlled" drug delivery systems." *Journal of Controlled Release* no. 132 (3):153–163.

Horcajada, Patricia, Christian Serre, María Vallet-Regí, Muriel Sebban, Francis Taulelle, and Gérard Férey. 2006. "Metal–organic frameworks as efficient materials for drug delivery." *Angewandte Chemie* no. 118 (36):6120–6124.

Hu, Zhonghua, and M.P. Srinivasan. 1999. "Preparation of high-surface-area activated carbons from coconut shell." *Microporous and Mesoporous Materials* no. 27 (1):11–18.

Hu, Zhonghua, and M.P. Srinivasan. 2001. "Mesoporous high-surface-area activated carbon." *Microporous and Mesoporous Materials* no. 43 (3):267–275.

Jani, Abdul Mutalib Md., Dusan Losic, and Nicolas H. Voelcker. 2013. "Nanoporous anodic aluminium oxide: Advances in surface engineering and emerging applications." *Progress in Materials Science* no. 58 (5):636–704.

Kakran, Mitali, and Lin Li. 2012. Carbon nanomaterials for drug delivery. Paper read at Key engineering materials.

Kaplan, David, W. Wade Adams, Barry Farmer, and Christopher Viney. 1993. *Silk Polymers: Materials Science and Biotechnology*. ACS Publications, Washington, DC.

Kaur, Jashandeep, Gurlal Singh Gill, and Kiran Jeet. 2019. "Applications of carbon nanotubes in drug delivery: A comprehensive review." *Characterization and Biology of Nanomaterials for Drug Delivery*, pp. 113–135. DOI: 10.1016/B978-0-12-814031-4.00005-2.

Khurana, Inderpreet Singh, Satvinder Kaur, Harpreet Kaur, and Rajneet Kaur Khurana. 2015. "Multifaceted role of clay minerals in pharmaceuticals." *Future Science OA* no. 1 (3):1–9.

Krajišnik, Danina, Aleksandra Daković, Jela Milić, and Marija Marković. 2019. "Zeolites as potential drug carriers." In Mariano Mercurio, Binoy Sarkar, Alessio Langella (eds.) *Modified Clay and Zeolite Nanocomposite Materials*, 27–55. Elsevier, Amsterdam.

Kresge, C.T., M.E. Leonowicz, W.J. Roth, J.C. Vartuli, and J.S. Beck. 1992. "Ordered mesoporous molecular sieves synthesized by a liquid-crystal template mechanism." *Nature* no. 359 (6397):710–712.

Kumar, B. Pavan, I. Sarath Chandiran, B. Bhavya, and M. Sindhuri. 2011. "Microparticulate drug delivery system: A review." *Indian Journal of Pharmaceutical Science & Research* no. 1 (1):19–37.

Kumeria, Tushar, Manpreet Bariana, Tariq Altalhi, Mahaveer Kurkuri, Christopher T Gibson, Wenrong Yang, and Dusan Losic. 2013. "Graphene oxide decorated diatom silica particles as new nano-hybrids: Towards smart natural drug microcarriers." *Journal of Materials Chemistry B* no. 1 (45):6302–6311.

Li, Bin, Hui-Min Wen, Yuanjing Cui, Wei Zhou, Guodong Qian, and Banglin Chen. 2016. "Emerging multifunctional metal–organic framework materials." *Advanced Materials* no. 28 (40):8819–8860.

Li, Zhu-Zhu, Li-Xiong Wen, Lei Shao, and Jian-Feng Chen. 2004. "Fabrication of porous hollow silica nanoparticles and their applications in drug release control." *Journal of Controlled Release* no. 98 (2):245–254.

Liu, Zhuang, Joshua T Robinson, Xiaoming Sun, and Hongjie Dai. 2008. "PEGylated nanographene oxide for delivery of water-insoluble cancer drugs." *Journal of the American Chemical Society* no. 130 (33):10876–10877.

Losic, Dusan, and Spomenka Simovic. 2009. "Self-ordered nanopore and nanotube platforms for drug delivery applications." *Expert Opinion on Drug Delivery* no. 6 (12):1363–1381.

Losic, Dusan, Yang Yu, Moom Sinn Aw, Spomenka Simovic, Benjamin Thierry, and Jonas Addai-Mensah. 2010. "Surface functionalisation of diatoms with dopamine modified iron-oxide nanoparticles: Toward magnetically guided drug microcarriers with biologically derived morphologies." *Chemical Communications* no. 46 (34):6323–6325.

Mainardes, Rubiana M., and Luciano P. Silva. 2004. "Drug delivery systems: Past, present, and future." *Current Drug Targets* no. 5 (5):449–455.

Meinel, Lorenz, Vassilis Karageorgiou, Sandra Hofmann, Robert Fajardo, Brian Snyder, Chunmei Li, Ludwig Zichner, Robert Langer, Gordana Vunjak-Novakovic, and David L. Kaplan. 2004. "Engineering bone-like tissue in vitro using human bone marrow stem cells and silk scaffolds." *Journal of Biomedical Materials Research Part A: An Official Journal of the Society for Biomaterials, The Japanese Society for Biomaterials, and The Australian Society for Biomaterials and the Korean Society for Biomaterials* no. 71 (1):25–34.

Melke, Johanna, Swati Midha, Sourabh Ghosh, Keita Ito, and Sandra Hofmann. 2016. "Silk fibroin as biomaterial for bone tissue engineering." *Acta Biomaterialia* no. 31:1–16.

Montellano, Alejandro, Tatiana Da Ros, Alberto Bianco, and Maurizio Prato. 2011. "Fullerene C 60 as a multifunctional system for drug and gene delivery." *Nanoscale* no. 3 (10):4035–4041.

Numata, Keiji, Juliana Hamasaki, Balajikarthick Subramanian, and David L. Kaplan. 2010. "Gene delivery mediated by recombinant silk proteins containing cationic and cell binding motifs." *Journal of Controlled Release* no. 146 (1):136–143.

Numata, Keiji, and David L Kaplan. 2010. "Silk-based delivery systems of bioactive molecules." *Advanced Drug Delivery Reviews* no. 62 (15):1497–1508.

Rani, Kirti, and Saurabh Paliwal. 2014. "A review on targeted drug delivery: Its entire focus on advanced therapeutics and diagnostics." *Scholars Journal of Applied Medical Sciences* no. 2 (1C):328–31.

Sahoo, Nanda Gopal, Hongqian Bao, Yongzheng Pan, Mintu Pal, Mitali Kakran, Henry Kuo Feng Cheng, Lin Li, and Lay Poh Tan. 2011. "Functionalized carbon nanomaterials as nanocarriers for loading and delivery of a poorly water-soluble anticancer drug: A comparative study." *Chemical Communications* no. 47 (18):5235–5237.

Salis, Andrea, Enrico Sanjust, Vincenzo Solinas, and Maura Monduzzi. 2003. "Characterisation of Accurel MP1004 polypropylene powder and its use as a support for lipase immobilization." *Journal of Molecular Catalysis B: Enzymatic* no. 24:75–82.

Santos, Abel, Moom Sinn Aw, Manpreet Bariana, Tushar Kumeria, Ye Wang, and Dusan Losic. 2014. "Drug-releasing implants: Current progress, challenges and perspectives." *Journal of Materials Chemistry B* no. 2 (37):6157–6182.

Santos, Hélder A. 2012. *Porous-Based Biomaterials for Tissue Engineering and Drug Delivery Applications*. Taylor & Francis, London.

Sharma, Sameer, Praveen Sher, Shraddha Badve, and Atmaram P. Pawar. 2005. "Adsorption of meloxicam on porous calcium silicate: Characterization and tablet formulation." *Aaps Pharmscitech* no. 6 (4):E618–E625.

Sher, Praveen, Ganesh Ingavle, Surendra Ponrathnam, and Atmaram P. Pawar. 2007. "Low density porous carrier: Drug adsorption and release study by response surface methodology using different solvents." *International Journal of Pharmaceutics* no. 331 (1):72–83.

Shi, Jinjin, Yan Liu, Lei Wang, Jun Gao, Jing Zhang, Xiaoyuan Yu, Rou Ma, Ruiyuan Liu, and Zhenzhong Zhang. 2014. "A tumoral acidic pH-responsive drug delivery system based on a novel photosensitizer (fullerene) for in vitro and in vivo chemo-photodynamic therapy." *Acta Biomaterialia* no. 10 (3):1280–1291.

Shivanand, Padmaja, and Omar L. Sprockel. 1998. "A controlled porosity drug delivery system." *International Journal of Pharmaceutics* no. 167 (1–2):83–96.

Sing, Kenneth S.W. 1985. "Reporting physisorption data for gas/solid systems with special reference to the determination of surface area and porosity (Recommendations 1984)." *Pure and Applied Chemistry* no. 57 (4):603–619.

Solano Umaña, Víctor, and José Vega Baudrit. 2015. "Micro, meso and macro porous materials on medicine." *Journal of Biomaterials and Nanobiotechnology* no. 6:247–256. http://dx.doi.org/10.4236/jbnb.2015.64023

Song, S.-W., K. Hidajat, and S. Kawi. 2005. "Functionalized SBA-15 materials as carriers for controlled drug delivery: Influence of surface properties on matrix– drug interactions." *Langmuir* no. 21 (21):9568–9575.

Streubel, A., J. Siepmann, and R. Bodmeier. 2002. "Floating microparticles based on low density foam powder." *International Journal of Pharmaceutics* no. 241 (2):279–292.

Streubel, A., J. Siepmann, and R. Bodmeier. 2003. "Floating matrix tablets based on low density foam powder: Effects of formulation and processing parameters on drug release." *European Journal of Pharmaceutical Sciences* no. 18 (1):37–45.

Sun, Xiaoming, Zhuang Liu, Kevin Welsher, Joshua Tucker Robinson, Andrew Goodwin, Sasa Zaric, and Hongjie Dai. 2008. "Nano-graphene oxide for cellular imaging and drug delivery." *Nano Research* no. 1 (3):203–212.

Trofimov, Alexey D., Anna A. Ivanova, Mikhail V Zyuzin, and Alexander S Timin. 2018. "Porous inorganic carriers based on silica, calcium carbonate and calcium phosphate for controlled/modulated drug delivery: Fresh outlook and future perspectives." *Pharmaceutics* no. 10 (4):167.

Uthappa, U.T., Varsha Brahmkhatri, G. Sriram, Ho-Young Jung, Jingxian Yu, Nikita Kurkuri, Tejraj M. Aminabhavi, Tariq Altalhi, Gururaj M. Neelgund, and Mahaveer D. Kurkuri. 2018. "Nature engineered diatom biosilica as drug delivery systems." *Journal of Controlled Release* no. 281:70–83.

Uthappa, U.T., Madhuprasad Kigga, G. Sriram, Kanalli V. Ajeya, Ho-Young Jung, Gururaj M. Neelgund, and Mahaveer D. Kurkuri. 2019. "Facile green synthetic approach of bio inspired polydopamine coated diatoms as a drug vehicle for controlled drug release and active catalyst for dye degradation." *Microporous and Mesoporous Materials* no. 288:109572.

Uthappa, U.T., Mahaveer D. Kurkuri, and Madhuprasad Kigga. 2019. "Nanotechnology advances for the development of various drug carriers." In Prasad, R., Kumar, V., Kumar, M., Choudhary, D. (eds) *Nanobiotechnology in Bioformulations*, 187–224. Springer, Cham.

Uthappa, U.T., G. Sriram, O.R. Arvind, Sandeep Kumar, Gururaj M. Neelgund, Dusan Losic, and Mahaveer D. Kurkuri. 2020. "Engineering MIL-100 (Fe) on 3D porous natural diatoms as a versatile high performing platform for controlled isoniazid drug release, Fenton's catalysis for malachite green dye degradation and environmental adsorbents for Pb^{2+} removal and dyes." *Applied Surface Science* no. 528:146974.

Wang, Chaoyang, Chengyi He, Zhen Tong, Xinxing Liu, Biye Ren, and Fang Zeng. 2006. "Combination of adsorption by porous $CaCO_3$ microparticles and encapsulation by polyelectrolyte multilayer films for sustained drug delivery." *International Journal of Pharmaceutics* no. 308 (1–2):160–167.

Williams, Lynda B., and Shelley E. Haydel. 2010. "Evaluation of the medicinal use of clay minerals as antibacterial agents." *International Geology Review* no. 52 (7–8):745–770.

Yang, Lei, Brian W. Sheldon, and Thomas J. Webster. 2010. "Nanophase ceramics for improved drug delivery." *American Ceramic Society Bulletin* no. 89 (2):24–32.

Yao, Shuncheng, Zhirong Liu, and Linlin Li. 2021. "Recent progress in nanoscale covalent organic frameworks for cancer diagnosis and therapy." *Nano-Micro Letters* no. 13 (1):1–20.

Yuasa, Hiroshi, Yuki Takashima, and Yoshio Kanaya. 1996. "Studies on the development of intragastric floating and sustained release preparation. I. Application of calcium silicate as a floating carrier." *Chemical and Pharmaceutical Bulletin* no. 44 (7):1361–1366.

Zhang, De-Xiang, Chiaki Yoshikawa, Nicholas G. Welch, Paul Pasic, Helmut Thissen, and Nicolas H. Voelcker. 2019. "Spatially controlled surface modification of porous silicon for sustained drug delivery applications." *Scientific Reports* no. 9 (1):1–11.

Zhou, Cuisong, Tao Chen, Cuichen Wu, Guizhi Zhu, Liping Qiu, Cheng Cui, Weijia Hou, and Weihong Tan. 2015. "Aptamer $CaCO_3$ nanostructures: A facile, pH-responsive, specific platform for targeted anticancer theranostics." *Chemistry–An Asian Journal* no. 10 (1):166–171.

Part B

Natural Porous Materials

Chapter 2

Silk Fibroin-Based Drug Delivery Systems

Tafadzwa Justin Chiome and Asha Srinivasan

JSS Academy of Higher Education & Research

CONTENTS

2.1 INTRODUCTION

A drug delivery system is defined as a device or formulation which enables the efficient introduction of a therapeutic compound or substance or molecules into the body. Furthermore, the system is designed in such a way that

DOI: 10.1201/9781003217114-4

it improves the compound's efficacy by manipulating rate, release time and drug dumping site. A stepwise process is followed whereby the active compound is introduced into the body via a suitable route after which the compound is then released from the formulation allowing it to diffuse through biological membranes towards the target site. During the development of drug formulations, the major challenge faced by pharmaceutical scientists and engineers is designing a drug delivery system capable of efficiently reaching a specific target site. In order for the drugs to be effective, the plasma drug concentration is to be maintained within the therapeutic window. The concentration should remain above the minimum effective concentration while avoiding crossing the maximum effective concentration as this will lead to drug-induced toxicity or side effects. To have an effective formulation, the system should be able to maintain the drug concentration within the therapeutic window for a prolonged period of time (hours/days/weeks/months). In order to have such an effect, a well-designed drug delivery system is important; hence, it led to the evolution of drug delivery systems based on different materials and intending for greater therapeutic efficacy.

2.2 DRUG DELIVERY SYSTEMS

The use of therapeutic agents is not a new concept as it dates back for centuries. One of the oldest known records of medical practice known as *Ebers papyrus* can be traced back to the Egyptian era which is believed to have been written around 1500 BC but having material dating further back to 3400 BC. Seven scrolls have been discovered, and amongst these, the *Ebers papyrus* stands out the most. This is due to the fact that it contains over 900 remedies/drugs which were administered in the form of eye drops, ointments, inhalations, plugs, lozenges, infusions, suppositories, pills and liquid mixtures. As a vehicle for administration, water, honey, oil, fat, milk, wine and beer were used with water being the most common followed by honey. Routes of administration exploited included oral, vaginal, rectal and topical route. With 70% of the drugs being administered topically in one area, it was envisioned to have its effect transferred to the intended site through afferent ducts. Regardless of the vast amount of knowledge, from a current-day perspective the Egyptian drug therapy is viewed to be ineffective. Out of the 260 remedies found in the Hearst Papysrus, 28% of them are already known to have an activity towards the condition it was being used for, while the other third of the remedies will inevitably cause severe gastric irritation leading to a purgative effect (Cameron, 2005).

Down the line, vaccines came into the picture followed by the introduction of the controlled release concept in the 1960s. Such a concept allowed for a slow and timely release of the active compound from the delivery system, hence stretching the longevity of the drug's effectiveness. Seeing the efficiency of such systems, this has led to great strides being made in the development of drug delivery systems as novel formulations now incorporate advanced materials, biodegradables and even nanomaterials. In an attempt to push forward the therapeutic efficiency of pharmaceutical compounds, this has led to the evolution of drug delivery systems each with the sole objective of creating highly successful pharma therapies.

For years, small molecules have been the centre of attention when it comes to drug design and development with most delivery systems designed and fabricated specifically for them. Taking the properties of the molecules into consideration when designing the delivery systems, it made it possible for the manipulation of the compound's solubility, release rate, bioavailability and amplifying its effectiveness while optimizing their pharmacokinetics (Serajuddin, 1999).

Technological advancement became the springboard for numerous other innovations. Therapies no longer relied solely on small molecules but rather exploited the use of live cells, nucleic acids, peptides, proteins and monoclonal antibodies for the development of new therapies. With the exploitation of larger therapeutic molecules, this has led to a shift in the landscape of drug delivery systems as the strategy and technology changes based on the molecule's characteristics. Regardless of already having existing delivery systems which were designed for small molecules, such systems were not compatible for the delivery of the larger molecules. Efficient for small molecules, the systems had their own pitfalls when it came to large molecules which prompted the evolution of the existing delivery systems in order to address the new challenges.

As a way to resolve the challenges, novel drug delivery systems were optimized through modification of the active compound itself, manipulating the immediate environment as well as allowing interaction of the drug and its surrounding environment in a restricted manner. Having these core fundamentals, each class of therapeutic compound had to be altered accordingly to overcome the challenges of conventional systems through the introduction of novel drug delivery systems (Figure 2.1).

2.3 THE IDEAL DELIVERY SYSTEM

Drug delivery systems are designed in such a way that they are able to have the active compound incorporated into their matrix or on the surface of the vehicle particle. Such a complex structure should be able to allow for drugs to be absorbed into the biological environment and produce the intended effect. In order to design such an efficient system, in-depth knowledge is required when it comes to biological microenvironment, target cell/tissue and the surface receptors present to allow for targeted delivery is essential (Groneberg et al., 2006). As the disease progresses, it is accompanied by relative molecular changes such that it is important for pharmaceutical engineers to be aware of these cellular changes, for instance cell surface

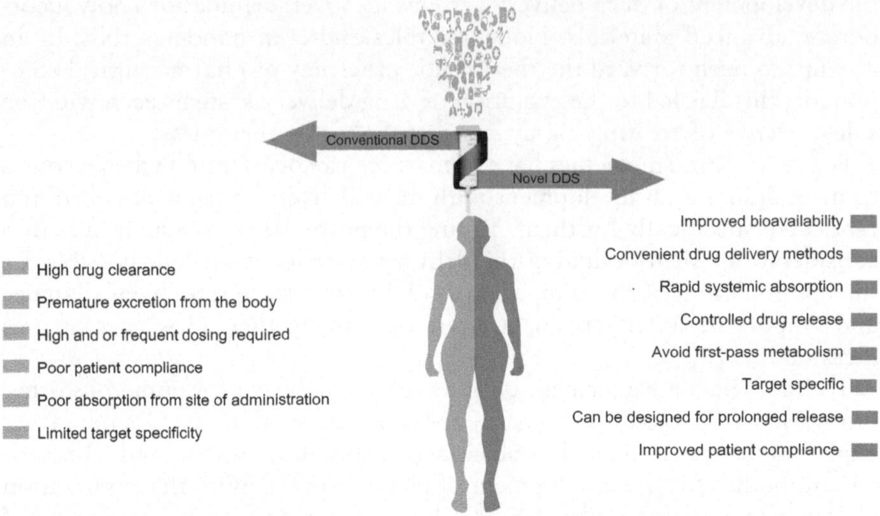

Figure 2.1 Conventional drug delivery systems vs Novel drug delivery systems.

receptor changes. In other cases, the progression of some cancers has been linked to excessive DNA methylation which leads to the ineffectiveness of anti-neoplastic agents like cisplatin and doxorubicin (Grady, 2005). As one fully understands the pathobiology and molecular mechanisms involved, this plays a huge role in the determination of routes of administration which influences the drug's retention time henceforth affecting the bioavailability.

Each delivery system is designed taking into account the physicochemical properties of the drugs. Some of the drug barriers include stability and solubility of the therapeutic agent which tend to influence bioavailability of the compound in the cellular environment directly affecting the drug's efficacy. Drug availability heavily relies on the intrinsic factors which are molecule based, and these include solubility, receptor affinity and compound's molecular weight, therefore influencing cellular uptake/permeability (Savjani et al., 2012). On the other hand, extrinsic factors like enzyme activity and pH of the microenvironment make the compound susceptible to degradation. Taking into account the route of administration used, the compound interacts with other substances during the distribution process with such interactions resulting in synergistic or antagonistic interactions which directly affect the drug's potency (Foucquier and Guedj, 2015). In-depth knowledge of drug interactions is vital during the development of delivery systems as the drug can be rendered ineffective due to factors like high drug efflux rate by the cell, instability of the active compound leading to degradation, and modification of cell receptors and pathways as the disease progresses. The characteristics of an ideal delivery system are shown in Figure 2.2.

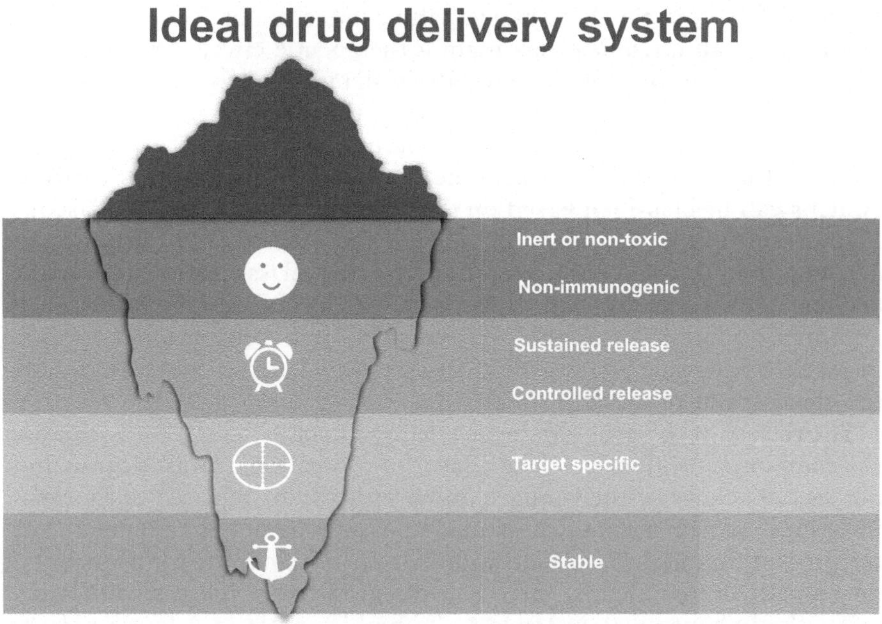

Figure 2.2 Characteristics of an ideal delivery system.

In order for a drug to have the intended therapeutic effect, the active compound must be able to overcome all barriers during the distribution process and still have an adequate amount of the drug reaching the target sites. One of the main challenges faced is ensuring that an optimum amount of the drug/molecule/compound is released at the right time. With the development of each system, the delivery should also be reproducible and precise.

Despite the immense advancements that have taken place over the past decades in relation to drug delivery, a vast number of drugs to this day still induce undesirable side effects, which can be traced back to the compound's unintended interaction with other biological components. Regardless of the drug reaching its target, on-target toxicity is still an issue as the same interaction produces both efficacious and toxic effects. On the other hand, off-target toxicity is a result of the drug binding to an alternative target; for instance, when terfenadine binds to H1 receptor, the result is an antihistamine effect, but when it binds to the human ether-à-go-go-related gene (hERG) channel, it ends up causing arrhythmias (Guengerich, 2011).

Conventional drug delivery systems are often characterized by having high plasma drug concentration as a result of repeated dosing. As the concentration passes the maximum threshold concentration, it ends up leading to drug-induced toxicity hence the side effects. The severity of these effects differs from patient to patient taking into account dosage and dosing frequency in an attempt to maintain a therapeutic effect. Therefore, it is important to develop effective and safer systems.

An ideal system helps to ensure that the drug is delivered to the intended site with its concentration maintained within the therapeutic window for intended/extended time periods. To achieve this, delivery systems can be classified based on their dosage form to include gaseous, liquid, semisolid and solid forms (Perrie and Rades, 2012). Taking into account the route of administration, further classification into intravenous, intramuscular, subcutaneous, intradermal and intraperitoneal administrations are available. As we shift from conventional to more novel delivery systems, immediate and modified release systems are now the epicentre of research.

The release of the drug can be in a delayed manner, such that by coating the compound it offers the drug a layer of protection against degradation due to the acidity of the stomach and eventually be released in the small intestines. Such a mechanism is made possible due to the polymer coating present that makes the matrix dissolve in a higher pH environment in an immediate manner. As there is a pH gradient in the gastrointestinal tract, the polymer matrix tends to be highly stable at a lower pH and disintegrates at higher pH levels. Having this feature allows the drug to be responsive to its surrounding environment with pH as a stimulus to induce drug release. Therefore, as the pH gradually increases as the drug moves away from the stomach, there is partial disintegration of the polymer matrix in response to the pH change with complete collapse of the matrix once the set pH is reached in the small intestines, therefore leading to an immediate release of the drug. The encapsulation of compounds within a protective matrix helps to reduce physiochemical and enzymatic disruptions which might be encountered during the distribution process in turn increasing bioavailability while minimizing the development of undesirable effects.

On the other hand, extended-release systems are designed in a way to increase the period in which the drug is available after ingestion henceforth reducing dosing frequency while improving stability, safety and the efficacy of the compound. The controlled release system helps to regulate the concentration of the drug in the body while a sustained-release system just regulates the rate at which the drug is released from the present dosage form (Chien, 1992). In order to produce more efficient delivery systems, it is important to fully understand the mechanism of drug uptake, intracellular trafficking, drug retention and drug interactions, as this allows for efficacy enhancement of the encapsulated therapeutic agent. To achieve this, more complex systems using large molecules for the development of drug delivery systems are proving to be fruitful alternatives and worthwhile factors to be considered.

2.3.1 Protein-Based Delivery Systems

As drug delivery systems evolve, the use of protein-based biopolymers for the delivery of therapeutic compounds has gained a lot of attention from researchers. In comparison to synthetic polymers which are widely accepted, protein-based biopolymers have proved to be advantageous due to their characteristic features like water solubility, biodegradable and biocompatible while being non-toxic in nature (Garrait et al., 2014). Natural proteins have been widely accepted due to ease of extraction under mild conditions without compromising their activity such that high biocompatibility, structural properties and therapeutic activity are preserved. The barriers to protein delivery and ideal non-invasive routes are shown in Figure 2.3.

In comparison, synthetic biomaterials are advantageous as they are reproducible, scalable and available on demand. With minor changes applied to their structure, degradation rate, size, compositions and shape, they make it possible to tailor the material to suit its end application. The main drawback of synthetic materials is that they lack cell adhesion sites while having biocompatibility that is questionable.

Animal and plant-based proteins are being used in the development of delivery systems due to their favourable characteristics. Animal proteins are the most common with silk, collagen, elastin and keratin being the most investigated as they are inexpensive and rather sustainable alternatives to synthetic polymers. On the other hand, plant-based proteins like zein, soy protein and gliadin are highly explored for various delivery applications for materials like vaccines, peptides, proteins and DNA (Peng et al., 2016). The upside of using animal and plant-based proteins is that such proteins and peptides along with their hydrolysates can be easily extracted from

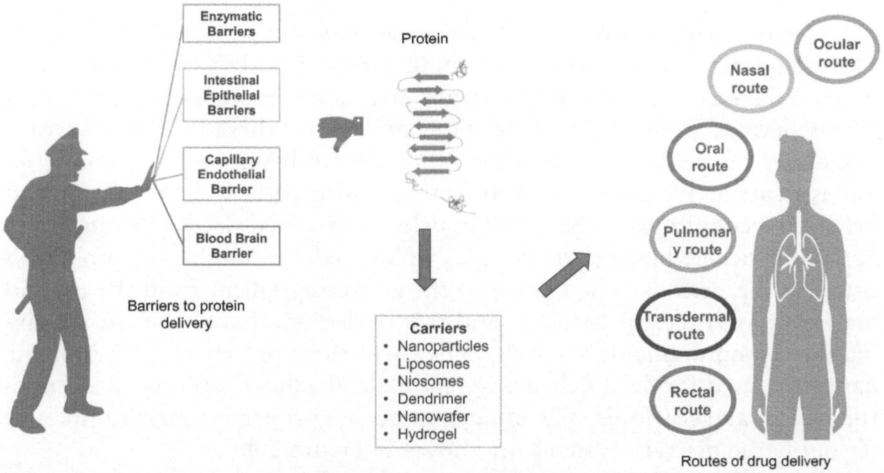

Figure 2.3 Barriers to protein delivery and ideal non-invasive delivery routes.

waste material from sectors like agriculture allowing for their repurposing in higher priority fields such as drug delivery, biomedical engineering and pharmaceutics (Ferraro et al., 2016).

Looking from a therapeutic perspective, the use of proteins for the development of therapeutic compounds is considered as a highly successful endeavour as proteins enhance specificity and potency, while offering extended duration of effectiveness due to decrease in clearance and also by having lower intrinsic toxicity (Yin et al., 2015). Regardless of having the above-mentioned upsides, proteins-based systems should also overcome the common barriers such as short half-life, immunogenicity, instability and limited biological membrane permeability due to their high molecular weight (Kintzing et al., 2016). To overcome these protein therapeutic drawbacks, several strategies are being implemented, and these include moiety covalent attachments, fragment crystallizable fusions (Fc-fusions) or conjugation with other polymers such as poly(ethylene glycol) (Schellenberger et al., 2009). After overcoming these drawbacks, protein therapeutics exhibit superior upsides as compared to small molecules as they are able to undertake scrupulous and multifarious functions with enhanced specificity making them explicit and exclusive. Looking from an economical perspective, it takes a shorter amount of time for the FDA to approve protein-based drugs as compared to small molecule-based therapies, therefore making therapeutic proteins more attractive to the pharmaceutical industry (Pisal et al., 2010). With this in mind, it makes protein-based delivery systems worth pushing forward as part of the novel drug delivery systems.

2.3.2 Silk

Silk is a naturally occurring protein whose value has been realized in fields like tissue engineering, biomedical applications, ligand repair, wound healing and ligament repair (Mobini et al., 2013). Silk proteins are most commonly derived from silkworm cocoons and spider threads with silkworm silk derived from *Bombyx mori*, *Eri* and *Tussah* being the most common. Silk is an attractive material due to low processing costs and unsophisticated processing conditions. When used in delivery systems, silk is biocompatible and has tuneable biodegradable rates which make it suitable for prolonged drug-eluting periods. The release of the active ingredient from the protein matrix is governed by diffusion and rate of degradation of the matrix giving them programmable solubility. Owing to these properties, silk proteins have been used for drug delivery in materials like films, nanoparticles, microparticles and scaffolds. The important fibroin properties and examples of fibroin-based delivery systems are shown in Figure 2.4

Unlike silk obtained from cocoons, spider silk is well known for having excellent mechanical properties such as elasticity and high tensile strength.

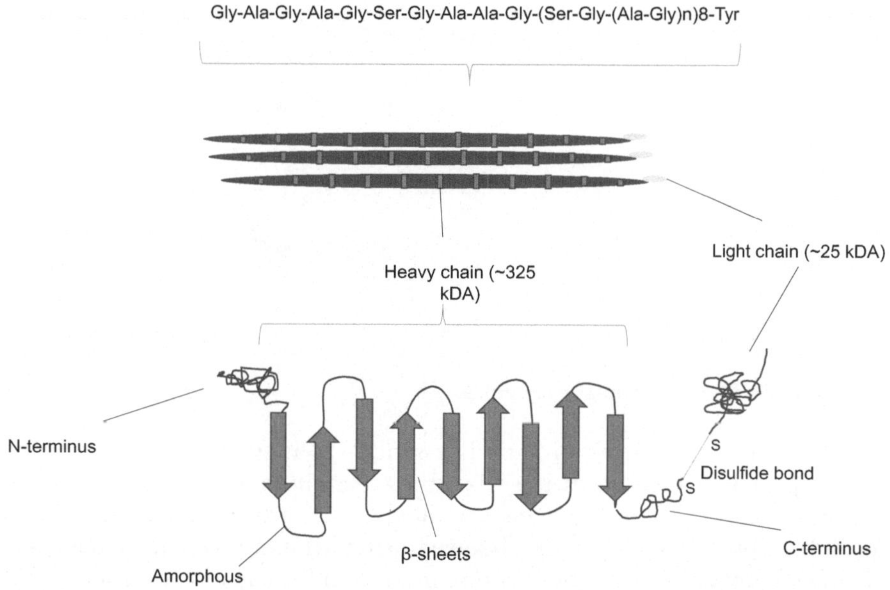

Figure 2.4 Important fibroin properties and examples of fibroin-based delivery systems.

Such advantages have been met with developmental difficulties as spiders are territorial creatures. Under controlled environments, only limited amounts of silk protein can be produced as it is difficult to assemble the silk protein into fibres having native-sized protein of 250–320 kDa. Exploring gene recombinant technology makes it possible for the production of favourable silk proteins in both silkworms and spiders having properties that are customizable. With this manipulation, the strength and elasticity of the fibres can be amplified to exceed the extent observed in the native silk. With this bioengineering approach, it is possible to customize silk fibres to better suit their intended application in fields like drug delivery, biomaterial, wound healing, tissue engineering and ligament repair with the aid of strong and lightweight silk fibres.

2.3.3 Silk Fibroin

Looking at the composition of silk fibres, fibroin protein accounts for 65%–85% of the total protein present (Numta and Kaplan, 2010). The fibroin secondary structure is shown in Figure 2.5. In the majority of the cases, silk fibroin is extracted from silkworms like *Bombyx mori* and *Antheraea mylitta* either from the silkworm cocoons or directly from the silk glands. Silk proteins extracted from different silkworm species are known to have different structure as well as properties. In order to access the silk fibroin

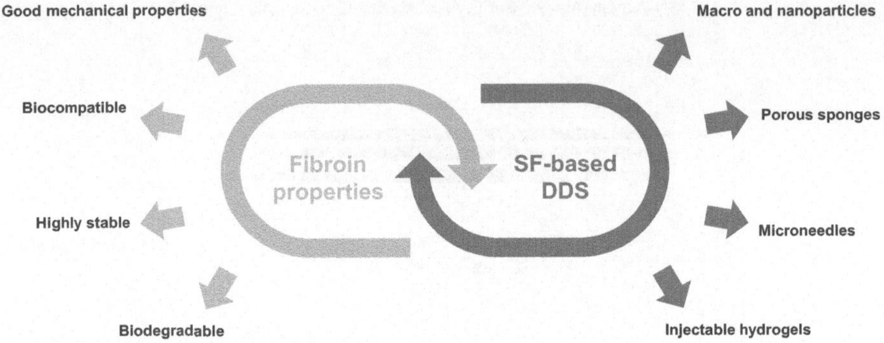

Figure 2.5 Silk fibroin secondary structure.

solution, the degumming process is essential as it strips off the external sericin protein which coats the silk fibres. Sericin is a water-soluble protein which can be extracted using thermochemical processes leaving behind insoluble fibroin which can be dissolved using lithium bromide or with the aid of calcium chloride to give fibroin in solution form also known as regenerative fibroin.

Having a heavy and light chain, silk fibroin protein is an example of a semi-crystalline structure whose heavy chain is comprised of 45% glycine (Gly), 30% alanine (Ala) and 12% serine (Ser), while the light chain is made up of 15% Asp, 14% Ala, 11% Gly, 11% Ser and traces of cysteine (Ki et al., 2009). The heavy chain is ~325kDa, while the light chain is ~25 kDa (Figure 2.5). The fibroin chains are held together by sericin protein which is glue-like in nature with a size range of 20–310 kDa. Just like in amphiphilic block copolymers, fibroin heavy chains have regions which are hydrophobic and hydrophilic alternating. The hydrophobic blocks make up for the protein's crystalline structure allowing it to fold into intermolecular β-sheets with the aid of intermolecular hydrogen bonds and Van der Waals' forces. As compared to the hydrophobic regions, the hydrophilic blocks are smaller in size while also lacking repetitiveness in their sequence.

Looking at the amino acid composition of fibroin, it provides vast opportunities for chemical modifications to be made with amines, carboxyl groups, alcohols and thiols being explored as potential reactive sites for modification. Modifications to the carboxylic acid side groups have been explored to enhance cell adhesion while altering tyrosine residues change the protein's hydrophilicity (Zhou et al., 2001). Fibroin's elasticity is attributed to the light chain being more hydrophilic and hence less water resistant. The reason behind the protein's popularity in research is due to its high mechanical strength, elasticity, biocompatibility, biodegradability, immunogenicity and cheaper processing costs leading to its application in biomaterial synthesis. On the other hand, sericin has similar properties, but it is frowned upon as it induces an immune response (Wang et al., 2015). With a variety of possible modification sites, fibroin offers the opportunity for the introduction of specific functional groups which aids in the interaction between drug molecules and the protein. By exploiting this property, it allows for the loading of a variety of drugs in different quantities into a protein matrix having distinct release kinetics properties. Proper functionalization makes it possible for precise cell adhesion and signalling pathway targeting which are all attributes of an ideal delivery system.

2.4 FIBROIN PROPERTIES EXPLOITED IN DELIVERY SYSTEMS

2.4.1 Mechanical Properties

Due to the unique properties of silk fibroin, the biopolymer tends to exhibit properties of both natural and synthetic polymers when it comes to physical and biological characteristics. Like two sides of a coin, fibroin in the textile industry gives softness to the material, while in biomedical applications, it is a robust material due to its high tensile strength and elasticity. The high mechanical strength of fibroin makes it applicable in bone regeneration biomaterial as high mechanical performance is a prerequisite (Luo et al., 2015a).

In tissue engineering, it is important that the stiffness of the biomaterial should match that of the target tissue. In order to enhance the stiffness of polymers such as collagen, crosslinking is done, but the process is linked to cell toxicity and inducing an immune response (Bhat et al., 2021). Due to the presence of β-sheets, fibroin already has high tensile strength, therefore eliminating the need for any form of crosslinking. The high tensile strength of this material makes it suitable for tissue engineering and drug delivery applications.

2.4.2 Biocompatibility

Backed by decades of research, silk fibroin is deemed to be a highly biocompatible material with little to non-immunogenic response observed as observed to other commonly used polymers like collagen, polylactide and even silk sericin itself (Meinel et al., 2004). Fibroin has been found to be highly compatible with multiple cell lines such as fibroblast, mesenchymal stem cells and osteoblasts. Cytotoxicity of fibroin has been linked to the use of organic solvents during the extraction of fibroin as the reagents induce a structural transformation from α- to ß-sheets to make the fibres soluble leading to an inflammatory response being observed (Meinel et al., 2005). The shift from organic solvent to using less hush salts to solubilize fibroin has been observed to eliminate the element of cytotoxicity effect.

In vivo studies have also shown the biocompatibility of fibroin when it was used to make scaffolds which were implanted into rats and even after a year the scaffolds were well tolerated. The only immune response observed was very low and localized (Wang et al., 2008).

2.4.3 Stability

In order for utilization of biopolymers, both synthetic and natural materials should be highly stable in order to be used in pharmaceutical formulations. The major problem observed when it comes to silk fibroin is its stability as it tends to aggregate or turn into a gel during both processing and storage. When the protein contains a high amount of α-helix and random coils, it will be in solution form while a shift to high β-sheet content renders it insoluble. The storage condition of fibroin plays a major role in determining its stability as the humid condition induces an α- to β-sheet conversion leading to protein gelation (Min et al., 2006). The low content of β-sheets in untreated fibroin allows it to be more hygroscopic, making it highly sensitive to humidity in the surrounding environment. Therefore, the storage of silk fibroin in a humid environment changes the structural conformation of the protein.

2.4.4 Degradability

A properly designed drug delivery system should be degradable in nature such that it will allow for the release of the payload. In order to have efficient delivery, the system should be designed in such a way that the degradation rate/kinetics should be responsive to the evolving surrounding environment. Looking at conventional drug delivery systems, the degradation rate tends to be fast leading to the immediate release of the drug (Langer and Vacanti, 1993). Such an approach is advantageous when an immediate therapeutic effect is the goal, but when it comes to tissue engineering where the structural integrity of the biomaterial is to be maintained for load-bearing purpose, this becomes a problem.

Silk fibroin tends to be prone to proteomic enzyme degradation when it comes to some clinical applications. To protect the protein from degradation, modifications to the molecular weight and crosslinking of the protein can be done. Collagenase IA has been reported to lead to the conversion of Silk II to Silk I, while protease XIV converts the sheets to Silk I while the latter had a much lower degradation rate (Li et al., 2003). Therefore, there is a link between protein degradation and loss of mechanical strength.

2.5 SILK FIBROIN-BASED DRUG DELIVERY SYSTEMS

In order for the drug molecules to be delivered in a controlled and sustained manner, attention must be given to the delivery system's size, composition and manner of administration. With polymers being the most common material to develop such systems, it is essential for mild processing conditions to be used so as to preserve the material's mechanical and physical properties as well as the integrity of the active ingredient. Silk fibroin possesses the necessary properties for its application in the development of drug delivery systems and due to the capability of modifying properties like release kinetics, degradation, solubility, stability and other mechanical properties to suit its intended application. With this in mind, fibroin has been used to develop silk fibroin-based drug delivery systems with some of the systems discussed below.

2.5.1 Fibroin Particles

The most common method that is used in developing a drug delivery system is by encapsulating the drug compound. This is mostly done by premixing the drug and the polymer prior to processing, but care should be taken to ensure that the drug activity is preserved during processing. In other cases, it is possible for the drug compound to be incorporated after processing through the process of adsorption or covalent bonds with the already processed fibroin system. The latter method is advantageous as it allows for prolonged stability of the drug compound with its potency elevated when incorporated into the matrix just before use such that the drug's stability and potency are well maintained.

Thebilityy of silk fibroin to bind with drugs is owed to its physiochemical properties, for instance the hydrophobic moieties found in fibroin's heavy chain (Wenk et al., 2008). The use of fibroin for drug delivery purposes has led to the development of materials such as microparticles, nanoparticles, microspheres, coatings and nanolayers, especially for the development of controlled release delivery systems. Microparticles are the most commonly used, but micro and nanoparticles offer a processing advantage as they can be produced through chemical-free methods allowing them to be used as matrix reinforcement in scaffolds, therefore improving the material's mechanical and biological properties (Kundu et al., 2013).

The use of fibroin for the development of silk fibroin-based nanoparticles has been found to be biocompatible in nature, having a highly desirable degradation rate and a stimuli-responsive drug release mechanism. Due to the nanoscale size of fibroin-based nanoparticles, this has been a useful feature in the development of anticancer drugs due to their stability and non-toxicity nature. The use of fibroin as an encapsulation matrix makes it possible for the loading of small molecules, proteins and nucleic acids through surface adsorption, physical encapsulation and covalent binding all aimed at preventing drug degradation. With additional protective effects, such a delivery system will help optimize the drug's pharmacokinetics while enhancing the cellular uptake of the drug by biological systems (Zhao et al., 2015).

The major challenge observed when it comes to fibroin-based delivery systems is the ability to combine and enhance both functional properties of the material while upholding the drug delivery purpose. As the functionality of the particles heavily depends on the type of processing method used, the main objective is to develop monodisperse-sized particles, and this is difficult to achieve when the milling method is used as a processing step.

In drug delivery, it has been observed that the application of a magnetic field can enhance drug penetration when it comes to transdermal delivery. In this regard, alternating fields enhance percutaneous penetration as compared to the stationary type while a combination of both field types produces the best results. Methotrexate-loaded fibroin magnetic nanoparticles showed enhanced permeation flux under stationary magnetic field, but an alternating field gave much better drug permeation. On the other hand, the combination of both field types showed a better effect giving the best results (Chen et al., 2015).

2.5.2 Porous Sponges

Spongy fibroin scaffolds are three-dimensional structures which can be prepared using regenerative fibroin through processes like freeze drying and salt leaching. The resulting structural and morphological characteristics of the sponges will depend on protein concentration, salt size and salt concentration as well as the type of solvent used in the process (Wang et al., 2006).

The catabolic degradation of fibroin is by proteolytic enzymes to which the degradation rate depends on collective factors like chemical, physical and even biological factors. To this, enzymes, molecular weight and processing methods employed also affect the rate and extent of degradation. The processing solvent and process used can affect the functional groups of the protein chains such that the rate of degradation can be accelerated through hydrolysis of part of the protein leading to decrease in molecular weight as well as mechanical properties of the protein (Zuo et al., 2006).

It should also be noted that the pore size of the sponge plays a role in the degradation of the biomaterial, henceforth affecting the drug delivery pharmacokinetics. A larger pore size distribution has been linked to an accelerated degradation rate on exposure of collagenase IA sponges to protease. While on the other hand, inter-pore walls having smaller pore sizes took longer to degrade as the morphological and structural features of the material remained intact for about twice as long (Luo et al., 2015b).

Silk fibroin has gained a lot of attention, especially in tissue engineering where it has been used to regenerate nerves, cartilage, ligaments and vascular. Intervertebral disc tissue engineering is another application where fibroin hyaluronic acid composite gels have been used to regenerate the nucleus pulposus. As nucleus pulposus properties are in tier with those of the cartilage tissue when it comes to biocomposition, biomechanical function and cellular type, fibroin-based porous scaffolds provide an ideal microenvironment which supports nucleus pulposus cell growth, cell infiltration and secretion of extracellular matrix (Zeng et al., 2014).

A vast number of studies have been carried out using fibroin-based porous sponges with some in applications like vascular grafts (Zhu et al., 2014), bone tissue engineering (Zeng et al., 2015) and bone regeneration (Nisal et al., 2018). In this application, the spongy material is used as a system for the delivery of therapeutic agents, for example recombinant human bone morphogenetic protein 2 and dexamethasone for bone regeneration (Yao et al., 2020), bone morphogenetic protein 1 (Karageorgiou et al., 2006), curcumin for wound healing (Li et al., 2015), cell loading using chondrocytes (Han et al., 2014) and simvastatin for bone tissue regeneration (Wang et al., 2015).

2.5.3 Microneedles

When it comes to drug delivery routes, transdermal delivery is an attractive alternative to parenteral administration as it tends to bypass the hepatic first-pass metabolism and intestinal drug degradation which are responsible for low bioavailability. Transdermal delivery on its own has a downside when it comes to drug molecule size as drugs lower than 400 Da are the ones that can successfully cross the skin barrier (Schaefer and Schaefer, 1997). In order to overcome such a limitation, techniques such as microdermabrasion, radiofrequency, laser ablation and thermal abrasion have been used to improve drug penetration through the skin. Not only are such methods painful, but some of them also tend to inflict serious damage to the patient's skin.

Use of microneedles has proved to be advantageous as the needles are able to penetrate the skin and deliver therapeutic agents like vaccines, enzymes, peptides and drugs in a pain-free manner as they do not stimulate the dermal nerves (Donnelly et al., 2010). Microneedles form a good delivery system for local, regiospecific and systemic delivery. Delivery of drugs is made possible through various methods with direct transport pathways where the needles of the device form small holes on the application, and after its removal, a drug-containing patch is applied over the punctured area. The punctures will create a direct path allowing for the drug to cross the skin barrier. In another method, the drug is coated onto the microneedle surface, to which the device is scrapped onto the application site depositing the drug in the process along the formed abrasions (Dugam et al., 2021).

For transdermal delivery, the structural and morphological properties of the needles play an important role. Looking at hollow needles, it is possible to load a drug solution into the hollow space of the needles. On the other hand, it is possible to coat the microneedles with a drug solution, and after insertion at the local site, the drug will dissolve from the coated surface. With the working principle of microneedles in mind, they have been used for the delivery of compounds in unique regions like ocular delivery (Moffatt et al., 2017), nail (Chiu et al., 2015), inner ear (Aksit et al., 2020), brain (Kearney et al., 2016), sensor-based application (Gowers et al., 2019) and in cosmetics as well (Hirobe et al., 2017).

Fibroin-based microneedles with 500 µm length, 200 µm base diameter and 5 µm tip radius were developed having rapid dissolving capabilities, allowing for the release of methylene blue after implantation under the skin with the dissolved fibroin creating a non-inflammatory amino acid degradation product incorporated in cell metabolic functions (You et al., 2011). The degradation rate and diffusion rate of loaded material rely on post-processing conditions applied during microneedle synthesis. Fabrication at room temperature and use of aqueous-based micro-moulding allowed for bulk loading of a compound like tetracycline whose release rate was reduced by 5.6-fold by tempering with fibroin's secondary structure as increase in annealing time amplified β-sheet content. This allowed for a 10-fold decrease in bacterial density during in vitro studies (Tsioris et al., 2011).

Further work has been done using fibroin-based microneedles for the delivery of anti-programmed cell death protein 1 (anti-PD-1) (Wang et al., 2016), B16F10 tumour lysates (Ye et al., 2017), insulin (Chen et al., 2018) and contraception (Li et al., 2019). Yavuz et al. (2020) were able to develop levonorgestrel-loaded microneedle patches whose drug release lasted up to 100 days when the drug was loaded directly inside the needles, while on the other hand preloading the drug into microparticles before incorporation into the microneedles resulted in a prolonged release of more than a year creating a feasible long-acting contraceptive patch.

Use of microneedles for drug delivery makes it possible for the synthesis of hybrid materials. Poly(ethylene glycol) diacrylate/sucrose microneedles patches having fibroin scaffold had high mechanical strength which allowed for easy skin penetration by using simple thumb force. With such a hybrid material, it was possible to encapsulate Rhodamine B (RHB), indocyanine green, and doxorubicin in the microneedles with the release kinetics of the drugs capable of being manipulated by adjusting the sucrose concentration of the material (Gao et al., 2019).

2.5.4 Injectable Hydrogels

In recent years, hydrogels have been recognized as a promising biomaterial when it comes to biomedical applications. Owing to fibroin's biocompatibility, minimum inflammatory response, good tunable mechanical properties and biodegradability, fibroin-based hydrogels have promising clinical translational potential. Such a biomaterial has been successful in bone regeneration, cancer therapy, drug delivery and bioprinting. The fact that fibroin-based hydrogels are injectable, thixotropic and exhibit in situ gelation has led to their implication in drug delivery. Dual drug loading of doxorubicin and curcumin has been successful in fibroin/hydroxypropyl cellulose hydrogels, which showed long-term sustained release, thixotropic behaviour and in situ gelation with potential use in cancer therapy (Cao et al., 2019). Extensive work has been done using injectable fibroin hydrogels for the delivery of doxorubicin, and it should be noted that such an approach proved superior in the delivery of the anticancer agent as compared to intravenous administration as the delivery system is pH responsive, therefore allowing for targeted delivery (Wu et al., 2016; Zhu et al., 2019).

Angiogenetics is the driving factor for neovascularization as it induces cell migration and angiogenesis, but the drawback for the delivery of such compounds is that they have poor absorption, low stability and aggregation issues leading to decline in therapeutic efficacy. For delivery of such compounds, fibroin-based hydrogels have the capacity to induce endothelial cell adhesion, growth, migration and tubulogenesis. In vitro hydrogel implantation led to enhancement of vascularization and epimerization for epidermal repair through stimulation of collagen deposition while upregulating the expression of angiogenesis-related proteins and genes making it suitable for vascular growth and tissue regeneration (Wang et al., 2021).

Treatment of deep-seated cancer tumours is problematic, while injectable magnetic fibroin-based hydrogels and iron oxide nanocubes offer a promising alternative. After injection, the hydrogels were able to remain in position throughout the treatment near the tumour where they had been injected. With a magnetic field as a stimulus, the ferromagnetic material could efficiently generate a hyperthermia effect leading to ablation of deep-seated tumours (Qian et al., 2020). He et al. (2019) fabricated conversion nanoparticles and nanographene oxide composite having luminesce imaging and photothermal properties with fibroin forming a hydrogel matrix. In vitro studies showed that the material had excellent biocompatibility with the capability to successfully obliterate cancer cells through photothermal effect.

Following the unique properties of injectable hydrogels, promising work has been done for the delivery of adult stem cells (Ciocci et al., 2018), ciprofloxacin for wound healing (Dong et al., 2021), brain tissue engineering applications, insulin delivery (Maity et al., 2020), mesenchymal stem cells delivery for tissue regeneration (Boudreau and Jeong, 2021) and glucosamine delivery for the regeneration of degenerated disc tissue (Murab et al., 2015).

2.6 CONCLUSION AND FUTURE PROSPECTS

Over the years, many efforts have been put towards the development of formulations having good therapeutic efficacy when it comes to several biomedical applications with emphasis on drug delivery systems. Silk fibroin has received lots of attention in drug delivery applications due to its unique characteristics such as good mechanical properties, biocompatible, biodegradable, surface functionalization, swelling capabilities and tunable degradation rate, all of which make it a good candidate for drug delivery applications.

Regardless of such good properties, fibroin stability provides a limitation to its application as it easily changes conformation. As a way to overcome such limitations, efforts have gone into developing fibroin-based biomaterials like nanoparticles, microneedles, sponges, hydrogels and also nanofibres, all of which are recognized as suitable vehicles for the delivery of active drug compounds. Silk fibroin is consistent with other naturals as well as synthetic polymers which makes it possible for drug encapsulations as well as other therapeutic agents within the biomaterials. The porosity and adjustable degradation rate make it possible for a controlled and sustained release of the therapeutic agents making silk fibroin-based material very attractive. With room for modifications and functionalization, this makes efficient drug binding to the system during the loading process while creating the possibility of site-specific drug targeting. A lot of work has been carried out using silk fibroin-based drug delivery systems, but there are still some gaps in research which are still to be further explored, creating unlimited possibilities for combined/advanced drug delivery systems having distinct release kinetics.

ACKNOWLEDGEMENT

We would like to acknowledge JSS Academy of Higher Education and Research, Mysore, India, for the unwavering support to ensure the completion of this manuscript in a successful manner.

REFERENCES

Aksit, Aykut, Shruti Rastogi, Maria L. Nadal, Amber M. Parker, Anil K. Lalwani, Alan C. West, and Jeffrey W. Kysar. "Drug delivery device for the inner ear: Ultra-sharp fully metallic microneedles." *Drug Delivery and Translational Research*, no. 1 (June 2, 2020), 214–26. https://doi.org/10.1007/s13346-020-00782-9.

Bhat, Shrinath, U. T. Uthappa, Tariq Altalhi, Ho-Young Jung, and Mahaveer D. Kurkuri. "Functionalized porous hydroxyapatite scaffolds for tissue engineering applications: A focused review." *ACS Biomaterials Science & Engineering* (September 9, 2021). https://doi.org/10.1021/acsbiomaterials.1c00438.

Boudreau, Ryann D., and Kyung Jae Jeong. "Injectable gelatin-silk fibroin composite hydrogels for in situ cell encapsulation." *University of New Hampshire Scholar's Repository* (2021).

Cameron, Ian A. "History of medicine days: Calgary 2004 W. A. Whitelaw." *Canadian Bulletin of Medical History*, no. 2 (October 2005), 418–19. https://doi.org/10.3138/cbmh.22.2.418.

Cao, Han, Yu Duan, Qinrui Lin, Yuhong Yang, Zuguang Gong, Yiming Zhong, Xin Chen, and Zhengzhong Shao. "Dual-loaded, long-term sustained drug releasing and thixotropic hydrogel for localized chemotherapy of cancer." *Biomaterials Science*, no. 7 (2019), 2975–85. https://doi.org/10.1039/c9bm00540d.

Chen, Ai-Zheng, Lin-qing Chen, Shi-bin Wang, Ya-qiong Wang, and Jun-zhe Zha. "Study of magnetic silk fibroin nanoparticles for massage-like transdermal drug delivery." *International Journal of Nanomedicine* (July 2015), 4639. https://doi.org/10.2147/ijn.s85999.

Chen, Bo Zhi, Mohammad Ashfaq, Dan Dan Zhu, Xiao Peng Zhang, and Xin Dong Guo. "Controlled delivery of insulin using rapidly separating microneedles fabricated from genipin-crosslinked gelatin." *Macromolecular Rapid Communications*, no. 20 (May 2, 2018), 1800075. https://doi.org/10.1002/marc.201800075.

Chien, Yie. *"Novel Drug Delivery Systems" Drugs and the Pharmaceutical Sciences*. 2nd ed. New York: CRC Press (1992).

Chiu, Wing Sin, Natalie A. Belsey, Natalie L. Garrett, Julian Moger, Gareth J. Price, M. Begoña Delgado-Charro, and Richard H. Guy. "Drug delivery into microneedle-porated nails from nanoparticle reservoirs." *Journal of Controlled Release* (December 2015), 98–106. https://doi.org/10.1016/j.jconrel.2015.10.026.

Ciocci, Matteo, Ilaria Cacciotti, Dror Seliktar, and Sonia Melino. "Injectable silk fibroin hydrogels functionalized with microspheres as adult stem cells-carrier systems." *International Journal of Biological Macromolecules* (March 2018), 960–71. https://doi.org/10.1016/j.ijbiomac.2017.11.013.

Dong, Meiping, Yi Mao, Zhiwei Zhao, Jinbo Zhang, Lipeng Zhu, Linlu Chen, and Liexiang Cao. "Novel fabrication of antibiotic containing multifunctional silk fibroin injectable hydrogel dressing to enhance bactericidal action and wound healing efficiency on burn wound: In vitro and in vivo evaluations." *International Wound Journal*, no. 3 (August 20, 2021), 679–91. https://doi.org/10.1111/iwj.13665.

Donnelly, Ryan F., Martin J. Garland, Desmond I.J. Morrow, Katarzyna Migalska, Thakur Raghu Raj Singh, Rita Majithiya, and A. David Woolfson. "Optical coherence tomography is a valuable tool in the study of the effects of microneedle geometry on skin penetration characteristics and in-skin dissolution." *Journal of Controlled Release*, no. 3 (November 2010), 333–41. https://doi.org/10.1016/j.jconrel.2010.08.008.

Dugam, Shailesh, Rahul Tade, Rani Dhole, and Sopan Nangare. "Emerging era of microneedle array for pharmaceutical and biomedical applications: Recent advances and toxicological perspectives." *Future Journal of Pharmaceutical Sciences*, no. 1 (January 13, 2021). https://doi.org/10.1186/s43094-020-00176-1.

Ferraro, Vincenza, Marc Anton, and Véronique Santé-Lhoutellier. "The 'Sisters' α-helices of collagen, elastin and keratin recovered from animal by-products: Functionality, bioactivity and trends of application." *Trends in Food Science & Technology* (May 2016), 65–75. https://doi.org/10.1016/j.tifs.2016.03.006.

Foucquier, Julie, and Mickael Guedj. "Analysis of drug combinations: Current methodological landscape." *Pharmacology Research & Perspectives*, no. 3 (May 20, 2015), e00149. https://doi.org/10.1002/prp2.149.

Gao, Ya, Mengmeng Hou, Ruihao Yang, Lei Zhang, Zhigang Xu, Yuejun Kang, and Peng Xue. "Highly porous silk fibroin scaffold packed in PEGDA/sucrose microneedles for controllable transdermal drug delivery." *Biomacromolecules*, no. 3 (January 31, 2019), 1334–45. https://doi.org/10.1021/acs.biomac.8b01715.

Garrait, Ghislain, Eric Beyssac, and Muriel Subirade. "Development of a novel drug delivery system: Chitosan nanoparticles entrapped in alginate microparticles." *Journal of Microencapsulation*, no. 4 (2014), 363–72. https://doi.org/10.3109/02652048.2013.858792.

Gowers, Sally A. N., David M. E. Freeman, Timothy M. Rawson, Michelle L. Rogers, Richard C. Wilson, Alison H. Holmes, Anthony E. Cass, and Danny O'Hare. "Development of a minimally invasive microneedle-based sensor for continuous monitoring of β-lactam antibiotic concentrations in vivo." *ACS Sensors*, no. 4 (April 5, 2019), 1072–80. https://doi.org/10.1021/acssensors.9b00288.

Grady, W.M. "Epigenetic events in the colorectum and in colon cancer." *Biochemical Society Transactions*, no. 4 (August 1, 2005), 684–88. https://doi.org/10.1042/bst0330684.

Groneberg, David A., Klaus F. Rabe, and Axel Fischer. "Novel concepts of neuropeptide-based drug therapy: Vasoactive intestinal polypeptide and its receptors." *European Journal of Pharmacology*, no. 1–3 (March 2006), 182–94. https://doi.org/10.1016/j.ejphar.2005.12.055.

Guengerich, F. Peter. "Mechanisms of drug toxicity and relevance to pharmaceutical development." *Drug Metabolism and Pharmacokinetics*, no. 1 (2011), 3–14. https://doi.org/10.2133/dmpk.dmpk-10-rv-062.

Han, Qianqian, Chao Li, Boon Chin Heng, Gang Wu, and Zigang Ge. "Dynamic distribution of cells in porous scaffolds during cell loading." *Journal of Medical and Biological Engineering*, no. 2 (2014), 130–36. https://doi.org/10.5405/jmbe.1445.

He Wei, Li Po, Zhu Yue, Liu Mingming, Huang Xiaonan, and Qi Hui. "An injectable silk fibroin nanofiber hydrogel hybrid system for tumuor upconversion luminescence imaging and optothermal therapy." *New Journal of Chemistry*, no. 5 (2019). https://doi.org/10.1039/C8NJ05766D.

Hirobe, Sachiko, Risa Otsuka, Hiroshi Iioka, Ying-Shu Quan, Fumio Kamiyama, Hideo Asada, Naoki Okada, and Shinsaku Nakagawa. "Clinical study of a retinoic acid-loaded microneedle patch for seborrheic keratosis or senile lentigo." *Life Sciences* (January 2017), 24–27. https://doi.org/10.1016/j.lfs.2015.12.051.

Karageorgiou, Vassilis, Michael Tomkins, Robert Fajardo, Lorenz Meinel, Brian Snyder, Katherine Wade, Jake Chen, Gordana Vunjak-Novakovic, and David L. Kaplan. "Porous silk fibroin 3-D scaffolds for delivery of bone morphogenetic protein-2in vitro andin vivo." *Journal of Biomedical Materials Research Part A*, no. 2 (2006), 324–34. https://doi.org/10.1002/jbm.a.30728.

Kearney, Mary-Carmel, Ester Caffarel-Salvador, Steven J. Fallows, Helen O. McCarthy, and Ryan F. Donnelly. "Microneedle-mediated delivery of donepezil: Potential for improved treatment options in Alzheimer's disease." *European Journal of Pharmaceutics and Biopharmaceutics* (June 2016), 43–50. https://doi.org/10.1016/j.ejpb.2016.03.026.

Ki, Chang Seok, Young Hwan Park, and Hyoung-Joon Jin. "Silk protein as a fascinating biomedical polymer: Structural fundamentals and applications." *Macromolecular Research*, no. 12 (December 2009), 935–42. https://doi.org/10.1007/bf03218639.

Kintzing, James R., Maria V. Filsinger Interrante, and Jennifer R. Cochran. "Emerging strategies for developing next-generation protein therapeutics for cancer treatment." *Trends in Pharmacological Sciences*, no. 12 (December 2016), 993–1008. https://doi.org/10.1016/j.tips.2016.10.005.

Kundu, Banani, Rangam Rajkhowa, Subhas C. Kundu, and Xungai Wang. "Silk fibroin biomaterials for tissue regenerations." *Advanced Drug Delivery Reviews*, no. 4 (April 2013), 457–70. https://doi.org/10.1016/j.addr.2012.09.043.

Langer, Robert, and Joseph P. Vacanti. "Tissue engineering." *Science*, no. 5110 (May 14, 1993), 920–26. https://doi.org/10.1126/science.8493529.

Li, Mingzhong, Masayo Ogiso, and Norihiko Minoura. "Enzymatic degradation behavior of porous silk fibroin sheets." *Biomaterials*, no. 2 (January 2003), 357–65. https://doi.org/10.1016/s0142-9612(02)00326-5.

Li Wei, Tang Jie, Terry N Richard, Li Song, Brunie Aurelie, Callahan L Rebecca, Noel K Richard, Rodriguez A Carlos, Schwendeman P Steven, and Prausnitiz R Mark. "Long-acting reversible contraception by effervescent microneedle patch." *Science Advances*, vol. 5, no. 11 (2019). https://doi.org/10.1126/sciadv.aaw8145.

Li, X., J. Qin, and J. Ma. "Silk fibroin/poly (Vinyl Alcohol) blend scaffolds for controlled delivery of curcumin." *Regenerative Biomaterials*, no. 2 (May 26, 2015), 97–105. https://doi.org/10.1093/rb/rbv008.

Luo, Kunyuan, Yuhong Yang, and Zhengzhong Shao. "Physically crosslinked biocompatible silk-fibroin-based hydrogels with high mechanical performance." *Advanced Functional Materials*, no. 6 (December 23, 2015a), 872–80. https://doi.org/10.1002/adfm.201503450.

Luo, Zuwei, Qin Zhang, Meijing Shi, Yang Zhang, Wei Tao, and Mingzhong Li. "Effect of pore size on the biodegradation rate of silk fibroin scaffolds." *Advances in Materials Science and Engineering*, no. 2015 (2015b), 1–7. https://doi.org/10.1155/2015/315397.

Maity, Biswanath, Sourav Samanta, Shradhya Sarkar, Shadab Alam, and Thimmaiah Govindaraju. "Injectable silk fibroin-based hydrogel for sustained insulin delivery in diabetic rats." *ACS Applied Bio Materials*, no. 6 (April 23, 2020), 3544–52. https://doi.org/10.1021/acsabm.0c00152.

Meinel, Lorenz, Sandra Hofmann, Vassilis Karageorgiou, Carl Kirker-Head, John McCool, Gloria Gronowicz, Ludwig Zichner, Robert Langer, Gordana Vunjak-Novakovic, and David L. Kaplan. "The inflammatory responses to silk films in vitro and in vivo." *Biomaterials*, no. 2 (January 2005), 147–55. https://doi.org/10.1016/j.biomaterials.2004.02.047.

Meinel, Lorenz, Vassilis Karageorgiou, Sandra Hofmann, Robert Fajardo, Brian Snyder, Chunmei Li, Ludwig Zichner, Robert Langer, Gordana Vunjak-Novakovic, and David L. Kaplan. "Engineering bone-like Tissuein vitro using human bone marrow stem cells and silk scaffolds." *Journal of Biomedical Materials Research*, no. 1 (2004), 25–34. https://doi.org/10.1002/jbm.a.30117.

Min, Byung-Moo, Lim Jeong, Kuen Yong Lee, and Won Ho Park. "Regenerated silk fibroin nanofibers: Water vapor-induced structural changes and their effects on the behavior of normal human cells." *Macromolecular Bioscience*, no. 4 (April 12, 2006), 285–92. https://doi.org/10.1002/mabi.200500246.

Mobini, Sahba, Mehran Sola-Hashjun, H. Pelrovi, Noor Azuan A Osman, Mazaher Gholipoumalekabadi, Mahmmood Barati, and Ali Samadiluchaksarael. "Bioactivity and biocompatibility studies on silk-based scaffold for bone tissue engineering." *Journal of Medical and Biological Engineering*, no. 2 (2013), 207. https://doi.org/10.5405/jmbe.1065.

Moffatt, Kurtis, Yujing Wang, Thakur Raghu Raj Singh, and Ryan F. Donnelly. "Microneedles for enhanced transdermal and intraocular drug delivery." *Current Opinion in Pharmacology* (October 2017), 14–21. https://doi.org/10.1016/j.coph.2017.07.007.

Murab, Sumit, Juhi Samal, Akshay Shrivastava, Alok Ranjan Ray, Abhay Pandit, and Sourabh Ghosh. "Glucosamine loaded injectable silk-in-silk integrated system modulate mechanical properties in bovine ex-vivo degenerated intervertebral disc model." *Biomaterials* (July 2015), 64–83. https://doi.org/10.1016/j.biomaterials.2015.03.032.

Nisal, Anuya, Raeesa Sayyad, Prachi Dhavale, Bhakti Khude, Rucha Deshpande, Vidhyashri Mapare, Swati Shukla, and Premnath Venugopalan. "Silk fibroin micro-particle scaffolds with superior compression modulus and slow bioresorption for effective bone regeneration." *Scientific Reports*, no. 1 (May 8, 2018). https://doi.org/10.1038/s41598-018-25643-x.

Numata, Keiji, and David L. Kaplan. "Silk-based delivery systems of bioactive molecules." *Advanced Drug Delivery Reviews*, no. 15 (December 2010), 1497–1508. https://doi.org/10.1016/j.addr.2010.03.009.

Peng, Zhili, Shanghao Li, Xu Han, Abdulrahman O. Al-Youbi, Abdulaziz S. Bashammakh, Mohammad S. El-Shahawi, and Roger M. Leblanc. "Determination of the composition, encapsulation efficiency and loading capacity in protein drug delivery systems using circular dichroism spectroscopy." *Analytica Chimica Acta* (September 2016), 113–18. https://doi.org/10.1016/j.aca.2016.08.014.

Perrie, Yvonne, and Thomas Rades. *FASTtrack Pharmaceutics*. 2nd ed. London: Pharmaceutical Press, 2012.

Pisal, Dipak S., Matthew P. Kosloski, and Sathy V. Balu-Iyer. "Delivery of therapeutic proteins." *Journal of Pharmaceutical Sciences*, no. 6 (June 2010), 2557–75. https://doi.org/10.1002/jps.22054.

Qian, Kun-Yu, Yonghong Song, Xu Yan, Liang Dong, Jingzhe Xue, Yunjun Xu, Bao Wang, et al. "Injectable ferrimagnetic silk fibroin hydrogel for magnetic hyperthermia ablation of deep tumor." *Biomaterials* (November 2020), 120299. https://doi.org/10.1016/j.biomaterials.2020.120299.

Savjani, Ketan T., Anuradha K. Gajjar, and Jignasa K. Savjani. "Drug solubility: Importance and enhancement techniques." *ISRN Pharmaceutics* (July 5, 2012), 1–10. https://doi.org/10.5402/2012/195727.

Schaefer, Hans, and Thomas E. Redelmeier. *Skin Barrier: Principles of Percutaneous Absorption*. S Karger Ag, Berlin (1997). https://doi.org/10.1001/archderm.1997.03890430146031.

Schellenberger, Volker, Chia-Wei Wang, Nathan C. Geething, Benjamin J. Spink, Andrew Campbell, Wayne To, Michael D. Scholle, et al. "A recombinant polypeptide extends the in vivo half-life of peptides and proteins in a tunable manner." *Nature Biotechnology*, no. 12 (November 15, 2009), 1186–90. https://doi.org/10.1038/nbt.1588.

Serajuddin, Abu T.M. "Solid dispersion of poorly water-soluble drugs: Early promises, subsequent problems, and recent breakthroughs." *Journal of Pharmaceutical Sciences*, no. 10 (October 1999), 1058–66. https://doi.org/10.1021/js980403l.

Tsioris, Konstantinos, Waseem K. Raja, Eleanor M. Pritchard, Bruce Panilaitis, David L. Kaplan, and Fiorenzo G. Omenetto. "Fabrication of silk microneedles for controlled-release drug delivery." *Advanced Functional Materials*, no. 2 (December 2, 2011), 330–35. https://doi.org/10.1002/adfm.201102012.

Wang, Chao, Yanqi Ye, Gabrielle M. Hochu, Hasan Sadeghifar, and Zhen Gu. "Enhanced cancer immunotherapy by microneedle patch-assisted delivery of anti-PD1 antibody." *Nano Letters*, no. 4 (March 24, 2016), 2334–40. https://doi.org/10.1021/acs.nanolett.5b05030.

Wang, Lianlian, Zhijie Chen, Yufei Yan, Chuan He, and Xinming Li. "Fabrication of injectable hydrogels from silk fibroin and angiogenic peptides for vascular growth and tissue regeneration." *Chemical Engineering Journal* (August 2021), 129308. https://doi.org/10.1016/j.cej.2021.129308.

Wang, Lu, Chunxiang Lu, Yonghong Li, Feng Wu, Bin Zhao, and Xiaozhong Dong. "Green fabrication of porous silk fibroin/graphene oxide hybrid scaffolds for bone tissue engineering." *RSC Advances*, no. 96 (2015), 78660–68. https://doi.org/10.1039/c5ra12173f.

Wang, Yongzhong, Hyeon-Joo Kim, Gordana Vunjak-Novakovic, and David L. Kaplan. "Stem cell-based tissue engineering with silk biomaterials." *Biomaterials*, no. 36 (December 2006), 6064–82. https://doi.org/10.1016/j.biomaterials.2006.07.008.

Wang, Yongzhong, Darya D. Rudym, Ashley Walsh, Lauren Abrahamsen, Hyeon-Joo Kim, Hyun S. Kim, Carl Kirker-Head, and David L. Kaplan. "In vivo degradation of three-dimensional silk fibroin scaffolds." *Biomaterials*, no. 24–25 (August 2008), 3415–28. https://doi.org/10.1016/j.biomaterials.2008.05.002.

Wenk, Esther, Anne J. Wandrey, Hans P. Merkle, and Lorenz Meinel. "Silk fibroin spheres as a platform for controlled drug delivery." *Journal of Controlled Release*, no. 1 (November 2008), 26–34. https://doi.org/10.1016/j.jconrel.2008.08.005.

Wu, Hongchun, Shanshan Liu, Liying Xiao, Xiaodan Dong, Qiang Lu, and David L. Kaplan. "Injectable and PH-responsive silk nanofiber hydrogels for sustained anticancer drug delivery." *ACS Applied Materials & Interfaces*, no. 27 (June 27, 2016), 17118–26. https://doi.org/10.1021/acsami.6b04424.

Yao, Jihang, Yilong Wang, Wendi Ma, Wenying Dong, Mei Zhang, and Dahui Sun. "Erratum to 'dual-drug-loaded silk fibroin/PLGA scaffolds for potential bone regeneration applications.'" *Journal of Nanomaterials* (September 1, 2020), 1–2. https://doi.org/10.1155/2020/7373065.

Ye, Yanqi, Chao Wang, Xudong Zhang, Quanyin Hu, Yuqi Zhang, Qi Liu, Di Wen, et al. "A melanin-mediated cancer immunotherapy patch." *Science Immunology*, no. 17 (November 17, 2017). https://doi.org/10.1126/sciimmunol.aan5692.

Yin, Liusong, Xiaoying Chen, Paolo Vicini, Bonita Rup, and Timothy P. Hickling. "Therapeutic outcomes, assessments, risk factors and mitigation efforts of immunogenicity of therapeutic protein products." *Cellular Immunology*, no. 2 (June 2015), 118–26. https://doi.org/10.1016/j.cellimm.2015.03.002.

You, Xueqiu, Jong-hyeon Chang, Byeong-Kwon Ju, and James Jungho Pak. "Rapidly dissolving fibroin microneedles for transdermal drug delivery." *Materials Science and Engineering: C*, no. 8 (December 2011), 1632–36. https://doi.org/10.1016/j.msec.2011.06.010.

Zeng, Chao, Qiang Yang, Meifeng Zhu, Lilong Du, Jiamin Zhang, Xinlong Ma, Baoshan Xu, and Lianyong Wang. "Silk fibroin porous scaffolds for nucleus pulposus tissue engineering." *Materials Science and Engineering: C*, no. 37 (April 2014), 232–40. https://doi.org/10.1016/j.msec.2014.01.012.

Zeng, Shuguang, Lei Liu, Yong Shi, Junqi Qiu, Wei Fang, Mingdeng Rong, Zehong Guo, and Wenfeng Gao. "Characterization of silk fibroin/chitosan 3D porous scaffold and in vitro cytology." *PLOS ONE*, no. 6 (June 17, 2015), e0128658. Edited by Feng Zhao https://doi.org/10.1371/journal.pone.0128658.

Zhao, Zheng, Yi Li, and Mao-Bin Xie. "Silk fibroin-based nanoparticles for drug delivery." *International Journal of Molecular Sciences*, no. 3 (March 4, 2015), 4880–4903. https://doi.org/10.3390/ijms16034880.

Zhou, Cong-Zhao, Fabrice Confalonieri, Michel Jacquet, Roland Perasso, Zhen-Gang Li, and Joel Janin. "Silk fibroin: Structural implications of a remarkable amino acid sequence." *Proteins: Structure, Function, and Genetics*, no. 2 (2001), 119–22. https://doi.org/10.1002/prot.1078.

Zhu, Caihong, Zhaozhao Ding, Qiang Lu, Guozhong Lu, Liying Xiao, Xiaoyi Zhang, Xiaodan Dong, Changhai Ru, and David L. Kaplan. "Injectable silk–vaterite composite hydrogels with tunable sustained drug release capacity." *ACS Biomaterials Science & Engineering*, no. 12 (November 5, 2019), 6602–9. https://doi.org/10.1021/acsbiomaterials.9b01313.

Zhu, Meifeng, Kai Wang, Jingjing Mei, Chen Li, Jiamin Zhang, Wenting Zheng, Di An, et al. "Fabrication of highly interconnected porous silk fibroin scaffolds for potential use as vascular grafts." *Acta Biomaterialia*, no. 5 (May 2014), 2014–23. https://doi.org/10.1016/j.actbio.2014.01.022.

Zuo, B., L. Dai, and Z. Wu. "Analysis of structure and properties of biodegradable regenerated silk fibroin fibers." *Journal of Materials Science*, no. 11 (April 12, 2006), 3357–61. https://doi.org/10.1007/s10853-005-5384-z.

Chapter 3

Surface Bioengineering of Nanostructured Diatom Biosilica and Their Applications in Drug Delivery

Shaheer Maher
The University of Adelaide
and
Assiut University

Dusan Losic
The University of Adelaide

CONTENTS

3.1 INTRODUCTION

There has been an extensive development of new nanomaterials using nanotechnology in the last two decades, which significantly impacted various aspects of biomedical research including the emerging field of nanomedicine and its applications for drug delivery. On the other hand, from drug discovery research driven by pharmaceutical chemistry, many new drug molecules have been developed through the remarkable advances in molecular biotechnology. However, the efficacy of many of these drugs based on conventional drug delivery systems has many limitations and disadvantages challenged by many factors such as their limited stability (e.g., enzymes, proteins), undesirable low solubility (e.g., hydrophobic

DOI: 10.1201/9781003217114-5

drugs), and uncontrolled distribution throughout the body causing toxicity causing their low efficiency. As a result, there has been an unprecedented need for innovative drug delivery systems (DDS), which paved a foundation to merge these two fields to develop new and advanced DD systems.

The main objectives of these new systems are to deliver the drug to its desired site of action (i.e., targeted drug delivery), at required concentration for required time, and to reduce the undesired adverse effects together with enhancing their physicochemical properties (e.g., solubility and stability). In order to achieve these requirements, drug carrier materials employed in such DDS should possess many desirable properties including being non-toxic and biocompatible while easily excreted from the body after delivering their cargo. In addition, they should be easily produced at large scale with low cost. At the same time, they are required to provide sufficient drug loading and release kinetics for the desired period of treatment to minimize the frequency of administration and patient discomfort. To attain the aforementioned properties, a large variety of synthetic materials are broadly explored for developing micro and nanocarriers such as liposomes, niosomes, polymeric and magnetic nanoparticles, micelles, carbon nanomaterials (CNT, graphene), silicon and silica porous nanoparticles, quantum dots, etc., and only a few are clinically approved and used for real applications [1–6].

In this context, silica and silicon (Si)-based systems are considered attractive alternatives to polymeric and other DDS owing to their exceptional chemical, physical, and optical properties. In particular, synthetic silica manufactured through sol–gel process or porous silicon (pSi) prepared by electrochemical etching of Si wafers have attracted considerable research as innovative drug carriers because of their unique physical, chemical, and optical properties, including high surface area which permits high drug loading capacity, tunable pore size, stability, and controlled drug release profiles [7,8]. Despite their desired properties and success in many biomedical applications such as biosensors for DNA and bacterial detection [9,10], tissue engineering [11], cell culture [12] as well as drug carrier purposes [13–16], silica and silicon-based nanomaterials are challenged by their complicated synthesis procedure that involves several time-consuming steps. In addition, the scalability of silica/silicon drug nanocarriers is limited by the fabrication cost associated with the use of silicon wafers, chemicals, and expensive equipment (e.g., etching cells, power supplies, safety equipment). Furthermore, using highly toxic chemicals, such as hydrofluoric acid (HF), requires specific safety precautions during handling and is environmentally unfriendly [17]. Moreover, the use of toxic chemicals during the synthesis process may eventually lead to residual toxicity in the prepared materials, limiting the applicability of this system for real biomedical applications [18,19]. For example, in a study performed by Koynov et al., they proved the presence of residual toxic SiF_4 and H_2SiF_6 which are formed during the fabrication of pSi particles using the commonly used etching technique [20]. To overcome limitations of these synthetic silica/silicon drug carriers and avoid costly and environmentally unfriendly manufacturing processes, nanostructured silica/silicon can be sourced from nature with minimal cost and less processing without the use of hazardous chemicals.

Nature through millions of years has developed elegant three-dimentional (3D) biologically based silica material with hierarchical porous structures obtained from unicellular photosynthetic algae [21], i.e., diatom (DE). There are more than 200 living DE genera with more than 110,000 estimated species with different shapes and sizes (from 2 µm to 2 mm). Diatoms, as a natural source of silica, can be easily mass-produced by cultivation or found naturally. Furthermore, diatomite is considered a less expensive source of diatoms silica, a compound of sedimentation process of accumulated dead DE on the ocean beds or lakes bottom and mining sites [22]. Silica nanoparticles (SiO_2NPs) can be manufactured from these inexpensive (≈$200 per tonne) and abundant natural resources using scalable, reproducible, and cost-effective processes. The unique properties of DE, such as ordered micro/nanoporous network, large surface area (up to 200 m^2/g), high porosity, amorphous silica composition, low density, controllable surface chemistry, and biocompatibility, render them an appealing replacement for synthetic silica in many fields, such as water purification, chromatography, drug delivery applications, tissue engineering, sensing and biosensing, biosensing energy storage, solar cells, composites, and many more [7,23].

This chapter aims to present the recent progress in the applications of DE silica in drug delivery applications. The structural and physicochemical properties of DE structures and their critical drug delivery characteristics for controlled and triggered drug release are discussed including their surface functionalization methods in order to enhance the biocompatibility and cellular uptake of diatomite DDS for targeting therapeutic molecules. The most appealing examples of using diatom structures for drug delivery applications showing their advantages and limitations are discussed. Finally, a general overview on recent trends in this field presenting key challenges and future perspectives has been concluded.

3.2 DIATOMS: STRUCTURE, PROPERTIES AND MODIFICATIONS

Diatoms are unicellular eukaryotic algae which are present in almost every aquatic environment including oceans, rivers, soils, etc. producing ~25% of atmospheric oxygen and represent almost 30% of biomass. They are considered nature's silica nanofabrication factories. Despite the great variety of DE frustules, these unicellular algae share common structural features.

DE encapsulate themselves within a rigid silica shell, which is called frustules, made of two perforated valves called thecae (epithecae and hypthecae) sealed together by girdle bands to hold the valves together as illustrated in Figure 3.1a. The frustules are created with a magnificent 3D precision of tens of nanometers which was optimized through evolution over millions of years to provide a variety of functions including mechanical protection against predators, nutrients uptake, and light harvesting. The valve consists of hexagonal chambers divided by silica plates. The plates have uniform pores with ascending or descending diameters from the outside to the inside which act as sieves to collect food and light (Figure 3.1b–d).

Each species of DE features a specific frustule shape decorated with a unique pattern of nanosized features such as pores, ridges, and spines with specific functions and properties, hollow pill-box structure, and aerodynamic shape with variety of sizes (500 nm to 50 μm) [25,26]. Their shapes and sizes vary from circular to triangular and from approximately

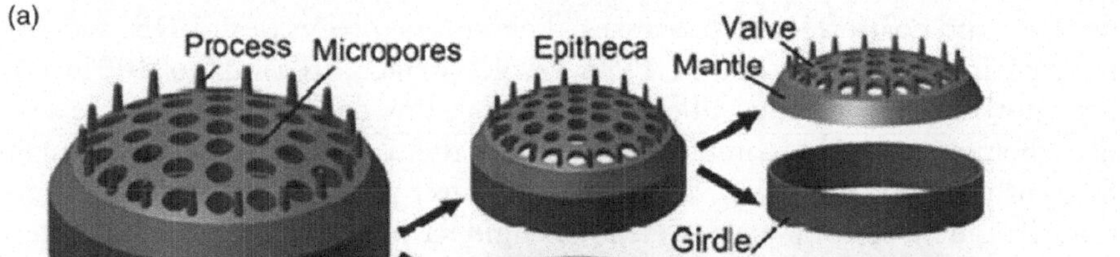

Figure 3.1 (a) Schematic illustration of DE structure. SEM image of a *Coscinodiscus* sp. frustule with images of pore structures on these layers; (b) arrays of foramen and second-level pores, scale bar 1 μm; (c) array of sieve pores, scale bar 2 μm; and (d) array of nanopores on girdle band, scale bar 1 μm. (Published from ref. [24] with permission of Springer.)

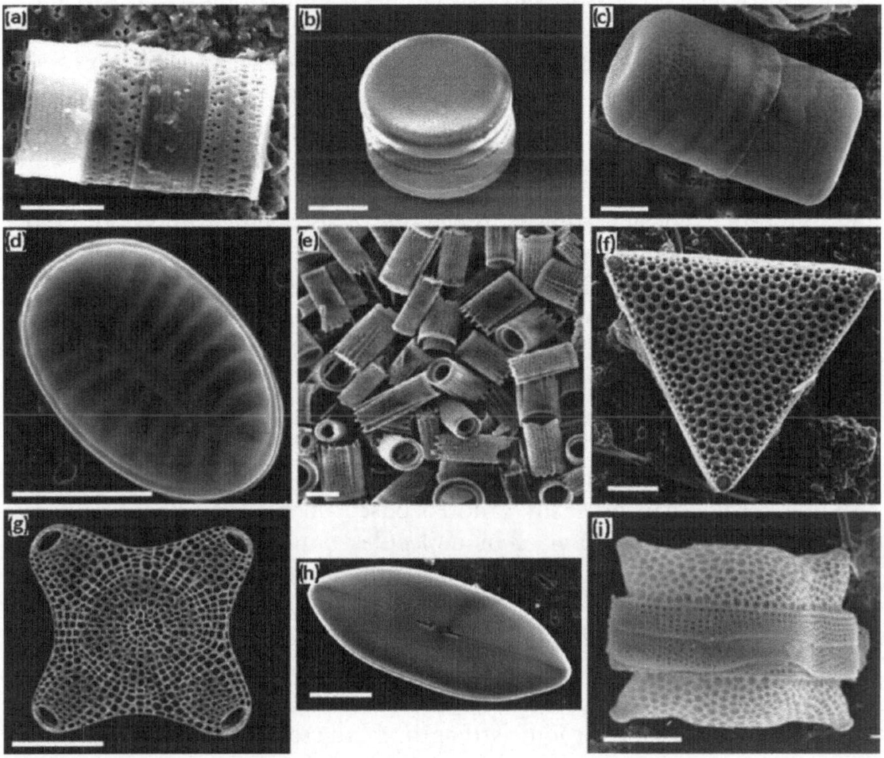

Figure 3.2 SEM images of different shapes and structures of diatoms species. Scale bar = 10 µm. (Reproduced with permission from ref. [25].)

five micrometers to a few hundred micrometers (Figure 3.2). The large species-specific variation in shape, size, geometry, organization, and density of pore structures represent subtle changes in the material structure to optimize movement and interactions in a complex biological environment. DE frustules inspire the design and production of novel nanostructured materials and have recently led to new nanomaterials through the maintenance of the DE's nanostructure with modification of the material chemistry [27].

3.3 SURFACE MODIFICATION STRATEGIES

Prior to their use in biomedical applications, raw and calcinated diatomite (supplied as rocks or powder) are usually purified to remove any impurities (e.g., alkaline metals and organic debris) attached to the silica frustules which could interfere with surface properties of diatoms required for specific applications. The processing of raw diatoms from diatomite minerals starts with crushing of large parts to obtain micron to submicron DE powders [28]. This is followed by numerous physical and chemical purification steps. Physical purification involves the calcination of raw diatoms powder at high temperature (>600°C); however, it leads to crystallization of the silica making them unsuitable for some commercial applications [29]. On the other hand, chemical purification of cultured diatoms by acid treatment (e.g., piranha solution) is considered more preferable, eco-friendly, simple, and rapid [30–33]. In this context, many studies were conducted to explore the effect of acid type, its concentration, and treatment time on the properties of the produced DEs. It is worth mentioning that our team (Losic et al.) refined the purification process to obtain pure intact DE frustules by combining sedimentation and filtration steps that are scalable and could provide DE silica material in large quantities needed for pharmaceutical industry [7,27,34].

After obtaining purified nonporous microparticles of DE, the surface chemistry of the purified porous silica structures (made of silicon dioxide building blocks) can be easily tailored based on the intended biomedical application. Immobilization of biomolecules onto the surface of DE can be achieved through two approaches: (i) non-covalent interaction, and (ii) covalent interactions. Since silica DE have negatively charged surface, non-covalent binding (e.g., electrostatic interaction and physical adsorption) is considered a simple and rapid loading technique; however, it is relatively weak and usually affected by various conditions such as solution pH, size of the biomolecule, or ionic strength. At the same time, it is sometimes difficult to control the amount of biomolecules loaded or released, which depends mainly on available surface area and release environment (e.g., pH or temperature). On the other hand, covalent binding (e.g., chemisorption interactions) is more stronger and easy to be controlled. Thus, from stability and reproducibility perspectives, the covalent binding of biomolecules to the surface of diatoms is more favored [35].

Chemical surface modification of DE has been continuously progressing during the last two decades [36]. Initially, alkene-thiols were used to form self-assembled monolayers on the surface. However, the long-term stability of the produced layers is compromised as a result of oxidation of sulfur (S) atom which leads to layer breakdown [37]. On the contrary, the presence of reactive silanol (SiOH) groups on frustules surface facilitates easy functionalization with reactive groups (e.g., $-NH_2$, –COOH, –SH, and –CHO) for the subsequent conjugation of biomolecules (e.g., drugs, enzymes, proteins, antibodies, peptides, DNA, and aptamer) [38,39]. SiOH allows strong coupling points for the attachment of biological or chemical moieties via the formation of self-assembled layer through Si–O–Si covalent bonds [40–42]. As a result, silanization is the most commonly applied process for the surface chemical modification of DE in order to prepare advanced DDS [37,-41–45]. Figure 3.3 represents an overview of common surface modification

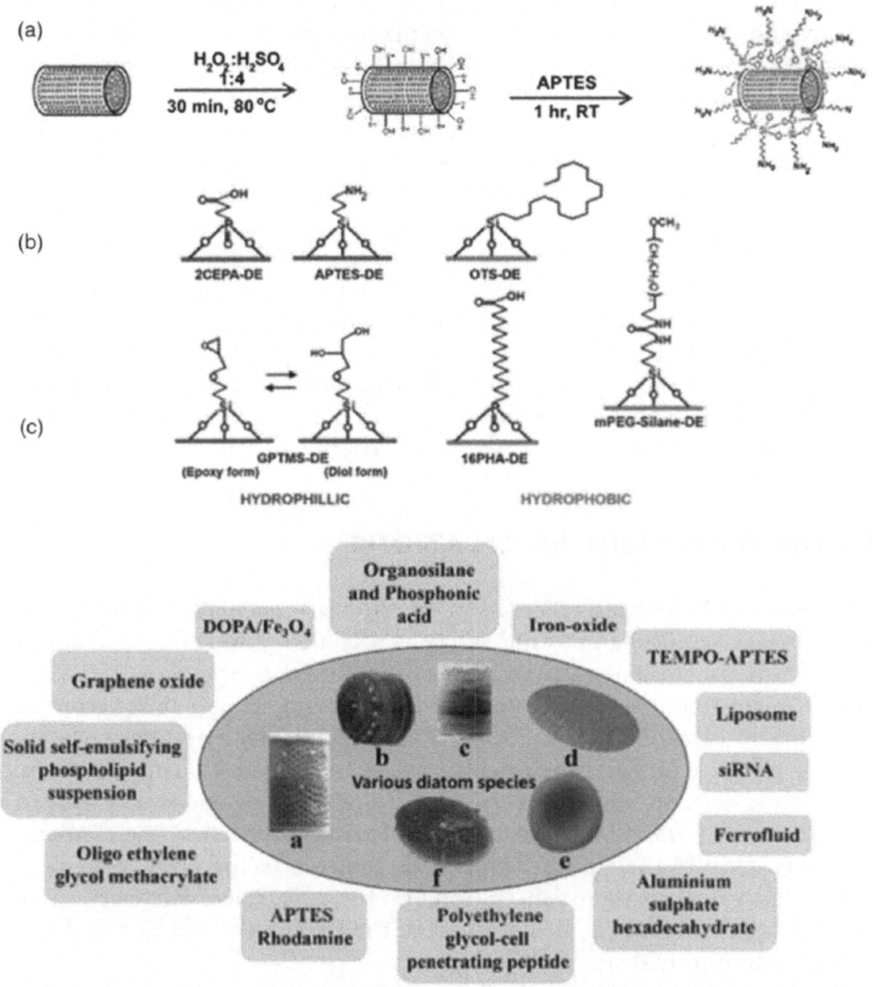

Figure 3.3 (a) Scheme representing surface functionalization of diatoms using 3-aminopropyl triethoxysilane (APTES). (Reproduced with permission [47], Copyright 2016, SpringerLink.) (b) Schematic illustration of DE functionalization using organosilans and phosphonic acids with hydrophobic and hydrophilic properties. (Reproduced with permission from ref. [48].)(c) An overview of different species of diatoms and their surface modification strategies for drug delivery applications. (a) *Aulacoseira* sp.: Dopa/Fe_3O_4, organosilane and phosphonic acid (hydrophobic and hydrophilic silane), graphene oxide, solid self-emulsifying phospholipid suspension (SEPS), oligo ethylene-glycol methacrylate. (b) *Thalassiosira weissflogii* sp.: TEMPO-APTES. (c) *Thalassiosira pseudonoma* sp.: Liposomes. (d) *Nitzschia* sp.: Ferrofluid. (e) Calcined diatomite sp.: Polyethylene glycol – cell-penetrating peptide, APTES Rhodamine, siRNA. (f) Kolubara coal basin diatomite: aluminum sulfate hexadecahydrate. (Reproduced by permission from ref. [46].)

strategies employed for drug delivery applications and shows a schematic illustration of typical surface functionalization of DE microcapsules using organosilanes via the formation of self-assembled layer through Si–O–Si covalent bonds [46,47].

Apart from the aforementioned surface modification of diatoms silica frustules, chemical modification of the living DE was achieved through the incorporation of alkoxysilane and organoalkoxysilane precursors in the culture media of DE [49]. Based on the biomineralization process which occurs within specialized units inside DE known as the silica deposition vesicle (SDV) cells, Lang et al. demonstrated the successful incorporation of thiol moieties into *Thalassiosira weissflogii* species during frustule synthesis as illustrated in Figure 3.4. Thus, owing to the ability to grow diatoms in large quantities in the laboratory, this live chemical modification strategy could open the door to endless alterations to the surface chemistry of living diatoms frustules organisms for a broad variety of applications.

3.4 DRUG DELIVERY APPLICATIONS

The delivery of therapeutic agents at an effective concentration to diseased body tissues while maintaining safety is a challenging task especially for drugs with a narrow therapeutic index (e.g., anticancer agents) [50,51]. In addition, the majority of new and existing drug molecules suffer from low solubility in physiologic conditions, inadequate cellular uptake, or lack of desired pharmacokinetic properties leading to limited biodistribution and therapeutic activity. Thus, a great pool of improved drug carriers has been investigated to improve their physicochemical properties (e.g., enhance stability), modify their distribution and retention in the body, control the release, and increase their penetration into the cells. These advanced carrier systems have been recognized to improve the therapeutic efficacy in desired tissues with minimal side effects [52–54].

As mentioned above, porous silica and silicon-based materials have been widely investigated as effective drug carriers [55–57]. However, their applications are confronted by high cost and time-consuming fabrication procedures, which also involve toxic solvents that may leave residue in the final products [25,58]. Since the expansion of nanotechnology as a separate science, there have been various reviews focusing on the unique DE biosilica structures that prompted to introduce new research field of DE nanotechnology [27,33,46,59–61]. Many inspiring research studies were generated from this field showing the application of DE across many disciplines and addressing many problems in water purification, microfluidics, biosensing, and energy storage [25,62,63]. For example, the surface of silica DE was modified to adsorb mercury ions from contaminated water for purification applications. This was achieved by attaching a layer of 3-mercaptopropyl-trimethoxysilane

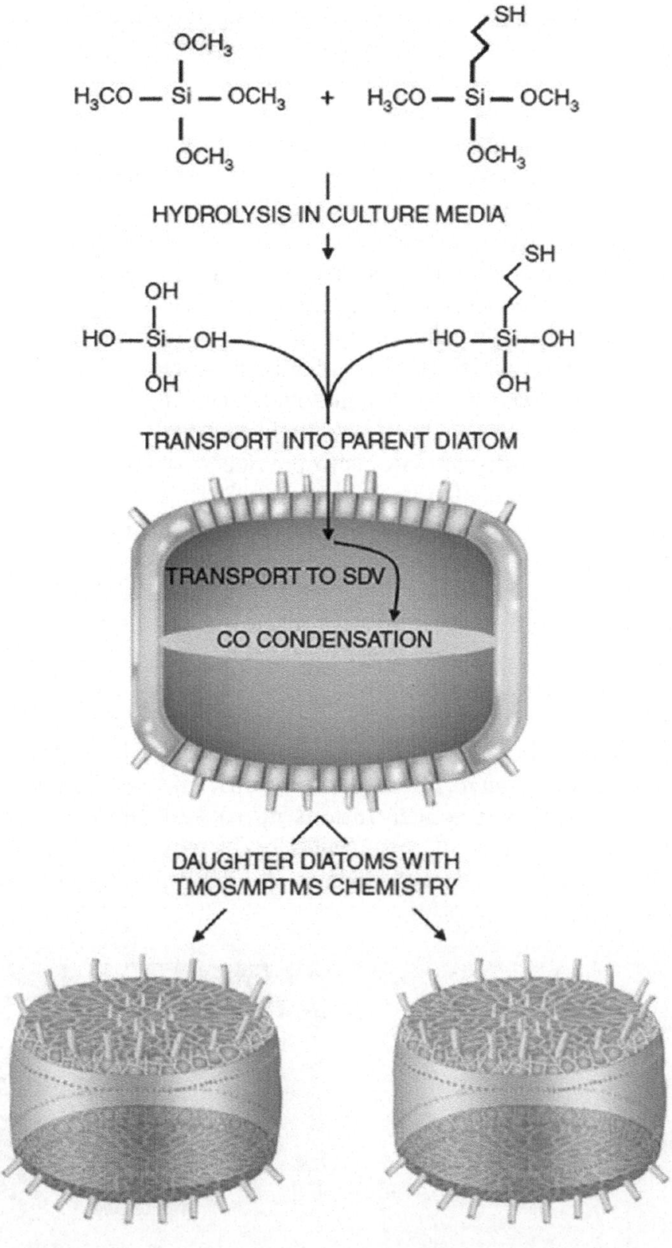

Figure 3.4 Thiol-functionalization of *Thalassiosira weissflogii*. Proposed hydrolysis of alkoxysilane tetramethoxysilane (TMOS) and 3-mercaptopropyltrimethoxysilan (MPTMS) in the culture media, transport into diatom, subsequent co-condensation within the silica deposition vesicle and incorporation into the frustule. (Reproduced with permission from ref. [49].)

(MPTMS), 3-aminopropyl-trimethoxysilane (APTES), and n-(2-aminoethyl)-3-aminopropyl-trimethoxysilane (AEAPTMS) on the surface of the frustules [63]. Silica DE was also used to immobilize active butyrylcholinesterase which showed much higher activity than its free form for biosensing applications [64]. A broad range of nature-inspired nanotechnology applications initiated by Morse et al. proposed the use of the 3D structure of DE as a new material owing to the genetically controlled precision of their nanoscale architecture that surpasses the conventional engineering capabilities [65]. The first attempt to use diatoms as a carrier was first demonstrated by Rosi et al. in which gold nanoparticles were loaded and subsequently released from DE [66]. The first demonstration of the concept of drug delivery by DE with an idea to encapsulate therapeutic agents within DE microcapsules for oral delivery was performed by Losic et al., which is schematically presented in Figure 3.5 [43,67]. Idea was to use a high surface area of hollow DE capsule for loading drugs and their nanopores to achieve slow and sustainable drug release. This study by Aw et al. confirmed the ability of diatoms to provide a prolonged release of indomethacin for 14 days with a loading efficacy of ~22%. During this experiment, indomethacin loading was achieved by sonication of the drug solution with DE followed by complete evaporation of the solvent. A two-phase release profile was observed; a burst release for the first 6 hours which resulted from the dissolution of the drug adsorbed on the surface followed by a sustained zero-order release as a result of the drug entrapped inside DE porous structure.

This idea is further explored by others showing the sustained delivery of other drugs such as prednisone and mesalamine that was achieved through their loading onto silica DE by physical adsorption [66]. In a study, Zhang et al. evaluated the *in vitro* toxicity of diatoms, and results confirmed the safety of DE frustules at concentrations up to 1,000 µg/mL. In addition, the uptake of both drugs by Caco-2/HT-29 cells when co-cultured together was significantly enhanced compared to the drugs alone (i.e., not loaded

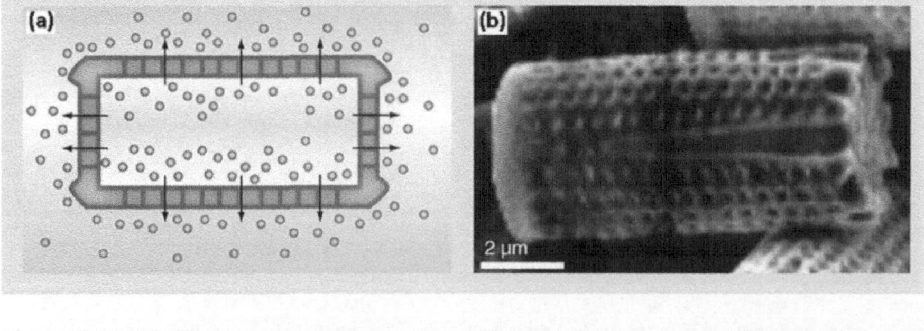

Figure 3.5 (a) Scheme of drug release from diatom silica structure. (b) Scanning electron microscopy image of typical DE structure in the form of microcapsules obtained from natural and purified diatomaceous earth. (Reproduced with permission from ref. [43].)

on diatoms) [68]. In another study, Janicijevic et al. prepared inorganically modified diatoms for sustained drug release applications where food-grade diatomite was modified by steering in aluminum sulfate hexadecahydrate solution followed by loading nonsteroidal anti-inflammatory agent, ibuprofen. High-loading efficiency (201 mg/g) and sustained drug release were obtained. In addition, the analgesic properties of ibuprofen-loaded diatoms were superior to that of an equivalent dose of ibuprofen alone when tested in rats [69].

As we mentioned above, hydroxyl groups present on the surface of DE silica could be effectively utilized to modify their surface properties to allow better control over the drug loading and release profiles. The effect of chemical functionalization of DE surface on drug loading and release of indomethacin as an example of poorly water-soluble drug was demonstrated [70]. In this study, organosilane 3-aminopropyltriethoxysilane (APTES) and N-(3-(trimethoxysilyl)propyl)ethylenediamine (AEAPTMS) and phosphonic acids (2-carboxyethyl-phosphonic acid and 16-phosphono-hexadecanoic acid) were utilized to render the of diatoms hydrophilic and hydrophobic, respectively (Figure 3.3b). Results showed that hydrophilic functionalization could increase the drug loading up to 24% wt compared to 15% in the case of hydrophobic surface. Moreover, the hydrophilic surface provided sustained release of loaded medications for 2 weeks in contrast to hydrophobic surface which caused a faster release over 6 days. Likewise, Bariana et al. [48] used methoxy-poly-(ethylene-glycol)-silane (mPEG-silane), 7-octadecyltrichlorosilane (OTS), 3-(glycidyloxypropyl) trimethoxysilane (GPTMS), and two phosphonic acids, namely, 2-carboxyethyl-phosphonic acid (2 CEPA) and 16-phosphono-hexadecanoic acid (16 PHA), to tune drug loading and release properties of poorly insoluble drug (indomethacin) and soluble drug (gentamicin). Successful insertion of these functional groups was confirmed with X-ray photoelectron spectroscopy (XPS) and Fourier transform infrared spectroscopy (FTIR) analysis. Again, different functional groups on the surface of diatom microparticles showed variations in drug loading capacity ranging from 14%wt up to 24%wt. In addition, the presence of hydrophilic moieties (polar carboxyl (e.g., 2 CEPA), amine (APTES), or hydrolyzed epoxy group (GPTMS)) on diatoms surface favored the prolonged release of indomethacin, while long chain hydrocarbons (e.g., OTS) surface-coated diatoms provided an extended release for gentamicin [48,71].

In the same context, self-emulsifying drug delivery system (SEDDS) is prepared by loading self-emulsifying phospholipid suspension (SEPS) of water-insoluble drug, carbamazepine, onto diatoms microparticles (Figure 3.6). In vitro study data showed enhanced dissolution of carbamazepine SSEPS after loading onto silica DE compared to free drug owing to the high porous surface of diatoms which provides a larger contact area with the dissolution medium [72].

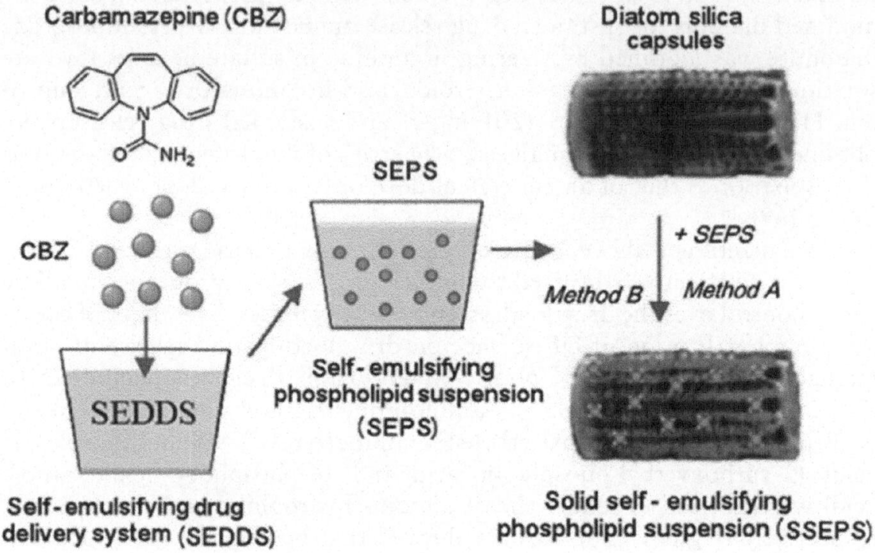

Figure 3.6 Scheme representing the SEPS technique for SEDDS. (Reproduced with permission from ref. [72].)

Cicco et al. also explored the bactericidal activity of diatoms loaded with reactive oxygen species (ROC) scavengers and antibiotics (ciprofloxacin) for fibroblasts and osteoblast-like cells growth applications. The surface of the diatoms was chemically modified by covalent attachment of ROC scavenger, cyclic nitroxide 2,6,6-tetramethylpiperid ine-N-oxyl (TEMPO), followed by the attachment of ciprofloxacin. The results confirmed that the prepared diatoms could be effectively used as substrates for bone cells' growth while providing antibacterial activity against infection [45].

Additional functions like drug targeting and triggered drug release could be achieved through surface functionalization. In this aspect, Losic et al. designed magnetically guided DE for drug targeting purposes by attaching dopamine-modified iron-oxide nanoparticles on DE surface. The fabricated magnetized diatoms provided a sustained release for 2 weeks of water-insoluble drug (indomethacin) [42]. This concept opens the door to fabricate targeted drug delivery systems offering many benefits compared with conventional drug delivery systems. Javalkote et al. investigated the anticancer activity of curcumin-loaded magnetically active diatom frustules. The results depicted that the prepared targeted drug delivery system could be useful to deliver different anticancer agents for efficient chemotherapy [73]. In another study, Todd and coworkers investigated in vivo magnetic targeting of iron-oxide-decorated diatoms [74]. Upon application of the magnetic field, a significant accumulation of drug-loaded diatoms was observed at the tumor site compared to control (i.e., no magnetic field applied).

Drug targeting was also achieved through a novel concept which was introduced to genetically control the properties of cultured diatom in laboratory settings and apply them as targeted drug carriers for different therapies. This concept is based on the fascinating self-assembly genetically controlled system of DE to produce silica-building blocks from silicic acid in water. Thus, regulating the process of gene expression in DE could result in DE species with unique properties [61,75]. Genetically engineered DEs, displaying IgG-binding domain of protein G (GB1-bioselica) on their surface, were developed to deliver anticancer agents (Camptothecin and 7-ethyl-10-hydroxy Camptothecin), [58]. First, IgG antibodies (e.g., antibody specific for the p75 neurotrophin receptor (p75NTR) (anti-p75NTR)) were attached to GB1-bioselica to specifically target neuroblastoma and B-lymphoma cells. After that, the cytotoxic agents were loaded onto diatoms by electrostatic interaction. In vivo study in SH-SY5Y neuroblastoma tumor-bearing BALB/c nude mice showed a significant reduction in tumor growth after drug-loaded diatoms were administered as shown in Figure 3.7.

Targeted drug delivery was also achieved by Uthappa et al. by generating a polydopamine (PDA) functionalized DE for curcumin delivery. First, curcumin was loaded onto DE followed by PDA coating. To improve the affinity of the drug-loaded DEs, folic acid ligands were also attached to the surface as shown in Figure 3.8. Curcumin release from the fabricated delivery system showed pH-dependent behavior. At the same time, dopamine formed a barrier controlling curcumin release [76].

Recently, Delasoie et al. prepared targeted DDS composed of DE coated with vitamin B_{12} as tumor-targeting ligand. Anticancer agent, a tris-tetraethyl[2,2′-bipyridine]-4,4′-diamine–ruthenium(II) complex, was then loaded as illustrated in Figure 3.9. An unprecedented release profile was recorded for ruthenium(II) complex for up to 5 days in aqueous media. The adherence of vitamin B_{12} coated diatoms was three folds higher compared to uncoated DE when tested with colorectal cancer cell line HT-29 and breast cancer cell line MCF-7 [77]. Most recently, the same group explored similar vitamin B_{12} diatoms DDS but with the incorporation of chemical photosensitizer (porphyrins) for photodynamic therapy or a photo-triggered CO-releasing molecule ((2,20-bipyridine)-3,40-dicarbox ylic acid manganese tricarbonyl complex) [78]. This multifunctional system offered dual anticancer activity; chemotherapy and spatio-temporal controlled activity allowed by the photoactivation. Two folds increase in the cytotoxic activity was observed upon light activation which confirms the ability of DE to fabricate multifunctional therapeutic systems with enhanced selectivity and activity.

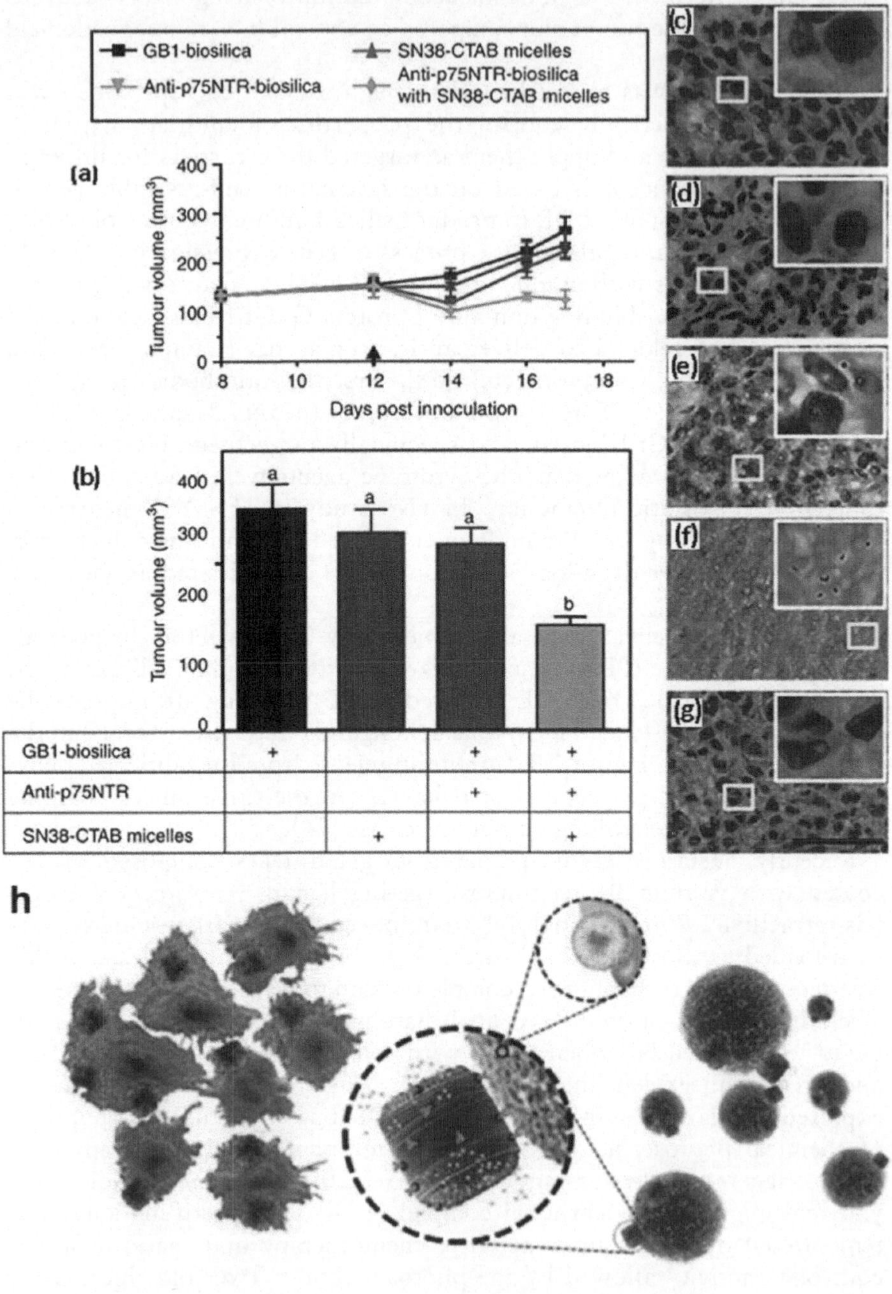
GB1-biosilica
SN38-CTAB micelles
Anti-p75NTR-biosilica
Anti-p75NTR-biosilica with SN38-CTAB micelles
(a)
Tumour volume (mm^3)
400
300
200
100
0
8
10
12
14
16
18
Days post innoculation
(b)
a
a
a
b
GB1-biosilica
Anti-p75NTR
SN38-CTAB micelles
+
(c)
(d)
(e)
(f)
(g)
h

(Continued)

Figure 3.7 (Continued) Antibody-labeled DE biosilica loaded with SN38 reduces neuroblastoma SH-SY5Y tumor growth and histochemical analysis of SH-SY5Y xenografts. (a) Average tumor volumes measured over 17 days in immunodeficient Balb/c nude mice that were implanted with SH-SY5Y neuroblastoma cells and treated with a single dose of different DE biosilica-based materials. (b) Comparison of average tumor volumes after 17 days of treatment with anti-p75NTR–GB1–SN38, GB1–biosilica, SN38–CTAB micelles, and anti-p75NTR–GB1–biosilica. Arrow indicates the day on which the intraperitoneal injection was administered. (c) Untreated tumor control. Tumor treated with (d) GB1–biosilica, (e) anti-p75NTR–GB1-labeled biosilica, (f) anti-p75NTR–GB1–biosilica–SN38–CTAB micelles, and (g) SN38–CTAB micelles. Treatments via intraperitoneal injection occurred 12 days after tumor cell inoculation. Images are representative of tissue sections selected from four independent experiments. Insets: dark spots show the DE biosilica. Scale bar, 50 mm (h) Schematic representation of genetically engineered DE biosilica containing liposome-encapsulated drug molecules can be targeted to both adherent neuroblastoma cells and lymphocyte cells in suspension by functionalizing the biosilica surface with cell-specific antibodies. Liposome-encapsulated drug molecules are released from the biosilica carrier in the immediate vicinity of the target cells (inset). (Reproduced with permission [58], Copyright 2015, Springer Nature.)

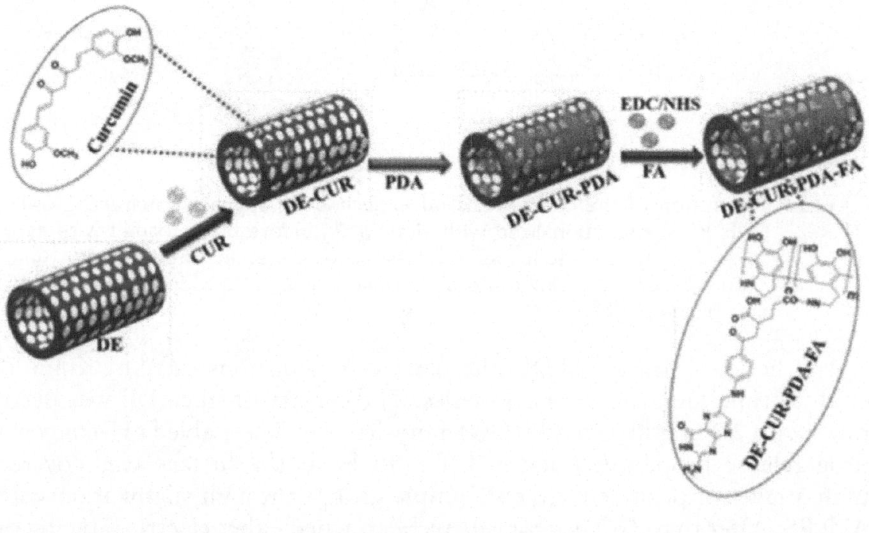

Figure 3.8 Schematic illustration for the synthesis of curcumin-loaded polydopamine-coated diatoms. DE: Diatoms, CUR: Curcumin, PDA: polydopamine, and FA: folic acid. (Reproduced by permission from ref. [76] with modifications.)

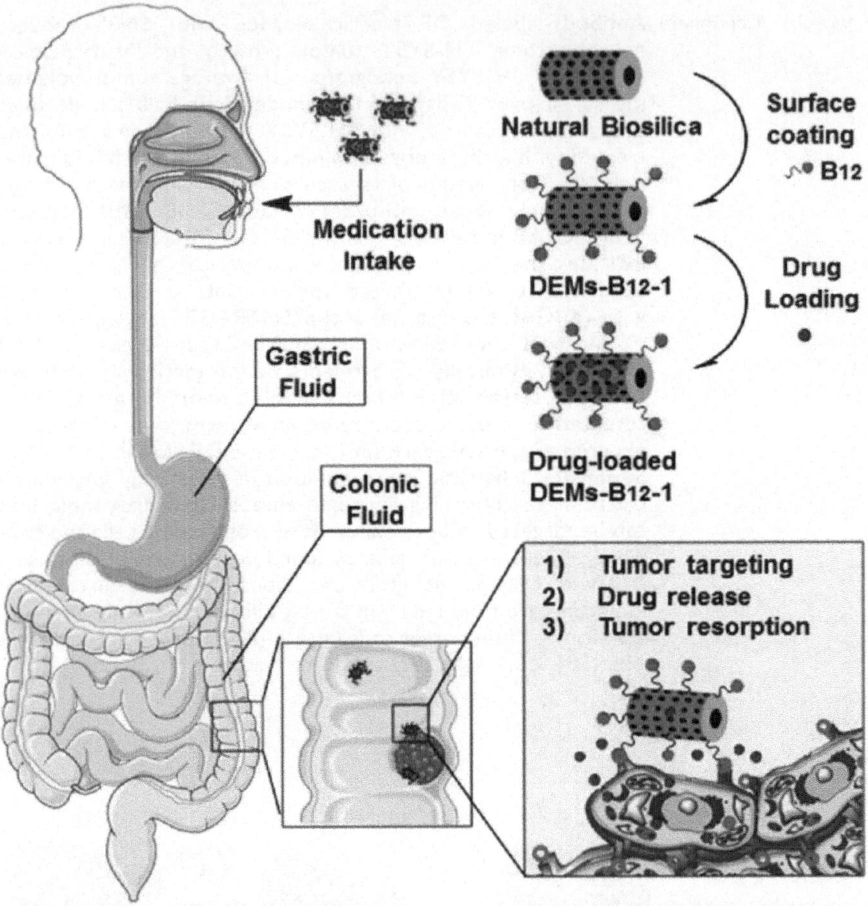

Figure 3.9 Illustration of the conceptual and experimental approach. Natural biosilica "DEMs" are functionalized with vitamin B_{12} before being loaded with cytotoxic drug agent. The loaded micro-shuttles target and interact with tumor tissues before releasing the drug in their vicinity. (Reproduced with permission from ref. [77].)

Another modification of DE silica surface was demonstrated by Kumeria et al. to tune the drug release kinetics. The surface of silica DE was decorated with 2D graphene oxide (GO) nanosheets which enabled pH-triggered drug release properties (Figure 3.10a–d). First, the surface was covered with a layer of positively charged amine groups through silanization with APTES. After that, GO nanosheets were attached either electrostatically or covalently to the surface of DE. Results confirmed the pH-dependent drug release of nonsteroidal anti-inflammatory drug, indomethacin, after loading on GO nanosheets in buffers with different pH values [78].

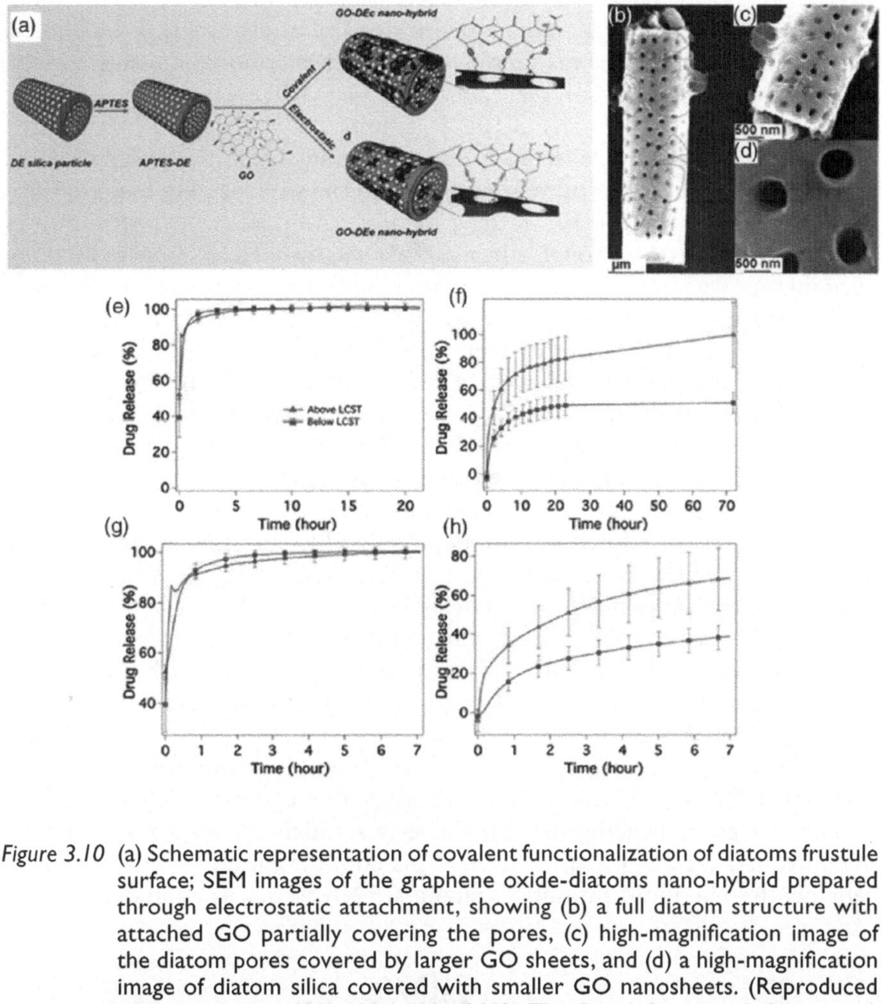

Figure 3.10 (a) Schematic representation of covalent functionalization of diatoms frustule surface; SEM images of the graphene oxide-diatoms nano-hybrid prepared through electrostatic attachment, showing (b) a full diatom structure with attached GO partially covering the pores, (c) high-magnification image of the diatom pores covered by larger GO sheets, and (d) a high-magnification image of diatom silica covered with smaller GO nanosheets. (Reproduced with permission [80], Copyright 2013, The Royal Society of Chemistry.) (e–f) Release curves of levofloxacin drug from the diatom microcapsules below and above the lower critical solution temperature of the (O(EG)MA) copolymer. (e) Total release and (f) first 7 hours of release from unmodified microcapsules, (g) total release, and (h) first 7 hours of release from (O(EG)MA)-modified microcapsules. (Reproduced with permission [79], Copyright 2015, The Royal Society of Chemistry.)

Triggered drug release of antibacterial agent levofloxacin was demonstrated and explored by Vasani et al. Surface-initiated atom transfer radical polymerization (ATRP) was employed to graft thermo-responsive copolymers, oligo(ethylene-glycol) methacrylates (O(EG)MA), onto the surface of the DEs. As shown in Figure 3.10e–h, results showed a strong correlation between levofloxacin release and temperature in which the polymer acted as a physical actuator to pump the drug into the surrounding media [79].

In addition to the control of drug loading and release, incorporation of polymers or peptides onto DE silica surface was applied to improve biocompatibility, prevent aggregation, increase cellular uptake, and enhance stability. In one study, DE frustules were tested for the delivery of anticancer agent, sorafenib. First, DE frustules were crushed into nanoparticles followed by surface functionalization with APTES. After that, polyethylene glycol (PEG) was attached to the surface through the formation of amide bond between amino groups (-NH_2) of APTES on DE surface and the carboxylic groups (-COOH) of PEG by 1-ethyl-3-[3-dimethylaminopropyl] carbodiimide hydrochloride/N-hydroxysuccinimide (EDC/NHS). Following PEG coating, a layer of cell-penetrating peptide (CPP) was added to enhance the drug delivery of the anticancer agent as illustrated in Figure 3.11 [81]. The stability of the prepared nanoparticles in aqueous solution and their biocompatibility with RBCs were confirmed to be stable. Moreover, CPP significantly enhanced sorafenib cellular penetration. It is worth mentioning that the loading capacity of PEG-coated diatoms nanoparticles was double that of uncoated ones.

Besides drug molecules, silica DE were also explored for delivering small interfering RNA (siRNA) for gene therapy applications. siRNA could be applied for gene silencing of defective genes which are responsible for the uncontrolled growth of cancer cells. This could eventually result in cancer cells death. The main limitation facing siRNA is that they undergo rapid

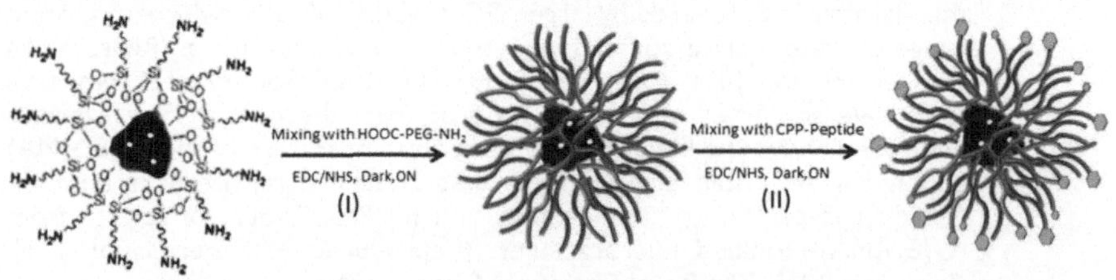

Figure 3.11 Schematic representation of the DNPs functionalization. Reaction I, the PEGylation of DNPs-APT (I) via EDC/NHS, under stirring ON at RT. Reaction II, CPP-peptide bio-conjugation of DNPs-APT-PEG via EDC/NHS, under stirring ON at RT. The dual bio-functionalization is based on a covalent binding between the NPs' surface and the biomolecules promoted by EDC/NHS chemistry. (Reproduced with permission [81], Copyright 2015, The Royal Society of Chemistry.)

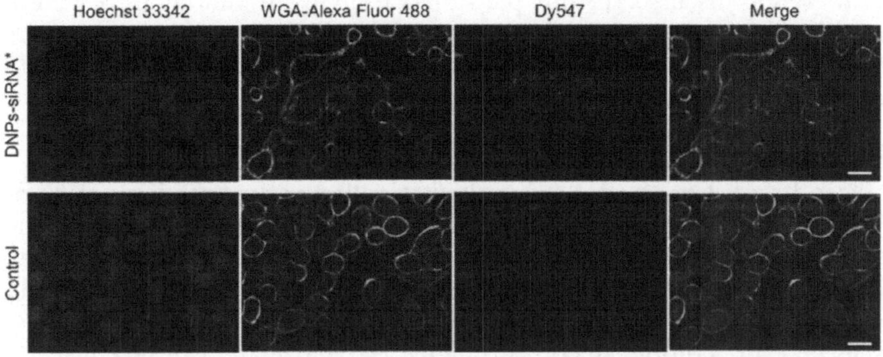

Figure 3.12 Confocal microscopy on cells treated with siRNA-modified diatomite nanovectors (first line) and untreated cells as control (second line). Cell nuclei and membranes were stained with Hoechst 33342 and WGA-Alexa Fluor 488, respectively. siRNA was labeled with Dy547. Scale bar corresponds to 20 μm. (Reproduced with permission [84], Copyright 2015, Elsevier.)

degradation by nucleases once introduced into the body before reaching their site of action (i.e., cancer cells). Thus, they should be protected by encapsulating them within a carrier (e.g., liposomes or polymeric nanoparticles) till they reach their targets [82,83]. In this context, poly d-arginine peptide/siRNA complex was effectively delivered into the cytoplasm of human epidermoid cancer cells (H1355) after being covalently linked to APTES surface modified diatom (Figure 3.12) [84].

3.5 BIODEGRADABLE DIATOMS DRUG CARRIERS

All the aforementioned studies have confirmed the capacity of silica diatoms frustules to provide controlled and sustained release of a wide variety of therapeutic agents for many clinical applications. Despite being more biocompatible and environmentally friendly than synthetic silica particles, silica DE are made of silica-building blocks which show limited biodegradation in biological environment (e.g., blood or interstitial tissue fluids) [85–90]. Upon repeated administration of silica drug-based carriers, accumulation of such particles is expected to take place, especially in case of organs with limited blood flow (e.g., vitreous body). In one study, silica particles accumulated in the lungs air sacs and kidney glomerulus of rats after systemic administration [91]. Thus, it is preferable for drug carriers to degrade into non-toxic products which can be easily cleared outside the body.

To overcome the biodegradation limitations of silica-based materials, synthetic porous silicon (pSi) was explored as an attractive alternative [17].

However, as discussed before, pSi suffers from major limitations related to its fabrication process based on electrochemical etching of silicon wafers which is a time-consuming synthesis procedure involving several steps and applies many toxic chemicals (*vide supra*) [17].

Thus, converting silica DE frustules into biodegradable silicon (Si) DE is recognized as a new approach of low-cost and non-toxic source of silicon-based drug carrier materials that will overcome the limitations of both silica and synthetic pSi nanoparticles. This approach is based on the fact that silicon is an essential trace element found in the human body (around 5 ppm in human plasma), and its degradation product, silicic acid (H_4SiO_4), is absorbed by the human body and is found in different tissues [92]. In addition, silicon is fully biodegradable and can be efficiently excreted by kidneys [13,85,93–99].

Fabrication of silicon replicates of diatoms silica is industrially scalable, cost-effective, and time-efficient process without the use of toxic chemicals. Furthermore, these replicates are biodegradable and non-toxic for biomedical applications. Magnesiothermic reduction reaction was applied for the first time by Bao et al. to convert silica DE frustules to pure silicon DE replicas which were then tested as gas sensors [100,101].

During magnesiothermic reduction, silica DE are totally converted to silicon replicas while the structure and morphology of the diatoms are completely preserved. This approach paved the way to prepare silicon micro/nanoparticles from naturally occurring DE frustules for advanced drug carrier applications. The first report of a novel self-reporting drug carriers (i.e., the drug carrier itself reports the amount of drug left or released at a specific time point) based on biodegradable and luminescent silicon diatoms with 3D biological morphology was demonstrated by the Losic group as illustrated in Figure 3.13a [34,102]. For the first time, the photoluminescence (PL) properties of silicon diatoms replicates were demonstrated to develop a novel self-reporting biodegradable system. Silicon DE microparticles showed significantly high surface area compared to pristine silica diatoms. This was confirmed by reduction of the silica-building blocks volume forming the frustules during the fabrication process of SiO_2 to Si. Moreover, the silicon replicas displayed a pH degradation rate which was faster under physiologic pH 7.4 compared to acidic pH conditions. The fabricated silicon DE replicas were also loaded with daunorubicin (DNR) for the treatment of proliferative vitreoretinopathy (PVR). The in vitro release data confirmed the ability of DNR-loaded particles to provide a sustained drug release for 30 days. At the same time, silicon diatoms served as self-reporting drug carriers to monitor the process of drug release (Figure 3.13b–d) [102].

Apart from self-monitoring applications of silicon DEs, studies showed that porous silicon nanoparticles tend to accumulate in tumor tissues owing to the poor lymphatic drainage and leaky vasculature within these tissues through enhanced permeation and retention (EPR) effect

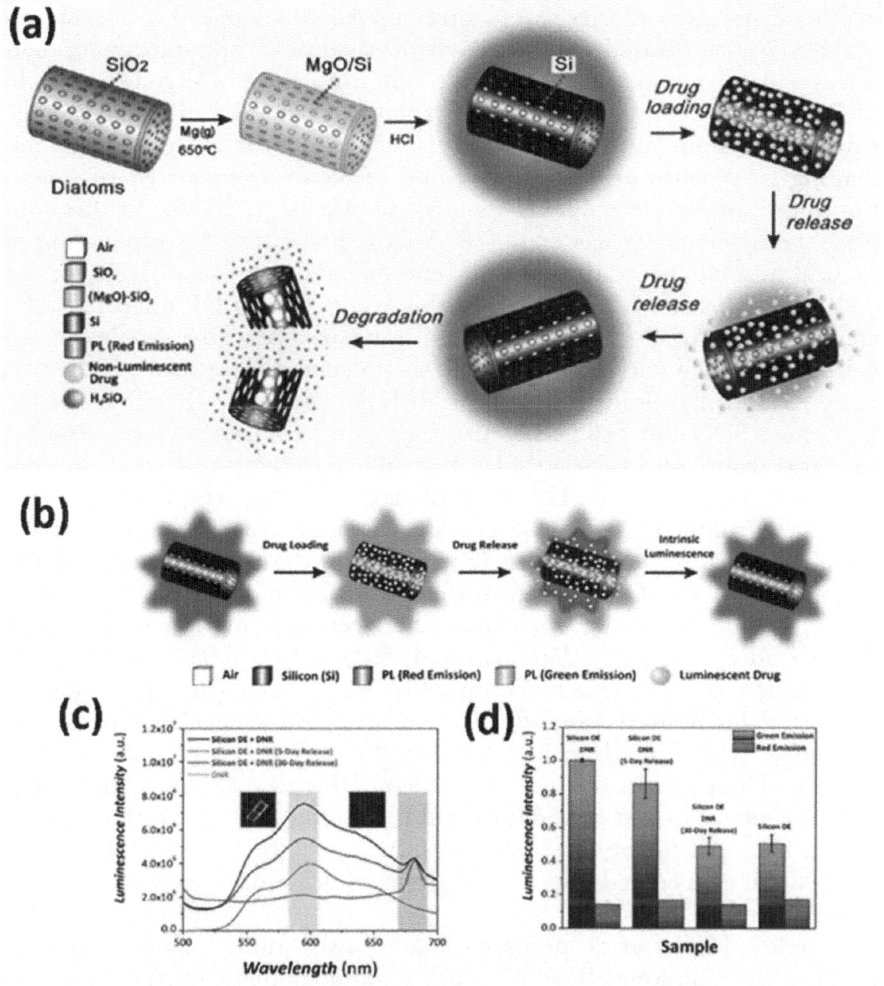

Figure 3.13 (a) Schematic illustration of the gas/silica displacement method based on the magnesiothermic reduction process employed to convert silica diatoms 3D structure into luminescent silicon replicas as a new biodegradable microcarrier with self-reporting function with unique biological-derived shape desirable for high drug loading and sustainable release for broad drug delivery applications. (b) Schematic illustration showing DNR loading onto silicon DE replicas and the change in luminescence properties at the different stages of the release process. (c) Photoluminescence spectra of silicon DE replicas after DNR loading, after 5 and 30 days of release (inset showing confocal microscope images in green (594 nm) and red (682 nm) regions). (d) Bar chart showing the intensity of luminescence measured from confocal microscope images after the different stages of the process. (Reproduced with permission [102], copyright 2015, WILEY-VCH.)

[103,104]. Nevertheless, it is worthwhile mentioning that drug-loaded synthetic pSi nanocarriers were investigated to reduce the side effects and toxicity associated with different therapeutics while improving their release. For example, the efficacy of the anticancer drug doxorubicin (DOX) is limited by its narrow therapeutic index, including bone marrow suppression and cardiotoxicity [105,106]. Studies confirmed that loading DOX onto drug carriers could result in its localized release at the tumor site while reducing its adverse effects [107,108]. In this context, the Losic group has explored, for the first time, the application of natural and biodegradable silicon diatoms nanoparticles (SiNPs) for the controlled release of DOX [34]. In this study, silicon DE microparticles were crushed by ultrasonication into nanosized silicon particles which were then loaded with DOX. During the in vitro release study, DOX was released over a prolonged period of 30 days confirming the ability of the fabricated SiNPs to provide a sustained and localized delivery of anticancer therapy. The nanoparticles were able to retain the loaded anticancer agent at physiologic pH (7.4) while releasing the drug in the tumor's acidic environment (pH 5.5). The drug release was dependent on the diffusion of DOX molecules entrapped within the nanoporous structure of DE and on the degradation of the silicon-building blocks which was demonstrated by strong correlation between degradation and release. Furthermore, this study demonstrated, for the first time, that such silicon DE nanoparticles are biocompatible. At the same time, DOX-loaded nanoparticles showed a significantly higher cytotoxic effect compared to free DOX when tested against MDA-MB-231-TXSA breast cancer cells in vitro. These results confirm that silicon DE-based carriers can be prepared from cheap and abundant natural resources using scalable process and grant a promising alternative to existing synthetic silicon materials for designing advanced micro/nanocarriers for a broad range of biomedical applications.

Recently, Maher et al. prepared magnetically guided microspheres by encapsulating diatom silicon NPs (SiNPs) and magnetic bacterial nanowires (BacNWs) with pH-sensitive biodegradable matrix using microfluidics technology to target colorectal cancer as illustrated in Figure 3.14a–c [109]. In this composite system, SiNPs and BacNWs were loaded with 5-flourouracil (5FU) and curcumin (CUR), respectively. BacNWs provided a magnetic field-assisted targeting and retention of the microspheres at the desired site of action (i.e., colon). The use of pH-sensitive polymer prevented premature release of loaded medications in the acidic pH of the stomach. Results revealed the ability of the microcapsules to selectively rupture at desired pH (Figure 3.14e), allowing 5FU and CUR to be released locally. In vitro data also showed a strong synergistic cytotoxic activity between 5FU and CUR when challenged against colon cancer cells (SW480).

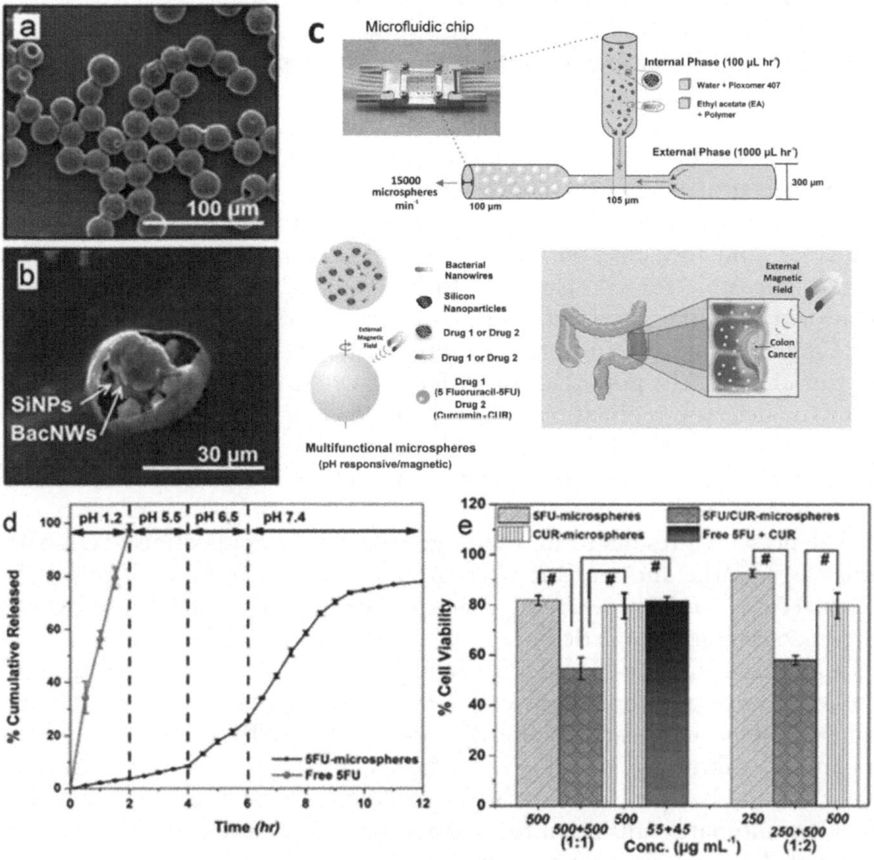

Figure 3.14 SEM images showing (a) 5FU-monodisperse polymer microspheres as prepared and (b) single microsphere encapsulated with 5FU-loaded diatom SiNPs and BacNWs. (c) Schematic illustration of the microfluidic system for monodisperse droplet preparation of pH-sensitive microspheres with SiNPs and BacNWs containing anticancer drug (5-fluorouracil or curcumin) and proposed application for intestinal combination therapy of colorectal cancer. (d) Typical pH-dependent drug release of 5FU loaded microspheres with diatom SiNPs tested at different pH conditions and (e) the viability of VSW480 cells after exposure to either single (i.e., only one type of microspheres used containing either 5FU or CUR) or multiple drug-loaded microspheres with SiNPs (i.e., both 5FU-microspheres and CUR-microspheres were added simultaneously). Error bars represent SD ($n=3$). Statistical analysis was calculated by ANOVA, followed by Bonferroni's multiple comparison test. The level of significance was set at a p value<0.05 for * in comparison to control group ($n \geq 3 \pm SD$). (Reproduced with permission from [109], Copyright 2017, The Royal Society of Chemistry.)

3.6 CONCLUSION AND PERSPECTIVES

Diatoms can be considered as natural biofactories for mass-scale production of micro- and nanoporous silica structures with unique structures which are not accessible by conventional synthetic porous silica materials. They are characterized by hierarchical 3D-porous structure offering a unique set of physical and chemical characteristics including high surface area, tunable surface chemistry, biocompatibility, high drug loading capacity, and low cost with efficient optical features. These properties make it feasible for DE frustules to be explored as an attractive cheap platform to replace synthetic silica/silicon materials for the preparation of a great variety of innovative nanomedicine and drug delivery systems. In this chapter, the potential use of DEs as whole or fragmented frustules for drug delivery applications was presented. The fabrication of DE carriers, surface functionalization, and ability to control drug release together with their capacity to enable targeting of therapeutic molecules inside the body were also discussed.

The presented results from recent progress on the application of DE frustules as versatile and realistic alternative to synthetic porous silica for the engineering of new generation of smart drug delivery systems and devices are encouraging. In particular, studies confirmed that DE could be used as a platform to design multifunctional DDS by combining targeting, controlled release with enhanced cellular uptake is significant. Furthermore, while diatomaceous earth is already approved by the EPA, USDA, and FDA as an anti-caking agent in livestock feed and used in chemical pesticides, their use in pharmaceutical industry could face some approval challenges for their ultimate translation for real applications that need to be explored. Nevertheless, the substantial number of in vitro and in vivo animal studies on DE and their replicas are a promising indication of their biocompatibility but still more extensive research in vivo studies are needed to assess any potential associated side effects with diatoms-based systems followed by testing their clinical efficiency to make the journey along the regulatory pathway for approval.

ACKNOWLEDGMENTS

The authors acknowledge the financial support provided to S.M. by Australian Research Council (ARC) (IH 15000003) grant, the Australian Government Training Program Scholarship, and Forrest George and Sandra Lynne Young Supplementary Scholarship. The authors are grateful to the School of Chemical Engineering at the University of Adelaide for support of this research.

REFERENCES

1. Yan L., Chen X. 7-nanomaterials for drug delivery. In: Tjong S.-C., editor. *Nanocrystalline Materials* (Second Edition). Oxford: Elsevier; 2014, pp. 221–268.
2. Wenzel J.G.W., Balaji K.S.S., Koushik K., et al. Pluronic® F127 gel formulations of Deslorelin and GnRH reduce drug degradation and sustain drug release and effect in cattle. *Journal of Controlled Release*, 2002; 85(1–3):51–59. doi: 10.1016/S0168-3659(02)00271-7.
3. Nokhodchi A., Tailor A. In situ cross-linking of sodium alginate with calcium and aluminum ions to sustain the release of theophylline from polymeric matrices. *Il Farmaco*, 2004; 59(12):999–1004. doi: 10.1016/j.farmac.2004.08.006.
4. Natarajan J.V., Nugraha C., Ng X.W., et al. Sustained-release from nanocarriers: A review. *Journal of Controlled Release*, 2014; 193:122–138. doi: 10.1016/j.jconrel.2014.05.029.
5. de Jesus M.B., Zuhorn I.S. Solid lipid nanoparticles as nucleic acid delivery system: Properties and molecular mechanisms. *Journal of Controlled Release*, 2015; 201:1–13. doi: 10.1016/j.jconrel.2015.01.010.
6. Farokhzad O.C., Langer R. Nanomedicine: Developing smarter therapeutic and diagnostic modalities. *Advanced Drug Delivery Reviews*, 2006; 58(-14):1456–1459. doi: 10.1016/j.addr.2006.09.011.
7. Maher S., Kumeria T., Aw M.S., et al. Diatom silica for biomedical applications: Recent progress and advances. *Advanced Healthcare Materials*, 2018;7(19):e1800552. doi: 10.1002/adhm.201800552. PubMed PMID: 30118185; eng.
8. Uthappa U.T., Sriram G., Brahmkhatri V., et al. Xerogel modified diatomaceous earth microparticles for controlled drug release studies. *New Journal of Chemistry*, 2018;42(14):11964–11971. doi: 10.1039/C8NJ01238E.
9. Archer M., Fauchet P.M. Electrical sensing of DNA hybridization in porous silicon layers. *Physica Status Solidi (a)*, 2003;198(2):503–507. doi: 10.1002/pssa.200306641.
10. Bonanno L.M., Segal E. Nanostructured porous silicon–polymer-based hybrids: From biosensing to drug delivery. *Nanomedicine*, 2011;6(10):1755–1770. doi: 10.2217/nnm.11.153.
11. Fan D., De Rosa E., Murphy M.B., et al. Mesoporous silicon-PLGA composite microspheres for the double controlled release of biomolecules for orthopedic tissue engineering. *Advanced Functional Materials*, 2012;22(2):282–293. doi: 10.1002/adfm.201100403.
12. Low S.P., Williams K.A., Canham L.T., et al. Evaluation of mammalian cell adhesion on surface-modified porous silicon. *Biomaterials*, 2006;27(-26):4538–4546. doi: 10.1016/j.biomaterials.2006.04.015.
13. Näkki S., Rytkönen J., Nissinen T., et al. Improved stability and biocompatibility of nanostructured silicon drug carrier for intravenous administration. *Acta Biomaterialia*, 2015;13:207–215. doi: 10.1016/j.actbio.2014.11.019.
14. Hernandez-Montelongo J., Naveas N., Degoutin S., et al. Porous silicon-cyclodextrin based polymer composites for drug delivery applications. *Carbohydrate Polymers*, 2014;110:238–252. doi: 10.1016/j.carbpol.2014.04.002.

15. Lee H.J., Son Y., Kim D., et al. A new thin silicon microneedle with an embedded microchannel for deep brain drug infusion. *Sensors and Actuators, B: Chemical Sensors and Materials.* 2015;209:413–422. doi: 10.1016/j.snb.2014.11.132.
16. Peng F., Su Y., Ji X., et al. Doxorubicin-loaded silicon nanowires for the treatment of drug-resistant cancer cells. *Biomaterials*, 2014;35(19):5188–5195. doi: 10.1016/j.biomaterials.2014.03.032.
17. Guo M., Zou X., Ren H., et al. Fabrication of high surface area mesoporous silicon via magnesiothermic reduction for drug delivery. *Microporous and Mesoporous Materials*, 2011;142(1):194–201. doi: 10.1016/j.micromeso.2010.11.036.
18. Vallet-Regi M., Ruiz-Gonzalez L., Izquierdo-Barba I., et al. Revisiting silica based ordered mesoporous materials: Medical applications. *Journal of Materials Chemistry*, 2006;16(1):26–31. doi: 10.1039/B509744D.
19. Vallet-Regí M., Izquierdo-Barba I., Rámila A., et al. Phosphorous-doped MCM-41 as bioactive material. *Solid State Sciences*, 2005;7(2):233–237. doi: 10.1016/j.solidstatesciences.2004.10.038.
20. Koynov S., Pereira R.N., Crnolatac I., et al. Purification of nano-porous silicon for biomedical applications. *Advanced Engineering Materials*, 2011;13(6):B225–B233. doi: 10.1002/adem.201080091.
21. Round F.E., Crawford R.M., Mann D.G. *Diatoms: Biology and Morphology of the Genera*. Cambridge University Press, Cambridge, 1990.
22. Anderson M.W., Holmes S.M., Hanif N., et al. Hierarchical pore structures through diatom zeolitization. *Angewandte Chemie*, 2000;112(15):2819–2822. doi: 10.1002/1521-3757(20000804)112:15<2819::AID-ANGE2819>3.0.CO;2-Z.
23. Rea I., Terracciano M., De Stefano L. Synthetic vs natural: Diatoms bioderived porous materials for the next generation of healthcare nanodevices. *Advanced Healthcare Materials*, 2017;6(3):1601125. doi: 10.1002/adhm.201601125.
24. Zhang D., Wang Y., Cai J., et al. Bio-manufacturing technology based on diatom micro- and nanostructure. *Chinese Science Bulletin*, 2012;57(30):3836–3849. doi: 10.1007/s11434-012-5410-x.
25. Losic D., Mitchell J.G., Voelcker N.H. Diatomaceous lessons in nanotechnology and advanced materials. *Advanced Materials*, 2009;21(29):2947–2958. doi: 10.1002/adma.200803778.
26. Sumper M., Brunner E. Learning from diatoms: Nature's tools for the production of nanostructured silica. *Advanced Functional Materials*, 2006;16(1):17–26. doi: 10.1002/adfm.200500616.
27. Gordon R., Losic D., Tiffany M.A., et al. The glass menagerie: Diatoms for novel applications in nanotechnology. *Trends in Biotechnology*, 2009;27(2):116–127. doi: 10.1016/j.tibtech.2008.11.003.
28. Sun Z., Yang X., Zhang G., et al. A novel method for purification of low grade diatomite powders in centrifugal fields. *International Journal of Mineral Processing*, 2013;125:18–26. doi: 10.1016/j.minpro.2013.09.005.
29. Zhang X., Liu X., Meng G. Sintering kinetics of porous ceramics from natural diatomite. *Journal of the American Ceramic Society*, 2005;88(7):1826–1830. doi: 10.1111/j.1551-2916.2005.00288.x.

30. Şan O., Gören R., Özgür C. Purification of diatomite powder by acid leaching for use in fabrication of porous ceramics. *International Journal of Mineral Processing*, 2009;93(1):6–10. doi: 10.1016/j.minpro.2009.04.007.
31. Goren R., Baykara T., Marsoglu M.A. study on the purification of diatomite in hydrochloric acid. *Scandinavian Journal of Metallurgy*, 2002;31(2):115–119. doi: 10.1034/j.1600-0692.2002.310205.x.
32. Goren R., Baykara T., Marsoglu M. Effects of purification and heat treatment on pore structure and composition of diatomite. *British Ceramic Transactions*, 2002;101(4):177–180. doi: 10.1179/096797802225003361.
33. Phogat S., Saxena A., Kapoor N., et al. Diatom mediated smart drug delivery system. *Journal of Drug Delivery Science and Technology*, 2021;63:102433. doi: 10.1016/j.jddst.2021.102433.
34. Maher S., Kumeria T., Wang Y., et al. From the mine to cancer therapy: Natural and biodegradable theranostic silicon nanocarriers from diatoms for sustained delivery of chemotherapeutics. *Advanced Healthcare Materials*, 2016;5(20):2667–2678. doi: 10.1002/adhm.201600688.
35. Son S.J., Reichel J., He B., et al. Magnetic nanotubes for magnetic-field-assisted bioseparation, biointeraction, and drug delivery. *Journal of the American Chemical Society*, 2005;127(20):7316–7317. doi: 10.1021/ja0517365. PubMed PMID: 15898772; eng.
36. Howarter J.A., Youngblood J.P. Optimization of silica silanization by 3-aminopropyltriethoxysilane. *Langmuir*, 2006;22(26):11142–11147. doi: 10.1021/la061240g. PubMed PMID: 17154595; eng.
37. Townley H.E., Parker A.R., White-Cooper H. Exploitation of diatom frustules for nanotechnology: Tethering active biomolecules. *Advanced Functional Materials*, 2008;18(2):369–374. doi: 10.1002/adfm.200700609.
38. Terracciano M., Rea I., Politi J., et al. Optical characterization of aminosilane-modified silicon dioxide surface for biosensing. *Journal of the European Optical Society Rapid Publication*, 2013;8:13075.
39. De Stefano L., Oliviero G., Amato J., et al. Aminosilane functionalizations of mesoporous oxidized silicon for oligonucleotide synthesis and detection. *Journal of The Royal Society Interface*, 2013;10(83). doi: 10.1098/rsif.2013.0160.
40. Nashat A.H., Moronne M., Ferrari M. Detection of functional groups and antibodies on microfabricated surfaces by confocal microscopy. *Biotechnology and Bioengineering*, 1998;60(2):137–146. doi: 10.1002/(SICI)1097-0290(19981020)60:2<137::AID-BIT1>3.0.CO;2-O.
41. Aw M.S., Bariana M., Yu Y., et al. Surface-functionalized diatom microcapsules for drug delivery of water-insoluble drugs. *Journal of Biomaterials Applications*, 2013;28(2):163–174. doi: 10.1177/0885328212441846.
42. Losic D., Yu Y., Aw M.S., et al. Surface functionalisation of diatoms with dopamine modified iron-oxide nanoparticles: Toward magnetically guided drug microcarriers with biologically derived morphologies. *Chemical Communications*, 2010;46(34):6323–6325. doi: 10.1039/c0cc01305f.
43. Aw M.S., Simovic S., Addai-Mensah J., et al. Silica microcapsules from diatoms as new carrier for delivery of therapeutics. *Nanomedicine*, 2011;6(-7):1159–1173. doi: 10.2217/nnm.11.29.

44. Bayramoglu G., Akbulut A., Aricaa M.Y. Immobilization of tyrosinase on modified diatom biosilica: Enzymatic removal of phenolic compounds from aqueous solution. *Journal of Hazardous Materials*, 2013;244:528–536.
45. Cicco S.R., Vona D., De Giglio E., et al. Chemically modified diatoms biosilica for bone cell growth with combined drug-delivery and antioxidant properties. *ChemPlusChem*, 2015;80(7):1104–1112. doi: 10.1002/cplu.201402398.
46. Uthappa U.T., Brahmkhatri V., Sriram G., et al. Nature engineered diatom biosilica as drug delivery systems. *Journal of Controlled Release*, 2018;281:70–83. doi: 10.1016/j.jconrel.2018.05.013.
47. Rea I., Terracciano M., Chandrasekaran S., et al. Bioengineered silicon diatoms: Adding photonic features to a nanostructured semiconductive material for biomolecular sensing. *Nanoscale Research Letters*, 2016;11:405. doi: 10.1186/s11671-016-1624-1. PubMed PMID: PMC5025415.
48. Bariana M., Aw MS., Kurkuri M., et al. Tuning drug loading and release properties of diatom silica microparticles by surface modifications. *International Journal of Pharmaceutics*, 2013;443(1–2):230–241. doi: 10.1016/j.ijpharm.2012.12.012. PubMed PMID: 23287775; eng.
49. Lang Y., del Monte F., Collins L., et al. Functionalization of the living diatom Thalassiosira weissflogii with thiol moieties. *Nature Communications*, 2013;4:2683. doi: 10.1038/ncomms3683. PubMed PMID: 24177724; eng.
50. Wagner V., Dullaart A., Bock A.K., et al. The emerging nanomedicine landscape. *Nature Biotechnology*, 2006;24(10):1211–1217. doi: 10.1038/nbt1006-1211. PubMed PMID: 17033654; eng.
51. Ferrari M. Cancer nanotechnology: Opportunities and challenges. *Nature Reviews Cancer*, 2005;5(3):161–171. doi: 10.1038/nrc1566. PubMed PMID: 15738981; eng.
52. Erhardt P.W., Proudfoot J.R. 1.02- drug discovery: Historical perspective, current status, and outlook A2- Taylor, John B. In: Triggle D.J., editor. *Comprehensive Medicinal Chemistry II*. Oxford: Elsevier; 2007, pp. 29–96.
53. El-Aneed A. An overview of current delivery systems in cancer gene therapy. *Journal of Controlled Release*, 2004;94(1):1–14. doi: 10.1016/j.jconrel.2003.09.013.
54. van der Meel R., Vehmeijer L.J., Kok R.J., et al. Ligand-targeted particulate nanomedicines undergoing clinical evaluation: Current status. *Advanced Drug Delivery Reviews*, 2013;65(10):1284–1298. doi: 10.1016/j.addr.2013.08.012. PubMed PMID: 24018362; eng.
55. Ezzati Nazhad Dolatabadi J., Omidi Y., Losic D. Carbon nanotubes as an advanced drug and gene delivery nanosystem. *Current Nanoscience*, 2011;7(18):297–314.
56. Shahbazi M.A., Herranz B., Santos H.A. Nanostructured porous Si-based nanoparticles for targeted drug delivery. *Biomatter*, 2012;2(4):296–312. doi: 10.4161/biom.22347. PubMed PMID: 23507894; PubMed Central PMCID: PMCPMC3568114. eng.
57. Tran P.A., Zhang L., Webster T.J. Carbon nanofibers and carbon nanotubes in regenerative medicine. *Advanced Drug Delivery Reviews*, 2009;61(-12):1097–114. doi: 10.1016/j.addr.2009.07.010. PubMed PMID: 19647768; eng.

58. Delalat B., Sheppard V.C., Rasi Ghaemi S., et al. Targeted drug delivery using genetically engineered diatom biosilica. *Nature Communications*, 2015;6. doi: 10.1038/ncomms9791.
59. Tiwari A., Melchor-Martínez E.M., Saxena A., et al. Therapeutic attributes and applied aspects of biological macromolecules (polypeptides, fucoxanthin, sterols, fatty acids, polysaccharides, and polyphenols) from diatoms - A review. *International Journal of Biological Macromolecules*, 2021;171:398–413. doi: 10.1016/j.ijbiomac.2020.12.219. PubMed PMID: 33422516; eng.
60. Neethirajan S., Gordon R., Wang L. Potential of silica bodies (phytoliths) for nanotechnology. *Trends Biotechnology*, 2009;27(8):461–467. doi: 10.1016/j.tibtech.2009.05.002.
61. De Riso V., Raniello R., Maumus F., et al. Gene silencing in the marine diatom Phaeodactylum tricornutum. *Nucleic Acids Research*, 2009;37(14):e96. doi: 10.1093/nar/gkp448. PubMed PMID: PMC2724275.
62. Chao J.T., Biggs M.J., Pandit A.S. Diatoms: A biotemplating approach to fabricating drug delivery reservoirs. *Expert Opinion on Drug Delivery*, 2014;11(11):1687–1695. doi: 10.1517/17425247.2014.935336. PubMed PMID: 25146231.
63. Yang Y., Jonas A-M., Dusan L. Functionalized diatom silica microparticles for removal of mercury ions. *Science and Technology of Advanced Materials*, 2012;13(1):015008.
64. Luckarift H.R., Spain J.C., Naik R.R., et al. Enzyme immobilization in a biomimetic silica support. *Nature Biotechnology*, 2004;22(2): 211–213.
65. Morse D. Silicon biotechnology: Harnessing biological silica production to construct new materials. *Trends in Biotechnology*, 1999;17(6):230–232.
66. Rosi N.L., Thaxton C.S., Mirkin C.A. Control of nanoparticle assembly by using DNA-modified diatom templates. *Angewandte Chemie International Edition*, 2004;43(41):5500–5503. doi: 10.1002/anie.200460905.
67. Aw M.S., Simovic S., Yu Y., et al. Porous silica microshells from diatoms as biocarrier for drug delivery applications. *Powder Technology*, 2012;223:52–58. doi: 10.1016/j.powtec.2011.04.023.
68. Zhang H., Shahbazi M.A., Makila E.M., et al. Diatom silica microparticles for sustained release and permeation enhancement following oral delivery of prednisone and mesalamine. *Biomaterials*, 2013;34(36):9210–9219. doi: 10.1016/j.biomaterials.2013.08.035. PubMed PMID: 24008036; eng.
69. Janićijević J., Milić J., Čalija B., et al. Potentiation of the ibuprofen antihyperalgesic effect using inorganically functionalized diatomite. *Journal of Materials Chemistry B*, 2018;6(36):5812–5822. doi: 10.1039/C8TB01376D.
70. Aw M.S., Bariana M., Yu Y., et al. Surface-functionalized diatom microcapsules for drug delivery of water-insoluble drugs. *Journal of Biomaterials Applications*, 2012;28(2):163–174. doi: 10.1177/0885328212441846.
71. Bariana M., Aw M.S., Losic D. Tailoring morphological and interfacial properties of diatom silica microparticles for drug delivery applications. *Advanced Powder Technology*, 2013;24(4):757–763. doi: 10.1016/j.apt.2013.03.015.
72. Milović M., Simović S., Lošić D., et al. Solid self-emulsifying phospholipid suspension (SSEPS) with diatom as a drug carrier. *European Journal of Pharmaceutical Sciences*, 2014;63:226–232. doi: 10.1016/j.ejps.2014.07.010.

73. Javalkote V.S., Pandey A.P., Puranik P.R., et al. Magnetically responsive siliceous frustules for efficient chemotherapy. *Materials Science and Engineering: C*, 2015;50:107–116. doi: 10.1016/j.msec.2015.01.079.
74. Todd T., Zhen Z., Tang W., et al. Iron oxide nanoparticle encapsulated diatoms for magnetic delivery of small molecules to tumors. *Nanoscale*, 2014;6(4):2073–2076. doi: 10.1039/c3nr05623f. PubMed PMID: 24424277; PubMed Central PMCID: PMCPMC3974590. eng.
75. Lavaud J., Materna A.C., Sturm S., et al. Silencing of the violaxanthin de-epoxidase gene in the diatom phaeodactylum tricornutum reduces diatoxanthin synthesis and non-photochemical quenching. *PLoS One*, 2012;7(5):e36806. doi: 10.1371/journal.pone.0036806.
76. Uthappa U.T., Kigga M., Sriram G., et al. Facile green synthetic approach of bio inspired polydopamine coated diatoms as a drug vehicle for controlled drug release and active catalyst for dye degradation. *Microporous and Mesoporous Materials*, 2019;288:109572. doi: 10.1016/j.micromeso.2019.109572.
77. Delasoie J., Rossier J., Haeni L., et al. Slow-targeted release of a ruthenium anticancer agent from vitamin B12 functionalized marine diatom microalgae. *Dalton Transactions*, 2018;47(48):17221–17232. doi: 10.1039/C8DT02914H.
78. Delasoie J., Schiel P., Vojnovic S., et al. Photoactivatable surface-functionalized diatom microalgae for colorectal cancer targeted delivery and enhanced cytotoxicity of anticancer complexes. *Pharmaceutics*, 2020;12(5):480. PubMed PMID: doi:10.3390/pharmaceutics12050480.
79. Vasani R.B., Losic D., Cavallaro A., et al. Fabrication of stimulus-responsive diatom biosilica microcapsules for antibiotic drug delivery. *Journal of Materials Chemistry B*, 2015;3(21):4325–4329. doi: 10.1039/C5TB00648A.
80. Kumeria T., Bariana M., Altalhi T., et al. Graphene oxide decorated diatom silica particles as new nano-hybrids: Towards smart natural drug microcarriers. *Journal of Materials Chemistry B*, 2013;1(45):6302–6311. doi: 10.1039/c3tb21051k.
81. Terracciano M., Shahbazi M.A., Correia A., et al. Surface bioengineering of diatomite based nanovectors for efficient intracellular uptake and drug delivery. *Nanoscale*, 2015;7(47):20063–20074. doi: 10.1039/c5nr05173h. PubMed PMID: 26568517; eng.
82. Yu-Wai-Man C., Tagalakis A.D., Manunta M.D., et al. Receptor-targeted liposome-peptide-siRNA nanoparticles represent an efficient delivery system for MRTF silencing in conjunctival fibrosis. *Scientific Reports*, 2016;6:21881. doi: 10.1038/srep21881.
83. Gomes M.J., Kennedy P.J., Martins S., et al. Delivery of siRNA silencing P-gp in peptide-functionalized nanoparticles causes efflux modulation at the blood–brain barrier. *Nanomedicine*, 2017;12(12):1385–1399. doi: 10.2217/nnm-2017-0023.
84. Rea I., Martucci N.M., De Stefano L., et al. Diatomite biosilica nanocarriers for siRNA transport inside cancer cells. *Biochimica et Biophysica Acta*, 2014;1840(12):3393–3403. doi: 10.1016/j.bbagen.2014.09.009. PubMed PMID: 25224732; eng.
85. Cauda V., Schlossbauer A., Bein T. Bio-degradation study of colloidal mesoporous silica nanoparticles: Effect of surface functionalization with organo-silanes and poly(ethylene glycol). *Microporous and Mesoporous Materials*, 2010;132(1–2):60–71. doi: 10.1016/j.micromeso.2009.11.015.

86. Lauwers A.M., Heinen W. Bio-degradation and utilization of silica and quartz. *Archives of Microbiology*, 1974;95(1):67–78. doi: 10.1007/BF02451749. English.
87. Hao N., Liu H., Li L., et al. In vitro degradation behavior of silica nanoparticles under physiological conditions. *Journal of Nanoscience and Nanotechnology*, 2012;12(8):6346–6354. PubMed PMID: 22962747; eng.
88. Martinez J.O., Chiappini C., Ziemys A., et al. Engineering multi-stage nanovectors for controlled degradation and tunable release kinetics. *Biomaterials*, 2013;34(33):8469–8477. doi: 10.1016/j.biomaterials.2013.07.049.
89. Neethirajan S., Gordon R., Wang L. Potential of silica bodies (phytoliths) for nanotechnology. *Trends Biotechnology*, 2009;27(8):461–467. doi: 10.1016/j.tibtech.2009.05.002. PubMed PMID: 19577814; eng.
90. Vrieling E.G., Sun Q., Beelen T.P., et al. Controlled silica synthesis inspired by diatom silicon biomineralization. *Journal of Nanoscience and Nanotechnology*, 2005;5(1):68–78. PubMed PMID: 15762163; eng.
91. Borak B., Biernat P., Prescha A., et al. In vivo study on the biodistribution of silica particles in the bodies of rats. *Advances in Clinical and Experimental Medicine*, 2012;21(1):13–18.
92. Jugdaohsingh R. Silicon and bone health. *The Journal of Nutrition, Health and Aging*, 2007;11(2):99–110. PubMed PMID: 17435952; PubMed Central PMCID: PMCPMC2658806. eng.
93. Park J-H., Gu L., von Maltzahn G., et al. Biodegradable luminescent porous silicon nanoparticles for in vivo applications. *Nature Materials*, 2009;8(4):331–336. doi: http://www.nature.com/nmat/journal/v8/n4/suppinfo/nmat2398_S1.html.
94. Jaganathan H., Godin B. Biocompatibility assessment of Si-based nano- and micro-particles. *Advanced Drug Delivery Reviews*, 2012;64(15):1800–1819. doi: 10.1016/j.addr.2012.05.008.
95. Low S.P., Voelcker N.H., Canham L.T., et al. The biocompatibility of porous silicon in tissues of the eye. *Biomaterials*, 2009;30(15):2873–2880. doi: 10.1016/j.biomaterials.2009.02.008.
96. Tzur-Balter A., Shatsberg Z., Beckerman M., et al. Mechanism of erosion of nanostructured porous silicon drug carriers in neoplastic tissues. *Nature Communications*, 2015;6:6208. doi: 10.1038/ncomms7208. PubMed PMID: 25670235; PubMed Central PMCID: PMCPmc4339882. eng.
97. Borak B., Biernat P., Prescha A., et al. In vivo study on the biodistribution of silica particles in the bodies of rats. *Advances in Clinical and Experimental Medicine: Official Organ Wroclaw Medical University*, 2012;21(1):13–18.
98. Popplewell J.F., King S.J., Day J.P., et al. Kinetics of uptake and elimination of silicic acid by a human subject: A novel application of 32Si and accelerator mass spectrometry. *Journal of Inorganic Biochemistry*, 1998;69(3):177–180. doi: 10.1016/S0162-0134(97)10016-2.
99. Anderson S.H.C., Elliott H., Wallis D.J., et al. Dissolution of different forms of partially porous silicon wafers under simulated physiological conditions. *Physica Status Solidi (A)*, 2003;197(2):331–335. doi: 10.1002/pssa.200306519.
100. Bao Z., Ernst E.M., Yoo S., et al. Syntheses of porous self-supporting metal-nanoparticle assemblies with 3D morphologies inherited from biosilica templates (Diatom Frustules). *Advanced Materials*, 2009;21(4):474–478. doi: 10.1002/adma.200801499.

101. Bao Z., Weatherspoon M.R., Shian S., et al. Chemical reduction of three-dimensional silica micro-assemblies into microporous silicon replicas. *Nature*, 2007;446(7132):172–175. http://www.nature.com/nature/journal/v446/n7132/suppinfo/nature05570_S1.html.
102. Maher S., Alsawat M., Kumeria T., et al. Luminescent silicon diatom replicas: Self-reporting and degradable drug carriers with biologically derived shape for sustained delivery of therapeutics. *Advanced Functional Materials*, 2015;25(32):5017–5116. doi: 10.1002/adfm.201501249.
103. Maeda H., Wu J., Sawa T., et al. Tumor vascular permeability and the EPR effect in macromolecular therapeutics: A review. *Journal of Controlled Release*, 2000;65(1–2):271–284. PubMed PMID: 10699287; eng.
104. Maeda H. The enhanced permeability and retention (EPR) effect in tumor vasculature: The key role of tumor-selective macromolecular drug targeting. *Advances in Enzyme Regulation*, 2001;41:189–207. PubMed PMID: 11384745; eng.
105. Thorn C.F., Oshiro C., Marsh S., et al. Doxorubicin pathways: Pharmaco dynamics and adverse effects. *Pharmacogenetics and Genomics*, 2011;21(-7):440–446. doi: 10.1097/FPC.0b013e32833ffb56. PubMed PMID: 21048526; PubMed Central PMCID: PMCPmc3116111. eng.
106. Shalviri A., Raval G., Prasad P., et al. pH-Dependent doxorubicin release from terpolymer of starch, polymethacrylic acid and polysorbate 80 nanoparticles for overcoming multi-drug resistance in human breast cancer cells. *European Journal of Pharmaceutics and Biopharmaceutics*, 2012;82(3):587–597. doi: 10.1016/j.ejpb.2012.09.001. PubMed PMID: 22995704; eng.
107. Osminkina L.A., Tamarov K.P., Sviridov A.P., et al. Photoluminescent biocompatible silicon nanoparticles for cancer theranostic applications. *Journal of Biophotonics*, 2012;5(7):529–535. doi: 10.1002/jbio.201100112. PubMed PMID: 22438317; eng.
108. Wang C-F., Sarparanta M.P., Mäkilä E.M., et al. Multifunctional porous silicon nanoparticles for cancer theranostics. *Biomaterials*, 2015;48:108–118. doi: 10.1016/j.biomaterials.2015.01.008.
109. Maher S., Santos A., Kumeria T., et al. Multifunctional microspherical magnetic and pH responsive carriers for combination anticancer therapy engineered by droplet-based microfluidics. *Journal of Materials Chemistry B*, 2017;5(22):4097–4109. doi: 10.1039/C7TB00588A.

Chapter 4

Different Classes of Nanoclay Materials (Halloysite, Montmorillonite, and Kaolinite) and Its Applications in Controlled Drug Release and Targeted Drug Delivery

Sharon George
Jain (Deemed-to-be University)

Remya Pakkukalayil Narayanan
Global Academy of Technology

Baiju Kizhakekilikoodail Vijayan
Kannur University

Shajesh Palantavida
Jain (Deemed-to-be University)

CONTENTS

DOI: 10.1201/9781003217114-6

ABBREVIATION

Al^{3+}:	Aluminium (III) ion
$Al_2Si_2O_5(OH)_4$:	Kaolinite, Aluminium silicate
DNA:	Deoxyribonucleic acid
Fe^{2+}:	Iron (II) ion
Fe^{3+}:	Iron (III) ion
Mg^{2+}:	Magnesium (II) ion
Si^{4+}:	Silicon (IV) ion

4.1 INTRODUCTION

The use of clay minerals in therapeutic roles dates far back to the prehistoric period and continues to the present day. The therapeutic value of clay minerals in skin care, wound healing and gastrointestinal problems was known even to Neanderthals, and they are still valuable ingredients of therapeutic creams and pharmaceutical formulations. Clays exhibit crystalline micro and nanostructures along with permanent structural charge that provides them with high surface area, high surface reactivity and rich electrochemical properties benefits for therapeutic applications. Their proton absorption capacity makes them suitable as antacids, while their interactions with glycoproteins help in stabilizing the protective mucosal barrier and large surface area allow them to adhere and form a protective covering on skin (Dawson and Oreffo 2013). Hence the excipient and active ingredient roles of clay in pharmaceutical products. In the 1960s, the decreased bioavailability of drugs co-administered with clay-based formulations was noticed by practitioners, and the realization of the positive effects of delayed delivery led to the rise of clay-based delivery systems (Aguzzi et al. 2007). With the advent of the nanostructured drug carriers and targeted therapy, the prominence of clay materials and minerals increased progressively. Modified drug delivery systems are required to minimize temporal variations in drug concentration and avoid over-dosing or under-dosing windows (Azar 2021, Uthappa, Sriram, et al. 2018, Uthappa, Brahmkhatri, et al. 2018, Uthappa et al. 2019, Kurkuri and Aminabhavi 2004). As efficient and low-toxicity drug carriers, nanoclay minerals can induce stronger therapeutic effects by providing higher and longer-lasting drug concentrations by virtue of their adsorption capacity, ion-exchange property, biostability, degradability and excellent biocompatibility. Further nanoclay–polymer composites have found important biomedical applications apart from drug delivery, such as anti-microbial coatings, bone healing implants and cosmetic formulations. Particularly, significant scientific interest can be seen in case of clay minerals like halloysite, montmorillonite and kaolinite for such applications.

The structure and charge of clay materials play an important role in their properties. The joint nomenclature committees of the Association Internationale pour l'Etude des Argiles and the clay minerals society define clay as naturally occurring and composed of fine-grained minerals that are plastic when mixed with water and harden as they dry out. Clay minerals, on the other hand, are mostly formed of hydrated phyllosilicate minerals. Clay minerals are characterized by a layered structure with layer thickness in the range of 0.7–1 nm, anisotropy of the layers and presence of external, edge and interlayer surfaces. As Bergaya points out, the classification of clay materials can encompass a large family of materials, and the common perception of clay materials as layered silicates should be expanded to include all (Bergaya and Lagaly 2013). Accordingly, clay materials can be considered as (hydr)oxides of silicon, aluminium or magnesium and the closely related family of layered double hydroxides as (hydr)oxides of metals. The structures of these materials can be generally considered as being made up of tetrahedral and octahedral sheets, combined in a 1:1 or 2:1 proportion. Naturally occurring double hydroxides are made of octahedral sheets. Kaolinite montmorillonite and halloysite are naturally occurring clay minerals and have significant industrial applications as nanosorbents, catalysts, nanofillers in polymer composites, paints and anti-corrosion and flame-retardant coatings (Kryuchkova et al. 2016). The industrial use of these materials is based on the exfoliation of these minerals into nanoparticles of ~1 nm thickness and width in hundreds of nanometres. Colloidal states of these materials can be characterized as particles formed from assemblies of layers and aggregates from particles, allowing accessible volume between layers (interlayer), particles (interparticle) and aggregates (interaggregate). The electrochemical properties of the material are dictated by the layer charge density and nature of the balancing charges.

4.2 STRUCTURE OF CLAY

The model of 1:1 and 2:1 clay mineral is given in Figure 4.1. The tetrahedral sheets in phyllosilicates are formed from corner-sharing oxygen tetrahedra with the cation at the centre. Three oxygen atoms of a tetrahedra are shared with other tetrahedra in the same plane forming a layer of basal plane oxygen atoms. The apical oxygen that is out of the basal plane is shared with the next octahedral sheet. The octahedron is formed with the octahedral cation at the centre and oxygen at the corners. Octahedral layer is formed by the edge sharing of these octahedra. The commonly encountered

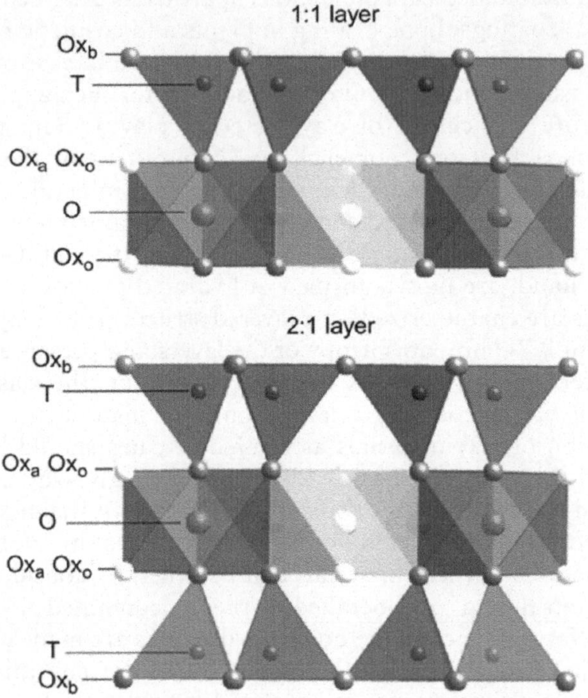

Figure 4.1 Models of 1:1 and 2:1 layer structures. Ox_b, basal oxygen atoms; T, tetrahedral cations; O, octahedral cations; Ox_a, apical oxygen atoms; Ox_o, octahedral anions (OH, F, Cl) (Brigattia, Galan, and Theng 2013).

tetrahedral cations are Si^{4+}, Al^{3+} and Fe^{3+}, while the octahedral cations are Al^{3+}, Mg^{2+}, $Fe^{3+}$and Fe^{2+}. The layers of a 1:1 structure is formed from the basal layer oxygen atoms from the tetrahedral sheet on one side and the unshared oxygen (mostly hydroxyl) from the octahedral sheet on the other side. In a 2:1 structure, a single layer is made up of two tetrahedral and one octahedral sheet. The octahedral side of the 1:1 layer is covered by an inverse-oriented tetrahedral sheet, and two-thirds of the hydroxyls on the octahedral layer are now replaced by the tetrahedral oxygen. The interlayer space in the 2:1 structure can host alkaline or alkaline earth cations with or without the presence of water depending on the mineral. Si^{4+} is the common tetrahedral cation. The charges are balanced, and the layers are neutral when divalent cations occupy all the octahedral sites (called *trioctahedral*). If trivalent cations occupy the octahedral sites, then a vacancy in every third octahedra (called *dioctahedral*) will maintain charge neutrality. When this arrangement is not followed, by the presence of trivalent cations (Al^{3+}) in tetrahedral site or in divalent octahedral sites, a negative charge for the layer remains. The net charge of the formula unit is the charge of the layer and is neutralized by the cations in the interlayer. Commonly 1:1 layer is neutral, and 2:1 layer exhibits charge density per unit in the range of 0.2–2. The extent of hydration and nature of interlayer cations depend on the magnitude and dispersion of this charge. The extent of this permanent charge is not affected by experimental conditions like pH and ionic strength.

4.3 STRUCTURE OF KAOLINITE

The kaolinite and halloysite minerals are polytypes of the 1:1 dioctahedral mineral group and the kaolin group and have the general formula $Al_2Si_2O_5(-OH)_4$. While kaolinite is dehydrated, halloysite exhibits layer thickness of 7 Å when dehydrated and 10 Å when hydrated. The kaolinite structure contains four types of hydroxyl bonds, and three of them are on the outer layer surface and one inside the layer. Kaolinite microstructure resembles a closed booklet from the stacked pseudohexagonal platelets of about 2 μm in size (Figure 4.2). Each platelet is an arrangement of several layers, each of which consists of the tetrahedral silica sheet (the siloxane surface) and the octahedral alumina sheet bearing hydroxyl groups (aluminol surface). Each kaolinite layer is considered a strong dipole due to the negatively charged siloxane surface and positively charged aluminol surface, and the interlayers are laced with hydrogen bonds between Al hydroxyls and Si oxygens. The siloxane layer is more hydrophobic, and the aluminol surface hydrophilic and the edges of these layers contain O atoms and OH groups. The hydroxyl groups ionize in solution depending on the pH (pKa ~3.6) and add additional charges to the kaolinite surface. But the limited substitutions in the kaolinite structure render low ion-exchange capacity, and also the closed structure provides low specific area (Figure 4.3).

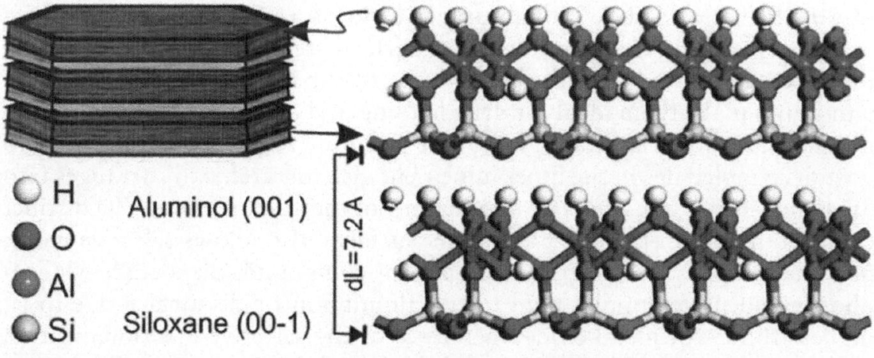

Figure 4.2 Molecular simulation model of kaolinite structure (Awad et al. 2017).

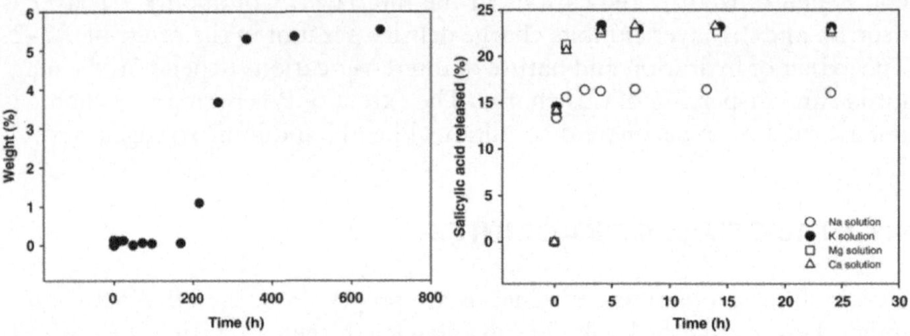

Figure 4.3 Absorption (a) and release (b) of iron-salicylic acid complex from kaolinite (Bonina et al. 2007). Adopted and rearranged from reference.

4.3.1 Structure of Halloysite

The structure and composition of halloysite resemble that of kaolinite, but a monolayer of water molecules separates its unit layers. The water layer is weakly held, and the hydrated halloysite can be dehydrated by heating. The hydrated water can be trapped in the tetrahedral layer (hole water), hydrogen bonded to tetrahedral oxygens or as a discontinuous layer (associated water) with intermolecular hydrogen bonds. Halloysite particles exhibit various shapes like tubes, spheres and plates, of which the most commonly encountered is the tubular morphology. The morphological variations are influenced by the crystal structure, degree of alteration, composition and effects of dehydration (Joussein et al. 2005). The tubular structure of halloysite is formed by the rolling of silica tetrahedral layer ending up in an outer silica layer and inner alumina layer. The silica surface of halloysite is negatively charged at neutral pH while the inner surface, made up of Al octahedra, is positively charged. Naturally occurring tubular halloysite clays have inner diameter in the range of 10–100 nm and outer diameter in the range of 30–190 nm and show a high aspect ratio of ≈19. Though it is considered a low-activity clay due to the low surface area and exchange capacity, the accessibility and considerable volume of the inner lumen of halloysite nanotubes make them ideal for drug loading and delivery applications. The unique charge distribution in halloysite nanotubes not only allows them to host drug molecules in the inner lumen but also hierarchically arranges into 3D higher-order structures by interactions of the outer surface. The distinct chemical nature of the inner and outer surfaces also allows selective modification of the surfaces. Organophosphorus compounds like octadecylphosphonic acid preferentially bind to the aluminium oxide surface due to its higher affinity for metal oxide, thereby allowing selective functionalization of the inner lumen (Yah, Takahara, and Lvov 2012). The approach has been used to bind bromo-N-[2-(3,4-dihydroxyphenyl)ethyl]-isobutyryl amide specifically to the inner lumen and use it as a surface initiator for atom transfer radial polymerization to grow polymethylmethacrylate brushes inside the lumen (Yah et al. 2012). Functionalizing sequentially, first with octadecylphosphonic acid and then with organosilanes yields nanotubes with hydrophobic inner lumen and anchoring groups for biofunctionalization like amines on the outer silica surface of the tubes.

4.3.2 Structure of Montmorillonite

Montmorillonite, on the other hand, is a 2:1 dioctahedral clay mineral with a net negative layer charge. The octahedral Al^{3+} cations are substituted by Mg^{2+} cations in some positions resulting in the net permanent negative charge. The general formula for the structure would be $M_y^+ \cdot n\mathrm{H_2O}\left(\mathrm{Al}_{(2-y)}^{3+}\mathrm{Mg}_y^{2+}\right)\mathrm{Si}_4^{4+}\mathrm{O}_{10}\left(\mathrm{OH}\right)_2$, where M is the monovalent interlayer cation which is hydrated. The exchange of the interlayer cation is a common step in their utilization in delivery or packaging applications. The charges of the layers can also arise from broken oxide bonds in the layer edges. The dangling M-O-M bonds in the layer edges terminate as hydroxyl groups and can ionize depending on pH leading to variable surface charge. The cation exchange capacity of layered clays is expressed as centimoles per kilogram of dry clay, and the exchange process is diffusion controlled and stoichiometric. Like inorganic cations, organic cations can also replace interlayer cations. Non-ionic polar organic molecules, on the other hand, can replace the water in the interlayers or adsorbed on clay surfaces. The surface characteristics of the clay change upon the adsorption of such molecules.

4.4 INTERACTIONS OF CLAY WITH DRUG MOLECULES

Various interactions that can occur between clay particles and organic drugs are provided in Table 4.1. The exact nature of the interaction depends on the type of clay and the nature of the organic molecule. Permanently charged clay-like montmorillonite can be loaded with cationic drugs like the ones bearing amine groups using cation exchange. The release is achieved by subsequent exchange of the drugs by physiological ions. Anionic drugs and larger drugs interact weakly and show fast release kinetics. Adsorption and dipole interactions play a role in the bonding of acidic and non-ionic molecules on montmorillonite. Interaction studies with kaolin clay indicated that anionic species are adsorbed on its edge faces while cationic ones interact with the basal planes (Aguzzi et al. 2007). The extent of possible interactions and the point of interactions with carrier clay multiply many folds when we consider the case of biomolecules like proteins and DNA. Hydrophobic and van der Walls' interactions are prominent along with

Table 4.1 Interactions between Clay and Organic Compounds

Mechanism	*Minerals Examples*	*Interacting Functional Groups*
Hydrophobic interactions (van der Waals)	Any clay with neutral sites (e.g., kaolinite, smectites)	Uncharged, nonpolar (e.g., aromatic, alkyl C)
Hydrogen bonding	Any clay with oxygen surfaces (e.g., kaolinite)	Amines, carbonyl, carboxyl, phenyl hydroxyl, heterocycle N
Protonation	Aluminosilicate edge sites, Fe and Al oxides, allophane, imogolite	Amines, heterocycle N, carbonyl, carboxylate
Ligand exchange	Aluminosilicate edge sites, Fe and Al oxides, allophane, imogolite	Amines, heterocycle N, carbonyl, carboxylate
Cation exchange (permanent charge sites)	Smectite, vermiculite, illite	Amines, ring NH, heterocyclic N
pH-dependent charge sites (anion exchange usually, cation exchange rarely)	Aluminosilicate edge sites, Fe and Al oxides, allophane, imogolite	Carboxylate for anion exchange, amines, ring NH, heterocyclic N for cation exchange
Cation bridging	Smectite, vermiculite, illite	Carboxylate, amines, carbonyl, alcoholic OH

Source: Adopted from Aguzzi et al. (2007).

dominant electrochemical interactions in the case of clay-protein interaction. The extent of these interactions is also dictated by the higher-order structure of the proteins. The large number of possible contacts between the clay and protein molecule also result in high affinity for the interactions and slow to no desorption upon dilution (Dawson and Oreffo 2013). Studies on the interactions of short peptide sequences have shown that there is considerable diversity in the sequences exhibiting high affinity for the same clay surface. In phage display studies using different peptide sequences with montmorillonite, the highest affinity was shown by a cationic peptide sequence with two lysine residues and one without any positive charge. The former was attracted to the surface at pH7 by ion exchange, while the latter was attracted by alkali ion coordination and hydrogen bonding (Heinz 2012). DNA adsorption on montmorillonite clay occurs at the edges, and no intercalation is observed. Chromosomal DNA has the highest affinity compared to plasmid DNA and ribosomal RNA. Unlike the case of proteins where conformational change is observed on adsorption, DNA do not show any conformational changes on adsorption to clay surface (Dawson and Oreffo 2013). The strong electrochemistry of clay particles has been shown to inhibit tumour proliferation in vitro and in vivo. As healthy cells turn malignant, biophysical changes results in a change in membrane potential, and specific adhesion decreases along with an increase in non-specific adhesion. As a result, montmorillonite particles adhere to cancer cells strongly resulting in considerable tumour reduction and tumour cell necrosis (Abduljauwad and Ahmed 2019, Abduljauwad, Ahmed, and Moy 2021).

4.5 CLAY-POLYMER COMPOSITES

Many clay-based delivery systems utilize polymers as modifiers of clay surfaces to improve loading, increase drug compatibility or improve the dispersibility of clay. On the other hand, the addition of clay to polymer matrices yields conducive systems for these applications. Clay improves the biocompatibility of polymer matrices, and clay-polymer composites are widely investigated for drug delivery and scaffolding applications. Synthesis of these composites is achieved by mixing or through in situ polymerization of the monomer clay mixture. Three possible states of clay minerals can be expected in the composite. The polymer chains can penetrate into the clay layers and get intercalated or further cause exfoliation of the clay layers in the composite. Intercalation can change the interlayer spacing of the clay layers, while exfoliation delaminates the layers and disperses them to the extent that few interactions remain between the layers. Mutually interacting clay particles through edge interactions can also associate and flocculate in the polymer matrix. Delamination is rare, and intercalation and flocculation can appear simultaneously in a sample. Surface modification of clay is required to improve its compatibility with hydrophobic polymers. Kaolinite clay has low cation exchange capacity and strong interlayer hydrogen bonding that intercalation of molecules into its layers is difficult to achieve and is not considered good for nanocomposites. The hollow structure of halloysite allows it to interact with polymer chains and form strong bonding. Halloysite is more hydrophilic than other clays and is well dispersible in water making it more biocompatible than others. Montmorillonite is the most ideal among the three for preparing composites since the interlayer space increases with the penetration of polymer molecules and intercalation to exfoliation can be achieved in their composites (Murugesan and Scheibel 2020). Clay-polymer composites can be processed to different morphologies like films, fibres and hydrogels for drug release applications. Montmorillonite polymer composites possess higher strength and loading efficiencies than halloysite and kaolinite composites that free-standing films for delivery applications are mostly reported for these composites. Halloysite, on the other hand, provides large loading properties to the composites due to its hollow structure. Chitosan films are known for their mucoadhesivity and vapour and oxygen barrier properties suitable for bandaging and topical applications but lack mechanical strength and sustained drug delivery properties. Influence of the addition of halloysite clay to chitosan films on the mechanical and drug delivery properties of chitosan films has been reported by Čalija et al. (2020). The films were produced by direct solvent evaporation, and tetracyclin-loaded halloysite nanotubes dispersed in chitosan films improved the elastic modulus of the films ~1.5 times along with an increase in tensile strength. The effects were more marked when low molecular weight chitosan polymer was used. The drug release rates plummeted by ~75% when drug was released from the halloysite nanotubes dispersed in the films compared to native films. Drug release characteristics from halloysite dispersed in polyvinylalcohol films showed a release of 50% of the loaded sodium salicylate after 6 hours while the release from native films reached 70% within 3 hours (Bediako et al. 2018).

Fibre morphologies are extensively used to prepare membranes and scaffolds suitable in regenerative medicine due to their mechanical properties and similarity to extracellular matrices (Ruiz-Hitzky et al. 2010). Addition of clay particles to hydrogels increases their mechanical strength and recoverability and aids to overcome the soft nature of hydrogels for applications like scaffolding and improve the stimuli responsiveness of these systems (Gao et al. 2018).

On the other hand, simple surface modification of clay particles with polymers can improve the properties of clay particles and enhance drug delivery applications. Colloidal stability of clay particles is low in physiological conditions due to the high ionic strength and presence of polyelectrolytes like proteins. The dispersibility of these particles can be improved by coating them with polyethylene glycol polymer, and studies have reported the insensitivity of polyethylene glycol-coated clay particles towards ionic strength or polyelectrolytes. The extent of polyethylene glycol coating can be followed using zetapotential which plateaus at complete coverage. Drug molecules loaded in the clay prior to the polyethylene glycol modification exhibit sustained release from the composite system. A demonstration with pyrene as a model compound showed 60% release over a period of 30 days (Takahashi et al. 2005). Much of the clay drug complexes we will encounter later are intercalation complexes with cationic or polar molecules with an expanded layer spacing. Nonpolar drugs that are hydrophobic are incorporated without the formation of a complex (Takahashi and Yamaguchi 1991).

4.6 KAOLINITE IN DRUG DELIVERY

Even though kaolinite does not possess easily accessible interlayer regions, it has been used as a promising excipient or active ingredient in various pharmaceutical applications (Awad et al. 2017). Recent advances in the use of kaolinite and its derivatives as drug, gene and protein delivery systems are attributed to its high interaction capacities with organic and biochemical molecules.

The low ion-exchange capacity of kaolin leads to slow adsorption kinetics during loading as seen in the case of iron-salicylic acid complex with kaolin. Its adsorption by kaolin follows a slow kinetics and starts only after 4 days and finished after 19 days with a 5.5% adsorption of the complex (Bonina et al. 2007). The desorption from kaolin was gradual and took 10 hours to reach equilibrium.

The affinity of drug molecules can be improved by modifying kaolinite clay. A comparison of kaolinite and methoxy-modified kaolinite for the delivery of 5-flourouracyl has been studied. 5-Fluorouracyl gets attached to the surface of kaolinite through hydrogen bonding, and these anchored 5-fluorouracyl will form hydrogen-bonded aggregates with more 5-flourouracyl molecules. The 5-flourouracyl loading onto the methoxy-modified kaolinite was 147.3% more than that onto kaolinite and is attributed to the high affinity of 5-flourouracyl towards the methoxy-modified kaolinite. Also the interlayers of the methoxy-modified kaolinite provide additional sites for the intercalation of 5-flourouracyl (Tan et al. 2014). Methoxy-modified kaolinite was also used as a carrier for loading and release of the herbicide 3-amino-1,2,4-triazole (amitrole) (Tan et al. 2015). Cetrylammonium bromide can be used to decrease the interactions between kaolinite layers and increase the interaction area for guest molecules. It has been demonstrated that the FePt complex can be prepared in situ and adhere to these surfaces. Further doxorubicin can be loaded on to the FePt-Kaolinite system to yield magnetically guided delivery systems and MRI contrast agents (Chan et al. 2020).

Intercalation of urea in kaolinite has been shown to increase the loading capacity of chlorhexidine diacetate, an anti-bacterial agent to obtain kaolinite with anti-bacterial properties. Molecular modelling along with XRD analysis indicated that while urea is present in the interlayers, chlorhexidine occupies the tetrahedral side of the layer surface (Holešová et al. 2014). Intercalation of kaolinite with methanol increases the interlayer spacing, allowing the infusion of drugs like doxorubicin (DOX) between the interlayers. The methanol intercalation is achieved by suspending the clay particles in methanol. Intercalation increases the interlayer spacing and can be observed by the shift in the d_{001} reflection in the powder X-ray diffraction pattern. The interlayer spacing is reported to increase from 0.72 to 0.85 nm upon methanol intercalation (Zhang et al. 2016). The zetapotential values for kaolinite particles of size in the range of 150–200 nm are reported to be around −5.5 mV at pH 2.5 and −43 mV at pH 11. The high negative charge of kaolinite at physiological pH makes it an ideal host for positively charged drugs like doxorubicin. The zetapotential of methoxy intercalated kaolinite is lower than that of pure kaolinite, −38 mV at pH 11 indicating a decrease in the surface charge. Even then the increase in interlayer spacing permits loading of doxorubicin in the order of 55% by weight (Zhang et al. 2016). The

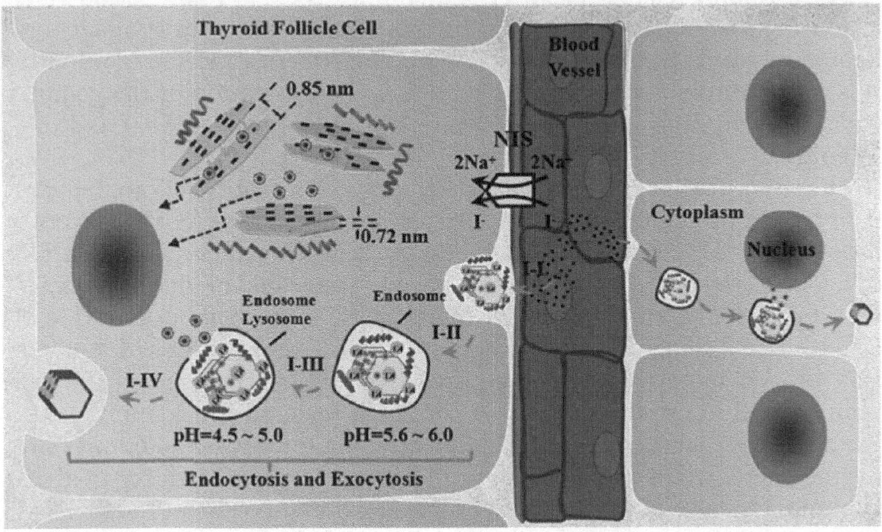

Figure 4.4 Illustration of mechanism of intracellular delivery of drug by potassium iodide functionalized kaolinite particles adopted from reference (Zhang et al. 2016).

strong interaction of the drug with the clay layers also ensures that the release kinetics is slow at physiological pH. A cumulative DOX release of 9.5% was seen over a period of 30 hours. On the other hand, in acidic pH of 5.5, the release rates increase and a cumulative release of 33% is observed in the same period. Intracellular pH in tumours is in the range of 6.5, and endosomes and lysosomes are 5.5. The DOX delivery in papillary thyroid cancer can be increased by adsorbing potassium iodide on DOX-loaded kaolinite. The potassium iodide modification allows the particles to cross the cell membrane, and the mechanism of endocytosis could be established for membrane crossing using bio-TEM analysis. An illustration of the mechanism is provided in Figure 4.4.

The complete exfoliation of kaolinite layers can be achieved by using cetrylammonium bromide under ultrasonication. The exfoliated kaolin can be used to form composites with polymers to yield delivery vehicles with high-loading capacity. Cellulose fibre-exfoliated kaolin composites have been seen to load and release oxaliplatin with high efficiency (Tian et al. 2020). Loading capacity of 670 mg/g and a release profile extending over 100 hours were observed for these composites in physiological buffers. First-order kinetics observed could be fit to Higuchi and Hixson-Crowell models indicating a diffusion with erosion mechanism involved in the release.

The adsorption and retention capacities for various proteins like α-lactalbumin (A-LA), bovine serum albumin (BSA) and β-lactoglobulin

(B-LG) of kaolinite, metakaolinite and silylated kaolinite were examined by Duarte-Silva et al. (2014). The affinity of a protein for a given surface depends on the surface properties of the adsorbent, the composition and structural stability of the protein and the pH and the ionic strength of the solution. The protein adsorption capacity and the selectivity show a clear dependence on the chemical nature of the adsorbent's surface and on the textural properties. Kaolinite acts as a strong adsorbent for the α-lactalbumin and bovine serum albumin and exhibits a very high affinity for β-lactoglobulin. Meta kaolinite shows good retention capacity for α-lactalbumin and β-lactoglobulin but does not retain significant amounts of the bovine serum albumin.

Kaolin is a common excipient in tablet formulations owing to its adsorbent properties. Tablet formulations of polymer composites containing kaolinite have proved to perform better with respect to drug release characteristics. Delivery of Zolpidem, – a model drug acting like the opioid fentanyl, using methacrylic acid-ethylacrylate copolymer, polyethylene glycol and alginate in metakaolin pellets – improves the delivery properties considerably (Jämstorp et al. 2012). Delayed release of fentanyl from kaolin-based geopolymers has also been observed (Forsgren et al. 2010). The drug release from pellets made of just the geopolymer and the one modified with copolymerization also were examined for the drug release. The delayed drug release occurs in both the intestinal track and gastric pH conditions. The release kinetics is aided at low pH by the improved solubility of the weakly basic drug and the degradation of the geopolymer at low pH (Jämstorp et al. 2010).

4.7 HALLOYSITE IN DRUG DELIVERY

Various studies have established the biocompatibility of halloysite nanotubes (Vergaro et al. 2010, Lai et al. 2013, Sandri et al. 2017). Functionalization of halloysite has shown some cytotoxicity, and dose-dependent cytotoxicity evaluations are necessary to determine safe dosages (Sánchez-Fernández et al. 2014, Sawicka et al. 2020). Drugs can be loaded inside the halloysite nanotubes from solutions and can be stored after drying. Efficiency of loading drugs in the nanotubes depends on the viscosity of the solvent, extent of wetting of the nanotube walls and solubility of the drug in the solvent. Low-viscosity solvents are preferred, and application of a vacuum will be required to remove the air trapped in the lumen to facilitate access of the drug to the lumen (Lvov, Aerov, and Fakhrullin 2014). Generally for drug loading, water, alcohol or acetone were often used. Upon hydration in the body fluids, the drug will be released.

Selective functionalization of the inner lumen can be used to improve specific drug loadings. Ferrocene loads preferentially to ferrocene

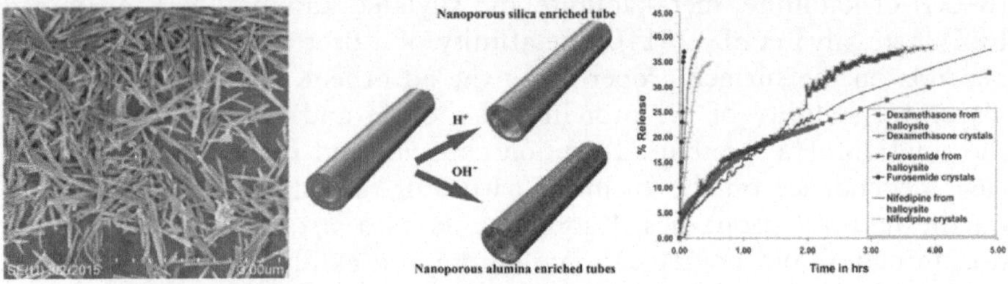

Figure 4.5 From left SEM image of halloysite nanotube. Schematic of etching of halloysite nanotubes with acid or alkali (pH 2 or 12). Drug release profile from loaded halloysite nanotubes (Lvov et al. 2016).

carboxylic acid in halloysite nanotubes with hydrophobized inner lumens (Yah, Takahara, and Lvov 2012). Controlled acid or base etching can be used to increase the lumen diameter from 12 to 24 nm. The removal of alumina or silica layer occurs during the process to increase the lumen volume (Figure 4.5). Lumen volume can be increased by up to 30% in this approach, and the loading capacity should double or triple. Consequently, the surface area also increases by up to six times. Since the etching process starts from the ends of the nanotubes, the expansion may not be uniform and the final tubes may have a more constricted middle region (Abdullayev et al. 2012). The adsorption capacity and the release of adsorbed drugs can also be influenced by simple acid treatments (Wang et al. 2014).

4.7.1 Drug Release Kinetics from Halloysite Nanotubes

Drug release studies indicate that most drugs are released from the halloysite nanotubes in 10–20 hours. Khellin, oxytetracycline, nicotinamide adenine dinucleotide, furosemide, nifedipine and dexamethasone are some of the drugs studied in the release from halloysite nanotubes (Price, Gaber, and Lvov 2001, Veerabadran, Price, and Lvov 2007, Bediako et al. 2018). The release rate studies show that the encapsulation increases the drug release time by about 50 times compared to direct release in water. Close to 40% of the drugs are usually released in the first 6 hours.

The release profile of drugs from halloysite nanotubes, in most cases, can be described by the semiempirical Peppa's model $M_t = K \times t^n$, where K and n are experimentally determined. A lower value of K indicates a lower rate of diffusion in the halloysite nanotubes. Kinetic studies on the release of furosemide, dexamethasone and nifedipine from halloysite nanotubes show a 10-fold decrease in K for furosemide and a 5–6-fold decrease for the rest compared to non-confined drugs. This indicates the slower diffusion of furosemide in the nanotubes and a stronger interaction of the molecules with the lumen walls. The magnitude of n provides information of the order of the rate of release. The value of n observed for furosemide and dexamethasone was 0.7 and indicates a close to zero-order kinetics while nifedipine had a value of 0.5 and was attributed to a Fickian mechanism for the diffusion. In contrast, the release of brilliant green from Cu-benzotriazole-coated halloysite happens in two steps, 60% in the first step and 40% in a slower second step. The release can be modelled by the first-order kinetics $M_t = M_\infty\left(1-e^{-\propto t}\right)$, where M_∞ is the amount of dye released at infinity and $\propto$ is the release rate constant. The release extended up to 75 hours in this study (Wei et al. 2014). Changing the pH of loading or changing the solvents can increase the charge compatibility of the drug molecule and the lumen walls and thereby increase the drug loading in the nanotubes. The kinetics of release can also be influenced by pH as seen in the case of polyelectrolyte-coated, ibuprofen-loaded halloysite nanotubes. Release kinetics at pH 7.4 was best fit with a first-order kinetics, while at pH 1.2 Peppa's model was a better fit (Li, Zhu, et al. 2016).

4.7.2 Halloysite-Drug Conjugates

Direct organosilane modification of halloysite nanotubes has also been seen to decrease the release rates (Yuan et al. 2012). Aminopropyltriethoxysilane modification of halloysite yielded a pH-dependent delivery system that showed higher release rates of anionic orange II dye at basic pH. Massaro and coworkers chemically grafted curcumin to halloysite nanotubes to create stimuli-responsive curcumin delivery systems. Curcumin was conjugated through imine bonds to amine functionalities on ormosil-modified halloysite. Further, the organic linker included a disulphide bond susceptible to glutathione. Glutathione concentration is higher in malignant cells compared to blood plasma (Kennedy et al. 2020). This provided a dual stimuli-responsive delivery system, responding to pH and glutathione concentration. The cumulative release increased four times at pH 7.4 in presence of glutathione and six times at pH 1 without glutathione compared to release at pH 7.4 without glutathione (Massaro et al. 2016). Triazolium functionalization of the halloysite nanotubes has also been attempted to obtain a synergistic effect with curcumin. Such nanotubes after curcumin loading showed pH-dependent release rates and activity against several tumour models (Riela et al. 2014). Triazolium-functionalized nanotubes were also tested for the delivery of long-chain model drug, cardanol. Cardanol has a 15-member carbon chain attached to the meta position of a phenolic head group. The functionalization doubled the loading capacity of the nanotubes and provided a pH-dependent release kinetics with the highest observed at lower pH (Massaro et al. 2015).

4.7.3 Polymer Coatings on Halloysite

Prolonging of drug release from halloysite nanotubes can be achieved by polymeric coatings that can work as clogs to the nanotubes. Coating halloysite nanotubes loaded with diltiazem-HCl with chitosan and poly(-ethyleneimine) reduced the release rate of the drug three times, and cross-linking with glutaraldehyde decreased the rates further at the expense of loading efficiency. The loading efficiency can be improved by the use of cyanoacrylate derivative coatings without compromising the retarded release rates (Levis and Deasy 2002, 2003). Poly(vinyl alcohol) can be used to create a similar coating with crosslinking using glutaraldehyde. Diphenhydramine hydrochloride–loaded nanotubes coated with cross-linked poly(vinyl alcohol) show pH-dependent release rates and retardation of rates by half compared to pristine halloysite nanotubes. Interestingly, the compositions with highest drug loading showed the slowest rates in acidic pH and fastest rates at pH 7 indicating the role of charge on the entrapped molecule in dictating rates (Ghebaur, Garea, and Iovu 2012). Curcumin-loaded halloysite nanotubes functionalized with chitosan shows better bioavailability of curcumin. The intracellular concentrations of free curcumin and curcumin loaded in chitosan-functionalized halloysite nanotubes were 70 μg /109 cells and 134 μg /109 cells after 4 hours incubation (Liu et al. 2016). Sixty-four percent of curcumin release occurred in 7 days in PBS. The release rates were considerably increased in cell lysate, an environment comparable to tumour microenvironment, 84% of release occurred in 48 hours. This indicates that the drug release in circulation is limited, and the delivery will happen mostly in the tumour region (Liu et al. 2016). Chitosan oligosaccharides can be grafted instead of the heavier chitosan polymer to improve the drug-loading efficiency. The oligosaccharides can be linked to the surface of the nanotubes through succinic anhydride modified aminopropyltriethoxysilane using EDS/NHS coupling. The drug entrapment efficiency was 55% in the oligosaccharide-modified nanotubes. The release kinetics show a release of 61% after 12 hours. The DOX-loaded-modified nanoparticles showed a better haemolysis ratio and showed enhanced toxicity to MCF7 cancer cells while did not show any obvious toxicity to L02 normal cells. The cytotoxicity is induced by multiple mechanisms and targets the nuclei and mitochondria. In vivo studies also showed the tumour inhibition effects of oligosaccharide-modified nanotubes (Yang et al. 2016). Due to the charged surface of the halloysite, nanotubes coatings can be achieved by layer-by-layer assembly of polycations like chitosan, polyethyleneimine, polylysine and polyallylamine hydrochloride and polyanions like polystyrene sulfonate, polyacrylic acid and heparin. The strong complexation of alternate layers yields slow release rates and inversion of surface charge of the tubes (Veerabadran et al. 2009). Higher ionic strength of the coating solution increased the adsorption thickness of polystyrene sulfonate-polyallylamine hydrochloride bilayer deposited on halloysite nanotubes. Higher retardation rate was observed for chitosan-gelatin triple coating of 12 nm on dexamethasone-loaded halloysite. The biodegradability of the coating is a determinant factor for the efficacy of the drug. Comparing the cytotoxicity of resveratrol-loaded halloysite nanotubes coated with polyethyleneimine-poly (sodium 4-styrene-sulfonate)/poly(allylaminehydrochloride) layer-by-layer coating and loaded nanotubes coated with protamine salt/dextran sulphate sodium salt, it was observed that the latter showed cytotoxicity in MCF7 cancer cells within 24 hours while the former did not. The protamine salt/dextran sulphate sodium salt coatings are digested by protease activity inside the cell (Vergaro, Lvov, and Leporatti 2012). Another interesting layered coating has been demonstrated using benzotriazole chelated to copper ions. Antiseptics-loaded halloysite nanotubes were washed with benzotriazole and then with copper sulphate to produce this coating. The release rates were seen to be influenced by the concentration of benzotriazole and copper ions. The release kinetics were retarded even after 200 hours, and only about 10% release was observed during this period. The loading efficiency was also improved by the coating (Wei et al. 2014). The polyelectrolyte coatings on halloysite nanotubes also provide the opportunity to design pH-responsive delivery systems. Ibuprofen-loaded halloysite coated with layers of chitosan and alginate shows different release kinetics and retardation rate at different pH. The release rates increase as the pH of the solution changed from 1.2 to 5.0 to 7.4. The tunability depends on the pKa of the polyelectrolyte groups and drug (Li, Zhu, et al. 2016). An interesting approach of creating hydrogels inside the halloysite lumen to trap drug molecules has been tested by Cavallaro et al. (2018). Cetyltrimethylammonium bromide–modified halloysite nanotubes were infused with sodium alginate and calcium chloride along with doxycycline in chloroform. The hydrogel is formed inside the halloysite by the coordination of calcium with the alginate. The formation of the hydrogel was confirmed using fluorescent probes. The release kinetics showed a marked decrease in the rate of release from hydrogel-infused nanotubes compared to just the nanotubes hosting the drug. Further, the release kinetics could be increased by the addition of ethylenediaminetetraacetic which chelates the calcium ions, thereby solubilizing the hydrogel in the inner lumen. The power law dependence of the kinetics conferred a Peppas release model.

Halloysite nanotubes coated with dextrin are unclogged by the cleavage of dextrin by the action of glycosyl hydrolase enzymes. This can be used to regulate the release of the drug inside the cell (Dzamukova et al. 2015). The external charge of halloysite nanotubes can be used to direct their higher-order colloidal assemblies, and further control on the release characteristics could be achieved. In the presence of oleic acid, halloysite nanotubes assemble into microspheres, and aspirin loaded in these microspheres shows controlled release in simulated intestinal fluid compared to simulated gastric fluid. The release of aspirin in the intestine instead of the stomach is recommended to increase the efficacy of the drug. The release profile could be further prolonged by the inclusion of chitosan in the assembly (Li, Yang, et al. 2016). The drug-loaded halloysite nanotubes can be admixed in polymeric matrices for much more prolonged release kinetics and are suggested for bone cement and dental filling applications (Kelly et al. 2004, Sánchez-Fernández et al. 2014, Shutava, Fakhrullin, and Lvov 2014). The release time extends to 250–300 hours in these studies, and a burst release can be observed under stress from the cracking of the structures. Polymethylmethacrylate composite cement with gentamicin-loaded halloysite nanotubes inhibited gram-negative and gram-positive bacterial strains indicating decreased risks of infections for such implants.

4.7.4 Biomolecule Loading in Halloysite

The positive charge of the inner lumen and the negative charge of the nanotube surface make the halloysite nanotubes suitable for loading negatively charged proteins specifically inside the nanotubes. Enhanced temperature and storage stability were observed for ⟨-amylase and urease loaded in halloysite nanotubes (Zhai et al. 2010). The isoelectric point of ⟨-amylase is pH 4.6 and that of urease is pH6. Hence immobilization at pH6 ensured charge compatibility for loading and strong ionic interactions between the enzymes and the inner surface of the lumen. The activity of the enzymes decreased by only about 10% after 15 days, while free enzymes were inactive after the same period of storage. Further, the enzymes retained about 50% of their activity even after seven continuous cycles. Layer-by-layer assembly of glucose oxidase–loaded halloysite nanotubes with polyethylene imine showed enzymatic activity upto 70% even after a month of storage (Lvov, Aerov, and Fakhrullin 2014). The inner pore size of halloysite nanotubes fits well for proteins of sizes 2–5 nm, and pepsin, lipase, urease, peroxidase and glucose oxidase have been loaded in halloysite nanotubes upto 6%–8% by weight. The loaded tubes could be dried and stored for months before testing for bioactivity and release. Release kinetics of pepsin-loaded halloysite nanotubes showed a fast release of 30–50 wt% within the first hour followed by slow release for further 4–5 hours. Significant amount of the enzymes still remained inside the tubes (Lvov, Aerov, and Fakhrullin 2014). The adsorption of DNA on to halloysite nanotubes has been used to create slow release system for doxorubicin. The interaction of DNA with the surface of the nanotubes is attributed to the phosphonate groups and influenced by the π-π interactions. Doxorubicin loading decreases the surface charge of DNA-modified nanotubes leading the authors to conclude that the drug is present on the surface of the nanotubes, either intercalated with the DNA or adsorbed on the hybrid structure. But Lvov has noted that the inclusion of the drug inside the lumen can also lead to a decrease in the outer surface charge. A constant release of the drug over the monitored period of 2 weeks was observed (Lvov et al. 2016, Lee et al. 2013).

4.7.5 Electrospun Composites

Electrospun composite nanofibre-based drug delivery system based on halloysite nanotubes presents an attractive system for scaffolding and bandaging applications. The typical release time of 10–20 hours for antibiotics loaded in halloysite nanotubes is extended to 2–3 weeks when incorporated into the electrospun matrix. The therapeutic effects on damaged sites can be extended by the use of such systems. Bone/tissue regeneration scaffolds should be biocompatible and provide mechanical and functional integrity, and the system should be able to withstand stress during surgical procedures (Agrawal and Ray 2001). Addition of halloysite nanotubes generally increases the mechanical properties of polymer composites (Gao 2004, Dong et al. 2011). The increase in mechanical properties of polycaprolactone fibres increased tensile strength and moduli by the inclusion of halloysite nanotubes have been seen to enhance human mesenchymal stem cell attachment, spreading and proliferation along with osteogenic differentiation and biomineralization (Ganesh Nitya et al. 2012). In an elaborate study using anti-bacterial agents chlorhexidine, povidone iodine, doxycycline, amoxicillin, potassium calvulanate and brilliant green, drug-infused halloysite nanotubes incorporated in polycaprolactone mats showed evidence to prolonged anti-bacterial effects. The drugs were loaded into the halloysite in ethanol. Polycaprolactone in chloroform solution was mixed with the nanotube solution to prepare the solution for electrospinning. Non-woven and oriented fibres could be prepared by using flat and U-shaped collectors, respectively. The addition of nanotubes up to 15% did not alter the fibre pattern or porosity. The addition of halloysite increases the hydrophilicity and hence wettability of the mats. While the drug release from halloysite nanotubes alone occurred within 5 hours, the drug release from scaffolds extended for over 9 days for amoxicillin and potassium calvulanate loaded and 1 day for brilliant green loaded ones. Zones of inhibition depended on the bacterial strain and bactericide and appeared within hours. The optimal weight percentage of 7.5% provided the balance between material properties and drug release kinetics. Burst release was observed for all compositions indicating the presence of surface adsorbed bactericidal molecules (Patel et al. 2016). Halloysite nanotubes encapsulating tetracycline hydrochloride mixed with poly(lactic-co-glycolic acid) were electrospun to form drug-loaded composite nanofibrous mats. The incorporation of nanotubes does not alter the morphology of the mats and did not influence viability and phenotype of cells. Sustained release of the drug was observed for the period of 30 days much retarded than fibres spun without halloysite (Qi et al. 2010). In vivo studies had shown the biocompatibility and biodegradation of polycaprolactone-gelatin matrix for cell proliferation and its ability to subdue inflammatory response with the inclusion of metronidazole (Xue et al. 2014). Metronidazole-loaded halloysite nanotubes electrospun with polycaprolactone-gelatin were proposed to prepare membranes with extended drug release profiles for guided tissue regeneration applications. Inclusion of halloysite nanotubes up to 20 wt% did not influence the morphology of electrospun fibres and doubled the tensile strength along the collector rotating direction. The surface of halloysite nanotubes had to be modified with aminopropyltriethosysilane to increase dispersibility in the electrospinning solvent, trifluoroethanol. About 5% drug-loaded membranes showed sustained release for 3 weeks preventing colonization of Fusobacterium throughout the period in in vitro studies. The addition of halloysite nanotubes increases the degradability of the matrix as observed from the weight loss of the samples during the observation time (Xue et al. 2015). Instead of loading the drug in the lumen, layer-by-layer assembly could be used to attach drugs to the surface of the nanotubes. Polyvinylpyrrolidone and polyacrylicacid-coated halloysite nanotubes show good absorption of methotrexate, and these halloysite nanotubes could be infused in nylon-6 to prepare composite mats that prevented osteosarcoma cell proliferation (Sun et al. 2016).

4.8 MONTMORILLONITE IN DRUG DELIVERY

Montmorillonite clay finds wide application as adsorbents, stabilizing and suspending agents as well as in drug formulations as drug carriers (Chang et al. 2003, Feng et al. 2009, Kevadiya, Thumbar, et al. 2012). Montmorillonite is widely considered a very good candidate for loading and controlled release of various categories of drugs such as antibiotics, anti-cancerous, anti-inflammatory antioxidant and anti-hypertensive drugs. It has been widely studied for drug delivery to the eye, transdermal delivery, targeted drug delivery to the colon and delivery to gastro-retentive system (Khatoon, Chu, and Zhou 2020). A list of drugs studied for delivery using montmorillonite is provided in Table 4.2. Montmorillonite nanoclays are promising in oral drug delivery since the drug molecules can get adsorbed on the alumino silicate layers and can release the drug in aqueous media. The Na^+ ions in the montmorillonite can easily be replaced with other inorganic and organic cations and allows easy modification for drug delivery. The rate of drug release is determined by the amount of nanoparticles dispersed (Cypes, Saltzman, and Giannelis 2003).

Table 4.2 Literature Review of Drugs Loaded in Montmorillonite

Class	*Drug*	*Ref*
Analgesic	Paracetamol	Anirudhan, Gopal, and Sandeep (2014)
	Tramadol hydrochloride	Chen et al. (2010) Adsorption
	Carboplatin	Iliescu et al. (2011) Ion exchange
Antibiotic	Tetracycline hydrochloride (Doxycycline)	Anirudhan, Sandeep, and Divya (2012) Sahoo et al. (2010)
	Doxorubicin	Anirudhan and Sandeep (2012)
Anti-inflammatory	Sodium diclofenac	Kaur and Datta (2014)
	Ibuprofen	Campbell, Craig, and McNally (2010)
	Naproxen	Mahkam, Rafi, and Gheshlaghi (2016)
	Triamcinolone actinide	Pinto et al. (2011)
	Docetaxel	Encapsulation (Feng et al. 2009)
Anti-cancerous	Exemestane	Filho (2019)
	Pomegranate	Golbashy et al. (2016)
Anti-hypertensive	Propranolol Hydrochloride	Seema and Datta (2013)
	Methyldopa and theophylline	Dornelas et al. (2011)
	Timolol maleate	Joshi et al. (2009) Intercalation
	Diltiazem hydrochloride	Anirudhan and Parvathy (2015)
	Venlafaxine Hydrochloride	Jain and Datta (2016) Encapsulation
Anti-depressant	Nortiptyline and Venlafaxine	Rajkumar, Kevadiya, and Bajaj (2015) Intercalation
Anti-septic	Chlorhexidine acetate	Saha, Butola, and Joshi (2014)
Anti-platelet drug	Clopidogrel bisulphate	Li et al. (2014)
Anti-metabolite	5-Fluorouracil	Lin et al. (2002) Intercalation
	Vitamins B1 and B6	Golubeva, Pavlova, and Yakovlev (2015)

4.8.1 Intercalation of Drugs in Montmorillonite

Intercalation of 5-fluorouracil in montmorillonite has been suggested as a method for improving its efficacy and lowering its toxicity in the treatment of colorectal cancer. Studies on intercalation of the drug in montmorillonite show that the intercalation happens by replacement of OH^- via ion exchange and some surface adsorption. The optimal loading conditions depend on pH, time and temperature. 5-Flourouracil loading at a pH 11.6 and 80°C for 2 hours resulted in a 88 mg/g loading (Lin et al. 2002). Salahuddin et al. studied the loading of a series of polyamides, prepared by the reaction of 5-phenyl-1,3,4-oxadiazole-2-thiol, 5-phenyl-1,3,4-oxadiazole-2-amine and 5-(4-chlorophenyl)-1,3,4-thiadiazole-2-thiol with ethyl chloroformate in montmorillonite (Salahuddin et al. 2014). The intercalation of the synthesized polyamide in to the interlayers of montmorillonite happens through the ion-exchange process between the amine hydrochloride in the polyamide and the sodium ions in the montmorillonite. Similarly, the anti-diabetic, cationic drug metformin intercalates into the interlayers of montmorillonite via ion exchange (Rebitski et al. 2018). Retention of about 93 meq of metformin per 100 g of montmorillonite could be achieved after water washing. Release studies in double-distilled water at pH≈5.5 showed a 15% release in 5 hours from a 25 mg/150 mg loaded sample. Increasing the loading concentration to 300 mg, increased the release to 25% in 3 hours. The study also simulated the fate of an oral delivery by studying the release of metformin in a sequence of pH. An initial pH of 1.2 for 2 hours (mimicking the stomach fluid) was changed to pH 6.8 for 2 hours (mimicking the small intestine fluid), and then to pH 7.4 (pH of the fluids in the colon) in the last 4 hours. A burst release of 40% happened at pH 1.2 from H^+ exchanging the metformin cations. In a neutral medium, pH 6.8 ion exchange occurs between intercalated metformin with Na^+ ions in the simulated track. The release profiles along with the intercalated structure are given in Figure 4.6.

Intercalated, weakly acidic drug ibuprofen is also released faster at pH 7.4 than at pH 1.2 at 37°C. Intercalation improves the thermal stability of the drug. The decomposition temperature increased to 47°C (Zheng et al. 2007). Tramadol, a common analgesic, can also be intercalated into montmorillonite via the cation exchange mechanism. A vertical monolayer arrangement of the drug is inferred from the intercalated basal spacing of 1.99 nm. An initial pH of 1.2 for 2 hours (mimicking the stomach fluid) was changed to pH 6.8 for 2 hours (mimicking the small intestine fluid), and then to pH 7.4 (pH of the fluids in the colon) in the last 4 hours (Chen

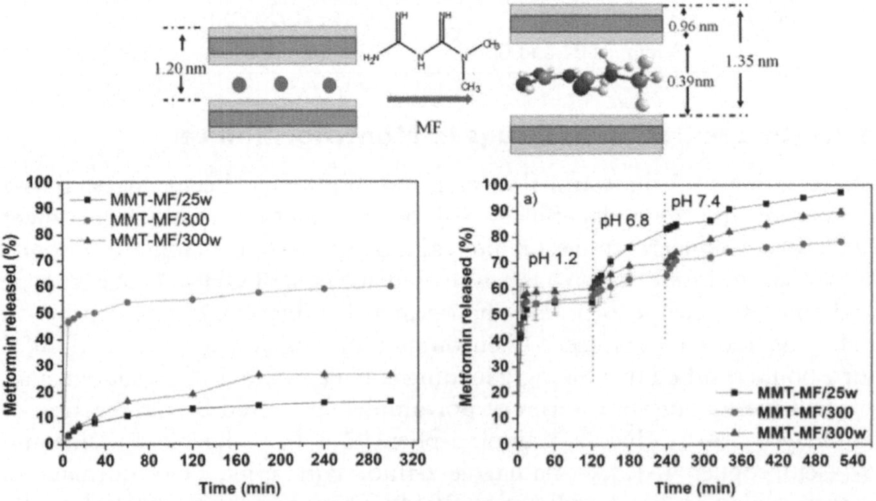

Figure 4.6 Mechanism of intercalation of metformin in montmorillonite interlayers (top). Release profile of metformin in aqueous medium (5.5 pH) (bottom left) and simulated gastrointestinal tract (Rebitski et al. 2018).

et al. 2010). Studies on the loading of timolol maleate, a non-selective β-adrenergic blocking agent, show that the extent of drug loading depends on pH and the loading capacity starts to decrease below pH 4 and above pH 7. As the pH approach the pKa of montmorillonite surface silanols or that of the drug molecule, then the electrostatic interaction that drives the ion exchange decreases. The study also reiterates that there is an optimal external concentration of the drug that is required to achieve maximum loading in montmorillonite. A maximum loading of 217 mg/g was achieved in this study. The controlled release tests in simulated gastric and intestinal fluids at 37°C±0.5°C using the timolol maleate absorbance at 294 nm showed slow and persistent release at pH 1.2 as well as at pH 7.4 fluids. ~50% of the loaded drug was released in 9 hours (Joshi et al. 2009).

A more elaborate understanding of adsorption and release of antibiotic metronidazole used in the treatment of amoebiasis from montmorillonite has been derived from systematic kinetic and equilibrium studies and XRD. The adsorption of the drug at pH 0.2 and 2.5 fits to a Freundlich model indicating multiple type of adsorption sites and changes to a Langmuir model, one nature of adsorption site at pH 5. The pKa of metronidazole is reported to be around 2.6, that the molecule will be neutral at around pH 5 (Cho et al. 1982). Hence, it can be safely argued that the drug molecules are intercalated in the interlayers at pH5, while it interacts with the charged lamella along with intercalation at lower pH. The Freundlich isotherm fits yielded the exponent values of 1 for pH 0.2 and <1 for pH 2.5. They could be interpreted as the presence of adsorption sites with similar energy at pH 0.2, while mutually interacting sites are present at pH 2.5. The progressive adsorption of metronidazole at pH 2.5 increases the sorption capacity of the solid further, probably by revealing new adsorption sites. At high pH the neutral nature of the drug presents the single option of intercalation for loading, while at pH 2.5 ion exchange and adsorption on the lumen surfaces are available. At a very low pH, the cationic drug competes with proton exchange as the silanol groups on the clay surface will also be protonated. Hence the general conclusion would be that the cationic form of the drug interacts with lamellar sites at highly acidic pH and cation exchange and lamellar sites at less acidic pH and intercalation at higher pH (Calabrese et al. 2013). Montmorillonite-tetracycline nanoclay has been suggested for the treatment of gastric infection caused by *Helicobacter pylori.* The reaction of montmorillonite and tetracycline occurs via an ion-exchange mechanism, in which all the Na^+ and Ca^{2+} cations in the clay are replaced by NHR_3^+ group of tetracycline resulting in an increase in the interlayer spacing. A comparatively strong tetracycline adsorption and a strong linking of drug fraction were observed at acidic pH compared to basic. Both acidic and basic nanocomposites showed good mucoadhesion properties to porcine mucin. Desorption of tetracycline also happens via the cation exchange process (Iannuccelli et al. 2015).

In an interesting approach, silylated (3-methacryloxypropyltrimethoxy silane) montmorillonite was used as anchor points for imprinting thiamine hydrochloride in a itaconic acid–based polymer matrix. This could yield specific binding and release system for thiamine hydrochloride with a maximum capacity of 100 mg/L. The silylation decreased the swelling of the polymer matrix and release profiles followed the Ritger–Peppas model, with 88% release in 8 hours at physiological pH (Anirudhan, Divya, and Nima 2013). Expanding the inter layers of montmorillonite is a preferable approach to intercalate larger molecules. The application of montmorillonite as a vector for gene delivery has been reported. Since the interlayer space in montmorillonite, 12 Å is not sufficient to accommodate DNA, the space was increased by intercalating a cationic expander hexadecyltrimethylammonium (HDTMA) prior to DNA intercalation. A suitable HDTMA intercalated montmorillonite with a spacing of 20.05 Å could be achieved using 1.5 CEC of HDTMA (Lin et al. 2006). After DNA intercalation in water at pH ~6, transfection of pGFP-C1vector was successfully carried out in a human fibroblast model. Montmorillonite has also been reported for the loading of enzyme insulin. Insulin was loaded in a montmorillonite titania composite carrier. Intercalation of insulin in montmorillonite is performed in acidic pH, below the IEP of insulin and the intercalation occur by cation exchange. Titania is co-condensed on to the intercalated montmorillonite from butoxide precursor resulting in titania-coated montmorillonite structures. The release was extended by 21 hours after the titania coating. The composite carrier prevents the digestive degradation of insulin and improves the drug passage time (Kamari, Ghiaci, and Ghiaci 2017).

4.8.2 Drug Loading in Polymer-Montmorillonite Composites

Multiple studies have shown that the inclusion of montmorillonite in biocompatible polymer matrices like alginate, chitosan, poly(lactic-co-glycolic acid), etc. yields drug delivery systems that have improved release characteristics than montmorillonite or polymer alone. The interactions of the montmorillonite clay with the polymer depend on the types of functional groups available on the polymer chain. Direct intercalation of the polymer or polymer-drug composite to polymer interactions with surface groups without intercalation has been exploited to obtain release matrices with varying characteristics. Among biocompatible polymer nanocomposites, chitosan intercalated with montmorillonite is highly promising due to its non-toxicity, high biocompatibility and non-antigenicity. Quaternized chitosan-montmorillonite nanocomposites can be prepared using hot intercalation technique. Compared to chitosan nanoparticles, quarternized chitosan-loaded montmorillonite nanocomposite exhibits enhanced efficiency in drug encapsulation and delayed drug release (Wang, Du, and

Luo 2008). A biocomposite based on montmorillonite-gelatin-lecithin microparticles has been reported for the controlled release of atorvastatin. Atorvastatin is a second-generation statin drug used in the lowering of cholesterol. The drug has low bioavailability on oral administration. Gelatin is a cationic polymer that can interact with the montmorillonite interlayers, and lecithin is a lipid molecule. The process involved the preparation of high molecular weight gelatin-lecithin composite with crosslinking and infusion of drugs into the composite. Montmorillonite is added to the composite in the final step, and the clay particles add on to the polymer particles. This arrangement is suggested to avoid the decrease in loading efficiency observed when montmorillonite is placed inside the polymer matrix. The lipid-polymer particles allow the encapsulation of drugs with low water solubility. A drug-loading efficiency of >67% was observed with release profiles extending through 48 hours (García Guzmán et al. 2018, 2019).

Ionotropic gelation of alginate in the presence of multivalent cations can be used to prepare gels that can encapsulate drugs and other bioactive agents. Drug release from these gels is pH dependent and occurs through diffusion on swelling and erosion of the matrix. The alginate system has low entrapment efficiency for water-soluble drugs due to leakage during cross-linking and undergoes fast disintegration in intestinal fluid leading to rapid drug release. Addition of montmorillonite into the alginate system provides resistance to solubility in water, increases loading capacity and decreases the release rate of the drug. The negatively charged alginate interacts electrostatically with the clay particles at the positively charged edges and interacts with the surface hydroxyls of clay to form 3D networks. The cationic drug irinotecan is a topoisomerase 1 inhibitor that prevents DNA unwinding and is used in the treatment of multiple cancers. Irinotecan-loaded montmorillonite alginate system has been studied for the release characteristics of the drug. The clay layers are exfoliated by the loading of irinotecan and can be observed by the disappearance of the characteristic XRD peaks of montmorillonite. The release profiles of drug loaded in montmorillonite and drug in montmorillonite in alginate showed that the release rates almost halved by the incorporation in alginate (Iliescu et al. 2014). Montmorillonite alginate-based drug delivery system was also tried for the extended release of venlafaxine hydrochloride. It is an effective third-generation drug that inhibits the reabsorption of norepinephrine, serotonin and dopamine. The water solubility of venlafaxine hydrochloride is high and results in the burst release of the drug with 100% cumulative release within 5.5 and 3.5 hours in the gastric and intestinal fluids, respectively, from pure alginate-based delivery. To maintain the concentration in the plasma, 2–3 times administration daily would be required. But the intercalation into montmorillonite minimized the burst release of drug and showed a controlled release of 20% in 26 hours in gastric fluid and 22% in 29 hours in an intestinal fluid (Jain and Datta 2016). Olanzapine is a drug that is used in the treatment of schizophrenia and has many side effects when administered orally. A hybrid system based on olanzapine/montmorillonite dispersed in a mixture of alginate and xanthan gum biopolymers obtained by incubation for 24 hours at pH 5.8 was studied for controlled drug release. A maximum intercalation of 47.37 mg per 100 mg of montmorillonite could be achieved by this method. The hybrid system prevents oxidation of the drug and improves controlled release. The hybrid showed a release of ~90% of drug after 8 hours and selective release at pH 7.4 (Oliveira, Alcântara, and Pergher 2017).

The delivery of the anti-depressant venlafaxine hydrochloride and dexamethasone, a glucocorticoid class of steroid drug by incorporating into montmorillonite-poly(lactic-co-glycolic acid) composite, has been reported. The intercalation process used was a w/o/w double emulsion technique followed by evaporation of the solvent. The process adopted for venlafaxine is provided in Figure 4.7. The intercalation of the polymer-drug composite is expected to happen between the drug layers. The intercalation resulted in extending the migration pathways of the drug in the composite. This inturn

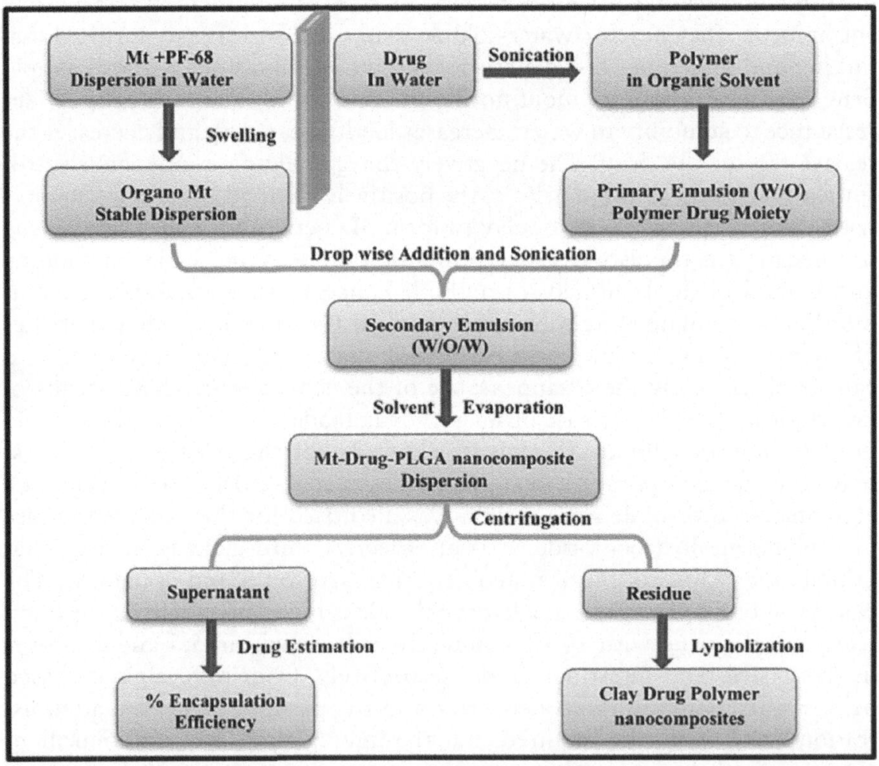

Figure 4.7 Synthetic process of drug -poly(lactic-co-glycolic acid)-montmorillonite used in (Jain and Datta 2014). PF-68 is the pluronic surfactant used to stabilize the emulsion.

reduced the burst effect and allowed a more controlled delivery compared to drug-polymer composite alone. The montmorillonite-poly(lactic-co-glycolic acid) drug nanocomposites thus yield effective longer delivery with less dosage (Jain and Datta 2014, 2015). A new curcumin-activated carboxymethyl cellulose-montmorillonite nanocomposite where carboxymethyl cellulose was used as an emulsifier for curcumin has also been reported. The water solubility of the carboxymethyl cellulose-curcumin intercalated in the montmorillonite clay was significantly high compared to normal curcumin. An effective release of curcumin, ~60% was achieved within 2.5 hours at 25°C at pH 5.4 (Madusanka, de Silva, and Amaratunga 2015).

A solvent displacement method was used to obtain poly(D, L-lactide)/montmorillonite nanocomposite via glass capillary microfluidics for the controlled delivery of acetaminophen. The co-flow glass capillary device delivered an organic phase into an aqueous flow. The polymer-montmorillonite drug composites were prepared by melt intercalation and then dissolved in tetrahydrofuran for use in the capillary device. The compatibility of montmorillonite with the polymer was improved by initially modifying it using quaternary ammonium surfactant N,N-Bis(2-hydroxyethyl)-N-methyl-N-tallow ammonium chloride. Nanoparticles are formed in the flow as the organic phase comes in contact with the aqueous phase, and tetrahydrofuran is displaced from the polymer-rich organic phase. The encapsulation efficiency, loading of the drug and release into a simulated intestinal fluid at pH 7.4 were improved by the introduction of montmorillonite into the polymer matrix (Othman et al. 2016). A schematic of the expected structure of the composite is given in Figure 4.8. Oral delivery vehicles

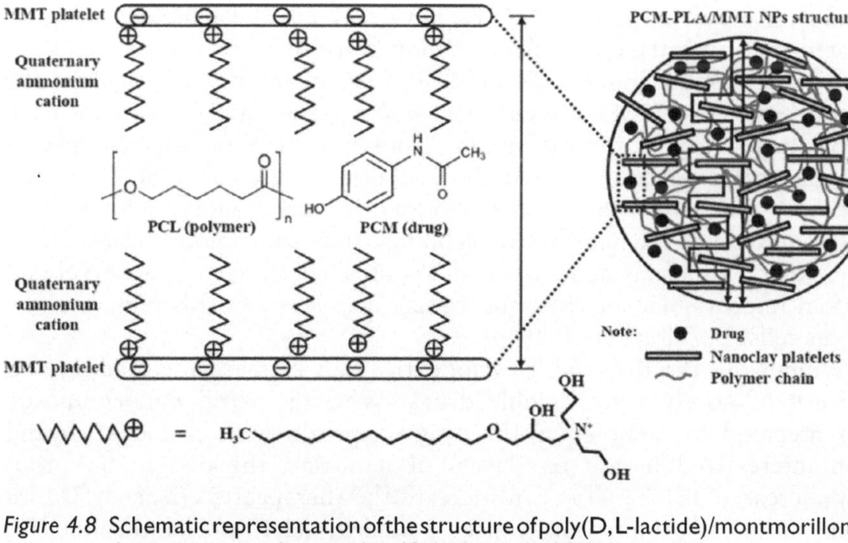

Figure 4.8 Schematic representation of the structure of poly(D, L-lactide)/montmorillonite drug composite discussed in (Othman et al. 2016).

for chemotherapeutic drugs are of significant interest since such a system can eliminate the need for hospital visits for chemotherapy. Composites of FDA-approved poly(lactic-co-glycolic acid) and poly(lactide) polymers with montmorillonite have been tested for such delivery using docetaxel as the model drug. Emulsification and solvent evaporation were used to synthesize the nanoparticles. An oil in water emulsion of polymer and drug in dichloromethane in water containing montmorillonite particles is initially prepared, and nanoparticles are separated after the evaporation of dichloromethane. The percentage of drug release from the poly(lactic-co-glycolic acid) composite particles in 10 days was close to 18% and that from the poly(lactide) composite was close to 25%. In vivo pharmacokinetic studies showed that the delivery systems maintained the drug plasma levels in the therapeutic window throughout the study (Feng et al. 2009). Three-week sustained chemotherapy was achieved when nanocomposite intercalated with 10 mg/mL of docetaxel was used compared to 22 hours of intravenous administration of Taxotere. The oral bioavailability was enhanced from 3.59% for Taxotere to 91.3% for selected composite.

Similarly, montmorillonite/poly-(e-caprolactone) composites have been reported for the controlled release of the anti-cancerous tamoxifen. The anti-cancerous tamoxifen is intercalated into the interlayers of montmorillonite and then compounded with poly-(e-caprolactone) to form tamoxifen-montmorillonite-poly-(e-caprolactone) nanocomposite for oral chemotherapy of breast cancer. The intercalation of tamoxifen in to the interlayers of montmorillonite followed a similar monolayer longitudinal mode through electrostatic interaction and marginally reduced the genotoxic effects of the drug. In vivo pharmacokinetics of formulations in rats showed that plasma levels of the drug were always within the therapeutic window (Kevadiya, Patel, et al. 2012; Silva et al. 2019). Paclitaxel was intercalated into an interlayer gallery of montmorillonite by an ion-exchange reaction. Optimum intercalation (58%) of paclitaxel molecules within the interlayer space of MMT was achieved with a pH of 6 at 3 hours for 120 mg of paclitaxel. The X-ray diffraction, Fourier transform infrared spectra and thermal analysis indicated the paclitaxel intercalated into the clay interlayer space and stabilized in the longitudinal monolayer by electrostatic interaction. The surface morphology showed a smooth layered surface. Nanocomposites demonstrated a controlled release of paclitaxel and 12-fold improvement in vitro anti-cancer activities towards human colon cancer cells (Bothiraja et al. 2014).

Complexing the drug with cyclodextrin can increase the loading and delivery of poorly water-soluble drugs. When a hybrid nanocomposite was prepared by complexing the drug oxaprozin with cyclodextrin and then intercalated in the interlayers of nanoclay, the dissolution property increased 100%. This can increase the therapeutic efficiency (Mura et al. 2016). Platinum anti-cancer complex, [(1,10-phenanthroline)(1S,

2S-diaminocyclohexane)platinum(II)]chloride can be loaded in montmorillonite within 1 hour. A maximum loading of 0.257 mmol/g of montmorillonite can be obtained with a 30 mM drug solution. The maximum loading occurs at a pH 6. The release of the anti-cancer complex is incomplete, both in dialysis and dispersion methods (Apps et al. 2014). Partial retention of loaded drugs in release studies is commonly observed in kinetic studies. Strong interaction of some of the drug molecules with the inner surface of the clay particles results in this retention.

4.8.3 Anti-microbial Applications

Anti-microbial properties can be improved by using the drug-metal ion complex, and the intercalation of such a complex in the montmorillonite clay will further facilitate prolonged anti-microbial effects (Mohanambe and Vasudevan 2005). Wu et al. have investigated the long-term, controlled release of chlorhexidine by complexing it with Cu(II) and then intercalating the drug complex into montmorillonite clay to form chlorhexidine–copper (II)/montmorillonite nanocomposites (Wu et al. 2013). Improved anti-bacterial property with higher thermal stability was obtained. The release of the drug followed a pseudo-second-order kinetics. Anti-bacterial property of montmorillonite intercalated with chlorhexidine acetate drug has also been reported. The intercalation happens via an ion-exchange route in which the cations in the clay are exchanged with the Ca^{2+} in the chlorhexidine acetate. The growth of different bacteria including gram-positive and gram-negative bacteria, like *E. coli* and *Staphylococcus aureus*, was inhibited by chlorhexidine acetate–montmorillonite intercalates. The kinetics of drug release shows an initial burst release followed by a sustained release (Saha, Butola, and Joshi 2014).

4.9 CONCLUSIONS

Drug delivery systems based on clay nanoparticles utilize the high surface area and rich electrochemical properties of clay materials. The high surface area, permanent charge on interlayers and ionizable groups on layer surfaces present rich interaction sites for guest molecules in clay materials.

Interactions of drug molecules with kaolinite occur with layer surfaces and newly exposed surfaces on exfoliation. The low drug-loading efficiency due to lack of permeant charge in kaolinite systems can be overcome through modification and exfoliation of kaolinite with small molecules like methanol or polymeric molecules. The loading capacities are influenced by the interaction of drug molecules with the modified kaolinite and intermolecular aggregation. Halloysite nanotubes, formed from the rolling of kaolinite, possess higher loading capacity due to the closed lumen formed from the rolling. Halloysite nanotubes possess chemically distinct inner and outer surfaces which allow specific modification of the inner and outer surfaces. The ionizable silanol groups on the outer surface provide variable charge to the outer surface depending on the pH. Modification of inner lumen with hydrophobic molecules permits the loading of hydrophobic drugs with high efficiency in these systems. The rich interactions possible for halloysite surfaces with polymer molecules allow the realization of multiple polymer-composite structures ideal for drug delivery and cell viability. Montmorillonite clays present myriad opportunity in drug delivery applications due to the permanent charge of interlayers and accessibility of the interlayers through ion exchange. The possibility of intercalation in montmorillonite presents the opportunity of expanding the interlayers and allows packing of large drug molecules. The modification of the nature of interlayers that can be achieved through ion exchange and intercalation also allows the packing of less soluble drugs in the interlayers.

The drug release kinetics from clay layers are significantly retarded compared to pure drugs in water. This helps in regulating the drug concentrations within the therapeutic window during the period of delivery. The packaging also ensures a longer lifetime for the drugs, increased bioavailability and release at the desired site of action. A complete analysis of the drug release kinetics allows the understanding of release mechanisms and rational design of the delivery system for better performance.

REFERENCES

Abduljauwad, S. N., and H.-R. Ahmed. 2019. "Enhancing cancer cell adhesion with clay nanoparticles for countering metastasis." *Scientific Reports* 9 (1):5935. doi: 10.1038/s41598-019-42498-y.

Abduljauwad, S. N., H.-R. Ahmed, and V. T. Moy. 2021. "Melanoma treatment via non-specific adhesion of cancer cells using charged nano-clays in pre-clinical studies." *Scientific Reports* 11 (1):2737. doi: 10.1038/s41598-021-82441-8.

Abdullayev, E., A. Joshi, W. Wei, Y. Zhao, and Y. Lvov. 2012. "Enlargement of halloysite clay nanotube lumen by selective etching of aluminum oxide." *ACS Nano* 6 (8):7216–7226. doi: 10.1021/nn302328x.

Agrawal, C. M., and R. B. Ray. 2001. "Biodegradable polymeric scaffolds for musculoskeletal tissue engineering." *Journal of Biomedical Materials Research* 55 (2):141–150.

Aguzzi, C., P. Cerezo, C. Viseras, and C. Caramella. 2007. "Use of clays as drug delivery systems: Possibilities and limitations." *Applied Clay Science* 36 (1):22–36. doi: 10.1016/j.clay.2006.06.015.

Anirudhan, T. S., P. L. Divya, and J. Nima. 2013. "Silylated montmorillonite based molecularly imprinted polymer for the selective binding and controlled release of thiamine hydrochloride." *Reactive and Functional Polymers* 73 (8):1144–1155. doi: 10.1016/j.reactfunctpolym.2013.05.004.

Anirudhan, T. S., and J. Parvathy. 2015. "Novel pH sensitive composite hydrogel based on functionalized chitosan/clay for the controlled release of a calcium channel blocker." *Designed Monomers and Polymers* 18 (5):413–423. doi: 10.1080/15685551.2015.1012622.

Anirudhan, T. S., and S. Sandeep. 2012. "Synthesis, characterization, cellular uptake and cytotoxicity of a multi-functional magnetic nanocomposite for the targeted delivery and controlled release of doxorubicin to cancer cells." *Journal of Materials Chemistry* 22 (25):12888–12899. doi: 10.1039/c2jm31794j.

Anirudhan, T. S., S. Sandeep, and P. L. Divya. 2012. "Synthesis and characterization of maleated cyclodextrin-grafted-silylated montmorillonite for the controlled release and colon specific delivery of tetracycline hydrochloride." *RSC Advances* 2 (25):9555–9564. doi: 10.1039/c2ra21093b.

Anirudhan, T. S., S. Saranya Gopal, and S. Sandeep. 2014. "Synthesis and characterization of montmorillonite/N-(carboxyacyl) chitosan coated magnetic particle nanocomposites for controlled delivery of paracetamol." *Applied Clay Science* 88–89:151–158. doi: 10.1016/j.clay.2013.11.039.

Apps, M. G., A. J. Ammit, A. Gu, and N. J. Wheate. 2014. "Analysis of montmorillonite clay as a vehicle in platinum anticancer drug delivery." *Inorganica Chimica Acta* 421:513–518 doi: 10.1016/j.ica.2014.07.009.

Awad, M. E., A. López-Galindo, M. Setti, M. M. El-Rahmany, and C. V. Iborra. 2017. "Kaolinite in pharmaceutics and biomedicine." *International Journal of Pharmaceutics* 533 (1):34–48. doi: 10.1016/j.ijpharm.2017.09.056.

Azar, Ahmad Taher, ed. 2021. *Modeling and Control of Drug Delivery Systems*. Academic Press, Cambridge, MA.

Bediako, E. G., E. Nyankson, D. Dodoo-Arhin, B. Agyei-Tuffour, D. Łukowiec, B. Tomiczek, A. Yaya, and J. K. Efavi. 2018. "Modified halloysite nanoclay as a vehicle for sustained drug delivery." *Heliyon* 4 (7):e00689. doi: 10.1016/j.heliyon.2018.e00689.

Bergaya, F., and G. Lagaly. 2013. "General introduction: Clays, clay minerals, and clay science." In *Developments in Clay Science*, 1–19. Elsevier. doi: 10.1016/S1572-4352(05)01001-9.

Bonina, F. P., M. L. Giannossi, L. Medici, C. Puglia, V. Summa, and F. Tateo. 2007. "Adsorption of salicylic acid on bentonite and kaolin and release experiments." *Applied Clay Science* 36 (1):77–85. doi: 10.1016/j.clay.2006.07.008.

Bothiraja, C., U. H. Thorat, A. P. Pawar, and K. S. Shaikh. 2014. "Chitosan coated layered clay montmorillonite nanocomposites modulate oral delivery of paclitaxel in colonic cancer." *Materials Technology* 29 (sup3):B120–B126. doi: 10.1179/1753555714y.0000000174.

Brigattia, M.F., E. Galan, and B.K.G. Theng. 2013. "Structure and mineralogy of clay minerals." In *Developments in Clay Science*, 21–81. Elsevier. doi: 10.1016/B978-0-08-098258-8.00002-X.

Calabrese, I., G. Cavallaro, C. Scialabba, M. Licciardi, M. Merli, L. Sciascia, and M. L. T. Liveri. 2013. "Montmorillonite nanodevices for the colon metronidazole delivery." *International Journal of Pharmaceutics* 457 (1):224–236. doi: 10.1016/j.ijpharm.2013.09.017.

Čalija, B., J. Milić, N. Milašinović, A. Daković, K. Trifković, J. Stojanović, and D. Krajišnik. 2020. "Functionality of chitosan-halloysite nanocomposite films for sustained delivery of antibiotics: The effect of chitosan molar mass." *Journal of Applied Polymer Science* 137 (8):48406. doi: 10.1002/app.48406.

Campbell, K. T., D. Q. M. Craig, and T. McNally. 2010. "Ibuprofen-loaded poly(-ε-caprolactone) layered silicate nanocomposites prepared by hot melt extrusion." *Journal of Materials Science: Materials in Medicine* 21 (8):2307–2316. doi: 10.1007/s10856-009-3963-2.

Cavallaro, G., G. Lazzara, S. Milioto, F. Parisi, V. Evtugyn, E. Rozhina, and R. Fakhrullin. 2018. "Nanohydrogel formation within the halloysite lumen for triggered and sustained release." *ACS Applied Materials & Interfaces* 10 (9):8265–8273. doi: 10.1021/acsami.7b19361.

Chan, M.-H., M.-R. Hsieh, R.-S. Liu, D.-H. Wei, and M. Hsiao. 2020. "Magnetically guided theranostics: Optimizing magnetic resonance imaging with sandwich-like kaolinite-based iron/platinum nanoparticles for magnetic fluid hyperthermia and chemotherapy." *Chemistry of Materials* 32 (2):697–708. doi: 10.1021/acs.chemmater.9b03552.

Chang, J.-H., Y. U. An, D. Cho, and E. P. Giannelis. 2003. "Poly(lactic acid) nanocomposites: Comparison of their properties with montmorillonite and synthetic mica (II)." *Polymer* 44 (13):3715–3720. doi: 10.1016/S0032-3861(03)00276-3.

Chen, Y., A. Zhou, B. Liu, and J. Liang. 2010a. "Tramadol hydrochloride/montmorillonite composite: Preparation and controlled drug release." *Applied Clay Science* 49 (3):108–112. doi: 10.1016/j.clay.2010.04.011.

Cho, M. J., R. R. Kurtz, C. Lewis, S. M. Machkovech, and D. J. Houser. 1982. "Metronidazole phosphate–a water-soluble prodrug for parenteral solutions of metronidazole." *Journal of Pharmaceutical Sciences* 71 (4):410–4. doi: 10.1002/jps.2600710409.

Cypes, S. H., W. Mark Saltzman, and E. P. Giannelis. 2003. "Organosilicate-polymer drug delivery systems: Controlled release and enhanced mechanical properties." *Journal of Controlled Release* 90 (2):163–169. doi: 10.1016/S0168-3659(03)00133-0.

Dawson, J. I., and R. O. C. Oreffo. 2013. "Clay: New opportunities for tissue regeneration and biomaterial design." *Advanced Materials* 25 (30):4069–4086. doi: 10.1002/adma.201301034.

Dong, Y., D. Chaudhary, H. Haroosh, and T. Bickford. 2011. "Development and characterisation of novel electrospun polylactic acid/tubular clay nanocomposites." *Journal of Materials Science* 46 (18):6148–6153. doi: 10.1007/s10853-011-5605-6.

Dornelas, C. B., A. M. da Silva, C. B. Dantas, C. R. Rodrigues, S. S. Coutinho, P. C. Sathler, H. C. Castro, L. R. Dias, V. P. de Sousa, and L. M. Cabral. 2011. "Preparation and evaluation of a new nano pharmaceutical excipients and drug delivery system based in polyvinylpyrrolidone and silicate." *Journal of Pharmacy and Pharmaceutical Sciences* 14 (1):17–35. doi: 10.18433/j3hc72.

Duarte-Silva, R., M. A. Villa-García, M. Rendueles, and M. Díaz. 2014. "Structural, textural and protein adsorption properties of kaolinite and surface modified kaolinite adsorbents." *Applied Clay Science* 90:73–80. doi: 10.1016/j.clay.2013.12.027.

Dzamukova, M. R., E. A. Naumenko, Y. M. Lvov, and R. F. Fakhrullin. 2015. "Enzyme-activated intracellular drug delivery with tubule clay nanoformulation." *Scientific Reports* 5:10560.

Feng, S. S., L. Mei, P. Anitha, C. W. Gan, and W. Zhou. 2009. "Poly(lactide)-vitamin E derivative/montmorillonite nanoparticle formulations for the oral delivery of Docetaxel." *Biomaterials* 30 (19):3297–306. doi: 10.1016/j.biomaterials.2009.02.045.

Filho, E. 2019. "Clays as biomaterials in controlled drug release: A scientific and technological short review." *Biomedical Journal of Scientific & Technical Research* 15. doi: 10.26717/bjstr.2019.15.002677.

Forsgren, J., E. Jämstorp, S. Bredenberg, H. Engqvist, and M. Strømme. 2010. "A ceramic drug delivery vehicle for oral administration of highly potent opioids**Johan Forsgren and Erik Jämstorp contributed equally to this work." *Journal of Pharmaceutical Sciences* 99 (1):219–226. doi: 10.1002/jps.21814.

Ganesh Nitya, G. T. N., U. Mony, K. P. Chennazhi, and S. V. Nair. 2012. "In vitro evaluation of electrospun PCL/nanoclay composite scaffold for bone tissue engineering." *Journal of Materials Science: Materials in Medicine* 23:1749–1761.

Gao, F. 2004. "Clay/polymer composites: The story." *Materials Today* 7 (11):50–55. doi: 10.1016/S1369-7021(04)00509-7.

Gao, G., L. Wang, Y. Cong, Z. Wang, Y. Zhou, R. Wang, J. Chen, and J. Fu. 2018. "Synergistic pH and temperature-driven actuation of Poly (NIPAM-co-DMAPMA)/clay nanocomposite hydrogel bilayers." *ACS Omega* 3 (12):17914–17921. doi: 10.1021/acsomega.8b02979.

García-Guzmán, P., L. Medina-Torres, F. Calderas, M. J. Bernad-Bernad, J. Gracia-Mora, X. Marcos, J. Correa-Basurto, D. M. Núñez-Ramírez, and O. Manero. 2019. "Rheological mucoadhesion and cytotoxicity of montmorillonite clay mineral/hybrid microparticles biocomposite." *Applied Clay Science* 180:105202. doi: 10.1016/j.clay.2019.105202.

García-Guzmán, P., L. Medina-Torres, F. Calderas, M. J. Bernad-Bernad, J. Gracia-Mora, B. Mena, and O. Manero. 2018. "Characterization of hybrid microparticles/Montmorillonite composite with raspberry-like morphology for Atorvastatin controlled release." *Colloids Surf B Biointerfaces* 167:397–406. doi: 10.1016/j.colsurfb.2018.04.020.

Ghebaur, A., S. A. Garea, and H. Iovu. 2012. "New polymer–halloysite hybrid materials—potential controlled drug release system." *International Journal of Pharmaceutics* 436 (1):568–573. doi: 10.1016/j.ijpharm.2012.07.014.

Golbashy, M., H. Sabahi, I. Allahdadi, H. Nazokdast, and M. Hosseini. 2016. "Synthesis the montmorillonite- pomegranate (Punicagranatum L.) peel polyphenols nanostructure as a drug delivery vehicle." *Biomedical and Pharmacology Journal* 9 (1): 385–392.

Golubeva, O. Y., S. V. Pavlova, and A. V. Yakovlev. 2015. "Adsorption and in vitro release of vitamin B1 by synthetic nanoclays with montmorillonite structure." *Applied Clay Science* 112–113:10–16. doi: 10.1016/j.clay.2015.04.013.

Heinz, H. 2012. "Clay minerals for nanocomposites and biotechnology: Surface modification, dynamics and responses to stimuli." *Clay Minerals* 47 (2):205–230. doi: 10.1180/claymin.2012.047.2.05.

Holešová, S., M. Valášková, D. Hlaváč, J. Madejová, M. Samlíková, J. Tokarský, and E. Pazdziora. 2014. "Antibacterial kaolinite/urea/chlorhexidine nanocomposites: Experiment and molecular modelling." *Applied Surface Science* 305:783–791. doi: 10.1016/j.apsusc.2014.04.008.

Iannuccelli, V., E. Maretti, M. Montorsi, C. Rustichelli, F. Sacchetti, and E. Leo. 2015. "Gastroretentive montmorillonite-tetracycline nanoclay for the treatment of Helicobacter pylori infection." *International Journal of Pharmaceutics* 493 (1):295–304. doi: 10.1016/j.ijpharm.2015.06.049.

Iliescu, R. I., E. Andronescu, C. D. Ghitulica, D. Berger, and A. Ficai. 2011. "Montmorillonite-alginate nanocompositebeads as drug carrier for oral administrationof carboplatin – preparation andcharacterization." *UPB Scientific Bulletin, Series B: Chemistry and Materials Science* 73 (3):3–16.

Iliescu, R. I., E. Andronescu, C. D. Ghitulica, G. Voicu, A. Ficai, and M. Hoteteu. 2014. "Montmorillonite–alginate nanocomposite as a drug delivery system – incorporation and in vitro release of irinotecan." *International Journal of Pharmaceutics* 463 (2):184–192. doi: 10.1016/j.ijpharm.2013.08.043.

Jain, S., and M. Datta. 2014. "Montmorillonite-PLGA nanocomposites as an oral extended drug delivery vehicle for venlafaxine hydrochloride." *Applied Clay Science* 99:42–47 doi: 10.1016/j.clay.2014.06.006.

Jain, S., and M. Datta. 2015. "Oral extended release of dexamethasone: Montmorillonite–PLGA nanocomposites as a delivery vehicle." *Applied Clay Science* 104:182–188. doi: 10.1016/j.clay.2014.11.028.

Jain, S., and M. Datta. 2016. "Montmorillonite-alginate microspheres as a delivery vehicle for oral extended release of Venlafaxine hydrochloride." *Journal of Drug Delivery Science and Technology* 33:149–156. doi: 10.1016/j.jddst.2016.04.002.

Jämstorp, E., T. Yarra, B. Cai, H. Engqvist, S. Bredenberg, and M. Strømme. 2012. "Polymer excipients enable sustained drug release in low pH from mechanically strong inorganic geopolymers." *Results Pharma Sciences* 2:23–8. doi: 10.1016/j.rinphs.2012.02.001.

Jämstorp, E., J. Forsgren, S. Bredenberg, H. Engqvist, and M. Strømme. 2010. "Mechanically strong geopolymers offer new possibilities in treatment of chronic pain." *Journal of Controlled Release* 146 (3):370–377. doi: 10.1016/j.jconrel.2010.05.029.

Joshi, G. V., B. D. Kevadiya, H. A. Patel, H. C. Bajaj, and R. V. Jasra. 2009. "Montmorillonite as a drug delivery system: Intercalation and in vitro release of timolol maleate." *International Journal of Pharmaceutics* 374 (1):53–57. doi: 10.1016/j.ijpharm.2009.03.004.

Joussein, E., S. Petit, J. Churchman, B. Theng, D. Righi, and B. Delvaux. 2005. "Halloysite clay minerals — a review." *Clay Minerals* 40 (4):383–426. doi: 10.1180/0009855054040180.

Kamari, Y., P. Ghiaci, and M. Ghiaci. 2017. "Study on montmorillonite/insulin/TiO_2 hybrid nanocomposite as a new oral drug-delivery system." *Materials Science and Engineering: C* 75:822–828.doi: 10.1016/j.msec.2017.02.115.

Kaur, M., and M. Datta. 2014. "Diclofenac sodium adsorption onto montmorillonite: Adsorption equilibrium studies and drug release kinetics." *Adsorption Science & Technology* 32 (5):365–387. doi: 10.1260/0263-6174.32.5.365.

Kelly, H. M., P. B. Deasy, E. Ziaka, and N. Claffey. 2004. "Formulation and preliminary in vivo dog studies of a novel drug delivery system for the treatment of periodontitis." *International Journal of Pharmaceutics* 274 (1):167–183. doi: 10.1016/j.ijpharm.2004.01.019.

Kennedy, L., J. K. Sandhu, M.-E. Harper, and M. Cuperlovic-Culf. 2020. "Role of glutathione in cancer: From mechanisms to therapies." *Biomolecules* 10 (10):1429. doi: 10.3390/biom10101429.

Kevadiya, B. D., R. P. Thumbar, M. M. Rajput, S. Rajkumar, H. Brambhatt, G. V. Joshi, G. P. Dangi, H. M. Mody, P. K. Gadhia, and H. C. Bajaj. 2012. "Mo ntmorillonite/poly-(ε-caprolactone) composites as versatile layered material: Reservoirs for anticancer drug and controlled release property." *European Journal of Pharmacology* 47 (1):265–72. doi: 10.1016/j.ejps.2012.04.009.

Kevadiya, B. D., T. A. Patel, D. D. Jhala, R. P. Thumbar, H. Brahmbhatt, M. P. Pandya, S. Rajkumar, P. K. Jena, G. V. Joshi, P. K. Gadhia, C. B. Tripathi, and H. C. Bajaj. 2012. "Layered inorganic nanocomposites: A promising carrier for 5-fluorouracil (5-FU)." *European Journal of Pharmaceutics and Biopharmaceutics* 81 (1):91–101. doi: 10.1016/j.ejpb.2012.01.004.

Khatoon, N., M. Q. Chu, and C. H. Zhou. 2020. "Nanoclay-based drug delivery systems and their therapeutic potentials." *Journal of Materials Chemistry B* 8 (33):7335–7351. doi: 10.1039/d0tb01031f.

Kryuchkova, M., A. Danilushkina, Y. Lvov, and R. Fakhrullin. 2016. "Evaluation of toxicity of nanoclays and graphene oxide in vivo: A Paramecium caudatum study." *Environmental Science: Nano* 3 (2):442–452. doi: 10.1039/C5EN00201J.

Kurkuri, M. D., and T. M. Aminabhavi. 2004. "Poly(vinyl alcohol) and poly(-acrylic acid) sequential interpenetrating network pH-sensitive microspheres for the delivery of diclofenac sodium to the intestine." *Journal of Controlled Release* 96 (1):9–20. doi: 10.1016/j.jconrel.2003.12.025.

Lai, X., M. Agarwal, Y. M. Lvov, C. Pachpande, K. Varahramyan, and F. A. Witzmann. 2013. "Proteomic profiling of halloysite clay nanotube exposure in intestinal cell co-culture." *Journal of Applied Toxicology: JAT* 33 (11):1316–1329. doi: 10.1002/jat.2858.

Lee, Y., G.-E. Jung, S. J. Cho, K. E. Geckeler, and H. Fuchs. 2013. "Cellular interactions of doxorubicin-loaded DNA-modified halloysite nanotubes." *Nanoscale* 5 (18):8577–8585. doi: 10.1039/C3NR02665E.

Levis, S. R., and P. B. Deasy. 2002. "Characterisation of halloysite for use as a microtubular drug delivery system." *International Journal of Pharmaceutics* 243 (1–2):125–34. doi: 10.1016/s0378-5173(02)00274-0.

Levis, S. R., and P. B. Deasy. 2003. "Use of coated microtubular halloysite for the sustained release of diltiazem hydrochloride and propranolol hydrochloride." *International Journal of Pharmaceutics* 253 (1):145–157. doi: 10.1016/S0378-5173(02)00702-0.

Li, H., X. Zhu, J. Xu, W. Peng, S. Zhong, and Y. Wang. 2016. "The combination of adsorption by functionalized halloysite nanotubes and encapsulation by polyelectrolyte coatings for sustained drug delivery." *RSC Advances* 6 (59):54463–54470. doi: 10.1039/C6RA09599B.

Li, W., L. Sun, L. Pan, Z. Lan, T. Jiang, X. Yang, J. Luo, R. Li, L. Tan, S. Zhang, and M. Yu. 2014. "Dendrimer-like assemblies based on organoclays as multi-host system for sustained drug delivery." *European Journal of Pharmaceutics and Biopharmaceutics* 88 (3):706–17. doi: 10.1016/j.ejpb.2014.09.014.

Li, X., Q. Yang, J. Ouyang, H. Yang, and S. Chang. 2016. "Chitosan modified halloysite nanotubes as emerging porous microspheres for drug carrier." *Applied Clay Science* 126:306–312 doi: 10.1016/j.clay.2016.03.035.

Lin, F. H., Y. H. Lee, C. H. Jian, J.-M. Wong, M.-J. Shieh, and C.-Y. Wang. 2002. "A study of purified montmorillonite intercalated with 5-fluorouracil as drug carrier." *Biomaterials* 23 (9):1981–1987. doi: 10.1016/S0142-9612(01)00325-8.

Lin, F. -H., C.-H. Chen, W. T. K. Cheng, and T.-F. Kuo. 2006. "Modified montmorillonite as vector for gene delivery." *Biomaterials* 27 (17):3333–3338. doi: 10.1016/j.biomaterials.2005.12.029.

Liu, M., Y. Chang, J. Yang, Y. You, R. He, T. Chen, and C. Zhou. 2016. "Functionalized halloysite nanotube by chitosan grafting for drug delivery of curcumin to achieve enhanced anticancer efficacy." *Journal of Materials Chemistry B* 4 (13):2253–2263. doi: 10.1039/C5TB02725J.

Lvov, Y., A. Aerov, and R. Fakhrullin. 2014. "Clay nanotube encapsulation for functional biocomposites." *Advances in Colloid and Interface Science* 207:189–198 doi: 10.1016/j.cis.2013.10.006.

Lvov, Y., W. Wang, L. Zhang, and R. Fakhrullin. 2016. "Halloysite clay nanotubes for loading and sustained release of functional compounds." *Advanced Materials* 28 (6):1227–1250. doi: 10.1002/adma.201502341.

Madusanka, N., K. M. Nalin de Silva, and G. Amaratunga. 2015. "A curcumin activated carboxymethyl cellulose–montmorillonite clay nanocomposite having enhanced curcumin release in aqueous media." *Carbohydrate Polymers* 134:695–699 doi: 10.1016/j.carbpol.2015.08.030.

Mahkam, M., A. A. Rafi, and L. M. Gheshlaghi. 2016. "Preparation of novel pH-sensitive nanocomposites based on ionic-liquid modified montmorillonite for colon specific drug delivery system." *Polymer Composites* 37 (1):182–187. doi: 10.1002/pc.23169.

Massaro, M., R. Amorati, G. Cavallaro, S. Guernelli, G. Lazzara, S. Milioto, R. Noto, P. Poma, and S. Riela. 2016. "Direct chemical grafted curcumin on halloysite nanotubes as dual-responsive prodrug for pharmacological applications." *Colloids and Surfaces B: Biointerfaces* 140:505–513. doi: 10.1016/j.colsurfb.2016.01.025.

Massaro, M., C. G. Colletti, R. Noto, S. Riela, P. Poma, S. Guernelli, F. Parisi, S. Milioto, and G. Lazzara. 2015. "Pharmaceutical properties of supramolecular assembly of co-loaded cardanol/triazole-halloysite systems." *International Journal of Pharmaceutics* 478 (2):476–485. doi: 10.1016/j.ijpharm.2014.12.004.

Mohanambe, L., and S. Vasudevan. 2005. "Anionic clays containing anti-inflammatory drug molecules: Comparison of molecular dynamics simulation and measurements." *The Journal of Physical Chemistry B* 109 (32):15651–15658. doi: 10.1021/jp050480m.

Mura, P., F. Maestrelli, C. Aguzzi, and C. Viseras. 2016. "Hybrid systems based on "drug - in cyclodextrin - in nanoclays" for improving oxaprozin dissolution properties." *International Journal of Pharmaceutics* 509 (1–2):8–15. doi: 10.1016/j.ijpharm.2016.05.028.

Murugesan, S., and T. Scheibel. 2020. "Copolymer/clay nanocomposites for biomedical applications." *Advanced Functional Materials* 30 (17):1908101. doi: 10.1002/adfm.201908101.

Oliveira, A. S., Ana C. S. Alcântara, and S. B. C. Pergher. 2017. "Bionanocomposite systems based on montmorillonite and biopolymers for the controlled release of olanzapine." *Materials Science and Engineering: C* 75:1250–1258. doi: 10.1016/j.msec.2017.03.044.

Othman, R., G. T. Vladisavljević, N. L. Thomas, and Z. K. Nagy. 2016. "Fabrication of composite poly(d,l-lactide)/montmorillonite nanoparticles for controlled delivery of acetaminophen by solvent-displacement method using glass capillary microfluidics." *Colloids and Surfaces B: Biointerfaces* 141:187–195. doi: 10.1016/j.colsurfb.2016.01.042.

Patel, S., U. Jammalamadaka, L. Sun, K. Tappa, and D. K. Mills. 2016. "Sustained release of antibacterial agents from doped halloysite nanotubes." *Bioengineering (Basel)* 3 (1). doi: 10.3390/bioengineering3010001.

Pinto, F. C. H., A. Silva-Cunha, G. A. Pianetti, E. Ayres, R. L. Oréfice, and G. R. Da Silva. 2011. "Montmorillonite clay-based polyurethane nanocomposite as local triamcinolone acetonide delivery system." *Journal of Nanomaterials* 2011:528628. doi: 10.1155/2011/528628.

Price, R. R., B. P. Gaber, and Y. Lvov. 2001. "In-vitro release characteristics of tetracycline HCl, khellin and nicotinamide adenine dineculeotide from halloysite; a cylindrical mineral." *Journal of Microencapsulation* 18 (6):713–22. doi: 10.1080/02652040010019532.

Qi, R., R. Guo, M. Shen, X. Cao, L. Zhang, J. Xu, J. Yu, and X. Shi. 2010. "Electrospun poly(lactic-co-glycolic acid)/halloysite nanotube composite nanofibers for drug encapsulation and sustained release." *Journal of Materials Chemistry* 20 (47):10622–10629. doi: 10.1039/C0JM01328E.

Rajkumar, S., B. D. Kevadiya, and H. C. Bajaj. 2015. "Montmorillonite/Poly (L-Lactide) microcomposite spheres as reservoirs of antidepressant drugs and their controlled release property." *Asian Journal of Pharmaceutical Sciences* 10 (5):452–458. doi: 10.1016/j.ajps.2015.06.002.

Rebitski, E. P., P. Aranda, M. Darder, R. Carraro, and E. Ruiz-Hitzky. 2018. "Intercalation of metformin into montmorillonite." *Dalton Transactions* 47 (9):3185–3192. doi: 10.1039/c7dt04197g.

Riela, S., M. Massaro, C. G. Colletti, A. Bommarito, C. Giordano, S. Milioto, R. Noto, P. Poma, and G. Lazzara. 2014. "Development and characterization of co-loaded curcumin/triazole-halloysite systems and evaluation of their potential anticancer activity." *International Journal of Pharmaceutics* 475 (1):613–623. doi: 10.1016/j.ijpharm.2014.09.019.

Ruiz-Hitzky, E., P. Aranda, M. Darder, and G. Rytwo. 2010. "Hybrid materials based on clays for environmental and biomedical applications." *Journal of Materials Chemistry* 20 (42):9306–9321. doi: 10.1039/C0JM00432D.

Saha, K., B. S. Butola, and M. Joshi. 2014. "Synthesis and characterization of chlorhexidine acetate drug–montmorillonite intercalates for antibacterial applications." *Applied Clay Science* 101:477–483. doi: 10.1016/j.clay.2014.09.010.

Sahoo, S., A. Sasmal, D. Sahoo, and P. Nayak. 2010. "Synthesis and characterization of chitosan-polycaprolactone blended with organoclay for control release of doxycycline." *Journal of Applied Polymer Science* 118 (6):3167–3175. doi: 10.1002/app.32474.

Salahuddin, N., A. Elbarbary, N. G. Allam, and A. F. Hashim. 2014. "Polyamide-montmorillonite nanocomposites as a drug delivery system: Preparation, release of 1,3,4-oxa(thia)diazoles, and antimicrobial activity." *Journal of Applied Polymer Science* 131 (23). doi: 10.1002/app.41177.

Sánchez-Fernández, A., L. Peña-Parás, R. Vidaltamayo, R. Cué-Sampedro, A. Mendoza-Martínez, V. C. Zomosa-Signoret, A. M. Rivas-Estilla, and P. Riojas. 2014. Synthesization, characterization, and in vitro evaluation of cytotoxicity of biomaterials based on halloysite nanotubes. *Materials (Basel, Switzerland)* 7 (12): 7770–7780. Accessed 2014/12. doi:10.3390/ma7127770.

Sandri, G., C. Aguzzi, S. Rossi, M. C. Bonferoni, G. Bruni, C. Boselli, A. I. Cornaglia, F. Riva, C. Viseras, C. Caramella, and F. Ferrari. 2017. "Halloysite and chitosan oligosaccharide nanocomposite for wound healing." *Acta Biomaterialia* 57:216–224 doi: 10.1016/j.actbio.2017.05.032.

Sawicka, D., L. Zapor, L. Chojnacka-Puchta, and K. Miranowicz-Dzierzawska. 2020. "The in vitro toxicity evaluation of halloysite nanotubes (HNTs) in human lung cells." *Toxicological Research* 37 (3):301–310. doi: 10.1007/s43188-020-00062-1.

Seema, and M. Datta. 2013. "Clay–polymer nanocomposites as a novel drug carrier: Synthesis, characterization and controlled release study of propranolol hydrochloride." *Applied Clay Science* 80–81:85–92. doi: 10.1016/j.clay.2013.06.009.

Shutava, T. G., R. F. Fakhrullin, and Y. M. Lvov. 2014. "Spherical and tubule nanocarriers for sustained drug release." *Current Opinion in Pharmacology* 18:141–148. doi: 10.1016/j.coph.2014.10.001.

Silva, D. T. C., I. E. S. Arruda, L. M. França, D. B. França, M. G. Fonseca, M. F. L. R. Soares, C. V. Iborra, and J. L. Soares-Sobrinho. 2019. "Tamoxifen/montmorillonite system – Effect of the experimental conditions." *Applied Clay Science* 180:105142. doi: 10.1016/j.clay.2019.105142.

Sun, L., C. Boyer, R. Grimes, and D. K. Mills. 2016. "Drug coated clay nanoparticles for delivery of chemotherapeutics." *Current Nanoscience* 12 (2):207–214. doi: 10.2174/1573413711666151008014051.

Takahashi, T., Y. Yamada, K. Kataoka, and Y. Nagasaki. 2005. "Preparation of a novel PEG–clay hybrid as a DDS material: Dispersion stability and sustained release profiles." *Journal of Controlled Release* 107 (3):408–416. doi: 10.1016/j.jconrel.2005.03.031.

Takahashi, T., and M. Yamaguchi. 1991. "Host-guest interactions between swelling clay minerals and poorly water-soluble drugs: II. Solubilization of griseofulvin by complex formation with a swelling clay mineral." *Journal of Colloid and Interface Science* 146 (2):556–564. doi: 10.1016/0021-9797(91)90219-X.

Tan, D., P. Yuan, F. Annabi-Bergaya, D. Liu, and H. He. 2014. "High-capacity loading of 5-fluorouracil on the methoxy-modified kaolinite." *Applied Clay Science* 100:60–65 doi: 10.1016/j.clay.2014.02.022.

Tan, D., P. Yuan, F. Annabi-Bergaya, D. Liu, and H. He. 2015. "Methoxy-modified kaolinite as a novel carrier for high-capacity loading and controlled-release of the herbicide amitrole." *Scientific Reports* 5 (1). doi: 10.1038/srep08870.

Tian, L., M. R. Abukhadra, A. S. Mohamed, A. Nadeem, S. F. Ahmad, and K. E. Ibrahim. 2020. "Insight into the loading and release properties of an exfoliated kaolinite/cellulose fiber (EXK/CF) composite as a carrier for oxaliplatin drug: Cytotoxicity and release kinetics." *ACS Omega* 5 (30):19165–19173. doi: 10.1021/acsomega.0c02529.

Uthappa, U. T., V. Brahmkhatri, G. Sriram, H.-Y. Jung, J. Yu, N. Kurkuri, T. M. Aminabhavi, T. Altalhi, G. M. Neelgund, and M. D. Kurkuri. 2018. "Nature engineered diatom biosilica as drug delivery systems." *Journal of Controlled Release* 281:70–83 doi: 10.1016/j.jconrel.2018.05.013.

Uthappa, U. T., M. Kigga, G. Sriram, K. V. Ajeya, H.-Y. Jung, G. M. Neelgund, and M. D. Kurkuri. 2019. "Facile green synthetic approach of bio inspired polydopamine coated diatoms as a drug vehicle for controlled drug release and active catalyst for dye degradation." *Microporous and Mesoporous Materials* 288:109572. doi: 10.1016/j.micromeso.2019.109572.

Uthappa, U. T., G. Sriram, V. Brahmkhatri, M. Kigga, H.-Y. Jung, T. Altalhi, G. M. Neelgund, and M. D. Kurkuri. 2018. "Xerogel modified diatomaceous earth microparticles for controlled drug release studies." *New Journal of Chemistry* 42 (14):11964–11971. doi: 10.1039/C8NJ01238E.

Veerabadran, N. G., D. Mongayt, V. Torchilin, R. R. Price, and Y. M. Lvov. 2009. "Organized shells on clay nanotubes for controlled release of macromolecules." *Macromolecular Rapid Communications* 30 (2):99–103. doi: 10.1002/marc.200800510.

Veerabadran, N. G., R. R. Price, and Y. M. Lvov. 2007. "Clay nanotubes for encapsulation and sustained release of drugs." *Nano* 02 (02):115–120. doi: 10.1142/s1793292007000441.

Vergaro, V., E. Abdullayev, Y. M. Lvov, A. Zeitoun, R. Cingolani, R. Rinaldi, and S. Leporatti. 2010. "Cytocompatibility and uptake of halloysite clay nanotubes." *Biomacromolecules* 11 (3):820–826. doi: 10.1021/bm9014446.

Vergaro, V., Y. M. Lvov, and S. Leporatti. 2012. "Halloysite clay nanotubes for resveratrol delivery to cancer cells." *Macromolecular Bioscience* 12 (9):1265–1271. doi: 10.1002/mabi.201200121.

Wang, Q., J. Zhang, Y. Zheng, and A. Wang. 2014. "Adsorption and release of ofloxacin from acid- and heat-treated halloysite." *Colloids and Surfaces B: Biointerfaces* 113:51–58. doi: 10.1016/j.colsurfb.2013.08.036.

Wang, X., Y. Du, and J. Luo. 2008. "Biopolymer/montmorillonite nanocomposite: Preparation, drug-controlled release property and cytotoxicity." *Nanotechnology* 19 (6):065707. doi: 10.1088/0957-4484/19/6/065707.

Wei, W., R. Minullina, E. Abdullayev, R. Fakhrullin, D. Mills, and Y. Lvov. 2014. "Enhanced efficiency of antiseptics with sustained release from clay nanotubes." *RSC Advances* 4 (1):488–494. doi: 10.1039/C3RA45011B.

Wu, Y., N. Zhou, W. Li, H. Gu, Y. Fan, and J. Yuan. 2013. "Long-term and controlled release of chlorhexidine–copper(II) from organically modified montmorillonite (OMMT) nanocomposites." *Materials Science and Engineering: C* 33 (2):752–757. doi: 10.1016/j.msec.2012.10.028.

Xue, J., M. He, H. Liu, Y. Niu, A. Crawford, P. D. Coates, D. Chen, R. Shi, and L. Zhang. 2014. "Drug loaded homogeneous electrospun PCL/gelatin hybrid nanofiber structures for anti-infective tissue regeneration membranes." *Biomaterials* 35 (34):9395–9405. doi: 10.1016/j.biomaterials.2014.07.060.

Xue, J., Y. Niu, M. Gong, R. Shi, D. Chen, L. Zhang, and Y. Lvov. 2015. "Electrospun microfiber membranes embedded with drug-loaded clay nanotubes for sustained antimicrobial protection." *ACS Nano* 9 (2):1600–1612. doi: 10.1021/nn506255e.

Yah, W. O., A. Takahara, and Y. M. Lvov. 2012. "Selective modification of halloysite lumen with octadecylphosphonic acid: New inorganic tubular micelle." *Journal of the American Chemical Society* 134 (3):1853–1859. doi: 10.1021/ja210258y.

Yah, W. O., H. Xu, H. Soejima, W. Ma, Y. Lvov, and A. Takahara. 2012. "Biomimetic dopamine derivative for selective polymer modification of halloysite nanotube lumen." *Journal of the American Chemical Society* 134 (29):12134–12137. doi: 10.1021/ja303340f.

Yang, J., Y. Wu, Y. Shen, C. Zhou, Y.-F. Li, R.-R. He, and M. Liu. 2016. "Enhanced therapeutic efficacy of doxorubicin for breast cancer using chitosan oligosaccharide-modified halloysite nanotubes." *ACS Applied Materials & Interfaces* 8 (40):26578–26590. doi: 10.1021/acsami.6b09074.

Yuan, P., P. D. Southon, Z. Liu, and C. J. Kepert. 2012. "Organosilane functionalization of halloysite nanotubes for enhanced loading and controlled release." *Nanotechnology* 23 (37):375705. doi: 10.1088/0957-4484/23/37/375705.

Zhai, R., B. Zhang, L. Liu, Y. Xie, H. Zhang, and J. Liu. 2010. "Immobilization of enzyme biocatalyst on natural halloysite nanotubes." *Catalysis Communications* 12 (4):259–263. doi: 10.1016/j.catcom.2010.09.030.

Zhang, Y., M. Long, P. Huang, H. Yang, S. Chang, Y. Hu, A. Tang, and L. Mao. 2016. "Emerging integrated nanoclay-facilitated drug delivery system for papillary thyroid cancer therapy." *Scientific Reports* 6 (1):33335. doi: 10.1038/srep33335.

Zheng, J. P., L. Luan, H. Y. Wang, L. F. Xi, and K. D. Yao. 2007. "Study on ibuprofen/montmorillonite intercalation composites as drug release system." *Applied Clay Science* 36 (4):297–301. doi: 10.1016/j.clay.2007.01.012.

Chapter 5

Naturally Obtained Zeolites for Drug Delivery Applications

R. Tiwari
Kali Charan Nigam Institute of Technology (KCNIT)

K. Kant
University of Vigo

CONTENTS

5.1 INTRODUCTION

Zeolites have unique structural traits such as high surface areas, controllable physicochemical properties, micro and mesoporous inorganic compounds, and biocompatibility (Servatan et al. 2018; Mohebbi et al. 2018; Zarrintaj, Ahmadi, Hosseinnezhad, et al. 2018). Zeolites have been extensively explored as drug delivery adjuncts in various forms, which include composites and host materials (Derakhshandeh et al. 2018; Nemati et al. 2018). In the biomedical the controlled drug delivery for the examination in drug release profile, zeolites have gained considerable attention due to their shape of pores, long-term biological robustness, and ability to change

DOI: 10.1201/9781003217114-7

immune system performance (Vilaça et al. 2013; Safari, Houshmand, and Nejad 2019). Due to the porous structures, ion-exchange abilities of zeolites have advantages over the controlled delivery of drugs (Hrenovic et al. 2012; Tavolaro et al. 2016; El-Maghrabi et al. 2018). Scientists have taken advantage of the large pore sizes, highly crystalline form, and ability to selectively adsorb help to use in the synthesis of hydrogels for biotechnological and therapeutic purposes (Sakaguchi, Matsui, and Mizukami 2005; Montalvo et al. 2012; Mastinu et al. 2019). The (Si/Al) ratio, pore size, and pore shape are used to classify zeolites. Nanoparticles are ideal candidates for drug delivery; one such example is mesoporous silica-based nanoparticles being one of the most promising choices in research (Uthappa, Sriram, et al. 2020). Zeolites have benefits due to their superior morphology, over the microbial flora in digestive tract, as well as the release of metabolically vital ions. It also helps in removal of unwanted ions and removal of toxic products of digestion. Additionally, zeolites can be absorbed by endocytosis, and they can also be utilized to transport DNA to cells. The cytotoxicity of zeolites has its disadvantage (e.g., erionite can cause cancer) but can also be employed in cancer treatment by using the antiproliferative and proapoptotic actions of zeolites (Serri et al. 2017). Zeolites also have advantages of low cost, abundance, and widespread availability (McCusker, Olson, and Baerlocher 2007).

The major disadvantage in drug development industry is of biological compatibility of drug molecules, and thus the development of nanoscience-based molecules has on progress to overcome compatibility issues (Fang et al. 2012; Rastin et al. 2017; Uthappa, Kurkuri, and Kigga 2019; Uthappa, Brahmkhatri, et al. 2018). The use of nanotechnology for medical applications has many advantages in drug release with poor water solubility, encapsulation and release of large molecular therapeutics, and release of several drugs with different release rates (Bagher et al. 2019; Kargozar, Ramakrishna, and Mozafari 2019; Zarrintaj, Ahmadi, Reza Saeb, et al. 2018).

NZ are non-toxic, exhibit long-term biological qualities, and may reversibly bind tiny molecules and cations, demonstrating that they can be used successfully in the pharmaceutical sector. NZs have some advantages over artificial zeolites in traditional therapeutics: reduced drug delivery-related side effects; more adaptability in conjugation of drugs, antibodies, peptides, DNA, carbohydrates, etc.; and can kill inflammatory or tumor cells using electrical, magnetic, or optical properties (e.g., magnetic or optical hyperthermia) to provide an effective response (Sadeghi-Kiakhani et al. 2018; Serri et al. 2016; Danilczuk et al. 2008; Bhat et al. 2021). Porous nano/microparticles are thought to be promising drug delivery carriers. NZs have been advanced as a functionally equivalent alternative to other nanostructured porous materials due to its (i) low cytotoxicity, limiting the negative effects on normal cells and tissues; (ii) customizable, high payload capacity that is beneficial to increase the loading content of various drugs due to the presence of zeolite pores; and (iii) enhanced intracellular targeting specificity and efficacy, which is advantageous for drug delivery applications (Uthappa, Arvind, et al. 2020).

NZ can be utilized as assistants to polymeric substances in a variety of forms for drug delivery due to their unique structural qualities, biocompatibility, vast surface areas, and capacity to alter their physicochemical properties (Uthappa et al. 2019; Krajišnik et al. 2010; Servatan et al. 2018; Sadeghi-Kiakhani et al. 2018). The hydrophilicity of zeolites limits their loading capacity, which is dependent on the zeolite's surface area (Uthappa, Sriram, et al. 2018; Serri et al. 2017; Salim and Malek 2016). However, NZ can be modified using surfactants to improve the hydrophobicity of the surface, resulting in a high affinity with drug molecules (Kurkuri and Aminabhavi 2004; Danilczuk et al. 2008; Vilaça et al. 2013; Cerri et al. 2016; Kontogiannidou et al. 2019). Natural zeolites were chosen for this investigation because of their nontoxicity, thermal stability, chemical tailorability, biocompatibility, and ability to adsorb diverse compounds into their micro- and mesopores, as shown in earlier research and presented in Figure 5.1. In this chapter, we explain the NZ and their types with focus on advancement in the use of natural zeolites in various biomedical applications feedbacks, especially drug delivery, and highlight the benefits of using zeolites in drug delivery applications. Due to their superior cytotoxicity, excipient activity, protein corona composition, and biological interactions, NZs become a potential candidate to be used as antidiarrheal agents, anticancer adjuvants, antimicrobial agents, drug carriers, and MRI contrast agents.

5.2 NATURAL ZEOLITES

Natural zeolites are found in sea salt and ash of activated volcanoes, and NZs usually are larger in particle size than synthetic zeolites (Figure 5.2). The classification of NZ is based on its origin and structure. So far, 200 types of synthetic zeolite and 10 types of natural zeolite shapes are identified. Various morphologies of these NZs are the differentiating part. The most commonly available natural zeolites are shown in Figure 5.2: (a) chabazite, (b) analzime, (c) clinoptilolite, (d) modernite, (e) smectite, (f) stilbite, (g) phillipsite, and (h) erionite. Application of NZ is dependent on physicochemical properties, which are representative of crystalline structure and chemical composition of zeolites.

5.3 APPLICATION AND TYPES OF NATURAL ZEOLITES

NZs can be used to deliver a variety of drugs. Because of the small size of the drugs, zeolites' porous nature helps in releasing drugs as per requirements.

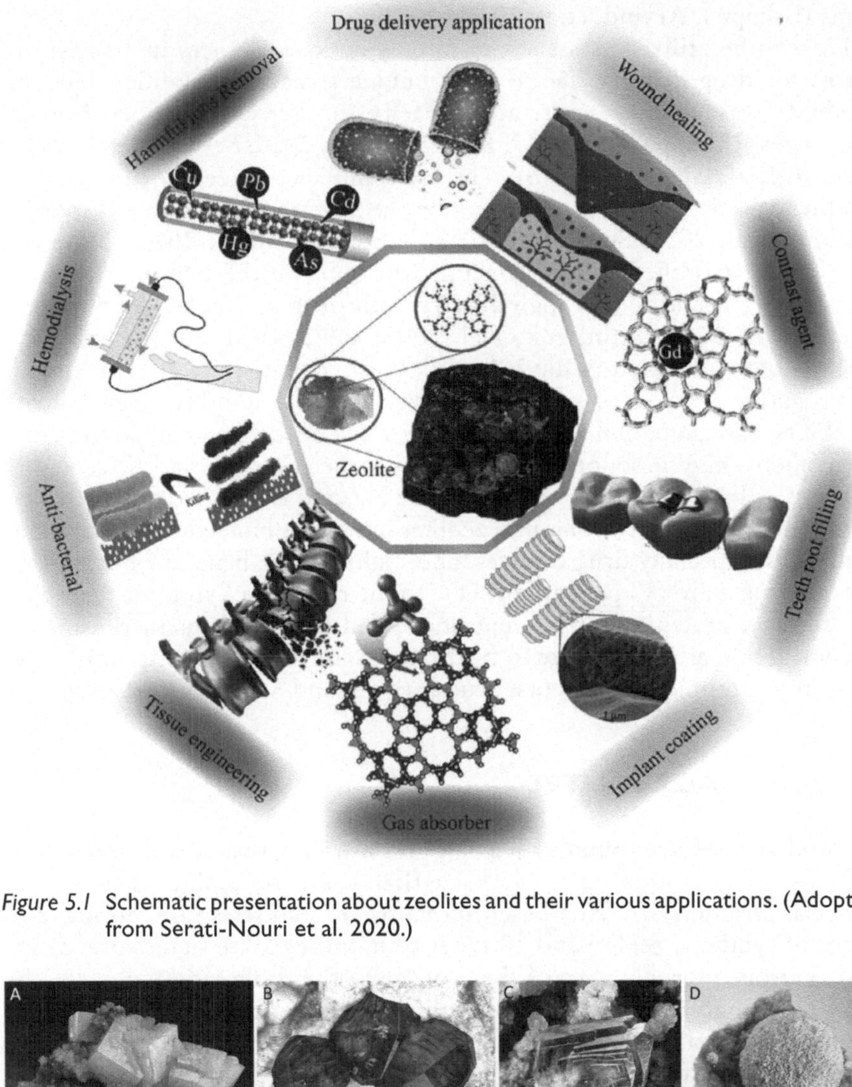

Figure 5.1 Schematic presentation about zeolites and their various applications. (Adopted from Serati-Nouri et al. 2020.)

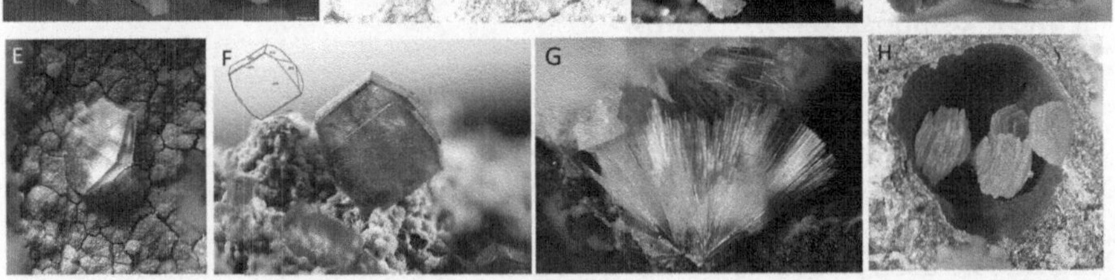

Figure 5.2 Various morphologies of commonly available NZs. (a) Chabazite. (b) Analzime. (c) Clinoptilolite. (d) Modernite. (e) Smectite. (f) Stilbite. (g) Phillipsite. (h) Erionite. (Adopted from Serati-Nouri et al. 2020.)

The desired drugs can be loaded/adsorbed into the zeolite pores, and pores are modified with polymers to hold the drugs. Drug-loading capabilities are altered with hydrophilicity between zeolites and medications, which can be solved by surface modification of zeolites. It is important to mention that surface modification of zeolite can be examined and altered as per the requirement of several kinds of drug delivery systems. Naturally occurring zeolites are basically known as clinoptilolite and mordenite.

5.3.1 Clinoptilolite

This type of zeolite is formed with volcanic glass shards in tufts and vesicle fills in basalts, andesites, and rhyolites are converted (as a glass) from a vitreous to a crystalline condition. The chemical formula for natural zeolite is (Na, K, and Ca) $Al_3(Al, Si)_2Si_{13}O_{36}.12H_2O$, with a microporous tetrahedral arrangement of silica and alumina. The physical appearance is as white to reddish tabular monoclinic tectosilicate crystals with a hardness of 3.5–4 Mohrs and 2.1–2.2 specific gravity (Mastinu et al. 2019; Colella 2011). Clinoptilolite type of NZ is commonly used in industry and academics due to its strong ion-exchange capabilities. It also has high affinity toward ammonium (NH_4^+), and this helps in its application in enzyme-based urea sensor, fertilizer as well as a deodorizer with pebble-sized chunks (McCusker, Olson, and Baerlocher 2007). These mesoporous zeolites also promote research on vitamin and mineral absorption on their pores and applied in human. Modification of zeolite with chitosan is widely used to control the drug release. Caffeic acid (CA) was also combined with chitosan via laccase leading to the continuous formation of hydrogen peroxide. This porous carrier of bentonite clinoptilolite NZ applied in slow release of vitamin E; thermodynamic investigations revealed the endothermic origin of the automatic encapsulation procedure and revealed that the release profile was within the recommended dietary allowance for humans (Tegl et al. 2018).

De Gennaro et al. treated the clinoptilolite with cetylpyridinium chloride and filled it with diclofenac sodium to examine the release behavior. Drug adsorption was controlled by boundary layer diffusion, and release mechanism was controlled by anionic exchange, with a quick final phase that resulted in long-term drug release (de Gennaro et al. 2015). Pasquino et al. modified the surface of clinoptilolite to use with nonsteroidal anti-inflammatory medicines (NSAIDs; e.g., ibuprofen and diclofenac). This presents that the molecular shape of drug molecules played a significant impact in their interaction with the zeolite and resulted in increased loading capacity (Pasquino et al. 2016). A rheology procedure was utilized to evaluate drug release performance, in which a gel-like solution was used with surfactant and a binding salt was used for relevant release. Such drugs function as a strong binding salt, causing the solution's viscosity to increase (Israelachvili, Mitchell, and Ninham 1976).

Serri et al. investigated diclofenac sodium (DS) in the oral delivery method, using cetylpyridinium chloride as surfactant-modified zeolites and analyzing release under pseudo-gastric fluid conditions. The DS-zeolite solution took almost 9 hours to release and perform as an effective technique in drug delivery (Serri et al. 2017). Pure form of clinoptilolite zeolites can be employed as effective porous materials in anti-diarrheic applications (Grce and Pavelic, n.d.). Clinoptilolite has also been employed in cancer adjuvant treatment, which resulted in decreased tumor size by reducing protein kinase B (c-Akt) expression (Grce and Pavelic, n.d.). NZs, particularly clinoptilolite, mostly attach to hydrogen ions and physiologically active amines and nitrates, which explain their gastroprotective action (Potgieter, Samuels, and Snyman 2014).

Ivkovic et al. reported the synthesis and processes of thermomechanically activated zeolites (e.g., clinoptilolite combined with synthetic and natural active chemicals) as a new approach for effective drug delivery. Ivkovic investigated anti-HIV, anti-diabetes, anti-hypertension, and anticancer drugs. Activated clinoptilolite blended with natural materials had collaborative advantages and enhanced biocompatibility due to their three-dimensional structure and suitable cellular activity (Ivkovic and Brezak 2008). Likewise, clinoptilolite's hemostatic qualities were compared to Quikclot, a commercially accessible therapy for external hemorrhage. The Quikclot group had a higher mortality rate (≈53%) than zeolite (≈20%). The zeolite finishes off the healing process, whereas Quikclot may cause necrotic tissue (Y. Li et al. 2012). Clinoptilolite improved health by modifying gut architecture, increasing villus height and villus to crypt depth, decreasing pH, and lowering *Salmonella* and *Escherichia coli* levels (L. Li et al. 2015; Wang et al. 2012).

5.3.2 Mordenite

Mordenite (MOR) is a zeolite mineral with the chemical formula (Ca, Na_2, K_2) $Al_2Si_{10}O_{24}.7H_2O$. It is a zeolite mineral with the chemical formula (Ca, Na_2, K_2) $Al_2Si_{10}O_{24}.7H_2O$. It is one of the six most prevalent zeolites, according to Ullmann's *Encyclopedia of Industrial Chemistry*, utilized commercially. MOR has an orthorhombic shape and colorless, white, or slightly yellow or pink in appearance. It has a Mohs hardness of 5 and a density of 2.1 g/cm^3. It produces hair-like crystals that are extremely long, thin, and fragile when fully shaped. MOR is made up of five-membered rings of attached silicate and aluminate tetrahedral molecules. MOR has a higher ratio of silicon to aluminum atoms, making it more acid resistant (Servatan et al. 2020). In a study, zeolite was discovered to soak up enhanced volumes of waste material into its porous cavities and decrease the concentration of unwanted soluble substances to less than <10 mg/L from an initial concentration of 45 mg/L (Li et al. 2013).

5.4 OTHER NATURAL ZEOLITE COMPOUNDS

5.4.1 Chabazite

Chabazite (Ca, Na_2, K_2, Mg) $Al_2Si_4O_{12}6H_2O$ is a tectosilicate mineral that is closely linked to geminate. Chabazite forms pseudo-cubic rhombohedral crystals in the triclinic crystal system. Twinning can be seen on the crystals, with both contact and penetration twinning. Colorless crystals, white crystals, orange crystals, brown crystals, pink crystals, green crystals, and yellow crystals are possibilities (Aly, Moustafa, and Abdelrahman 2012). It has specific gravity ranges from 2.0 to 2.2, and the hardness ranges from 3 to 5. Moreover, some natural materials have been unnoticed for such applications due to weak chemical and mineralogical characteristics in terms of cationic dispersion and cation exchange ability (Cappelletti et al. 2017). To better understand how chabazite releases DS, it was treated with a cationic surfactant called cetylpyridinium chloride (CP). According to the findings, film and particle diffusion mechanisms are primarily responsible for DS delivery, with film thickness and distribution coefficient being critical for film diffusion and effective diffusivity of exchanging ions being crucial for particle diffusion (Serri et al. 2016). NZs have the possibility to be utilized for nourishment and dietary purposes in animals to improve the quality of their products, such as eggs, meat, or milk, because they can increase drug targeting and nutrient transfer (Qiu Jue Wu et al. 2013). Likewise, Kececi et al. looked into the employment of porous inorganic zeolites in animals to mitigate the harmful effects of poisonous compounds consumed. Researcher monitored the capacity of zeolite and zeolite-containing composite containers to forage and soak up harmful compounds in body fluids when supplied directly to animals (Kececi et al. 2010). The three majorly available NZs are summarized in Table 5.1, on the basis of their structure and applications.

5.5 FUTURE DIRECTIONS

Regardless of the evident advantages of using zeolites as drug delivery carriers, there are some associated limitations in the exploration of such carriers. The pore size of zeolites is generally larger than drug molecules or particles, the drug molecules, or particles, help it to release drug rapidly. Additionally, some zeolites may have cytotoxic and carcinogenic properties. Erionite is a brittle, wool-like fibrous zeolite that possesses characteristics comparable to asbestos and causes lung cancer and malignant mesothelioma. Erionite's cytotoxicity affects the cytoplasm and causes cell necrosis at the nucleus level. Other fibrous zeolites, like offretite and skolecite, may also cause cytotoxicity, causing enlarged mitochondria and squared cells (Cangiotti et al. 2018; Turner et al. 2008). Zeolites have attracted significant research

Table 5.1 Types of NZ and Their Structures and Various Applications

No.	*Name*	*Structure*	*Applications*	*References*
1	Clinoptilolite	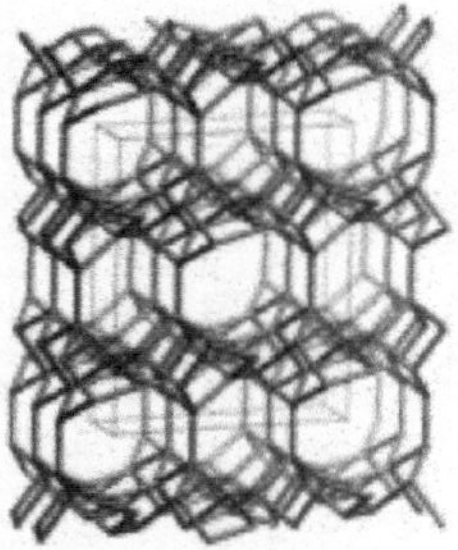	Environmental purification; removal of radioactive contaminants; detoxification of organisms; positive effects on nutrition and digestive tract; gastroprotective effects; drug delivery; construction of biosensors; antioxidant, antiapoptotic, anti-inflammatory, and antitumor activity	de Gennaro et al. (2015), Potgieter, Samuels, and Snyman (2014), Q. J. Wu et al. (2013), Qiu Jue Wu et al. (2013), Y. Wu et al. (2013), Valenzuela et al. (n.d.), Voronina et al. (2015)
2	Chabazite	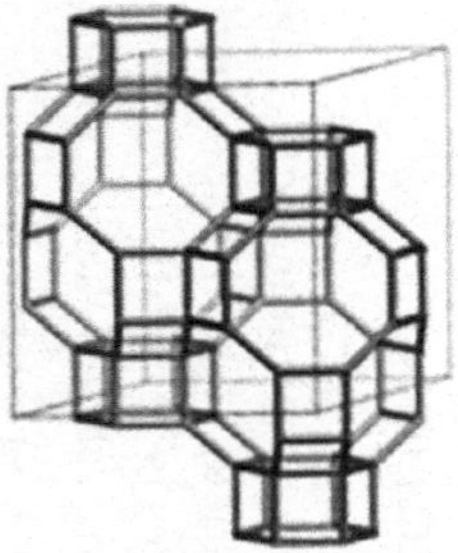	Optical imaging drug delivery	Cappelletti et al. (2017)
3	Mordenite	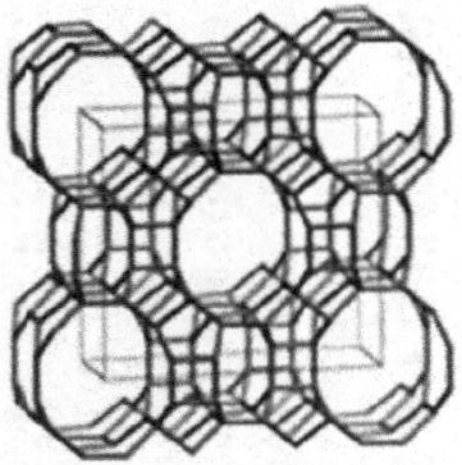	Drug delivering biomaterials	Martinho et al. (2015)

Source: Servatan et al. (2020).

attention in drug delivery systems, due to their porous structure, the ability to enhance their loading capacity, and control the drug release rate. Zeolites can transport a variety of medications and biological substances to specific tissues and organs. Zeolites can be surface modified to achieve some of the important desired properties when particularly focused on drug delivery. In the future, it is envisaged that zeolites' surface modification research will be extended, particularly for cancer therapy. Based on the nature of the materials utilized, some novel surface modifications not only improve delivery ability but also produce special therapeutic properties. Furthermore, altering the zeolites' particle size allows them to enter the live cells.

DECLARATION OF COMPETING INTEREST

The authors declare no conflict of interest.

ACKNOWLEDGMENTS

The authors thank to department of chemistry, Kali Charan Nigam Institute of Technology (KCNIT), Department of Chemistry Banda, Uttar Pradesh, India, and Universidade de Vigo, Departamento de Química Física, Campus Universitario, Lagoas, Marcosende, Vigo, Spain.

REFERENCES

Aly, Hisham M., Moustafa E. Moustafa, and Ehab A. Abdelrahman. 2012. "Synthesis of mordenite zeolite in absence of organic template." *Advanced Powder Technology* 23 (6): 757–60. https://doi.org/10.1016/J.APT.2011.10.003.

Bagher, Zohreh, Zhaleh Atoufi, Rafieh Alizadeh, Mohammad Farhadi, Payam Zarrintaj, Lorenzo Moroni, Mohsen Setayeshmehr, Ali Komeili, and S. Kamran Kamrava. 2019. "Conductive hydrogel based on chitosan-aniline pentamer/gelatin/agarose significantly promoted motor neuron-like cells differentiation of human olfactory ecto-mesenchymal stem cells." *Materials Science and Engineering:* C 101: 243–53. https://doi.org/10.1016/J.MSEC.2019.03.068.

Bhat, Shrinath, U. T. Uthappa, Tariq Altalhi, Ho Young Jung, and Mahaveer D. Kurkuri. 2021. "Functionalized porous hydroxyapatite scaffolds for tissue engineering applications: A focused review." *ACS Biomaterials Science & Engineering.* https://doi.org/10.1021/ACSBIOMATERIALS.1C00438.

Cangiotti, Michela, Sara Salucci, Michela Battistelli, Elisabetta Falcieri, Michele Mattioli, Matteo Giordani, and Maria Francesca Ottaviani. 2018. "EPR, TEM and cell viability study of asbestiform zeolite fibers in cell media." *Colloids and Surfaces B: Biointerfaces* 161: 147–55. https://doi.org/10.1016/J.COLSURFB.2017.10.045.

Cappelletti, Piergiulio, Abner Colella, Alessio Langella, Mariano Mercurio, Lilia Catalanotti, Vincenzo Monetti, and Bruno de Gennaro. 2017. "Use of surface modified natural zeolite (SMNZ) in pharmaceutical preparations part 1. Mineralogical and technological characterization of some industrial zeolite-rich rocks." *Microporous and Mesoporous Materials* 250: 232–44. https://doi.org/10.1016/J.MICROMESO.2015.05.048.

Cerri, Guido, Mauro Farina, Antonio Brundu, Aleksandra Daković, Paolo Giunchedi, Elisabetta Gavini, and Giovanna Rassu. 2016. "Natural zeolites for pharmaceutical formulations: Preparation and evaluation of a clinoptilolite-based material." *Microporous and Mesoporous Materials* 223: 58–67. https://doi.org/10.1016/J.MICROMESO.2015.10.034.

Colella, C. 2011. "A critical reconsideration of biomedical and veterinary applications of natural zeolites." *Clay Minerals* 46 (2): 295–309. https://doi.org/10.1180/CLAYMIN.2011.046.2.295.

Danilczuk, Marek, Karolina Dlugopolska, Tomasz Ruman, and Dariusz Pogocki. 2008. "Molecular sieves in medicine." *Mini Reviews in Medicinal Chemistry* 8 (13): 1407–17. https://doi.org/10.2174/138955708786369537.

de Gennaro, Bruno, Lilia Catalanotti, Piergiulio Cappelletti, Alessio Langella, Mariano Mercurio, Carla Serri, Marco Biondi, and Laura Mayol. 2015. "Surface modified natural zeolite as a carrier for sustained diclofenac release: A preliminary feasibility study." *Colloids and Surfaces B: Biointerfaces* 130 (June): 101–9. https://doi.org/10.1016/J.COLSURFB.2015.03.052.

Derakhshandeh, Mohammad Reza, Mohammad Javad Eshraghi, Masoumeh Javaheri, Sara Khamseh, Morteza Ganjaee Sari, Payam Zarrintaj, Mohammad Reza Saeb, and Masoud Mozafari. 2018. "Diamond-like carbon-deposited films: A new class of biocorrosion protective coatings." *Surface Innovations* 6 (4–5): 266–76. https://doi.org/10.1680/JSUIN.18.00002.

El-Maghrabi, Heba H., Ahmed Barhoum, Amr A. Nada, Yasser Mohamed Moustafa, Sara Mikhail Seliman, Ahmed M. Youssef, and Mikhael Bechelany. 2018. "Synthesis of mesoporous core-shell CdS@TiO_2 (0D and 1D) photocatalysts for solar-driven hydrogen fuel production." *Journal of Photochemistry and Photobiology A: Chemistry* 351: 261–70. https://doi.org/10.1016/J.JPHOTOCHEM.2017.10.048.

Fang, Xiaoliang, Zhaohui Liu, Ming Feng Hsieh, Mei Chen, Pengxin Liu, Cheng Chen, and Nanfeng Zheng. 2012. "Hollow mesoporous aluminosilica spheres with perpendicular pore channels as catalytic nanoreactors." *ACS Nano* 6 (5): 4434–44. https://doi.org/10.1021/NN3011703/SUPPL_FILE/NN3011703_SI_001.PDF.

Grce, Magdalena, and Kreimir Pavelic. n.d. "Zeolite research & scientific papers on clinoptilolite." *Microporous and Mesoporous Materials* 19: 165–69.

Hrenovic, Jasna, Jelena Milenkovic, Tomislav Ivankovic, and Nevenka Rajic. 2012. "Antibacterial activity of heavy metal-loaded natural zeolite." *Journal of Hazardous Materials* 201–202 (January): 260–64. https://doi.org/10.1016/J.JHAZMAT.2011.11.079.

Israelachvili, Jacob N., D. John Mitchell, and Barry W. Ninham. 1976. "Theory of self-assembly of hydrocarbon amphiphiles into micelles and bilayers." *Journal of the Chemical Society, Faraday Transactions 2: Molecular and Chemical Physics* 72: 1525–68. https://doi.org/10.1039/F29767201525.

Ivkovic, Slavko, and Danko Brezak. 2008. "Nanoparticles of the Thermo-Mechanically Activated Zeolite in the Design and Synthesis of New Drugs Generation." *TechConnect Briefs* 2: 375–378. Accessed December 9, 2021. https://briefs.techconnect.org/papers/nanoparticles-of-the-thermo-mechanically-activated-zeolite-in-the-design-and-synthesis-of-new-drugs-generation/.

Kargozar, Saeid, Seeram Ramakrishna, and Masoud Mozafari. 2019. "Chemistry of biomaterials: Future prospects." *Current Opinion in Biomedical Engineering* 10 (June): 181–90. https://doi.org/10.1016/J.COBME.2019.07.003.

Kececi, Tufan, Halis Oguz, Varol Kurtoglu, and O. Demet. 2010. "Effects of polyvinylpolypyrrolidone, synthetic zeolite and bentonite on serum biochemical and haematological characters of broiler chickens during aflatoxicosis." *British Poultry Science* 39 (3): 452–58. https://doi.org/10.1080/00071669889051.

Kontogiannidou, Eleni, Christina Karavasili, Maria G. Kouskoura, Maria Filippousi, Gustaaf Van Tendeloo, Ioannis I. Andreadis, Georgios K. Eleftheriadis, et al. 2019. "In vitro and ex vivo assessment of microporous faujasite zeolite (NaX-FAU) as a carrier for the oral delivery of danazol." *Journal of Drug Delivery Science and Technology* 51 (June): 177–84. https://doi.org/10.1016/J.JDDST.2019.02.036.

Krajišnik, Danina, Maja Milojević, Anelija Malenović, Aleksandra Daković, Svetlana Ibrić, Sneana Savić, Vera Dondur, et al. 2010. "Cationic surfactants-modified natural zeolites: Improvement of the excipients functionality." *Drug Development and Industrial Pharmacy* 36 (10): 1215–24. https://doi.org/10.3109/03639041003695121.

Kurkuri, Mahaveer D., and Tejraj M. Aminabhavi. 2004. "Poly(Vinyl Alcohol) and poly(Acrylic Acid) sequential interpenetrating network PH-sensitive microspheres for the delivery of diclofenac sodium to the intestine." *Journal of Controlled Release* 96 (1): 9–20. https://doi.org/10.1016/J.JCONREL.2003.12.025.

Li, Linfeng, Ping Li, Yueping Chen, Chao Wen, Su Zhuang, and Yanmin Zhou. 2015. "Zinc-bearing zeolite clinoptilolite improves tissue zinc accumulation in laying hens by enhancing zinc transporter gene MRNA abundance." *Animal Science Journal* 86 (8): 782–89. https://doi.org/10.1111/ASJ.12358.

Li, Xue Ying, Ning Ping, Guang Fei Qu, and Yi Lu Lin. 2013. "Experimental study on removing P from bovine urine wastewater by mordenite with static adsorption." *Journal of Yunnan University - Natural Sciences Edition* 35 (2): 177–82.

Li, Yunlong, Hui Li, Liping Xiao, Lin Zhou, Jianzhong Shentu, Xumin Zhang, and Jie Fan. 2012. "Hemostatic efficiency and wound healing properties of natural zeolite granules in a lethal rabbit model of complex groin injury." *Materials* 5 (12): 2586–96. https://doi.org/10.3390/MA5122586.

Martinho, Olga, Natália Vilaça, Paulo J.G. Castro, Ricardo Amorim, António M. Fonseca, Fátima Baltazar, Rui M. Reis, and Isabel C. Neves. 2015. "In vitro and in vivo studies of temozolomide loading in zeolite structures as drug delivery systems for glioblastoma." *RSC Advances* 5 (36): 28219–27. https://doi.org/10.1039/C5RA03871E.

Mastinu, Andrea, Amit Kumar, Giuseppina Maccarinelli, Sara Anna Bonini, Marika Premoli, Francesca Aria, Alessandra Gianoncelli, and Maurizio Memo. 2019. "Zeolite clinoptilolite: Therapeutic virtues of an ancient mineral." *Molecules* 24 (8): 1517. https://doi.org/10.3390/MOLECULES24081517.

McCusker, Lynne B., David H. Olson, and Christian Baerlocher. 2007. *Atlas of Zeolite Framework Types*. Elsevier. https://doi.org/10.1016/B978-0-444-53064-6.X5186-X.

Mohebbi, Shabnam, Mojtaba Nasiri Nezhad, Payam Zarrintaj, Seyed Hassan Jafari, Saman Seyed Gholizadeh, Mohammad Reza Saeb, and Masoud Mozafari. 2018. "Chitosan in biomedical engineering: A critical review." *Current Stem Cell Research & Therapy* 14 (2): 93–116. https://doi.org/10.2174/1574888X13666180912142028.

Montalvo, Silvio, Lorna Guerrero, Rafael Borja, Enrique Sánchez, Zhenia Milán, Isel Cortés, and M. Angeles de la la Rubia. 2012. "Application of natural zeolites in anaerobic digestion processes: A review." *Applied Clay Science* 58 (April): 125–33. https://doi.org/10.1016/J.CLAY.2012.01.013.

Nemati, Ali, Mahsa Saghafi, Sara Khamseh, Eiman Alibakhshi, Payam Zarrintaj, and Mohammad Reza Saeb. 2018. "Magnetron-sputtered TixNy thin films applied on titanium-based alloys for biomedical applications: Composition-microstructure-property relationships." *Surface and Coatings Technology* 349 (September): 251–59. https://doi.org/10.1016/J.SURFCOAT.2018.05.068.

Pasquino, Rossana, Marica Di Domenico, Francesco Izzo, Danila Gaudino, Veronica Vanzanella, Nino Grizzuti, and B. de Gennaro. 2016. "Rheology-sensitive response of zeolite-supported anti-inflammatory drug systems." *Colloids and Surfaces B: Biointerfaces* 146 (October): 938–44. https://doi.org/10.1016/J.COLSURFB.2016.07.039.

Potgieter, Wilna, Caroline Selma Samuels, and Jacques Renè Snyman. 2014. "Potentiated clinoptilolite: Artificially enhanced aluminosilicate reduces symptoms associated with endoscopically negative gastroesophageal reflux disease and nonsteroidal anti-inflammatory drug induced gastritis." *Clinical and Experimental Gastroenterology* 7 (1): 215. https://doi.org/10.2147/CEG.S51222.

Rastin, Hadi, Mohammad Reza Saeb, Milad Nonahal, Meisam Shabanian, Henri Vahabi, Krzysztof Formela, Xavier Gabrion, et al. 2017. "Transparent nanocomposite coatings based on epoxy and layered double hydroxide: Nonisothermal cure kinetics and viscoelastic behavior assessments." *Progress in Organic Coatings* 113 (December): 126–35. https://doi.org/10.1016/J.PORGCOAT.2017.09.003.

Sadeghi-Kiakhani, Mousa, Sara Khamseh, Akbar Rafie, Seyed Mohsen Fatemi Tekieh, Payam Zarrintaj, and Mohammad Reza Saeb. 2018. "Thermally stable antibacterial wool fabrics surface-decorated by TiON and TiON/Cu thin films." *Surface Innovations* 6 (4–5): 258–65. https://doi.org/10.1680/JSUIN.18.00001.

Safari, Fatemeh, Behzad Houshmand, and Azadeh Esmaeil Nejad. 2019. "Application of zeolite, a biomaterial agent, in dental science: A review article." *Regeneration, Reconstruction, and Restoration* 3 (4). https://doi.org/10.22037/RRR.V3I4.24267.

Sakaguchi, Kengo, Masayoshi Matsui, and Fujio Mizukami. 2005. "Applications of zeolite inorganic composites in biotechnology: Current state and perspectives." *Applied Microbiology and Biotechnology* 67 (3): 306–11. https://doi.org/10.1007/S00253-004-1782-4/FIGURES/1.

Salim, Mashitah Mad, and Nik Ahmad Nizam Nik Malek. 2016. "Characterization and antibacterial activity of silver exchanged regenerated NaY Zeolite from surfactant-modified NaY Zeolite." *Materials Science and Engineering: C* 59 (February): 70–77. https://doi.org/10.1016/J.MSEC.2015.09.099.

Serati-Nouri, Hamed, Amir Jafari, Leila Roshangar, Mehdi Dadashpour, Younes Pilehvar-Soltanahmadi, and Nosratollah Zarghami. 2020. "Biomedical applications of zeolite-based materials: A review." *Materials Science and Engineering: C* 116 (November): 111225. https://doi.org/10.1016/J.MSEC.2020.111225.

Serri, Carla, Bruno de Gennaro, Lilia Catalanotti, Piergiulio Cappelletti, Alessio Langella, Mariano Mercurio, Laura Mayol, and Marco Biondi. 2016. "Surfactant-modified phillipsite and chabazite as novel excipients for pharmaceutical applications?" *Microporous and Mesoporous Materials* 224 (April): 143–48. https://doi.org/10.1016/J.MICROMESO.2015.11.023.

Serri, Carla, Bruno de Gennaro, Vincenzo Quagliariello, Rosario Vincenzo Iaffaioli, Giuseppe De Rosa, Lilia Catalanotti, Marco Biondi, and Laura Mayol. 2017. "Surface modified zeolite-based granulates for the sustained release of diclofenac sodium." *European Journal of Pharmaceutical Sciences* 99 (March): 202–8. https://doi.org/10.1016/J.EJPS.2016.12.019.

Servatan, Morteza, Mohammad Ghadiri, Ahmad Taghizadeh Damanabi, Fateme Bahadori, Payam Zarrintaj, Zahed Ahmadi, Henri Vahabi, and Mohammad Reza Saeb. 2018. "Zeolite-based catalysts for exergy efficiency enhancement: The insights gained from nanotechnology." *Materials Today: Proceedings* 5 (7): 15868–76. https://doi.org/10.1016/J.MATPR.2018.05.086.

Servatan, Morteza, Payam Zarrintaj, Ghader Mahmodi, Seok Jhin Kim, Mohammad Reza Ganjali, Mohammad Reza Saeb, and Masoud Mozafari. 2020. "Zeolites in drug delivery: Progress, challenges and opportunities." *Drug Discovery Today* 25 (4): 642–56. https://doi.org/10.1016/J.DRUDIS.2020.02.005.

Tavolaro, Palmira, Silvia Catalano, Guglielmo Martino, and Adalgisa Tavolaro. 2016. "Zeolite inorganic scaffolds for novel biomedical application: Effect of physicochemical characteristic of zeolite membranes on cell adhesion and viability." *Applied Surface Science* 380 (September): 135–40. https://doi.org/10.1016/J.APSUSC.2016.01.279.

Tegl, Gregor, Viktoria Stagl, Anna Mensah, Daniela Huber, Walter Somitsch, Stefanie Grosse-Kracht, and Georg M. Guebitz. 2018. "The chemo enzymatic functionalization of chitosan zeolite particles provides antioxidant and antimicrobial properties." *Engineering in Life Sciences* 18 (5): 334–40. https://doi.org/10.1002/ELSC.201700120.

Turner, Kari K., Brian D. Nielsen, Cara O'Connor-Robison, Forrest H. Nielsen, and Michael William Orth. 2008. "Tissue response to a supplement high in aluminum and silicon." *Biological Trace Element Research* 121 (2): 134–48. https://doi.org/10.1007/S12011-007-8039-X/TABLES/6.

Uthappa, U. T., O. R. Arvind, G. Sriram, Dusan Losic, Ho-Young Jung, Madhuprasad Kigga, and Mahaveer D. Kurkuri. 2020. "Nanodiamonds and their surface modification strategies for drug delivery applications." *Journal of Drug Delivery Science and Technology* 60 (December): 101993. https://doi.org/10.1016/J.JDDST.2020.101993.

Uthappa, U. T., Varsha Brahmkhatri, G. Sriram, Ho-Young Jung, Jingxian Yu, Nikita Kurkuri, Tejraj M. Aminabhavi, Tariq Altalhi, Gururaj M. Neelgund, and Mahaveer D. Kurkuri. 2018. "Nature engineered diatom biosilica as drug delivery systems." *Journal of Controlled Release* 281 (July): 70–83. https://doi.org/10.1016/J.JCONREL.2018.05.013.

Uthappa, U. T., Madhuprasad Kigga, G. Sriram, Kanalli V. Ajeya, Ho-Young Jung, Gururaj M. Neelgund, and Mahaveer D. Kurkuri. 2019. "Facile green synthetic approach of bio inspired polydopamine coated diatoms as a drug vehicle for controlled drug release and active catalyst for dye degradation." *Microporous and Mesoporous Materials* 288 (November): 109572. https://doi.org/10.1016/J.MICROMESO.2019.109572.

Uthappa, U. T., Mahaveer D. Kurkuri, and Madhuprasad Kigga. 2019. "Nanotechnology advances for the development of various drug carriers." *Nanotechnology in the Life Sciences*, 187–224. https://doi.org/10.1007/978-3-030-17061-5_8.

Uthappa, U. T., G. Sriram, O. R. Arvind, Sandeep Kumar, Ho-Young Jung, Gururaj M. Neelgund, Dusan Losic, and Mahaveer D. Kurkuri. 2020. "Engineering MIL-100(Fe) on 3D porous natural diatoms as a versatile high performing platform for controlled isoniazid drug release, fenton's catalysis for malachite green dye degradation and environmental adsorbents for Pb^{2+} removal and dyes." *Applied Surface Science* 528 (October): 146974. https://doi.org/10.1016/J.APSUSC.2020.146974.

Uthappa, U. T., G. Sriram, Varsha Brahmkhatri, Madhuprasad Kigga, Ho-Young Jung, Tariq Altalhi, Gururaj M. Neelgund, and Mahaveer D. Kurkuri. 2018. "Xerogel modified diatomaceous earth microparticles for controlled drug release studies." *New Journal of Chemistry* 42 (14): 11964–71. https://doi.org/10.1039/C8NJ01238E.

Valenzuela, Cristian, Ruben Moraga, Carla Leon, Carlos T. Smith, Maria-Angelica Mondaca, and Victor L. Campos. n.d. "Arsenite oxidation by pseudomonas arsenicoxydans immobilized on zeolite and its potential biotechnological application." https://doi.org/10.1007/s00128-015-1495-7.

Vilaça, Natália, Ricardo Amorim, Ana F. Machado, Pier Parpot, Manuel F.R. Pereira, Mariana Sardo, João Rocha, António M. Fonseca, Isabel C. Neves, and Fátima Baltazar. 2013. "Potentiation of 5-fluorouracil encapsulated in zeolites as drug delivery systems for in vitro models of colorectal carcinoma." *Colloids and Surfaces B: Biointerfaces* 112 (December): 237–44. https://doi.org/10.1016/J.COLSURFB.2013.07.042.

Voronina, Anastasia V., Marina O. Blinova, Vladimir Sergeevich Semenishchev, and Dharmendra Kumar Gupta. 2015. "Returning land contaminated as a result of radiation accidents to farming use." *Journal of Environmental Radioactivity* 144 (June): 103–12. https://doi.org/10.1016/J.JENVRAD.2015.03.012.

Wang, L. C., T. T. Zhang, C. Wen, Z. Y. Jiang, Tian Wang, and Yan Min Zhou. 2012. "Protective effects of zinc-bearing clinoptilolite on broilers challenged withsalmonella pullorum." *Poultry Science* 91 (8): 1838–45. https://doi.org/10.3382/PS.2012–02284.

Wu, Q. J., L. C. Wang, Y. M. Zhou, J. F. Zhang, and T. Wang. 2013. "Effects of clinoptilolite and modified clinoptilolite on the growth performance, intestinal microflora, and gut parameters of broilers." *Poultry Science* 92 (3): 684–92. https://doi.org/10.3382/PS.2012-02308.

Wu, Qiu Jue, Yan Min Zhou, Ya Nan Wu, Li Li Zhang, and Tian Wang. 2013. "The effects of natural and modified clinoptilolite on intestinal barrier function and immune response to LPS in broiler chickens." *Veterinary Immunology and Immunopathology* 153 (1–2): 70–76. https://doi.org/10.1016/J.VETIMM.2013.02.006.

Wu, Yanan, Qiujue Wu, Yanmin Zhou, Hussain Ahmad, and Tian Wang. 2013. "Effects of clinoptilolite on growth performance and antioxidant status in broilers." *Biological Trace Element Research* 155 (2): 228–35. https://doi.org/10.1007/S12011-013-9777-6/TABLES/6.

Zarrintaj, Payam, Zahed Ahmadi, Mozhgan Hosseinnezhad, Mohammad Reza Saeb, Pascal Laheurte, and Masoud Mozafari. 2018. "Photosensitizers in medicine: Does nanotechnology make a difference?" *Materials Today: Proceedings* 5 (7): 15836–44. https://doi.org/10.1016/J.MATPR.2018.05.082.

Zarrintaj, Payam, Zahed Ahmadi, Mohammad Reza Saeb, and Masoud Mozafari. 2018. "Poloxamer-based stimuli-responsive biomaterials." *Materials Today: Proceedings* 5 (7): 15516–23. https://doi.org/10.1016/J.MATPR.2018.04.158.

Chapter 6

Porous Calcium Carbonates and Calcium Phosphates for Drug Delivery Applications

M. Hadden, C. Viray, G. Singh, and Yogambha Ramaswamy
University of Sydney

CONTENTS

DOI: 10.1201/9781003217114-8

6.1 INTRODUCTION

Bioceramics are commonly used for a range of biomedical applications such as prosthetic coatings, injectable cements, fillers, and scaffolds for bone defects. Ceramic-based drug delivery systems (DDSs) have garnered significant attention within the fields of biomedicine and drug development as vehicles for targeted and sustained drug release. Modern delivery systems using next-generation carriers are advantageous over conventional drug delivery methods because they provide a higher level of drug efficacy (Sayed et al. 2017). Drug carriers are biocompatible materials that can load biomolecules on their surfaces or encapsulate them within their structures for sustained release. A variety of drug carriers such as tissue engineering scaffolds, implant coatings, liposomes, polymeric micelles, microspheres, micro-fibers, and nanoparticles (NPs) have been explored (Y. Wu et al. 2020; R. Verma, Verma, and Kumar 2019; Maleki Dizaj et al. 2015; Bhat et al. 2021; Uthappa et al. 2020; Uthappa et al. 2018; Uthappa, Kurkuri, and Kigga 2019). Bioceramics such as calcium carbonates (CaC) and calcium phosphates (CaP) are considered to be excellent drug carriers due to their inherent biocompatibility, bioactivity, biodegradability, and environmental sensitivity to factors such as pH and temperature (Maleki Dizaj et al. 2015; Verron et al. 2010). These materials have been used as drug carriers in various forms such as scaffolds, microspheres, and NPs (Figure 6.1). Their diversity in scale, biocompatibility, and ease of fabrication have facilitated and expanded the use of both CaCs and CaPs for drug delivery applications.

Largely, DDSs are characterized by their drug-loading efficiency and sustained drug release kinetics over an extended period of time (Vallet-Regí, Balas, and Arcos 2007). Material porosity, defined as the total amount of empty space within a material, is directly correlated to these characteristics (Sayed et al. 2017). Higher porosity amounts to higher exposed surface area, which equals to greater drug-loading efficiency and a more controlled drug release profile (Vallet-Regí, Balas, and Arcos 2007). Furthermore, it has been proven that porosity can influence drug delivery, adhesion of proteins (which can affect cell-biomaterial interactions), and induce tissue regeneration. Pore size is a determining factor for these interactions, whereby macropores (diameters >80–$100\,\mu m$) allow for the loading of larger drug

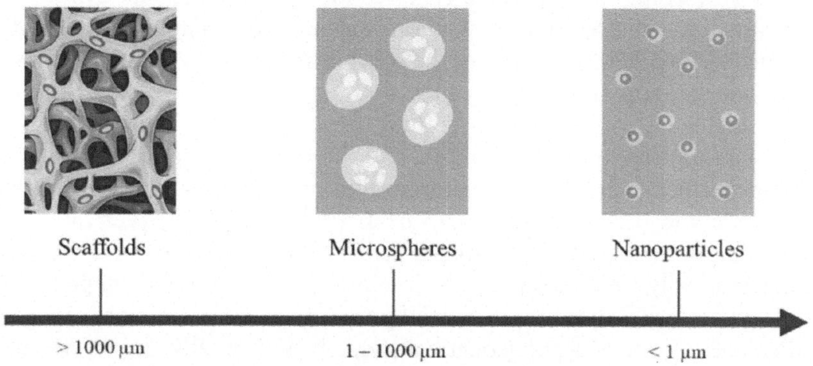

Figure 6.1 Calcium carbonate and calcium phosphate-based drug-eluting carriers for drug delivery applications. Ranging in size and scale (macro- to nano-), calcium-based carriers are widely used as drug delivery systems to suit a variety of applications, including anticancer treatments, vaccine adjuvants, and gene therapy.

molecules and the infiltration of cells, while micropores (diameters < 10 μm) increase the total surface area of the constructs and allow for the infiltration of fluids. Porosity as a material characteristic is highly tunable on the macroscale via various synthesis methods; however, it is more challenging to control on the micro- and nanoscale. CaCs and CaPs have inherently high micro- and nano-porosity after fabrication, making them ideal drug carriers. Indeed, they both possess several advantages as drug carriers such as improved pharmacokinetic profiles, the possibility to employ lipophilic drugs, higher circulation time, and a lower overall toxicity profile (Baeza, Ruiz-Molina, and Vallet-Regí 2017). Pore sizes of calcium-based carriers can be manipulated, allowing them to be used for the loading of a broader range of therapeutic agents, such as proteins, genetic materials (plasmids, mRNA, etc.), and low-molecular-weight drugs, thus increasing their uses within the biomedical and therapeutic industries.

Herein, we will outline the varying CaCs and CaPs used commercially, as well as describe the most recent advances in CaC and CaP-designed scaffolds, microspheres, and NPs for drug delivery applications. Each carrier will be investigated with reference to its desired design requirements, common synthesis methods, and most recent applications in drug delivery.

6.2 CALCIUM CARBONATES

CaC (chemical formula: $CaCO_3$) is one of the most abundant biominerals found on the Earth. It has far-reaching biomedical uses due to its general availability and incredible biocompatibility. CaC exists in six major forms: calcite (its most stable polymorph), aragonite, vaterite, monohydrocalcite, calcium carbonate hexahydrate (ikaite), and amorphous calcium carbonate (ACC) (Addadi, Raz, and Weiner 2003). Of these, the most commonly used polymorphs are calcite, vaterite, and aragonite, as shown in Figure 6.2. The crystallization of CaC occurs in a stepwise procedure: first through the formation of ACC, followed by its transformation to vaterite, and then either aragonite and/or calcite (Trofimov et al. 2018). These transformations are governed predominantly by temperature and pressure, which can be altered through the fabrication process to achieve the desired polymorph. Calcite is the most thermodynamically and mechanically stable polymorph. It exists as a rhomboidal-shaped crystal particle and is largely used for industrial purposes due to its stability. Aragonite (needle-shaped) and vaterite (spherical-shaped) will readily transform into a calcite polymorph under normal, stable conditions (Ševčík, Šašek, and Viani 2018).

Interestingly, for biomedical purposes, metastable vaterite is the most practical CaC polymorph because of its spherical shape, high microporosity, and biodegradability through pH-sensitive mechanisms (Trushina et al. 2014). Vaterite particles are considered excellent drug delivery carriers; however, difficulties remain in their stabilization. CaCs as drug carriers are most suited for microsphere or NP design owing to their structure and physical and chemical characteristics. Its applications in drug delivery are extensive and are highlighted in Figure 6.3.

6.3 CALCIUM PHOSPHATES

CaP systems are widely used in biomedical engineering owing to their varying degrees of stoichiometry, cellular biocompatibility, and similarities to native bone (Verron et al. 2010). CaPs can be sourced either biogenically (i.e., from calcined bovine, eggshell) or synthetically, with the most common synthesis method based on chemical precipitation (Canillas et al. 2017). Common examples of CaPs used in biomedical applications include hydroxyapatite (HA), β-tricalcium phosphate (β-TCP), and biphasic calcium phosphates (BCPs). These forms of CaPs can be synthesized as powders, granules, slurry, cement, or as coatings on medical devices. HA (chemical formula: $Ca_{10}(PO_4)_6(OH)_2$) is extensively used for various orthopedic applications due to its structural similarity to the mineral phase of bone (carbonated HA). HA is very stable under physiological conditions with low solubility and slow resorption kinetics (da Silva et al. 2007). TCP (chemical formula: $Ca_3(PO_4)_2$) belongs to the *whitlockites* family of minerals and has two common polymorphs: β- and α-TCP (Canillas et al. 2017). TCP, in general, is incredibly biodegradable in comparison to other CaPs. β-TCP has higher solubility when compared to HA or α-TCP and can be further stabilized with partial Ca substitution with strontium (Sr) and/or zinc (Zn) (Canillas et al. 2017). Both HA and β-TCP are

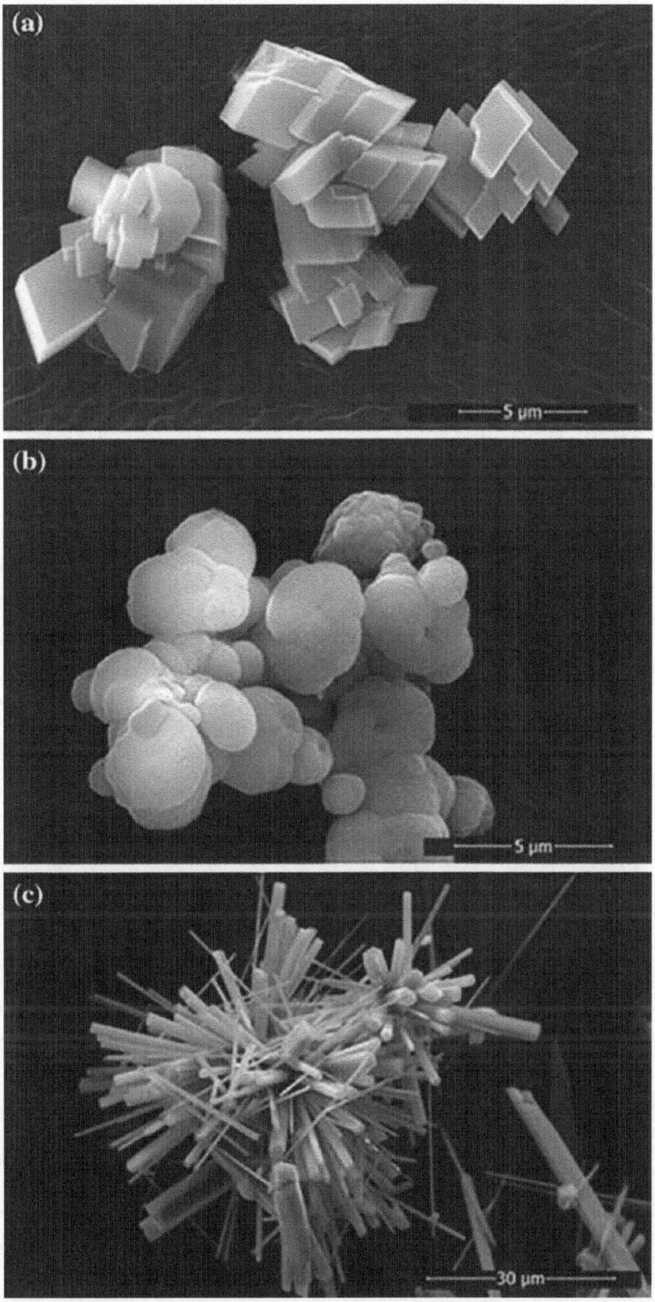

Figure 6.2 SEM images of common calcium carbonate isoforms. (a) Calcite. (b) Vaterite. and (c) Aragonite. (Sourced from Ševčík, Šašek, and Viani 2018.)

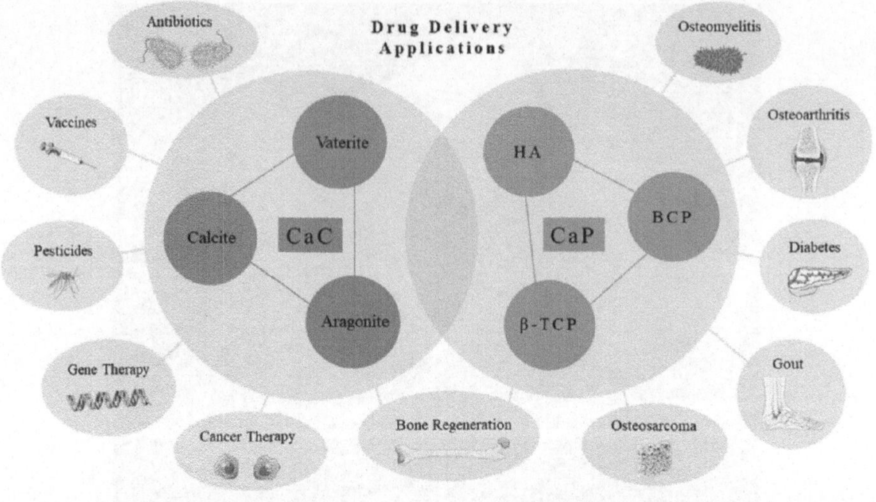

Figure 6.3 Common drug delivery applications of calcium carbonate and calcium phosphate. CaC exists in many polymorphs, with vaterite the most desirable for biomedical applications due to its shape and properties. CaC is being used as a carrier for drug delivery applications ranging from BTE, to cancer therapies (chemo-, radio-, and photo-therapies), to adjuvants in vaccine development. The most common forms of CaP used in biomedical applications are hydroxyapatite (HA), β-tricalcium phosphate (β-TCP), and biphasic calcium phosphate (BCP). As the mineral phase of native bone tissue is CaP, it is commonly used to treat bone pathologies as it also possesses superior bone-forming properties through its bioactive surface.

inherently bioactive, making them excellent promoters of new bone formation. Their bioresorbability and high porosity make them excellent vehicles for drug delivery with high-loading efficiency and prolonged drug release kinetics. Biphasic calcium phosphate (BCP) is the combination of HA and β-TCP at varying ratios and encompasses the best properties of both biomaterials. It utilizes HA's superior stability under physiological conditions and β-TCP's superior solubility, allowing tailorable degradability and drug release kinetics (Victor and Kumar 2008). Furthermore, by varying the HA/TCP ratio, BCP can alter its bioactivity, biodegradation, and mechanical properties to suit its application. For drug delivery purposes, BCP is emerging as the optimum CaP construct, with current applications including bone tissue regeneration, and treatments for osteomyelitis and osteosarcomas (Figure 6.3).

6.4 DRUG-LOADING APPROACHES

There are two common approaches for loading drugs or biomolecules into carrier systems for delivery applications: (i) surface adsorption or immobilization and (ii) encapsulation (Mouriño et al. 2013). They each have their advantages and disadvantages when explored in the context of drug delivery, with surface adsorption being the most approached method. The extent of these molecular interactions and the influence of outlying conditions such as bond strength or pH will determine the binding or the release of the cargo without any modifications during the fabrication and implantation processes (Mouriño et al. 2013). These loading techniques are employed by carrier systems of all shapes and sizes including the nanoscale. Release kinetics of a drug or biomolecule are heavily dependent on the loading approach and should be carefully considered alongside biomaterial resorption to achieve controlled and sustained drug release.

6.4.1 Surface Adsorption

Conventional surface adsorption involves immersing a pre-made carrier system in a saline solution containing the drug or biomolecule and is considered one of the simplest drug-loading strategies. Surface adsorption is predominantly facilitated by nonspecific binding mechanisms, such as hydrophobicity/hydrophilicity or electrostatic/van der Waals' interactions (Ziegler et al. 2002). These interactions depend heavily on the characteristics of both the drug (i.e., whether it is a protein, lipid, polymer, sugar, or nucleic acid) and the biomaterial properties (e.g., density, swelling ratio, porosity) (Saltzman and Olbricht 2002). CaCs and CaPs meet many requirements for this type of drug loading, given their inherent affinity for high protein absorption on their surfaces. The benefits of surface immobilization revolve around its simple methodology and easy loading strategy. Furthermore, incorporating the drug after the fabrication of relative carriers ensures the maintenance of the drug's composition and its stability and functionality during synthesis (Saltzman and Olbricht 2002). It is advantageous because the traditional fabrication of CaC and CaP biomaterials involves thermal treatments at temperatures >800°C which can denature biomolecules to be loaded onto the carrier. However, there is minimal control over the release kinetics of the drug due to the "burst release" scenario, where the greatest percentage of loaded drug is eluted very rapidly upon injection/implantation (Ziegler et al. 2002). This can result in an unpredictable release profile and long-term complications and systemic toxic effects due to the release of high drug concentrations at one time (Carragee, Hurwitz, and Weiner 2011). These drawbacks can be addressed by introducing functional groups on the biomaterial surface to bind the biomolecule or cargo covalently, thus reducing the characteristic "burst release" pattern (Mouriño et al. 2013).

6.4.2 Encapsulation

Encapsulation involves loading drugs or biomolecules directly into the matrix of a carrier system and allowing the degradation of that system to disperse the cargo (Langer 1998). Encapsulation relies heavily on the synthesis method with design considerations that protect the cargo during the manufacturing process, as this may affect its therapeutic properties. The drugs can be encapsulated in microspheres and NPs for targeted drug delivery and site-specific injection without any residual drug loss (Mouriño et al. 2013). Furthermore, delivery vehicles that encapsulate biomolecules within their matrices have tighter control over release kinetics when compared to surface adsorption (H. Sun et al. 2022). The release profile correlates the degradation or bioresorption of the vehicle, facilitating sustained drug delivery for an extended period of time. The use of biphasic or composite material can allow the delivery of multiple biomolecules at different rates, making such composite materials an attractive biomaterial for drug-eluting bone scaffolds to treat bone degeneration or osteosarcoma (Y. Chen et al. 2018; Y. Wu et al. 2020).

6.5 CALCIUM CARBONATE AND CALCIUM PHOSPHATE SCAFFOLDS

Biologically, the primary requirement of any scaffold is biocompatibility, a term often described as the ability of a foreign object to support normal cellular activity without any local or systemic toxic effect on the body (Williams 2008). Further biological considerations revolve around bioresorbability and biodegradability, meaning the biomaterial must degrade at a controlled rate and have nontoxic byproducts as a result of this degradation. Degradation rate will vary based on the application, biomaterial, and synthesis method, and is heavily tied to drug delivery (J. He et al. 2021). Scaffolds serve many functions in repairing tissue by providing mechanical support for growing cells and facilitating cell/matrix interaction (Bose and Tarafder 2012). Next-generation scaffolds improve the lives of patients suffering from tissue loss through the integration of advanced DDSs, providing both mechanical and biochemical support for enhanced tissue growth through the release of biomolecules that can direct cell behavior. This is particularly evident in BTE scaffolds, highlighted in Figure 6.4. Localized drug delivery through scaffolds has several advantages compared to systemic administration of the same drug, such as reduced side effects, reduced risk of overdose, and improved drug efficacy on target cells (Mouriño et al. 2013). However, challenge still remains in designing scaffolds that can satisfy the mechanical properties of specific tissues while also releasing stable drugs in a sustained and controlled manner (Baroli 2009; S.-H. Lee and Shin 2007). CaPs are extensively explored for BTE applications as they closely mimic the mineral phase of native bone and have the ability to deliver molecules that support successful integration and therapy. Current research is largely focused on

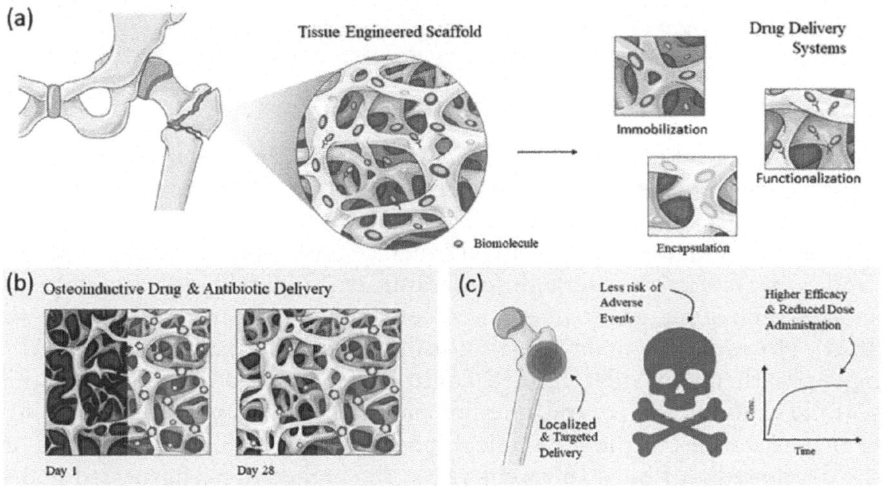

Figure 6.4 Bone tissue engineered scaffolds as next-generation drug delivery systems. (a) Schematic showing the varying kinds of drug delivery systems employed by bone tissue engineered scaffolds (surface immobilization, surface functionalization, and encapsulation). (b) Example of how next-generation drug delivery systems introduce osteoinductive drugs and antibiotics to sites of damage and infection, respectively. (c) Common advantages of these systems are localized and targeted drug delivery, less risk of adverse events, and higher drug efficacy.

improving drug incorporation within the scaffold and achieving their sustained and stable release upon implantation. The selection of appropriate biomaterial and cargo play significant roles in creating BTE scaffolds with drug-eluting capabilities.

6.5.1 Optimal Scaffold Properties for Drug Delivery

Scaffolds that incorporate DDSs must consider an additional set of requirements that revolve not only on the choice of biomaterials but also on the type of drugs or biological agents. These systems must consider the stability of the drug throughout the scaffold lifecycle, i.e., from the method of scaffold fabrication, the initial drug-loading stage, implantation site, its release from the scaffold into the surrounding tissue, and the uptake of the released drug by cells. Considerations must also include the release profile of the drug from the scaffold as the drug concentration will vary depending on the time frame and its affinity to the biomaterial. For example, low-affinity interactions between the drug and biomaterial will increase the release rate, while high-affinity interactions will reduce the release rate and, therefore, prolong the drug's effect. Furthermore, the release of the drug should be consistent and not get localized at certain points around the implant, thus avoiding side effects resulting from excessive drug activity.

6.5.2 Scaffold Fabrication Methods

There is a multitude of fabrication methods currently employed to synthesize drug-eluting calcium-based scaffolds. The fabrication method will ultimately control the total porosity of the scaffold and determine whether drug loading will occur via surface adsorption or encapsulation. Traditional fabrication methods for ceramic scaffolds include freeze-drying, sponge-templating, gas foaming, and conventional sintering (Collins et al. 2021). However, the main caveat of using traditional manufacturing techniques is that they offer limited control over the reproducibility of the scaffold's overall shape and internal pore structures, potentially leading to inconsistencies in the mechanical, physical, and biological functions of the developed scaffolds. In recent years, researchers have harnessed additive manufacturing technologies such as selective laser sintering, stereolithography, and three-dimensional (3D) printing for various biomedical applications (Eltom, Zhong, and Muhammad 2019). Additive manufacturing technologies enable the digital-assisted repeatable fabrication of 3D constructs via the precise, layer-by-layer deposition of material based on a computer-aided design (CAD) model. Among the various 3D printing approaches, extrusion-based printing has emerged as one of the most popular methods for creating CaP-based scaffolds for BTE due to its accessibility, versatility, ease of handling, and ability to produce high-fidelity shapes (H. Sun et al. 2022; Y. Wu et al. 2020). Studies have shown that drugs can be integrated with calcium phosphate ink prior to extrusion either by encapsulating it within the scaffold (H. Sun et al. 2022) or coated onto a complete scaffold as a post-processing method (Y. Wu et al. 2020).

6.5.3 Drug Delivery Applications

6.5.3.1 Bone Regeneration

Structurally, BTE scaffolds must be of a suitable mechanical strength to resist load, one that closely mimics native bone to avoid failure or stress shielding (Mouriño and Boccaccini 2010). They must be highly porous and interconnected to facilitate the ingrowth of newly formed tissue. Pore sizes above 80 μm (macroporosity) facilitate the migration of cells and blood vessels into the scaffold, while pore sizes below 10 μm (microporosity) facilitate the movement of nutrients and waste removal. Pore size is integral when considering the scaffold's structural integrity, drug binding, storage, and release (Mouriño and Boccaccini 2010). A highly interconnected, porous scaffold provides a larger overall surface area and can help with the mechanical interlocking between tissue and scaffold; however, it often comes at the expense of reduced mechanical strength. The surface area also dictates the concentration of drugs released into the environment. For example, when a drug is immobilized onto the surface of the scaffold, a larger surface area would see a higher concentration of drug bound and released upon implantation. Architecturally, their 3D geometry must imitate the macro- and micro-structure of cancellous or cortical bone, and their degradation rate must be tailored to match that of native bone regeneration as time progresses (Qu et al. 2019). The ideal BTE scaffold must possess osteogenic potential to support the formation of new bone. For this to occur, the biomaterial must be osteoconductive and osteoinductive. Osteoconduction is the ability of bone-forming cells to migrate across scaffold material and replace it with new bone, while osteoinduction refers to the ability of the biomaterial to stimulate the differentiation of cells toward osteogenic lineages. Materials such as calcium phosphates are inherently bioactive and osteogenic, while other biomaterials can be made osteogenic through the integration and release of growth factors and stimulating agents incorporated within their scaffold.

Incorporating drugs or growth factors into BTE scaffolds is an excellent way to increase their bioactivity, particularly their osteoinductive potential (i.e., their ability to induce osteogenic differentiation). The most commonly used osteoinductive proteins (bone morphogenic proteins (BMPs) and transforming growth factor-β (TGF-β)) can readily lose their bioactivity during fabrication, particularly if they are pre-encapsulated within the scaffold mixture (Ripamonti et al. 2016). Indeed, earlier studies have seen a multitude of growth factors adsorbed onto the surface of CaP-based scaffolds for enhanced bone regeneration. Therefore, osteoinductive, small molecular weight drugs have received attention as they remain relatively stable in harsh chemical and physical environments (see Table 6.1). Dexamethasone (DEX) is one such osteoinductive factor commonly used in bone tissue regeneration (Chou et al. 2001). In a recent study, He et al. combined polytrimethylene carbonate (PTMC) with β-TCP microspheres loaded with DEX to make a composite scaffold with high porosity and drug release capability (J. He et al. 2020). In this study, it was noted that the scaffolds had improved mechanical strength and creep resistance, as well as the sustained release of DEX over 30 days. However, the loading efficiency was only 30%, which was well below the theoretical value. Furthermore, Chen et al. fabricated a composite scaffold using collagen and BCP NPs loaded with DEX for improved osteoinductive properties (Y. Chen, Kawazoe, and Chen 2018). Nude mice studies showed ectopic bone tissue regeneration over 28 days, while DEX release was mapped over a 35-day period. The same group investigated their composite DEX-loaded scaffold on angiogenesis, revealing that DEX released promotes vascular ingrowth via concentration gradients (Y. Chen et al. 2018). Kim et al. investigated the release of DEX-loaded poly(lactic-co-glycolic acid) (PLGA) immobilized on the surface of negatively charged HA scaffolds for bone defects in dog model (J.M. Kim et al. 2012). The release profile was mapped over 4 weeks and observed an initial burst, characteristic of immobilized drug loading, followed by sustained release and new bone growth compared to untreated HA scaffolds. The challenge remains with all these studies, whereby the initial burst release of the drug followed by a relatively short, sustained release (>4 weeks).

Another osteoinductive drug commonly investigated in the literature is alendronate (ALN), a small molecular weight drug that inhibits bone resorption and induces osteogenic differentiation. Park et al. investigated the effect of ALN released from BCP scaffolds in rat tibial models, where they noticed that ALN concentrations maintained at the repair site for a duration that could facilitate cell migration and differentiation (Park et al. 2015). A similar study by Kim et al. investigated BCP scaffolds with ALN-eluting capacity via surface immobilization (S.E. Kim et al. 2015). They saw the sustained release of ALN over 28 days and noticed an increased expression of osteogenic markers for osteogenic differentiation and calcium deposition. In a more recent study, Sun et al. fabricated porous CaP scaffolds for large skull defects with the ability for controlled release of icariin, an osteogenic drug for bone regeneration (H. Sun et al. 2022). Icariin was loaded alongside HA slurry and 3D printed in the desired shape, with drug release measured over 700 hours. The personalized scaffold showed excellent biocompatibility, optimal mechanical properties, and a slow controlled release of icariin that continuously promoted new bone formation.

6.5.3.2 Treatment of Osteomyelitis

Infectious bone defects (such as periodontitis and osteomyelitis) remain a significant challenge in orthopedics, where conventional treatment involves a combination of systemic antibiotic administration, debridement surgery, and bone grafting (G. Qiu et al. 2021). Antibiotic administration has limited efficacy with low concentrations of antibiotics reaching the defect site. An ideal delivery method of antibiotics for bone infections would penetrate deep inside the tissue defect, provide support for the surrounding healthy tissue to start healing, and sustain high drug concentrations for an extended period to curb recurrence. Researchers are focused on addressing these requirements by integrating antibiotics within bone scaffolds to provide targeted and sustained treatments for bone infections and facilitate the healing process (S.-M. Liu, Chen, et al. 2021; Najafloo, Baheiraei, and Imani 2021; Prokopowicz et al. 2020; G. Qiu et al. 2021; S. Wu et al. 2021; Y. Zhang and Zhang 2002) (Table 6.1).

Several studies have explored CaP-based, antibiotic-loaded, BTE scaffolds. CaP powder has been used in composites to form a slurry or cement

Table 6.1 Applications and Examples of Calcium-Based Scaffolds as Drug Delivery Vehicles

Application	*Phase Type*	*Cargo*	*Synthesis Method*	*Cargo Loading Method*	*Construct*	*References*
Bone regeneration – Drug	HA	Icariin	3D printing	Encapsulation	Composite ALG / HA scaffold (32% porosity, pore size 400–500 μm)	H. Sun et al. (2022)
	β-TCP	Dexamethason	Emulsion/solvent sintering	Encapsulation	Composite PTMC/loaded TCP microsphere scaffold (50% porosity, pore size 120–180 μm)	J. He et al. (2020)
	BCP	Dexamethason	Emulsion/ hybridization	Encapsulation	Composite collagen scaffold with loaded BCP NPs (pore size 405–450 μm)	Y. Chen, Kawazoe, and Chen (2018)
	HA	Dexamethason	Emulsion/ polymeric template-coating	Encapsulation	Loaded PLGA microspheres coated on HA scaffold	J.M. Kim et al. (2012)
	BCP	Alendronate	–	Adsorption	Porous BCP scaffold	S.E. Kim et al. (2015); Park et al. (2015)
Bone regeneration – Biomolecule	BCP	Growth hormone	Machined from triosite blocks	Adsorption	Porous BCP scaffold (50% macroporosity, pore size 565 μm)	Guicheux et al. (1998)
	HA	BMP-2	Crystallization	Encapsulation	Cement slurry that formed loaded porous HA scaffold	Haddad et al. (2006)
	β-TCP	BMP-2	–	Encapsulation	Hand-rolled porous rod	Namikawa et al. (2005)
	BCP	TGF- β	–	Adsorption	Titanium scaffold with porous BCP coating	Turner et al. (2001)
	TCP	Insulin-like growth factor (IGF)	Double emulsion/ physical crosslinking	Encapsulation	Composite scaffold loaded with PLGA microspheres encapsulation IGF	Luginbuehl et al. (2005)

(*Continued*)

Table 6.1 (Continued) Applications and Examples of Calcium-Based Scaffolds as Drug Delivery Vehicles

Application	*Phase Type*	*Cargo*	*Synthesis Method*	*Cargo Loading Method*	*Construct*	*References*
Osteosarcoma treatment	BCP	5-Fluorouracil	3D printing	Encapsulation	Drug loaded in polymeric coating around porous BCP scaffold	Y. Wu et al. (2020)
	HA and β-TCP	Methotrexate (MTX)	–	Adsorption	Loading of MTX on scaffold block surface	Itokazu et al. (1998)
	HA	Paclitaxel	–	Encapsulation	Composite bead construct loaded with drug	Abe et al. (2008)
	HA	Cisplatin	Chemical precipitation/ hydrothermal	Adsorption	Composite powder loaded with drug	Sumathra et al. (2018)
Osteomyelitis	CaP	Doxycycline hyclate	Emulsion	Encapsulation	Loaded chitosan scaffold reinforced w/ CaP	G. Qiu et al. (2021)
	CaP	Doxycycline hyclate	Templating methods	Adsorption	Composite porous scaffold	Prokopowicz et al. (2020)
	β-TCP	Niosomal thymol	Lyophilization	Encapsulation	Composite collagen scaffold, molded to shape	Najafloo, Baheiraei, and Imani (2021)
	CaP	Gentamicin	–	Adsorption	Cement>loaded with hydrogel beads w/ drug on surface	S.-M. Liu, Chen, et al. (2021)
	CaP	Penicillin	Vapor diffusion methods	Encapsulation	Injectable microsphere slurry	S. Wu et al. (2021)
	β-TCP	Gentamicin sulfate	Phase separation technique	Adsorption	Composite scaffold with ALG	Y. Zhang and Zhang (2002)
	Vaterite -Calcite	Vancomycin	Particle crystallization	Adsorption	PHB fibrous scaffold coated with CaC	Chernozem et al. (2021)

for injection into the infected/defect site. These cements are advantageous for osteomyelitis treatment as they can fully occupy complex void morphologies upon injection, are minimally invasive, and solidify after injection to provide mechanical support similar to a preformed scaffold. Qiu et al. developed a chitosan-reinforced CaP cement that delivered encapsulated doxycycline hyclate to infectious bone defects that showed excellent mechanical properties and potent antibacterial activity over 21 days (G. Qiu et al. 2021). Liu et al. developed a composite CaP bone cement loaded with gelatin/alginate hydrogel beads immobilized with gentamicin on their surface (S.-M. Liu, Chen, et al. 2021). They saw an initial burst of gentamicin release which is a characteristic of drugs loaded via surface adsorption, followed by a weak but sustained release profile. Wu et al. reported composite CaP cement loaded with chitosan-alginate-penicillin microspheres and human umbilical cord mesenchymal stem cells (hUCMSCs) (S. Wu et al. 2021). The injectable scaffold had strong antibacterial effects against golden staph (*S. aureus*) with an inhibition zone greater than that of penicillin disk control *in vitro*.

CaP has also been combined with polymers to improve flexibility and increase compressive strength. These composite scaffolds allow for the tailorable delivery of drugs as well as support degradation. Prokopowicz et al. reported a novel biphasic composite of CaP and mesoporous silica (CaPMSi) with doxycycline hydrochloride (DOX) adsorbed onto its surface (Prokopowicz et al. 2020). The scaffold saw prolonged DOX release over 5 days and the conversion of CaP into bone-like apatite for enhanced bone regeneration in combination with preventative infection measures. Zhang et al. developed a composite scaffold of β-TCP and chitosan via phase separation and loaded gentamicin sulfate (GS) on its surface (Y. Zhang and Zhang 2002). Interestingly, the burst release of GS was reduced by incorporating CaP crystals that formed on the surface of the scaffold, followed by a sustained release of drug molecules over 5 weeks. Chernozem et al. uniformly coated their biodegradable piezoelectric polyhydroxybutyrate (PHB) fibrous scaffolds with biomineralized CaC particles and immobilized both enzyme alkaline phosphatase (ALP) and glycopeptide antibiotic vancomycin (VCM) on the surface (Chernozem et al. 2021). The calcium carbonate coating was formed via a simple synthesis method involving immersion in a mixture of calcium chloride and sodium carbonate salts twice or thrice under ultrasound exposure. At the same time, drug loading was performed at room temperature for 1 hour by immersion in both solutions. The CaC-coated scaffolds saw higher loading efficiency for VCM and demonstrated antibacterial effects against *S. aureus*, making it a promising scaffold for treating complicated infections.

6.6 CALCIUM CARBONATE AND CALCIUM PHOSPHATE MICROSPHERES

Microspheres (also called microparticles) are 3D, free-flowing spherical substances ranging in particle size from 1 to 1,000 μm (Mahale and Saudagar 2019). Microsphere DDSs are advantageous when compared to conventional drug delivery because they can: (i) protect the drug against hostile environments, (ii) enhance targeted delivery, (iii) possess a specifically tailored drug release profile to reduce drug toxicity and increase efficacy, and (iv) improve patient compliance in those that require frequent drug administration (R. Verma, Verma, and Kumar 2019). They offer higher injectability and flowability when compared to nano-carriers and are more suitable for drug delivery in areas of low-level blood circulation (e.g., infection sites, large bone defects, large areas of tissue loss). Furthermore, microspheres can achieve highly targeted drug release in response to various stimuli, such as pH, temperature, light, and ultrasound (R. Verma, Verma, and Kumar 2019).

CaCs and CaPs are among the most promising and well-studied bioceramic microspheres concerning drug delivery. Factors such as the polymorph of calcium, the total porosity, composition, surface chemistry, and microsphere size can be modified during the fabrication process to control the microsphere's drug-loading characteristics and release profiles. Recent advances in CaC and CaP research have investigated the utility of dual DDSs (Chemmalar et al. 2021; X. Liu, Li, et al. 2021; Sheng et al. 2021), vaccine adjuvants (Jia et al. 2017; Xianghui Li et al. 2021; Z. Liu et al. 2020), and even applications in treating cardiovascular disease (Pengzhong Shi et al. 2021) and type-1 diabetes (Sato, Seno, and Anzai 2014; D. Liu et al. 2017).

6.6.1 Optimal Microsphere Characteristics for Drug Delivery

Drug-delivering microspheres can be categorized as reservoir-type (i.e., the drug is encapsulated within the microsphere) or monolithic-type (i.e., the drug is dispersed throughout the microsphere matrix) depending on their synthesis method and application. Both methods can facilitate loading diverse cargo types, including drugs, nucleic acids (i.e., DNA and RNA), enzymes, and growth factors. Indeed, the most promising DDSs are characterized by high drug-loading capacity and sustained drug release kinetics. Numerous parameters strongly influence this, including the microsphere's surface morphology and internal architecture (Zarkesh et al. 2017). Microspheres with higher porosity and pore interconnectivity are highly desirable for successful drug delivery. This is because such microspheres possess greater surface areas and lower mass densities and therefore exhibit superior drug adsorption on their surfaces and drug release kinetics as compared to the corresponding bulk material (Hossain, Patel, and Ahmed 2015). Other characteristics which must be considered when engineering microspheres for drug delivery include biodegradability and surface interactions between drug and carrier as they directly correlate to effective drug release kinetics and drug loading, respectively.

The unique physical and chemical properties of CaC have attracted significant attention as microsphere constructs; however, their extended use is compromised due to its polymorphic characteristics (Fadia et al. 2021; Won et al. 2010). The most attractive crystalline CaC phase for microsphere design is its metastable vaterite form due to its spherical morphology and naturally porous interface (Figure 6.2). However, vaterite is the least stable polymorph of CaC and readily undergoes a phase transition to its more thermodynamically stable forms (i.e., calcite and/or aragonite), which do not present the same spherical porous morphology. The pH and temperature sensitivity of crystalline CaC allows for more tailorable drug release behavior as particles are taken up by the cells or exposed to the cancer microenvironment (Fadia et al. 2021). In order to stabilize calcium carbonate in its vaterite polymorph, inorganic or organic impurities such as ovalbumin (X. Wang et al. 2009), anionic starburst dendrimers (Naka, Tanaka, and Chujo 2002), and gold NPs (W.-Y. Cai et al. 2006) can be added.

Similar to CaCs, CaPs make superior biomaterials for microsphere fabrication due to their bioactivity, bioresorbability, high porosity, and good mechanical properties. Its similarity to native bone lends its applications to revolve primarily around BTE and subsequent drug delivery. CaPs, in general, are a large group of biomaterials, with HA, β-TCP, and BCP dominating the field in microsphere production (Dorozhkin 2012). HA is the most stable form of calcium phosphate and has inherent osteoinductive and osteoconductive properties but has a slow degradation rate. B-TCP, the more popular polymorph of tricalcium phosphate, is bioresorbable, making them excellent candidates for injectable bone cements. BCPs are a combination of HA and β-TCP, and by adjusting their ratio, one can maintain tight control of bioactivity and bioresorbability, which is a particular advantage when fabricating microspheres for drug delivery applications.

6.6.2 Particle Synthesis

The characteristics of a calcium-based microparticle or NP delivery vehicle are governed by the respective methods used to synthesize these particles. Calcium-based microspheres and NPs can be fabricated using several common synthesis approaches despite their distinct size-based definitions. These approaches can be broadly classified as dry synthesis, high-temperature synthesis, and wet chemical synthesis routes (Boyjoo, Pareek, and Liu 2014; A.Y. Cai, Zhu, and Qi 2020; Lin, Wu, and Chang 2014). A range of examples of the methods used to create various CaC and CaP microparticle and NPs and their applications are presented in Tables 6.2 and 6.3, and a discussion of the synthesis methods for particles of both dimension ranges will be addressed in this section.

Dry synthesis methods involve the use of dry precursor chemicals, which can be ball-milled without solvents, such as mechanochemical approaches (Nasiri-Tabrizi et al. 2009; Sargheini et al. 2012; Fadia et al. 2021) and solid-state synthesis, followed by high-temperature calcination (Xiaojun Guo, Yan, et al. 2013; Pramanik et al. 2007). The advantages of dry synthesis methods lie in their simplicity, including cost-effective materials and ease of scalability in manufacturing to produce a variety of particle structures with high crystallinity. However, dry synthesis methods usually suffer from heterogeneous particle sizes and morphologies, large aggregate formation, and low phase purity. High-temperature synthesis methods, such as spray pyrolysis (Ataol et al. 2015; Huber et al. 2005; Tsikourkitoudi et al. 2020) and spray drying methods (Mostafa et al. 2015; Vergaro et al. 2015; D.-H. Kim et al. 2014; Tateiwa et al. 2021), can produce calcium-based microspheres and NPs with superior crystallinity. However, high-temperature synthesis processes consume high energy, produce low yield, are challenging to scale up, and have inconsistent processing conditions (such as temperature and exposure time), which makes it difficult to regulate particle morphology and phase homogeneity.

Wet chemical synthesis methods are the conventional and most widely employed strategies for producing CaC and CaP microparticles and NPs and simply refer to techniques that utilize liquid solutions. These synthesis methods are straightforward to execute and offer exceptional versatility in the equipment and chemical reagents used (Boyjoo, Pareek, and Liu 2014; El-Toni et al. 2016; Sadat-Shojai et al. 2013). A variety of reaction parameters can be adjusted to control the growth of the microsphere or NP and its resulting physicochemical properties. Such parameters include the stoichiometric ratio of calcium ion to carbonate or phosphate ions, the types, concentrations, and molar ratios of additives used (including surfactants, synthetic polymers, biomolecules), pH, temperature, pressure, solvent ratio, reaction time, and the mixing mode (Xiaoyu Ma et al. 2016; Trushina, Bukreeva, and Antipina 2016; C. Wang, Chen, et al. 2020; Y. Wang et al. 2010).

The most popular wet synthesis methods for fabricating CaC and CaP microspheres and NPs are chemical precipitation and microemulsion (A.Y. Cai, Zhu, and Qi 2020; Konopacka-Łyskawa 2019; Lin, Wu, and Chang 2014). Chemical precipitation involves the combination of two aqueous reagents: one containing the calcium cation source and the other containing the carbonate or phosphate anion source. The interchange of ions in solution forms two new substances, typically resulting in one product forming a precipitate, i.e., CaC or CaP microspheres or NPs. In the case

Table 6.2 Applications and Examples of Calcium-based Microspheres as Drug Delivery Vehicles

Application	*Phase Type*	*Cargo*	*Synthesis Method*	*Cargo Loading Method*	*Construct*	*References*
Calcium carbonates						
Dual-drug delivery	Calcite+Vaterite	Rhodamine B+BSA	Chemical precipitation/emulsion	Adsorption	Dual-layered mesoporous microspheres (400–500 μm)	X. Liu, Li, et al. (2021)
	Vaterite	Methotrexate+Aspirin	Coprecipitation	Encapsulation	MTX-loaded CaC microspheres (~2 μm) encapsulated in Asp-loaded ALG	Sheng et al. (2021)
Bone regeneration	CaC	Bone morphogenic protein 2	Coprecipitation	Encapsulation	CaP microspheres loaded into TCS-P24 scaffold	Z. Wang, Liu, et al. (2020)
Cancer therapy	CaC	Doxorubicin hydrochloride	*Yeast* extract/calcination	Adsorption	Hollow, porous microspheres (~6 μm)	Wei et al. (2021)
	Vaterite	Doxorubicin hydrochloride	Coprecipitation	Encapsulation	Porous, monolithic-type microspheres doped with polyanions (1–8 μm)	Sudareva et al. (2021)
	Calcite	Doxorubicin Hydrochloride	Coprecipitation	Adsorption	Porous monolithic-type microspheres (~4–5 μm)	L. Li et al. (2020)
	Calcite+Vaterite	Camptothecin	Coprecipitation	Adsorption	Porous monolithic-type microspheres (2 μm)	N. Qiu et al. (2012)

(*Continued*)

Table 6.2 (Continued) Applications and Examples of Calcium-based Microspheres as Drug Delivery Vehicles

Application	*Phase Type*	*Cargo*	*Synthesis Method*	*Cargo Loading Method*	*Construct*	*References*
Radionuclide therapy	CaC	^{225}Ac	Coprecipitation + LbL Assembly	Encapsulation	Core-shell porous microspheres (~3.2 µm)	Muslimov et al. (2021)
	CaC	^{224}Ra	Coprecipitation	Encapsulation	Porous microspheres (1–15 µm)	Westrøm et al. (2018)
Photodynamic therapy	Vaterite	Photosens	Coprecipitation	Adsorption	Porous monolithic-type microspheres (3.6 µm)	Svenskaya et al. (2013)
Vaccine adjuvant	CaC	*Acanthopanax senticosus* polysaccharide	Coprecipitation + emulsion	Encapsulation	Porous monolithic-type microspheres (~6 µm)	Xianghui Li et al. (2021)
	CaC	Lentinan (LNT)	Coprecipitation	Encapsulation	Porous monolithic-type microspheres (~2-3 µm)	Z. Liu et al. (2020)
	CaC	Hepatitis B surface antigen (HBsAg)	Coprecipitation	Encapsulation	Porous monolithic-type microspheres (1–4 µm)	Jia et al. (2017)
Type-1 diabetes	Calcite + Vaterite	Insulin	Coprecipitation	Encapsulation	Dual-layered porous monolithic-type core microspheres (~5 µm)	Sato, Seno, and Anzai (2014)
Fungal infections	Vaterite	Naftifine hydrochloride	Coprecipitation	Encapsulation	Porous, monolithic-type microspheres (~2 µm)	Gusliakova et al. (2021)

(Continued)

Table 6.2 (*Continued*) Applications and Examples of Calcium-based Microspheres as Drug Delivery Vehicles

Application	*Phase Type*	*Cargo*	*Synthesis Method*	*Cargo Loading Method*	*Construct*	*References*
Cardiovascular research	CaC	Thrombin	Coprecipitation	Adsorption	Porous, monolithic-type microsphere (~10 μm)	Pengzhong Shi et al. (2021)
Pesticide delivery	Vaterite	Prochloraz	Coprecipitation	Adsorption	Porous, monolithic-type microspheres (~1.5 μm)	Xiao et al. (2021)
Herbicide delivery	Calcite	Prometryn (PMT)	Coprecipitation	Adsorption	Porous monolithic-type microspheres (~3 μm)	Xiang et al. (2018)
Calcium Phosphates						
Bone regeneration	HA	Bone morphogenic factor - 2	Flame spray/ sintering	Adsorption	Hollow, porous microsphere (~100 μm)	Xiong et al. (2015)
	HA / β-TCP	Bone morphogenic factor-2	Spray drying/ sintering	Adsorption	Porous monolithic-type microspheres (~70 μm)	Tateiwa et al. (2021)
	BCP	Dexamethasone (DEX) Bovine serum albumin (BSA)	Coprecipitation/templating	Adsorption	Porous monolithic-type microsphere w/ altered surface topographies (nano-sheets and rods)	Zarkesh et al. (2017)

(*Continued*)

Table 6.2 (Continued) Applications and Examples of Calcium-based Microspheres as Drug Delivery Vehicles

Application	*Phase Type*	*Cargo*	*Synthesis Method*	*Cargo Loading Method*	*Construct*	*References*
Osteosarcoma treatment	CaP	Doxorubicin	Coprecipitation	Adsorption	Hollow porous microspheres (~1 μm)	Zhou et al. (2017)
	CaP	Doxorubicin	Hydrothermal	Adsorption	Porous monolithic-type microspheres	Hu et al. (2021)
	CaP	Doxorubicin	Coprecipitation	Adsorption	Porous monolithic-type microspheres (~2 μm)	J.-F. Liu et al. (2018)
Antimicrobial treatment	BCP	Doxycycline	Hydrothermal/emulsion/ sintering	Adsorption	Porous monolithic-type microsphere (~1 μm)	Victor and Kumar (2008)
	BCP	Protamine	Ultrasonic spray pyrolysis	Adsorption	Hollow, porous microspheres (0.5– 2 μm)	Honda et al. (2017)
	β-TCP	Vancomycin hydrochloride (VH)	Double emulsion	Adsorption	Dual-layer porous microsphere w/ TCP shell (~1 μm)	J. He et al. (2021)
	HA	Gentamicin sulfate (GS)	Coprecipitation	Encapsulation	Porous monolithic-type microsphere bone scaffold	Cao et al. (2021)

Table 6.3 Applications and Examples of Calcium-based Nanoparticles as Delivery Vehicles

Application	*Phase Type*	*Cargo*	*Synthesis Method*	*Cargo Loading Method*	*Construct*	*References*
Calcium Carbonates						
Cancer therapy	ACC	Curcumin	Chemical precipitation	Encapsulation	Porous solid spheres (100 nm)	Rao et al. (2020)
	CC	EV peptide	Reverse microemulsion	Encapsulation	Spherical core, lipid shell (60–70 nm)	S.K. Kim, Foote, and Huang (2013)
	CC	Adriamycin	Reverse microemulsion	Adsorption	Porous solid spheres (69.4 nm)	Bai et al. (2017)
	Vaterite	Cisplatin	Chemical precipitation	Adsorption	Porous solid spheres (20–80 nm)	Dunuweera and Rajapakse (2017)
	CC	Cisplatin	Reverse microemulsion	Encapsulation	Platinum and Selenium-doped spherical core, lipid shell (120 nm)	P. Zhao, Li, et al. (2019)
	ACC	Mitoxantrone	Vapor diffusion	Encapsulation	Spherical solid core, lipid shell; (80 nm)	C. Wang, Han, et al. (2019)
	Aragonite	Gefitinib and Paclitaxel	Biogenic source (cockle shells)	Adsorption	Porous solid spheres (87.2 nm)	Chemmalar et al. (2021)
	Aragonite	Docetaxel	Biogenic source (cockle shells)	Adsorption	Porous solid spheres (37.11 nm)	Hammadi et al. (2017)
	Vaterite	Doxorubicin, superparamagnetic iron oxide NPs	Chemical precipitation	Adsorption	Porous solid spheres (800 nm)	Choukrani et al. (2020)
	CC	Epirubicin or Melittin	Reverse microemulsion	Adsorption	Globular, dimer mucin 1 aptamer surface functionalization (500 nm)	Yazdian-Robati et al. (2019)

(Continued)

Table 6.3 (Continued) Applications and Examples of Calcium-based Nanoparticles as Delivery Vehicles

Application	*Phase Type*	*Cargo*	*Synthesis Method*	*Cargo Loading Method*	*Construct*	*References*
	Vaterite	Photosens (photosensitizer)	Chemical precipitation	Adsorption	Porous solid spheres (650 nm)	Svenskaya et al. (2013)
	CC	Chlorin e6 (photosensitizer)	Vapor diffusion, biomineralization	Adsorption	Hollow CC-dopamine spheres, lipid + PEGylated shell (170 nm)	Dong et al. (2018)
Antimicrobial treatment	Vaterite	Ciprofloxacin	Reverse microemulsion	Encapsulation	Porous solid globules (116.09 nm)	Maleki Dizaj et al. (2017)
	Aragonite	Oxytetracycline	Biogenic source (cockle shells)	Adsorption	Porous solid spheres (62.4 nm)	Idris et al. (2019)
Vaccine (antigen) delivery	Vaterite	Ovalbumin	Chemical precipitation	Encapsulation	Spherical clusters (~500 nm)	S. Wang et al. (2018)
Pesticide	CC	Validamycin	Reverse microemulsion	Encapsulation	Solid sphere (57–387 nm)	Qian et al. (2011)
Calcium Phosphates						
Bone regeneration	ACP	Alendronate	Solvothermal	Adsorption	Porous globules (~5.6 nm)	R. Sun et al. (2020)
	HA	Zoledronate	Sol-gel	Adsorption	Porous solid spheres (100–130 nm)	Khajuria, Razdan, and Mahapatra (2015)
	BCP	Dexamethasone	Chemical precipitation	Encapsulation	Rod-like NPs incorporated into porous collagen scaffold (<50 nm)	Y. Chen, Kawazoe, and Chen (2018)

(Continued)

Table 6.3 (Continued) Applications and Examples of Calcium-based Nanoparticles as Delivery Vehicles

Application	*Phase Type*	*Cargo*	*Synthesis Method*	*Cargo Loading Method*	*Construct*	*References*
	HA	BMP-2	Hydrothermal	Adsorption	Porous rod-like NPs incorporated into silk fibroin/chitosan scaffold (length: 15–20 nm, width: 60–70 nm)	Y. Qiu et al. (2020)
	ACP	Ibuprofen	Spray drying	Encapsulation	Solid spheres (100–200 nm)	Mostafa et al. (2015)
	CDHA, BTCP	Tetracycline (antibiotic) and ibuprofen (anti-inflammatory)	Microwave-assisted chemical precipitation	Adsorption	Platelet (CDHA) and spherical (BTCP) (<100 nm)	Madhumathi et al. (2018)
Cancer therapy	ACP	Curcumin	Chemical precipitation	Encapsulation	Solid spheres (80–120 nm)	Xia Guo et al. (2018)
	HA	Doxorubicin	Chemical precipitation, hydrothermal	Encapsulation	Rods (length: 140 nm, diameter: 28 nm, height: 22 nm)	W. Sun, Fan, et al. (2018)
	HA	Doxorubicin, paclitaxel	Sol-gel	Adsorption	Porous hollow tubes (diameter: 140–350 nm, length: >1,000 nm)	Srivastav et al. (2019)
	CP	Doxorubicin and gadolinium-DPTA (MRI contrast agent)	Hydrothermal	Encapsulation	Spherical core, A54-peptide functionalized shell (38.10 nm)	N.-n. Zhang et al. (2018)
	CP	siRNA	Chemical precipitation	Encapsulation	Solid spherical core, alendronate-hyaluronic acid shell (170 nm)	C. Qiu et al. (2016)

(Continued)

Table 6.3 (Continued) Applications and Examples of Calcium-based Nanoparticles as Delivery Vehicles

Application	*Phase Type*	*Cargo*	*Synthesis Method*	*Cargo Loading Method*	*Construct*	*References*
	CP	siRNA	Reverse microemulsion	Encapsulation	Spherical core, reversible charge lipid shell (80 nm)	R.-Q. Cai et al. (2017)
Osteosarcoma	HA	Medronate (bisphosphonate) and JQ1 (antitumor)	Chemical precipitation	Encapsulation	Globular (~15 nm)	V.M. Wu, Mickens, and Uskoković (2017)
Rheumatoid arthritis	HA	Methylprednisolone acetate	Chemical precipitation	Adsorption	Porous globular (110 nm)	Jafari et al. (2016)
	HA	Methotrexate and teriflunomide	Chemical precipitation	Adsorption	Spherical core, hyaluronic acid shell (274.9 nm)	Pandey et al. (2021)
Diabetes	CP	Insulin	Reverse microemulsion	Encapsulation	Spherical core, vitamin B12/ chitosan layer-by-layer shell (212.6 nm)	A. Verma et al. (2016)
Gout	HA	Colchicine	Reverse microemulsion	Encapsulation, Adsorption	Globular (18.13 – 25.56 nm)	Zeng et al. (2021)
Amyotrophic lateral sclerosis (ALS)	CP	SOD1 (antisense oligonucleotide)	Reverse microemulsion	Encapsulation	Solid spherical core, lipid shell (31 nm)	Liyu Chen, Watson, et (al. 2017)
Antimicrobial treatment	CP	LL-37 peptide	Flame spray pyrolysis	Adsorption	Solid spheres (8–26 nm)	Tsikourkitoudi et al. (2020)
	HA	Ciprofloxacin	Chemical precipitation	Adsorption	Porous hollow (400 nm) and solid spheres (500 nm)	Munir et al. (2018)

of microemulsions, reverse or water-in-oil microemulsions can precipitate inorganic materials captured within spherical micelles by acting as micro- or nanoscale "reactors" (Malik, Wani, and Hashim 2012). Generally, this involves combining the reagents containing the calcium cation with a mixture of surfactants to form the microemulsion, followed by the dropwise addition of the carbonate ion- or phosphate ion-containing reagent to produce uniformly sized particles.

Other wet chemical approaches for fabricating calcium-based microparticles and NPs include hydrothermal (Y. Qiu et al. 2020; W. Sun, Fan, et al. 2018; N.-n. Zhang et al. 2018; Qi, Zhu, and Chen 2014), solvothermal (R. Sun et al. 2020), sol-gel (Khajuria, Razdan, and Mahapatra 2015; Srivastav et al. 2019; Yuan et al. 2010), microwave-assisted precipitation (Madhumathi et al. 2018; Reardon, Huang, and Tang 2015), sintering (Veljović et al. 2010), and vapor diffusion methods (Dong et al. 2018; C. Wang, Han, et al. 2019). Carbonation synthesis routes, which involve bubbling carbon dioxide gas through an aqueous mixture of calcium oxide or calcium hydroxide, can be used to produce CaC NPs successfully (Abeywardena et al. 2020; El-Sheikh et al. 2013). The abundance of calcium-based materials in nature has also prompted researchers to explore the feasibility of biogenic sources such as dolomite (Abeywardena et al. 2020), eggshells (Hassan et al. 2013), and cockle shells (Chemmalar et al. 2021; Hammadi et al. 2017) to fabricate CaC microparticles and NPs, fish bones (Asadollahzadeh, Rabiee, and Salimi-Kenari 2019), fish scales (Sathiskumar et al. 2019), and coral (Karacan, Ben-Nissan, and Sinutok 2019) to create CaP microparticles and NPs.

Calcium-based microparticles and NPs generated via the aforementioned synthesis methods are amenable to various drug-loading strategies, including encapsulation or surface loading via adsorption or covalent attachment to functional groups (N. Wang, Cheng, et al. 2019). There are specific synthesis approaches that can be utilized to improve drug-loading content and encapsulation efficiency. For example, hollow microspheres and NPs are useful for increasing the loading content and encapsulation efficiency of cargo and can enable a slower, more controlled degradation and release profile of the drug. The growth of the CaC or CaP crystals to form the particles can occur on the external surface of hard templates, including sacrificial calcium carbonate particles (Munir et al. 2018; Y.-J. Guo, Wang, et al. 2013), soft templates such as polymeric micelles (Dong et al. 2018), biological templates (Wei et al. 2021), or even template-free approaches (Dunuweera and Rajapakse 2017; Xiong et al. 2015; Zhou et al. 2017; Y. Wang et al. 2010). Microsphere drug adsorption can also be augmented by forming more nanopores on the surface of the particle. The porogen or template material can be added to the initial reaction mixture to be ingrained within the matrix during the precipitation reaction, and then broken down via thermal treatment (Zarkesh et al. 2017).

6.6.3 Drug Delivery Applications

6.6.3.1 *Cancer Therapies*

An emerging application for porous calcium microspheres is in the targeted treatment of cancer (Table 6.2). Current research has seen advances in using composite CaC microspheres for the delivery of chemotherapy agents (L. Li et al. 2020; N. Qiu et al. 2012; Sudareva et al. 2021; Wei et al. 2021), radionuclide therapy (Muslimov et al. 2021), and photodynamic therapy (Svenskaya et al. 2013). In a recent study, Wei et al. successfully prepared hybrid DOX-loaded CaC microspheres using yeast cells as templates (Wei et al. 2021). The hybrid CaC microspheres were biocompatible, biodegradable, and pH sensitive, allowing the controlled release of DOX in an acidic environment (i.e., tumor microenvironments). Sudareva et al. synthesized DOX-loaded CaC microspheres coated with polyanions which increased the stability and loading efficiency of DOX (Sudareva et al. 2021). Similarly, Li et al. found that stable gelatin/CaC composite microspheres showed promise as effective DOX carriers (L. Li et al. 2020). Recently, Qiu et al. fabricated camptothecin-loaded CaC microspheres using biogenic sources as carriers for the safe and efficient delivery of anticancer drugs of low aqueous solubility (N. Qiu et al. 2012).

Radionuclide therapy is another form of cancer therapy that requires delivering an effective dose of radiation directly to the tumor site to minimize damage to healthy cells (Gudkov et al. 2016). Depending on the type of nucleotide used, there are two common types of radionuclide therapy: α- and β-therapy. α-Emitters have a shorter effective therapeutic range but have higher capabilities to damage tumors, making them attractive for treatments (Kassis 2008). Muslimov et al. successfully encapsulated a potent α-emitter radionuclide (^{225}Ac) into CaC core-shell particles for targeted release of its daughter isotopes at tumor sites (Muslimov et al. 2021). In vitro studies proved that the loaded CaC microspheres retained the isotope, exhibited stability in biological environments, and achieved dose-dependent biocompatibility over 30 days. Interestingly, in vivo studies highlighted that radioactivity accumulation in kidneys and urine was significantly reduced in mice injected with the encapsulated isotope, suggesting the absence of radioisotope leakage from the CaC particles. Similarly, Westrom et al. successfully loaded CaC microspheres with ^{224}Ra isotopes for the targeted treatment of disseminated cancer in cavitary regions of the body (Westrøm et al. 2018).

6.6.3.2 *Vaccine Adjuvant*

Vaccines for immunization are one of the most powerful tools for preventing infectious and transmissible diseases, with current research focusing on improving immunogenicity. Conventional adjuvants, such as aluminum salts, display poor immunogenicity and can be associated with adverse reactions and weak cellular immunity, highlighting the need for new and more useful adjuvants in vaccine development (Zepp 2010). CaC microspheres have become an interesting subject surrounding vaccine development. They can act as efficient carriers for more effective adjuvants that would usually be cleared quickly by the body and fail to target an immune cell response, limiting their clinical application. Indeed, CaC microsphere vaccine administration is attractive because it can potentially facilitate the co-delivery of both adjuvant and antigen *in vivo* (Jia et al. 2017). One such example is the *Acanthopanax senticosus* polysaccharide (ASPS), a bioactive polymer reported as a potent immunopotentiator but cleared quickly from the body (Peiying Shi et al. 2020). Li et al. developed a core-shell microsphere system with a ASPS-loaded porous CaC core and a polyethylenimine (PEI) coating with porcine parvovirus antigen adsorbed onto its surface (Xianghui Li et al. 2021). The system elicited a higher immune response upon injection in mice, with upregulated cytokines (TNF-α, IL-1β), immune markers (CD86, MHCII), and macrophages near the injection site, compared to ASPS control. In a similar study, Liu et al. synthesized CaC microspheres as co-delivery vehicles for adjuvant and antigen (Z. Liu et al. 2020). In this study, Liu et al. encapsulated lentinan (LNT), a potent immunostimulator (sourced from *Lentinula edodes* (McCormack et al. 2010)) within CaC porous microspheres to high efficiency and adsorbed ovalbumin (OVA) onto their surface. They found that LNT-CaC microspheres loaded with OVA enhanced lymphocyte proliferation and boosted the secretion of antibodies and cytokines (IL-2, IL-4, IFN-γ, and TNF-α) in mice.

6.6.3.3 Other Applications

Calcium-based microspheres have been explored for tissue engineering applications and regenerative medicine, especially as dual-drug delivery vehicles (X. Liu, Li, et al. 2021; Sheng et al. 2021). CaP microspheres have been extensively used for bone regeneration (Tateiwa et al. 2021; Xiong et al. 2015; Zarkesh et al. 2017), osteosarcoma treatment (Hu et al. 2021; J.-F. Liu et al. 2018; Zhou et al. 2017), and osteomyelitis (Cao et al. 2021; J. He et al. 2021; Honda et al. 2017; Victor and Kumar 2008), due to their injectability, flowability, mechanical properties, ability to conform to irregular void shapes, and osteogenic capabilities. CaC microspheres loaded with insulin were developed as a possible treatment for type 1 diabetes (Sato, Seno, and Anzai 2014). Shi et al. developed a tannic acid-doped CaC microsphere construct loaded with low concentrations of thrombin to aid in the hemostasis mechanism with potential clinical application in cardiovascular medicine and could be a versatile and effective platform for hemorrhage control (Pengzhong Shi et al. 2021), while Gusliakova et al. developed a vaterite microsphere system loaded with naftifine hydrochloride antimycotic for the prolonged treatment of fungal infections (Gusliakova et al. 2021). Their CaC microspheres enhanced local drug concentration, prolonged release, and enabled deep penetration of the antimycotic drug during transfollicular delivery, which is a significant challenge in conventional treatments such as creams and gels.

6.7 CALCIUM CARBONATE AND CALCIUM PHOSPHATE NANOPARTICLES

Since the beginning of the twenty-first century, nanotechnology has rapidly evolved into one of the most promising frontiers of research and innovation across almost all scientific fields. The utility of NPs has been explored for various biomedical applications, including delivery vehicles for drugs and biological molecules. Akin to microspheres and microparticles, the use of NPs can address several limitations associated with the administration of bare drugs, such as poor solubility, aggregation, nonspecific distribution, and systemic toxic side effects due to high dosages (A.Y. Cai, Zhu, and Qi 2020; Parveen, Misra, and Sahoo 2012). NPs can serve as platforms that protect their cargo from degradation in vivo to ensure the prolonged, stable release of the drug, achieving increased bioavailability at specifically targeted sites (Mitchell et al. 2021). The distinct advantage of using NPs compared to microspheres is their superior intracellular uptake, including their ability to interact with and target organelles as a potential strategy for treating the disease (Azevedo, Macedo, and Sarmento 2018; Otto, Otto, and De Villiers 2015). In general, the design of an NP-based DDS must consider the interactions between the drug, the delivery vehicle, and the target cells to induce the desired biological responses (Rizvi and Saleh 2018). The interaction between the drug and delivery vehicle plays an important role in tailoring the drug-loading capacity, entrapment efficiency, and sustained and controlled release profile to limit the need for a large number of dosages and high concentration of NPs (Azevedo, Macedo, and Sarmento 2018; A.Y. Cai, Zhu, and Qi 2020). The delivery vehicle must also be designed to support a high therapeutic index by utilizing biocompatible components, including those which comprise the NP core and coating materials, to simultaneously enhance targeting specificity and uptake by the cells (Jiao et al. 2018; Yoo et al. 2019).

6.7.1 Nanoparticle Characteristics for Drug Delivery

Calcium-based nanomaterials offer exceptional versatility in their design, giving rise to opportunities for engineering multifunctional NPs as drug delivery vehicles, for diagnosis, imaging, and other therapeutic functions (Boyjoo, Pareek, and Liu 2014; A.Y. Cai, Zhu, and Qi 2020; Sokolova and

Epple 2021). The effectiveness of CaC and CaP NPs as drug delivery vehicles is influenced by the physicochemical and electrostatic properties of the nanomaterial. Key design characteristics considered for fabricating effective CaC and CaP NPs for DDSs include pore structures, particle size, degradation, and surface charge.

6.7.1.1 Pore Structures

The pore structures of a calcium-based NP are an essential design consideration as they influence drug-loading capacities and release kinetics (Vallet-Regí, Balas, and Arcos 2007). Calcium-based NPs should possess high porosities, which correlate with high-specific surface areas and pore volumes, to allow higher drug-loading contents and accommodate larger biomacromolecules such as proteins (Xiaomin Ma et al. 2018; Reardon, Huang, and Tang 2015). The critical requirement to ensure sustained release of drugs by NPs is their high porosity. Increased porosity and specific surface areas promote drug encapsulation within the NP's internal pore system to prevent the formation of a coating on its external surface and burst release of drug molecules (Peng, Zhao, and Gao 2010). As a result, the porosity and morphologies between the bare and drug-loaded forms of the porous NP will be virtually identical, as observed in several CaC NP systems (Dunuweera and Rajapakse 2017; Hammadi et al. 2017; R. Sun, Zhang, et al. 2018). However, pore volume and specific surface area in both CaP and CaC NPs have shown to generally increase in both CaP and CaC NPs with an increase in the encapsulated drug concentration as a result of exchange reactions (Hammadi et al. 2017; Xiaomin Ma et al. 2018).

6.7.1.2 Particle Size and Shape

Consideration must be given to the size of a calcium-based drug delivery NP as it directly affects biodistribution, cellular internalization, and clearance mechanisms (Auría-Soro et al. 2019; Otto, Otto, and De Villiers 2015). Improved circulation time in the blood and cellular uptake can be achieved by creating NPs with dimensions between 6 and 200 nm, as particles smaller than 6 nm will be cleared by the kidneys and particles larger than 200 nm will be removed by the reticuloendothelial system (RES) and accumulate in the liver and spleen (Som et al. 2016; Z. Zhao, Ukidve, et al. 2019). For calcium-based nanomaterials, the size of the particle also influences its rate of dissolution and downstream cellular behaviors. Smaller NPs have higher dissolution rates due to the larger surface area-to-volume ratio and can either lead to regulation or dysregulation of calcium ion homeostasis depending on the cell type (Horie et al. 2014; H. Wu et al. 2019). For example, studies have shown that smaller CaP NPs tend to cause apoptosis in cancer cells (Cui et al. 2016; Yuan et al. 2010) but support cell viability and proliferation in nontumor cell types (Y. Cai et al. 2007; H. Wu et al. 2019). In contrast, CaC NPs exhibit good biocompatibility across all cell types regardless of size (Horie et al. 2014; Lauth, Maas, and Rezwan 2017; C. Wang, Chen, et al. 2020). Ultimately, the size of the calcium-based NP will influence the drug release profile (Svenskaya et al. 2013).

NP morphology also influences its effectiveness as a drug delivery vehicle (Kapate, Clegg, and Mitragotri 2021). CaC and CaP NP morphologies can be produced into a multitude of morphologies such as solid, hollow spheres, rods, needles, and plates (Abeywardena et al. 2020; Dong et al. 2018; Lin, Wu, and Chang 2014; X. Zhao et al. 2013), and can be attributed to its polymorph composition and control of synthesis parameters (Boyjoo, Pareek, and Liu 2014; Khalifehzadeh and Arami 2020). For drug delivery applications, spherical NPs are favorable as they possess the "highest possible specific surface area for loading drugs" (Khalifehzadeh and Arami 2020). However, studies have shown that CaC particle shapes with higher aspect ratios such as ellipsoids have a higher cellular uptake frequency (Bahrom et al. 2019). Similarly, Srivastav et al. used hollow HA nanotubes, which demonstrated higher loading capacity and cell uptake than nanospheres (Srivastav et al. 2019). Furthermore, NP shape has been shown to influence cytotoxicity and is dependent on the cell type. Zhao et al. showed that needle-shaped and plate-shaped HA NPs demonstrated the highest cytotoxicity in normal bronchial epithelial cells compared to spherical and rod-like morphologies. In contrast, leukemia cells exhibited less sensitivity and insignificant cytotoxic effects across all NP shapes (X. Zhao et al. 2013).

6.7.1.3 Biodegradation

Long-term in vivo toxic effects can result from the unwanted accumulation of specific inorganic NPs within cells and tissues (Mohammadpour et al. 2019). This issue can be avoided by using CaC and CaP nanomaterials as they can degrade into their respective ionic constituents upon cell internalization (Lauth, Maas, and Rezwan 2017; Motskin et al. 2009). The use of calcium-based NPs is also advantageous in that a broad spectrum of dissolution rates can be achieved by adjusting the composition of its crystallographic phases, thus lending itself to a variety of delivery applications (Lauth, Maas, and Rezwan 2017; Uskoković and Desai 2013). For example, a highly crystalline drug-loaded calcium-based nanocarrier that degrades slowly over time can be chosen to deliver a sustained release profile (Maleki Dizaj et al. 2017). On the other hand, it may be desirable to use amorphous phases of CaCs or CaPs, which typically demonstrate higher dissolution rates to deliver drugs that are insoluble in aqueous solutions with greater efficiency (Xia Guo et al. 2018; R. Sun, Zhang, et al. 2018).

A unique feature of both CaC and CaP NPs is that they exhibit a pH-dependent degradation profile. At a physiological pH of 7.4, CaC (Dunuweera and Rajapakse 2017) and CaP NPs (Uskoković and Desai 2013) demonstrate limited solubility and correspondingly lower drug release levels. However, at lower pH values of less than 6.5, both exhibit a faster degradation and greater cumulative drug release (Dunuweera and Rajapakse 2017; Hammadi et al. 2017; Y. He et al. 2017; Rao et al. 2020; Svenskaya et al. 2013; N.-n. Zhang et al. 2018). However, it should be noted that the dissolution of both CaC and CaP NPs over time involves the transition of different phases. This can significantly alter their dissolution profile and thus release rate (Svenskaya et al. 2013).

6.7.1.4 Zeta Potential and Surface Charge

The zeta potential (ZP) of an NP is a crucial parameter that must be considered when designing a DDS. The zeta potential refers to the electrical potential measured at the slipping or shear plane, located at the interface between the diffuse layer and the liquid surrounding a mobile NP, and also gives insight into its surface charge (Bhattacharjee 2016; Xu 2008). Ideally, an NP for drug delivery should have a low positive zeta potential to prolong its blood circulation time, minimize the likelihood of clearance by the RES, and enhance cellular internalization by promoting electrostatic attractions between the anionic cell membrane (Duan and Li 2013). CaC and CaP nanomaterials inherently possess a negative zeta potential and surface charge (Chemmalar et al. 2021; H. Wu et al. 2019). However, the effect of zeta potential on cell internalization of these calcium-based NPs depends on the cell type. Chen et al. found that the internalization efficiency of surface-modified HA NPs in osteoblasts was significantly higher for positively charged NPs in comparison to negatively charged NPs (Liang Chen et al. 2011). In contrast, negatively charged CaC (Bai et al. 2017; Hammadi et al. 2017; C. Wang, Chen, et al. 2020) and CaP (Y. Sun et al. 2016; H. Wu et al. 2019; V.M. Wu, Mickens, and Uskoković 2017) NPs can be effectively internalized by various cancer cell types.

The surface charge of a NP also affects the binding affinity of the drug, affecting its ZP (Honary and Zahir 2013). Wu et al. showed that the ZPs and points of zero charge of drug-loaded HA NPs depended on the affinity of the binding drugs to either the phosphate anion or calcium cation on the NP's surface (V.M. Wu, Mickens, and Uskoković 2017). Finally, the release profile of a drug can be regulated by its ZP. Elbaz et al. fabricated curcumin-loaded CaC NP cores coated with multiple alternating layers of electrolytes of different zeta potentials, which demonstrated unique pH-dependent release profiles of curcumin for achieving targeted drug delivery to the stomach or small intestine (Elbaz et al. 2020). Other approaches for modifying the NP surface, such as PEGylation (Ramachandran, Paul, and Sharma 2009) and using charge-reversible coatings (R.-Q. Cai et al. 2017), have also shown promising results in tailoring the ZP of CaP NP delivery vehicles to improve tissue and intracellular targeting.

6.7.2 Drug Delivery Applications

6.7.2.1 *Cancer Therapies*

One of the most promising uses of porous calcium-based NPs is the delivery of drugs and biomolecules to treat various cancer types (Khalifehzadeh and Arami 2020; Maleki Dizaj et al. 2015). A myriad of chemotherapeutic drugs such as adriamycin (Bai et al. 2017), cisplatin (Dunuweera and Rajapakse 2017; P. Zhao, Li, et al. 2019), curcumin (Rao et al. 2020), docetaxel (Hammadi et al. 2017), doxorubicin (Srivastav et al. 2019; W. Sun, Fan, et al. 2018; N.-n. Zhang et al. 2018; Choukrani et al. 2020), gefitinib (Chemmalar et al. 2021), mitoxantrone (C. Wang, Han, et al. 2019), and paclitaxel (Chemmalar et al. 2021; Srivastav et al. 2019), as well as photosensitizers used for photodynamic therapy (Dong et al. 2018; Svenskaya et al. 2013), have been successfully loaded onto calcium-based NPs and demonstrated potent antitumor effects. Drug-loaded CaC (Bai et al. 2017; C. Wang, Han, et al. 2019; P. Zhao, Li, et al. 2019) and CaP NPs (W. Sun, Fan, et al. 2018; N.-n. Zhang et al. 2018) have demonstrated antitumor efficacy in several in vivo studies. Sun et al. fabricated doxorubicin-encapsulated HA nanorods and found that those with a folic acid surface coating showed improved tumor site targeting, as the average tumor volume in mice only increased by 2.5-fold in comparison to a 10-fold increase when free doxorubicin was administered without any delivery vehicle (W. Sun, Fan, et al. 2018). The utility of other biomolecules such as siRNA (R.-Q. Cai et al. 2017; C. Qiu et al. 2016) and peptides (W. Sun, Fan, et al. 2018; N.-n. Zhang et al. 2018) has also been explored for treating cancer.

Tumor microenvironments are typically acidic with a pH between 6.0 and 7.0, whereas normal physiological tissue has an extracellular pH of 7.4 (Dai et al. 2017). As a result, the pH-triggered decomposition of CaC and CaP NPs can be leveraged for cancer therapies (Elbaz et al. 2020; Som et al. 2016; Yazdian-Robati et al. 2019). In a recent study by Chemmalar et al., gefitinib and paclitaxel were adsorbed onto CaC NPs derived from cockle shells (Chemmalar et al. 2021). In vitro studies showed that the highest cumulative drug release concentration and highest alkalinization occurred in the lowest pH environment ($pH=5.6$) compared to higher pH values of 6.5 and 7.4. These results suggested that CaC NPs could provide enhanced targeting for greater drug release in a tumor microenvironment and reduce metastatic potential by increasing the extracellular pH. Research into the development of multifunctional calcium-based NPs has also recently gained traction. Delivering therapeutic agents, such NPs can act as magnetic resonance contrast agents for in vivo imaging (Dong et al. 2018; N.-n. Zhang et al. 2018), or facilitate magnetically targeted tumor drug delivery and provide highly localized thermo-chemotherapy (Choukrani et al. 2020).

6.7.2.2 Treatment of Musculoskeletal Disorders

CaP NPs are frequently utilized as nanovehicles to deliver drugs and biomolecules for the enhanced treatment of musculoskeletal diseases and promote bone regeneration. Bisphosphonates, such as alendronate (R. Sun et al. 2020) and zoledronate (Khajuria, Razdan, and Mahapatra 2015), are drugs used to treat osteoporosis by attenuating bone loss. An *in vivo* study by Khajuria et al. showed that the mechanical properties and microstructural integrity of the bones of osteoporosis-induced, ovariectomized rats were consistently higher in rats that received zoledronate-loaded HA NPs as compared to those which received an intravenous injection of pure zoledronate (Khajuria, Razdan, and Mahapatra 2015). Studies have also showed that CaP can be used to deliver anti-inflammatory drugs (Madhumathi et al. 2018; Mostafa et al. 2015) and antibiotics to treat bacterial infections (Madhumathi et al. 2018; Munir et al. 2018), such as osteomyelitis and periodontitis, that can lead to the destruction of bone tissue.

Rheumatoid arthritis is a chronic inflammatory autoimmune disease characterized by inflammation, swelling, and pain in the body's joints due to synovitis (Dolati et al. 2016). CaP NPs have been explored as delivery vehicles for antirheumatic drugs such as methotrexate and teriflunomide (Pandey et al. 2021), and corticosteroids such as methylprednisolone acetate (Jafari et al. 2016) in arthritic rat models. The histopathological analyses of rat knee joints revealed that the developed drug-loaded HA nanoformulations in the respective studies reduced cellular infiltration and joint inflammation, and markedly improved joint regeneration compared to pure or commercially available drugs (Pandey et al. 2021; Jafari et al. 2016).

6.7.2.3 Tissue Engineering

CaP NPs have been incorporated into scaffolds, particularly for BTE applications to deliver a range of cargo, including drugs, proteins, and genes. DEX is a drug capable of inducing the osteogenic differentiation of mesenchymal stem cells (Y. Chen, Li, et al. 2017). Chen et al. incorporated biphasic CaP NPs loaded with DEX into porous collagen scaffolds, which showed excellent bone regeneration *in vivo* (Y. Chen, Kawazoe, and Chen 2018). Qiu et al. found that the engineered silk fibroin/chitosan scaffolds containing porous, BMP-2-loaded nano-HA particles exhibited a sustained release of the protein and facilitated higher alkaline phosphatase activity and bone mineral deposition as compared to the scaffold with BMP-2 that was directly adsorbed on its surface displaying a burst release (Y. Qiu et al. 2020). Plasmid DNA loaded onto CaP NPs can also be used to transfect stem cells to express growth factors and proteins to cause chondrogenic (Gonzalez-Fernandez et al. 2016) and osteogenic differentiation (J.E. Lee et al. 2019). Consideration should also be given to the fundamental design of the nanomaterial platform, including its shape and size, to take advantage of any synergistic effects, as it has been found that porous CaC NPs with a fusiform morphology significantly promoted higher osteogenesis of mesenchymal stem cells compared to rhombohedron-like NPs (Xiaoning Li et al. 2018).

6.7.2.4 Other Applications

The feasibility of using CaC and CaP NPs to administer drugs with ease using unconventional methods has gained significant interest. Such examples include the oral delivery of insulin to treat diabetes (Ramachandran, Paul, and Sharma 2009; A. Verma et al. 2016) and cancer drugs for targeted delivery in the intestine to treat colon cancer (Elbaz et al. 2020), and the transdermal delivery of colchicine to treat gout (Zeng et al. 2021). Researchers have also investigated the therapeutic potential of calcium-based NPs for tackling other incurable diseases such as amyotrophic lateral sclerosis, a highly debilitating neurodegenerative disease affecting the brain and spinal cord's motor neurons that result in loss of muscle control and functionality. Lipid-coated CaP encapsulating the antisense oligonucleotide of superoxide dismutase I has demonstrated promising capabilities in targeting zebrafish's brain and spinal cord; however, future studies in small animal models will need to be conducted for further validation (Liyu Chen, Watson, et al. 2017).

6.8 CONCLUDING REMARKS

CaCs and CaPs-based materials are promising DDSs due to their inherent biocompatibility, bioactivity, porosity, and biodegradability in physiological conditions. They have been used successfully for various drug delivery applications in the form of macroscale (i.e., scaffolds, injectable cements), microscale (i.e., microspheres, coatings), and nanoscale (i.e., NPs, particulate systems) constructs. The last decade has witnessed an outstanding progression in manipulating these carrier systems to achieve not only targeted drug delivery, but controlled and sustained drug release, reducing systemic side effects of particularly toxic drugs and even reducing their required dosage. Indeed, recent advances have proven the utility of CaC and CaP as carriers for cancer therapies such as chemotherapy and radionuclide therapy, minimizing healthy cell death while only targeting diseased tissue through environmental sensitivity (i.e., pH, temperature). CaP drug delivery constructs have focused predominantly on bone tissue applications due to their close resemblance to native bone and their osteogenic properties. Next-generation bone scaffolds of CaP have shown local delivery of biomolecules to help bone regeneration, fight recurrent infections, and treat osteosarcomas. Ultimately, CaC and CaP demonstrate versatility in drug loading, with applications ranging from hemorrhage control, insulin delivery, and treatment of fungal skin infections. Future advances in this area include developing novel, multifunctional micro- and nano-constructs that can deliver drugs and serve other applications, including contrast agents for in vivo imaging and regenerative medicine. Dual-drug delivery models have also been investigated and show encouraging applications in treating diseases located in hostile environments within the body. The potential use of porous CaC and CaP as drug carriers and their clinical translation remains both a challenge and a promising future consideration for many biomedical applications.

REFERENCES

Abe, Tetsuya, Masataka Sakane, Toshiyuki Ikoma, Mihoko Kobayashi, Satoshi Nakamura, and Naoyuki Ochiai. 2008. "Intraosseous delivery of paclitaxel-loaded hydroxyapatitealginate composite beads delaying paralysis caused by metastatic spine cancer in rats." *Journal of Neurosurgery: Spine* 9 (5): 502–510.

Abeywardena, M.R., R.K.W.H.M.K. Elkaduwe, D.G.G.P. Karunarathne, H.M.T.G.A. Pitawala, R.M.G. Rajapakse, A. Manipura, and M.M.M.G.P.G. Mantilaka. 2020. "Surfactant assisted synthesis of precipitated calcium carbonate nanoparticles using dolomite: Effect of pH on morphology and particle size." *Advanced Powder Technology* 31(1): 269–278.

Addadi, Lia, Sefi Raz, and Steve Weiner. 2003. "Taking advantage of disorder: amorphous calcium carbonate and its roles in biomineralization." *Advanced Materials* 15(12): 959–970.

Asadollahzadeh, Morteza, Sayed Mahmood Rabiee, and Hamed Salimi-Kenari. 2019. "In vitro apatite formation of calcium phosphate composite synthesized from fish bone." *International Journal of Applied Ceramic Technology* 16(5): 1969–1978.

Ataol, Sibel, Ayşen Tezcaner, Ozgur Duygulu, Dilek Keskin, and Nesrin E. Machin. 2015. "Synthesis and characterization of nanosized calcium phosphates by flame spray pyrolysis, and their effect on osteogenic differentiation of stem cells." *Journal of Nanoparticle Research* 17(2): 1–14.

Auría-Soro, Carlota, Tabata Nesma, Pablo Juanes-Velasco, Alicia Landeira-Viñuela, Helena Fidalgo-Gomez, Vanessa Acebes-Fernandez, Rafael Gongora, María Jesus Almendral Parra, Raúl Manzano-Roman, and Manuel Fuentes. 2019. "Interactions of nanoparticles and biosystems: microenvironment of nanoparticles and biomolecules in nanomedicine." *Nanomaterials* 9 (10): 1365.

Azevedo, Cláudia, Maria Helena Macedo, and Bruno Sarmento. 2018. "Strategies for the enhanced intracellular delivery of nanomaterials." *Drug Discovery Today* 23 (5): 944–959.

Baeza, Alejandro, Daniel Ruiz-Molina, and María Vallet-Regí. 2017. "Recent advances in porous nanoparticles for drug delivery in antitumoral applications: inorganic nanoparticles and nanoscale metal-organic frameworks." *Expert Opinion on Drug Delivery* 14(6): 783–796.

Bahrom, Hani, Alexander A. Goncharenko, Landysh I. Fatkhutdinova, Oleksii O. Peltek, Albert R. Muslimov, Olga Yu Koval, Igor E. Eliseev, Andrey Manchev, Dmitry Gorin, and Ivan I. Shishkin. 2019. "Controllable synthesis of calcium carbonate with different geometry: Comprehensive analysis of particle formation, cellular uptake, and biocompatibility." *ACS Sustainable Chemistry & Engineering* 7(23): 19142–19156.

Bai, Jinghui, Jian Xu, Jian Zhao, and Rui Zhang. 2017. "Hyaluronan and calcium carbonate hybrid nanoparticles for colorectal cancer chemotherapy." *Materials Research Express* 4 (9): 095401.

Baroli, Biancamaria. 2009. "From natural bone grafts to tissue engineering therapeutics: brainstorming on pharmaceutical formulative requirements and challenges." *Journal of Pharmaceutical Sciences* 98 (4): 1317–1375.

Bhat, Shrinath, U.T. Uthappa, Tariq Altalhi, Ho-Young Jung, and Mahaveer D. Kurkuri. 2021. "Functionalized porous hydroxyapatite scaffolds for tissue engineering applications: A focused review." *ACS Biomaterials Science & Engineering.*

Bhattacharjee, Sourav. 2016. "DLS and zeta potential–what they are and what they are not?" *Journal of Controlled Release* 235: 337–351.

Bose, Susmita, and Solaiman Tarafder. 2012. "Calcium phosphate ceramic systems in growth factor and drug delivery for bone tissue engineering: A review." *Acta Biomaterialia* 8 (4): 1401–1421.

Boyjoo, Yash, Vishnu K. Pareek, and Jian Liu. 2014. "Synthesis of micro and nano-sized calcium carbonate particles and their applications." *Journal of Materials Chemistry A* 2(35): 14270–14288.

Cai, An-Yong, Ying-Jie Zhu, and Chao Qi. 2020. "Biodegradable inorganic nanostructured biomaterials for drug delivery." *Advanced Materials Interfaces* 7(20): 2000819.

Cai, Rong-Qiao, Dao-Zhou Liu, Han Cui, Ying Cheng, Miao Liu, Bang-Le Zhang, Qi-Bing Mei, and Si-Yuan Zhou. 2017. "Charge reversible calcium phosphate lipid hybrid nanoparticle for siRNA delivery." *Oncotarget* 8 (26): 42772.

Cai, Wen-Yi, Qin Xu, Xiao-Ning Zhao, Jun-Jie Zhu, and Hong-Yuan Chen. 2006. "Porous gold-nanoparticle–$CaCO_3$ hybrid material: preparation, characterization, and application for horseradish peroxidase assembly and direct electrochemistry." *Chemistry of materials* 18 (2): 279–284.

Cai, Yurong, Yukan Liu, Weiqi Yan, Qinghong Hu, Jinhui Tao, Ming Zhang, Zhongli Shi, and Ruikang Tang. 2007. "Role of hydroxyapatite nanoparticle size in bone cell proliferation." *Journal of Materials Chemistry* 17 (36): 3780–3787.

Canillas, Maria, Pilar Pena, H. Antonio, and Miguel A. Rodríguez. 2017. "Calcium phosphates for biomedical applications." *Boletín de la Sociedad Española de Cerámica y Vidrio* 56(3): 91–112.

Cao, Xing, Lingjun Dai, Shichang Sun, Rui Ma, and Xiangli Liu. 2021. "Preparation and performance of porous hydroxyapatite/poly (lactic-co-glycolic acid) drug-loaded microsphere scaffolds for gentamicin sulfate delivery." *Journal of Materials Science* 56(27): 15278–15298.

Carragee, Eugene J., Eric L. Hurwitz, and Bradley K. Weiner. 2011. "A critical review of recombinant human bone morphogenetic protein-2 trials in spinal surgery: Emerging safety concerns and lessons learned." *The Spine Journal* 11(6): 471–491.

Chemmalar, S., Abdul Razak Intan-Shameha, Che Azurahanim Che Abdullah, Nor Asma Ab Razak, Loqman Mohamad Yusof, Mokrish Ajat, N.S.K. Gowthaman, and Md Zuki Abu Bakar. 2021. "Synthesis and characterization of gefitinib and paclitaxel mono and dual drug-loaded blood cockle shells (Anadara granosa)-derived aragonite $CaCO_3$ nanoparticles." *Nanomaterials* 11(8): 1988.

Chen, Liang, Joseph M. Mccrate, James C.M. Lee, and Hao Li. 2011. "The role of surface charge on the uptake and biocompatibility of hydroxyapatite nanoparticles with osteoblast cells." *Nanotechnology* 22(10): 105708.

Chen, Liyu, Clare Watson, Marco Morsch, Nicholas J. Cole, Roger S. Chung, Darren N. Saunders, Justin J. Yerbury, and Kara L. Vine. 2017. "Improving the delivery of SOD1 antisense oligonucleotides to motor neurons using calcium phosphate-lipid nanoparticles." *Frontiers in Neuroscience* 11: 476.

Chen, Ying, Shangwu Chen, Naoki Kawazoe, and Guoping Chen. 2018. "Promoted angiogenesis and osteogenesis by dexamethasone-loaded calcium phosphate nanoparticles/collagen composite scaffolds with microgroove networks." *Scientific Reports* 8(1): 1–12.

Chen, Ying, Naoki Kawazoe, and Guoping Chen. 2018. "Preparation of dexamethasone-loaded biphasic calcium phosphate nanoparticles/collagen porous composite scaffolds for bone tissue engineering." *Acta Biomaterialia* 67: 341–353.

Chen, Ying, Jingchao Li, Naoki Kawazoe, and Guoping Chen. 2017. "Preparation of dexamethasone-loaded calcium phosphate nanoparticles for the osteogenic differentiation of human mesenchymal stem cells." *Journal of Materials Chemistry B* 5(33): 6801–6810.

Chernozem, Roman V., Maria A. Surmeneva, Anatolii A. Abalymov, Bogdan V. Parakhonskiy, Petra Rigole, Tom Coenye, Roman A. Surmenev, and Andre G. Skirtach. 2021. "Piezoelectric hybrid scaffolds mineralized with calcium carbonate for tissue engineering: Analysis of local enzyme and small-molecule drug delivery, cell response and antibacterial performance." *Materials Science and Engineering: C* 122: 111909.

Chou, Jenny Wen-Lin, Diane Decarie, Randall J. Dumont, and Mary H.H. Ensom. 2001. "Stability of dexamethasone in extemporaneously prepared oral suspensions." *The Canadian Journal of Hospital Pharmacy* 54 (2): 96–101.

Choukrani, Ghizlane, Bikendra Maharjan, Chan Hee Park, Cheol Sang Kim, and Arathyram Ramachandra Kurup Sasikala. 2020. "Biocompatible superparamagnetic sub-micron vaterite particles for thermo-chemotherapy: From controlled design to in vitro anticancer synergism." *Materials Science and Engineering: C* 106: 110226.

Collins, Maurice N., Guang Ren, Kieran Young, S. Pina, Rui L. Reis, and J. Miguel Oliveira. 2021. "Scaffold fabrication technologies and structure/function properties in bone tissue engineering." *Advanced Functional Materials* 31(21): 2010609.

Cui, Xinhui, Tong Liang, Changsheng Liu, Yuan Yuan, and Jiangchao Qian. 2016. "Correlation of particle properties with cytotoxicity and cellular uptake of hydroxyapatite nanoparticles in human gastric cancer cells." *Materials Science and Engineering: C* 67: 453–460.

da Silva, Rosane Vieira, Celso Aparecido Bertran, Elizabete Yoshie Kawachi, and José Angelo Camilli. 2007. "Repair of cranial bone defects with calcium phosphate ceramic implant or autogenous bone graft." *Journal of Craniofacial Surgery* 18 (2): 281–286.

Dai, Yunlu, Can Xu, Xiaolian Sun, and Xiaoyuan Chen. 2017. "Nanoparticle design strategies for enhanced anticancer therapy by exploiting the tumour microenvironment." *Chemical Society Reviews* 46 (12): 3830–3852.

Dolati, Sanam, Sanam Sadreddini, Davoud Rostamzadeh, Majid Ahmadi, Farhad Jadidi-Niaragh, and Mehdi Yousefi. 2016. "Utilization of nanoparticle technology in rheumatoid arthritis treatment." *Biomedicine & Pharmacotherapy* 80: 30–41.

Dong, Ziliang, Liangzhu Feng, Yu Hao, Muchao Chen, Min Gao, Yu Chao, He Zhao, Wenwen Zhu, Jingjing Liu, and Chao Liang. 2018. "Synthesis of hollow biomineralized $CaCO_3$–polydopamine nanoparticles for multimodal imaging-guided cancer photodynamic therapy with reduced skin photosensitivity." *Journal of the American Chemical Society* 140 (6): 2165–2178.

Dorozhkin, Sergey V. 2012. "Biphasic, triphasic and multiphasic calcium orthophosphates." *Acta Biomaterialia* 8 (3): 963–977.

Duan, Xiaopin, and Yaping Li. 2013. "Physicochemical characteristics of nanoparticles affect circulation, biodistribution, cellular internalization, and trafficking." *Small* 9 (9–10): 1521–1532.

Dunuweera, S.P., and R.M.G. Rajapakse. 2017. "Encapsulation of anticancer drug cisplatin in vaterite polymorph of calcium carbonate nanoparticles for targeted delivery and slow release." *Biomedical Physics & Engineering Express* 4 (1): 015017.

El-Sheikh, S.M., S. El-Sherbiny, A. Barhoum, and Yulin Deng. 2013. "Effects of cationic surfactant during the precipitation of calcium carbonate nanoparticles on their size, morphology, and other characteristics." *Colloids and Surfaces A: Physicochemical and Engineering Aspects* 422: 44–49.

El-Toni, Ahmed Mohamed, Mohamed A. Habila, Joselito Puzon Labis, Zeid A. ALOthman, Mansour Alhoshan, Ahmed A. Elzatahry, and Fan Zhang. 2016. "Design, synthesis and applications of core–shell, hollow core, and nanorattle multifunctional nanostructures." *Nanoscale* 8 (5): 2510–2531.

Elbaz, Nancy M., Andrew Owen, Steve Rannard, and Tom O. McDonald. 2020. "Controlled synthesis of calcium carbonate nanoparticles and stimuli-responsive multi-layered nanocapsules for oral drug delivery." *International Journal of Pharmaceutics* 574: 118866.

Eltom, Abdalla, Gaoyan Zhong, and Ameen Muhammad. 2019. "Scaffold techniques and designs in tissue engineering functions and purposes: A review." *Advances in Materials Science and Engineering* 2019. https://doi.org/10.1155/2019/3429527.

Fadia, Preksha, Simona Tyagi, Stuti Bhagat, Abhishek Nair, Pooja Panchal, Harsh Dave, Sadev Dang, and Sanjay Singh. 2021. "Calcium carbonate nano-and microparticles: synthesis methods and biological applications." *3 Biotech* 11(-11): 1–30.

Gonzalez-Fernandez, Tomas, Erica G. Tierney, Grainne M. Cunniffe, Fergal J. O'Brien, and Daniel J. Kelly. 2016. "Gene delivery of TGF-β3 and BMP2 in an MSC-laden alginate hydrogel for articular cartilage and endochondral bone tissue engineering." *Tissue Engineering Part A* 22 (9–10): 776–787.

Gudkov, Sergey V., Natalya Yu Shilyagina, Vladimir A. Vodeneev, and Andrei V. Zvyagin. 2016. "Targeted radionuclide therapy of human tumors." *International Journal of Molecular Sciences* 17(1): 33.

Guicheux, Jérôme, Olivier Gauthier, Eric Aguado, Paul Pilet, Séverine Couillaud, Dominique Jegou, Guy Daculsi, and Dominique Heymann. 1998. "Human growth hormone locally released in bone sites by calcium-phosphate biomaterial stimulates ceramic bone substitution without systemic effects: A rabbit study." *Journal of Bone and Mineral Research* 13 (4): 739–748.

Guo, Xia, Wenfeng Li, Heping Wang, Yan-Ying Fan, Huifang Wang, Xianghua Gao, Baolong Niu, and Xuechen Gong. 2018. "Preparation, characterization, release and antioxidant activity of curcumin-loaded amorphous calcium phosphate nanoparticles." *Journal of Non-Crystalline Solids* 500: 317–325.

Guo, Xiaojun, Hudong Yan, Shengguo Zhao, Zhang Li, Yutian Li, and Xiaohu Liang. 2013. "Effect of calcining temperature on particle size of hydroxyapatite synthesized by solid-state reaction at room temperature." *Advanced Powder Technology* 24 (6): 1034–1038.

Guo, Ya-Jun, Ying-Ying Wang, Ting Chen, Yi-Ting Wei, Lian-Feng Chu, and Ya-Ping Guo. 2013. "Hollow carbonated hydroxyapatite microspheres with mesoporous structure: hydrothermal fabrication and drug delivery property." *Materials Science and Engineering: C* 33 (6): 3166–3172.

Gusliakova, Olga, Roman Verkhovskii, Anatolii Abalymov, Ekaterina Lengert, Anastasiia Kozlova, Vsevolod Atkin, Olga Nechaeva, Anna Morrison, Valery Tuchin, and Yulia Svenskaya. 2021. "Transdermal platform for the delivery of the antifungal drug naftifine hydrochloride based on porous vaterite particles." *Materials Science and Engineering: C* 119: 111428.

Haddad, Albert J., Sean A.F. Peel, Cameron M.L. Clokie, and George K.B. Sándor. 2006. "Closure of rabbit calvarial critical-sized defects using protective composite allogeneic and alloplastic bone substitutes." *Journal of Craniofacial Surgery* 17(5): 926–934.

Hammadi, Nahidah Ibrahim, Yusuf Abba, Mohd Noor Mohd Hezmee, Intan Shameha Abdul Razak, Alhaji Zubair Jaji, Tijani Isa, Saffanah Khuder Mahmood, and Md Zuki Abu Bakar Zakaria. 2017. "Formulation of a sustained release docetaxel loaded cockle shell-derived calcium carbonate nanoparticles against breast cancer." *Pharmaceutical Research* 34 (6): 1193–1203.

Hassan, Tarig A., Vijay K. Rangari, Rohit K. Rana, and Shaik Jeelani. 2013. "Sonochemical effect on size reduction of $CaCO_3$ nanoparticles derived from waste eggshells." *Ultrasonics Sonochemistry* 20(5): 1308–1315.

He, Jian, Zhidong Lin, Xulin Hu, Luyao Xing, Gaofeng Liang, Dongliang Chen, Junling An, Chengdong Xiong, Xiangchun Zhang, and Lifang Zhang. 2021. "Biocompatible and biodegradable scaffold based on polytrimethylene carbonate-tricalcium phosphate microspheres for tissue engineering." *Colloids and Surfaces B: Biointerfaces* 204: 111808.

He, Jian, Yu Zhang, Xiaoyi Liu, Huiling Li, Chengdong Xiong, and Lifang Zhang. 2020. "Load-bearing PTMC-beta tri-calcium phosphate and dexamethasone biphasic composite microsphere scaffolds for bone tissue engineering." *Materials Letters* 260: 126939.

He, Yongju, Bowen Zeng, Shuquan Liang, Mengqiu Long, and Hui Xu. 2017. "Synthesis of pH-responsive biodegradable mesoporous silica–calcium phosphate hybrid nanoparticles as a high potential drug carrier." *ACS Applied Materials & Interfaces* 9 (51): 44402–44409.

Honary, Soheyla, and Foruhe Zahir. 2013. "Effect of zeta potential on the properties of nano-drug delivery systems-a review (Part 2)." *Tropical Journal of Pharmaceutical Research* 12 (2): 265–273.

Honda, M., Y. Kawanobe, H. Uchida, and M. Aizawa. 2017. "Inhibition of Bacterial Adhesion using Calcium Phosphate Microspheres Loaded with Protamine." *International Journal of Metallurgical and Materials Engineering* 3 (136): 2455–2372.

Horie, Masanori, Keiko Nishio, Haruhisa Kato, Shigehisa Endoh, Katsuhide Fujita, Ayako Nakamura, Shinichi Kinugasa, Yoshihisa Hagihara, Yasukazu Yoshida, and Hitoshi Iwahashi. 2014. "Evaluation of cellular influences caused by calcium carbonate nanoparticles." *Chemico-Biological Interactions* 210: 64–76.

Hossain, Kazi M Zakir, Uresha Patel, and Ifty Ahmed. 2015. "Development of microspheres for biomedical applications: A review." *Progress in Biomaterials* 4 (1): 1–19.

Hu, Jianping, Yingying Jiang, Shuo Tan, Kunpeng Zhu, Tao Cai, Taicheng Zhan, Shisheng He, Feng Chen, and Chunlin Zhang. 2021. "Selenium-doped calcium phosphate biomineral reverses multidrug resistance to enhance bone tumor chemotherapy." *Nanomedicine: Nanotechnology, Biology and Medicine* 32: 102322.

Huber, Matthias, Wendelin J. Stark, Stefan Loher, Marek Maciejewski, Frank Krumeich, and Alfons Baiker. 2005. "Flame synthesis of calcium carbonate nanoparticles." *Chemical Communications* 5: 648–650. https://doi.org/10.1039/b411725e.

Idris, Sherifat Banke, A. Arifah, F. Jesse, S. Ramanoon, M. Basit, Z. Zakaria, and M.Z.A.B. Zakaria. 2019. "Synthesis, characterization, and in vitro release of oxytetracycline loaded in pH-responsive $CaCO_3$ nanoparticles." *Journal of Applied Pharmaceutical Science* 9: 019–027.

Itokazu, Mansho, Tadashi Sugiyama, Takatoshi Ohno, Eiji Wada, and Yoshihiro Katagiri. 1998. "Development of porous apatite ceramic for local delivery of chemotherapeutic agents." *Journal of Biomedical Materials Research: An Official Journal of The Society for Biomaterials, The Japanese Society for Biomaterials, and the Australian Society for Biomaterials* 39 (4): 536–538.

Jafari, Samira, Nasrin Maleki-Dizaji, Jaleh Barar, Mohammad Barzegar-Jalali, Maryam Rameshrad, and Khosro Adibkia. 2016. "Methylprednisolone acetate-loaded hydroxyapatite nanoparticles as a potential drug delivery system for treatment of rheumatoid arthritis: In vitro and in vivo evaluations." *European Journal of Pharmaceutical Sciences* 91: 225–235.

Jia, Jilei, Qi Liu, Tingyuan Yang, Lianyan Wang, and Guanghui Ma. 2017. "Facile fabrication of varisized calcium carbonate microspheres as vaccine adjuvants." *Journal of Materials Chemistry B* 5 (8): 1611–1623.

Jiao, Mingxia, Peisen Zhang, Junli Meng, Yingying Li, Chunyan Liu, Xiliang Luo, and Mingyuan Gao. 2018. "Recent advancements in biocompatible inorganic nanoparticles towards biomedical applications." *Biomaterials Science* 6 (4): 726–745.

Kapate, Neha, John R. Clegg, and Samir Mitragotri. 2021. "Non-spherical micro- and nanoparticles for drug delivery: Progress over 15 years." *Advanced Drug Delivery Reviews* 177: 113807.

Karacan, Ipek, Besim Ben-Nissan, and Sutinee Sinutok. 2019. "Marine-based calcium phosphates from hard coral and calcified algae for biomedical applications." In Choi, A., and Ben-Nissan, B. (eds.) *Marine-Derived Biomaterials for Tissue Engineering Applications*, 137–153. Springer, Singapore.

Kassis, Amin I. 2008. "Therapeutic radionuclides: Biophysical and radiobiologic principles." *Seminars in Nuclear Medicine* 38(5):358–66.

Khajuria, Deepak Kumar, Rema Razdan, and Debiprosad Roy Mahapatra. 2015. "Development, in vitro and in vivo characterization of zoledronic acid functionalized hydroxyapatite nanoparticle based formulation for treatment of osteoporosis in animal model." *European Journal of Pharmaceutical Sciences* 66: 173–183.

Khalifehzadeh, Razieh, and Hamed Arami. 2020. "Biodegradable calcium phosphate nanoparticles for cancer therapy." *Advances in Colloid and Interface Science* 279: 102157.

Kim, Dong-Hyun, Ho Hwan Chun, Ju Dong Lee, and Seog-Young Yoon. 2014. "Evaluation of phase transformation behavior in biphasic calcium phosphate with controlled spherical micro-granule architecture." *Ceramics International* 40 (4): 5145–5155.

Kim, Jong Min, Tae Sung Han, Myoung Hwan Kim, Daniel S. Oh, Seong Soo Kang, Gonhyung Kim, Tae-Yub Kwon, Kyo-Han Kim, Kyu-Bok Lee, and Jun Sik Son. 2012. "Osteogenic evaluation of calcium phosphate scaffold with drug-loaded poly (lactic-co-glycolic acid) microspheres in beagle dogs." *Tissue Engineering and Regenerative Medicine* 9 (3): 175–183.

Kim, Sang Kyoon, Michael B. Foote, and Leaf Huang. 2013. "Targeted delivery of EV peptide to tumor cell cytoplasm using lipid coated calcium carbonate nanoparticles." *Cancer Letters* 334 (2): 311–318.

Kim, Sung Eun, Young-Pil Yun, Deok-Won Lee, Eun Young Kang, Won Jae Jeong, Boram Lee, Myeong Seon Jeong, Hak Jun Kim, Kyeongsoon Park, and Hae-Ryong Song. 2015. "Alendronate-eluting biphasic calcium phosphate (BCP) scaffolds stimulate osteogenic differentiation." *BioMed Research International* 2015: 320713.

Konopacka-Łyskawa, Donata. 2019. "Synthesis methods and favorable conditions for spherical vaterite precipitation: A review." *Crystals* 9 (4): 223.

Langer, Robert. 1998. "Drug delivery and targeting." *Nature* 392 (6679 Suppl): 5–10.

Lauth, V., M. Maas, and K. Rezwan. 2017. "An evaluation of colloidal and crystalline properties of $CaCO_3$ nanoparticles for biological applications." *Materials Science and Engineering: C* 78: 305–314.

Lee, Jung Eun, Yue Yin, Su Yeon Lim, E. Seul Kim, Jaeback Jung, Dahwun Kim, Ji Won Park, Min Sang Lee, and Ji Hoon Jeong. 2019. "Enhanced transfection of human mesenchymal stem cells using a hyaluronic acid/calcium phosphate hybrid gene delivery system." *Polymers* 11 (5): 798.

Lee, Soo-Hong, and Heungsoo Shin. 2007. "Matrices and scaffolds for delivery of bioactive molecules in bone and cartilage tissue engineering." *Advanced Drug Delivery Reviews* 59 (4–5): 339–359.

Li, Li, Yang Yang, Yirui Lv, Ping Yin, and Ting Lei. 2020. "Porous calcite $CaCO_3$ microspheres: Preparation, characterization and release behavior as doxorubicin carrier." *Colloids and Surfaces B: Biointerfaces* 186: 110720.

Li, Xianghui, Zhiqiang Zhang, Zhenhuan Guo, Xia Ma, Xueting Ban, Xinghui Song, Yonglu Liu, Li Zhao, Qiqi Liu, and Qigai He. 2021. "Acanthopanax senticosus polysaccharide-loaded calcium carbonate nanoparticle as an adjuvant to enhance porcine parvovirus vaccine immune responses." *Medicine in Drug Discovery* 11: 100094.

Li, Xiaoning, Xing Yang, Xujie Liu, Wei He, Qianli Huang, Shengrong Li, and Qingling Feng. 2018. "Calcium carbonate nanoparticles promote osteogenesis compared to adipogenesis in human bone-marrow mesenchymal stem cells." *Progress in Natural Science: Materials International* 28 (5): 598–608.

Lin, Kaili, Chengtie Wu, and Jiang Chang. 2014. "Advances in synthesis of calcium phosphate crystals with controlled size and shape." *Acta Biomaterialia* 10 (10): 4071–4102.

Liu, Depeng, Guohua Jiang, Weijiang Yu, Lei Li, Zaizai Tong, Xiangdong Kong, and Juming Yao. 2017. "Oral delivery of insulin using $CaCO_3$-based composite nanocarriers with hyaluronic acid coatings." *Materials Letters* 188: 263–266.

Liu, Jun-Feng, Lu Wei, Dilixiati Duolikun, Xiao-Dong Hou, Feng Chen, Jun-Jian Liu, and Long-Po Zheng. 2018. "Preparation of porous calcium phosphate microspheres with phosphate-containing molecules at room temperature for drug delivery and osteogenic differentiation.". *RSC Advances* 8 (45): 25480–25488.

Liu, Shih-Ming, Wen-Cheng Chen, Chia-Ling Ko, Hsu-Ting Chang, Ya-Shun Chen, Ssu-Meng Haung, Kai-Chi Chang, and Jian-Chih Chen. 2021. "In vitro evaluation of calcium phosphate bone cement composite hydrogel beads of cross-linked gelatin-alginate with gentamicin-impregnated porous scaffold." *Pharmaceuticals* 14(10): 1000.

Liu, Xujie, Xiaoning Li, Ranran Zhang, Liping Wang, and Qingling Feng. 2021. "A novel dual microsphere based on water-soluble thiolated chitosan/mesoporous calcium carbonate for controlled dual drug delivery." *Materials Letters* 285: 29142.

Liu, Zhenguang, Lin Yu, Pengfei Gu, Ruonan Bo, Adelijiang Wusiman, Jiaguo Liu, Yuanliang Hu, and Deyun Wang. 2020. "Preparation of lentinan-calcium carbonate microspheres and their application as vaccine adjuvants." *Carbohydrate Polymers* 245: 116520.

Luginbuehl, Vera, Esther Wenk, Annette Koch, Bruno Gander, Hans P. Merkle, and Lorenz Meinel. 2005. "Insulin-like growth factor I—Releasing alginate-tricalciumphosphate composites for bone regeneration." *Pharmaceutical Research* 22(6): 940–950.

Ma, Xiaomin, Zhe Sun, Wen Su, Zeng Yi, Xinxing Cui, Bo Guo, and Xudong Li. 2018. "Biologically inspired, catechol-coordinated, hierarchical organization of raspberry-like calcium phosphate nanospheres with high specific surface area." *Journal of Materials Chemistry B* 6 (22): 3811–3819.

Ma, Xiaoyu, Yaying Chen, Jiangchao Qian, Yuan Yuan, and Changsheng Liu. 2016. "Controllable synthesis of spherical hydroxyapatite nanoparticles using inverse microemulsion method." *Materials Chemistry and Physics* 183: 220–229.

Madhumathi, K., Y. Rubaiya, Mukesh Doble, R. Venkateswari, and T.S. Sampath Kumar. 2018. "Antibacterial, anti-inflammatory, and bone-regenerative dual-drug-loaded calcium phosphate nanocarriers—in vitro and in vivo studies." *Drug Delivery and Translational Research* 8 (5): 1066–1077.

Mahale, Manisha M., and R.B. Saudagar. 2019. "Microsphere: A review." *Journal of drug Delivery and Therapeutics* 9 (3-s): 854–856.

Maleki Dizaj, Solmaz, Mohammad Barzegar-Jalali, Mohammad Hossein Zarrintan, Khosro Adibkia, and Farzaneh Lotfipour. 2015. "Calcium carbonate nanoparticles as cancer drug delivery system." *Expert Opinion on Drug Delivery* 12(10): 1649–1660.

Maleki Dizaj, Solmaz, Farzaneh Lotfipour, Mohammad Barzegar-Jalali, Mohammad-Hossein Zarrintan, and Khosro Adibkia. 2017. "Ciprofloxacin HCl-loaded calcium carbonate nanoparticles: Preparation, solid state characterization, and evaluation of antimicrobial effect against Staphylococcus aureus." *Artificial Cells, Nanomedicine, and Biotechnology* 45(3): 535–543.

Malik, Maqsood Ahmad, Mohammad Younus Wani, and Mohd Ali Hashim. 2012. "Microemulsion method: A novel route to synthesize organic and inorganic nanomaterials: 1st Nano Update." *Arabian Journal of Chemistry* 5 (4): 397–417.

McCormack, Emmet, Jørn Skavland, Maja Mujić, Øystein Bruserud, and Bjørn Tore Gjertsen. 2010. "Lentinan: Hematopoietic, immunological, and efficacy studies in a syngeneic model of acute myeloid leukemia." *Nutrition and Cancer* 62 (5): 574–583.

Mitchell, Michael J., Margaret M. Billingsley, Rebecca M. Haley, Marissa E. Wechsler, Nicholas A. Peppas, and Robert Langer. 2021. "Engineering precision nanoparticles for drug delivery." *Nature Reviews Drug Discovery* 20(2): 101–124.

Mohammadpour, Raziye, Marina A. Dobrovolskaia, Darwin L. Cheney, Khaled F. Greish, and Hamidreza Ghandehari. 2019. "Subchronic and chronic toxicity evaluation of inorganic nanoparticles for delivery applications." *Advanced Drug Delivery Reviews* 144: 112–132.

Mostafa, Amany A., Mohamed H. Zaazou, Laurence C. Chow, Azza A. Mahmoud, Dalia Y. Zaki, Mona Basha, Mohamed A. Abdel Hamid, Maram E. Khallaf, Nehal F. Sharaf, and Tamer M. Hamdy. 2015. "Injectable nanoamorphous calcium phosphate based in situ gel systems for the treatment of periapical lesions." *Biomedical Materials* 10(6): 065006.

Motskin, M., D.M. Wright, K. Muller, N. Kyle, T.G. Gard, A.E. Porter, and J.N. Skepper. 2009. "Hydroxyapatite nano and microparticles: Correlation of particle properties with cytotoxicity and biostability." *Biomaterials* 30 (19): 3307–3317.

Mouriño, Viviana, and Aldo R Boccaccini. 2010. "Bone tissue engineering therapeutics: controlled drug delivery in three-dimensional scaffolds." *Journal of the Royal Society Interface* 7 (43): 209–227.

Mouriño, Viviana, Juan P. Cattalini, Judith A. Roether, Prachi Dubey, Ipsita Roy, and Aldo R. Boccaccini. 2013. "Composite polymer-bioceramic scaffolds with drug delivery capability for bone tissue engineering." *Expert Opinion on Drug Delivery* 10 (10): 1353–1365.

Munir, M Usman, Ayesha Ihsan, Yasra Sarwar, Sadia Zafar Bajwa, Khizra Bano, Bushra Tehseen, Neelam Zeb, Irshad Hussain, M Tayyab Ansari, and Madiha Saeed. 2018. "Hollow mesoporous hydroxyapatite nanostructures; smart nanocarriers with high drug loading and controlled releasing features." *International Journal of Pharmaceutics* 544(1): 112–120.

Muslimov, Albert R., Dmitrii Antuganov, Yana V. Tarakanchikova, Timofey E. Karpov, Mikhail V. Zhukov, Mikhail V. Zyuzin, and Alexander S. Timin. 2021. "An investigation of calcium carbonate core-shell particles for incorporation of 225Ac and sequester of daughter radionuclides: In vitro and in vivo studies." *Journal of Controlled Release* 330: 726–737.

Najafloo, Raziyeh, Nafiseh Baheiraei, and Rana Imani. 2021. "Synthesis and characterization of collagen/calcium phosphate scaffolds incorporating antibacterial agent for bone tissue engineering application." *Journal of Bioactive and Compatible Polymers* 36(1): 29–43.

Naka, Kensuke, Yasuyuki Tanaka, and Yoshiki Chujo. 2002. "Effect of anionic starburst dendrimers on the crystallization of $CaCO_3$ in aqueous solution: Size control of spherical vaterite particles." *Langmuir* 18 (9): 3655–3658.

Namikawa, Takashi, Hidetomi Terai, Eisuke Suzuki, Masatoshi Hoshino, Hiromitsu Toyoda, Hiroaki Nakamura, Shimpei Miyamoto, Naoyuki Takahashi, Tadashi Ninomiya, and Kunio Takaoka. 2005. "Experimental spinal fusion with recombinant human bone morphogenetic protein-2 delivered by a synthetic polymer and β-tricalcium phosphate in a rabbit model." *Spine* 30 (15): 1717–1722.

Nasiri-Tabrizi, B., Pezhman Honarmandi, R. Ebrahimi-Kahrizsangi, and Peyman Honarmandi. 2009. "Synthesis of nanosize single-crystal hydroxyapatite via mechanochemical method." *Materials Letters* 63(5): 543–546.

Otto, Daniel P., Anja Otto, and Melgardt M. De Villiers. 2015. "Differences in physicochemical properties to consider in the design, evaluation and choice between microparticles and nanoparticles for drug delivery." *Expert Opinion on Drug Delivery* 12 (5): 763–777.

Pandey, Shweta, Nishant Rai, Asiya Mahtab, Disha Mittal, Farhan Jalees Ahmad, Nidhi Sandal, Yub Raj Neupane, Anita Kamra Verma, and Sushama Talegaonkar. 2021. "Hyaluronate-functionalized hydroxyapatite nanoparticles laden with methotrexate and teriflunomide for the treatment of rheumatoid arthritis." *International Journal of Biological Macromolecules* 171: 502–513.

Park, Kwang-Won, Young-Pil Yun, Sung Eun Kim, and Hae-Ryong Song. 2015. "The effect of alendronate loaded biphasic calcium phosphate scaffolds on bone regeneration in a rat tibial defect model." *International Journal of Molecular Sciences* 16 (11): 26738–26753.

Parveen, Suphiya, Ranjita Misra, and Sanjeeb K. Sahoo. 2012. "Nanoparticles: A boon to drug delivery, therapeutics, diagnostics and imaging." *Nanomedicine: Nanotechnology, Biology and Medicine* 8(2): 147–166.

Peng, Caiyu, Qinghe Zhao, and Changyou Gao. 2010. "Sustained delivery of doxorubicin by porous $CaCO_3$ and chitosan/alginate multilayers-coated $CaCO_3$ microparticles." *Colloids and Surfaces A: Physicochemical and Engineering Aspects* 353 (2–3): 132–139.

Pramanik, Sumit, Avinash Kumar Agarwal, K.N. Rai, and Ashish Garg. 2007. "Development of high strength hydroxyapatite by solid-state-sintering process." *Ceramics International* 33(3): 419–426.

Prokopowicz, Magdalena, Adrian Szewczyk, Adrianna Skwira, Rafał Sądej, and Gavin Walker. 2020. "Biphasic composite of calcium phosphate-based mesoporous silica as a novel bone drug delivery system." *Drug Delivery and Translational Research* 10(2): 455–470.

Qi, Chao, Ying-Jie Zhu, and Feng Chen. 2014. "Microwave hydrothermal transformation of amorphous calcium carbonate nanospheres and application in protein adsorption." *ACS Applied Materials & Interfaces* 6(6): 4310–4320.

Qian, Kun, Tianyu Shi, Tao Tang, Shaoliang Zhang, Xili Liu, and Yongsong Cao. 2011. "Preparation and characterization of nano-sized calcium carbonate as controlled release pesticide carrier for validamycin against Rhizoctonia solani." *Microchimica Acta* 173 (1–2): 51–57.

Qiu, Chong, Wei Wei, Jing Sun, Hai-Tao Zhang, Jing-Song Ding, Jian-Cheng Wang, and Qiang Zhang. 2016. "Systemic delivery of siRNA by hyaluronan-functionalized calcium phosphate nanoparticles for tumor-targeted therapy." *Nanoscale* 8(26): 13033–13044.

Qiu, Gengtao, Mingguang Huang, Jin Liu, Ping Wang, Abraham Schneider, Ke Ren, Thomas W. Oates, Michael D. Weir, Hockin H.K. Xu, and Liang Zhao. 2021. "Antibacterial calcium phosphate cement with human periodontal ligament stem cell-microbeads to enhance bone regeneration and combat infection." *Journal of Tissue Engineering and Regenerative Medicine* 15(3): 232–243.

Qiu, Neng, Huabing Yin, Bozhi Ji, Norbert Klauke, Andrew Glidle, Yongkui Zhang, Hang Song, Lulu Cai, Liang Ma, and Guangcheng Wang. 2012. "Calcium carbonate microspheres as carriers for the anticancer drug camptothecin." *Materials Science and Engineering: C* 32 (8): 2634–2640.

Qiu, Yubei, Xiaodong Xu, Weizhong Guo, Yong Zhao, Jiehua Su, and Jiang Chen. 2020. "Mesoporous hydroxyapatite nanoparticles mediate the release and bioactivity of BMP-2 for enhanced bone regeneration." *ACS Biomaterials Science & Engineering* 6(4): 2323–2335.

Qu, Huawei, Hongya Fu, Zhenyu Han, and Yang Sun. 2019. "Biomaterials for bone tissue engineering scaffolds: A review." *RSC Advances* 9 (45): 26252–26262.

Ramachandran, Rukmani, Willi Paul, and Chandra P Sharma. 2009. "Synthesis and characterization of PEGylated calcium phosphate nanoparticles for oral insulin delivery." *Journal of Biomedical Materials Research Part B: Applied Biomaterials: An Official Journal of The Society for Biomaterials, The Japanese Society for Biomaterials, and The Australian Society for Biomaterials and the Korean Society for Biomaterials* 88(1): 41–48.

Rao, Chaohui, Min Li, Xiaoqing Sun, Meilin Li, Xiaojie Lian, Huifang Wang, Lan Jia, Baolong Niu, and Wenfeng Li. 2020. "Preparation and characterization of phosphate-stabilized amorphous calcium carbonate nanoparticles and their application in curcumin delivery." *Materials Chemistry and Physics* 255: 123552.

Reardon, Philip James Thomas, Jie Huang, and Junwang Tang. 2015. "Mesoporous calcium phosphate bionanomaterials with controlled morphology by an energy-efficient microwave method." *Journal of Biomedical Materials Research Part A* 103 (12): 3781–3789.

Ripamonti, Ugo, Ruqayya Parak, Roland M. Klar, Caroline Dickens, Thérèse Dix-Peek, and Raquel Duarte. 2016. "The synergistic induction of bone formation by the osteogenic proteins of the TGF-β supergene family." *Biomaterials* 104: 279–296.

Rizvi, Syed A.A., and Ayman M. Saleh. 2018. "Applications of nanoparticle systems in drug delivery technology." *Saudi Pharmaceutical Journal* 26(1): 64–70.

Sadat-Shojai, Mehdi, Mohammad-Taghi Khorasani, Ehsan Dinpanah-Khoshdargi, and Ahmad Jamshidi. 2013. "Synthesis methods for nanosized hydroxyapatite with diverse structures." *Acta Biomaterialia* 9 (8): 7591–7621.

Saltzman, W. Mark, and William L. Olbricht. 2002. "Building drug delivery into tissue engineering design." *Nature Reviews Drug Discovery* 1(3): 177–186.

Sargheini, J., A. Ataie, S.M. Salili, and A.A. Hoseinion. 2012. "One-step facile synthesis of $CaCO_3$ nanoparticles via mechano-chemical route." *Powder Technology* 219: 72–77.

Sathiskumar, Swamiappan, Sekar Vanaraj, Devaraj Sabarinathan, Somasundaram Bharath, Ganesan Sivarasan, Subramanian Arulmani, Kathirvel Preethi, and Vinoth Kumar Ponnusamy. 2019. "Green synthesis of biocompatible nanostructured hydroxyapatite from Cirrhinus mrigala fish scale–A biowaste to biomaterial." *Ceramics International* 45(6): 7804–7810.

Sato, Katsuhiko, Masaru Seno, and Jun-Ichi Anzai. 2014. "Release of insulin from calcium carbonate microspheres with and without layer-by-layer thin coatings." *Polymers* 6(8): 2157–2165.

Sayed, E., R. Haj-Ahmad, K. Ruparelia, M.S. Arshad, M.-W. Chang, and Z. Ahmad. 2017. "Porous inorganic drug delivery systems—A review." *Aaps Pharmscitech* 18(5): 1507–1525.

Ševčík, Radek, Petr Šašek, and Alberto Viani. 2018. "Physical and nanomechanical properties of the synthetic anhydrous crystalline $CaCO_3$ polymorphs: Vaterite, aragonite and calcite." *Journal of Materials Science* 53 (6): 4022–4033.

Sheng, Yanshan, Jun Gao, Zheng-Zhi Yin, Jing Kang, and Yong Kong. 2021. "Dual-drug delivery system based on the hydrogels of alginate and sodium carboxymethyl cellulose for colorectal cancer treatment." *Carbohydrate Polymers* 269: 118325.

Shi, Peiying, Yunjiao Xie, Rongfang Xie, Zuan Lin, Hong Yao, and Shuang Wu. 2020. "An integrated pharmacokinetic study of an acanthopanax senticosus extract preparation by combination of virtual screening, systems pharmacology, and multi-component pharmacokinetics in rats." *Frontiers in Pharmacology* 11: 1295.

Shi, Pengzhong, Daozhen Zhou, Yaxin Zhu, Bo Peng, Nannan Shao, and Xingjie Zan. 2021. "Thrombin-loaded TA-$CaCO_3$ microspheres as a budget, adaptable, and highly efficient hemostatic." *ACS Applied Bio Materials* 4(1): 1030–1037.

Sokolova, Viktoriya, and Matthias Epple. 2021. "Biological and medical applications of calcium phosphate nanoparticles." *Chemistry (Weinheim an der Bergstrasse, Germany)* 27(27): 7471.

Som, Avik, Ramesh Raliya, Limei Tian, Walter Akers, Joseph E. Ippolito, Srikanth Singamaneni, Pratim Biswas, and Samuel Achilefu. 2016. "Monodispersed calcium carbonate nanoparticles modulate local pH and inhibit tumor growth in vivo." *Nanoscale* 8(25): 12639–12647.

Srivastav, Ashu, Balasaheb Chandanshive, Prajakta Dandekar, Deepa Khushalani, and Ratnesh Jain. 2019. "Biomimetic hydroxyapatite a potential universal nanocarrier for cellular internalization & drug delivery." *Pharmaceutical Research* 36 (4): 1–12.

Sudareva, Natalia, Olga Suvorova, Natalia Saprykina, Helen Vlasova, and Alexander Vilesov. 2021. "Doxorubicin delivery systems based on doped $CaCO_3$ cores and polyanion drug conjugates." *Journal of Microencapsulation* 38(3): 164–176.

Sumathra, Murugan, Kishor Kumar Sadasivuni, S. Suresh Kumar, and Mariappan Rajan. 2018. "Cisplatin-loaded graphene oxide/chitosan/hydroxyapatite composite as a promising tool for osteosarcoma-affected bone regeneration." *ACS Omega* 3(11): 14620–14633.

Sun, Huan, Chenxi Zhang, Boqing Zhang, Ping Song, Xiujuan Xu, Xingyu Gui, Xinyue Chen, Gonggong Lu, Xiang Li, and Jie Liang. 2022. "3D printed calcium phosphate scaffolds with controlled release of osteogenic drugs for bone regeneration." *Chemical Engineering Journal* 427: 130961.

Sun, Rui, Michelle Åhlén, Cheuk-Wai Tai, Éva G. Bajnóczi, Fenne de Kleijne, Natalia Ferraz, Ingmar Persson, Maria Strømme, and Ocean Cheung. 2020. "Highly porous amorphous calcium phosphate for drug delivery and biomedical applications." *Nanomaterials* 10(1): 20.

Sun, Rui, Peng Zhang, Éva G. Bajnóczi, Alexandra Neagu, Cheuk-Wai Tai, Ingmar Persson, Maria Strømme, and Ocean Cheung. 2018. "Amorphous calcium carbonate constructed from nanoparticle aggregates with unprecedented surface area and mesoporosity." *ACS Applied Materials & Interfaces* 10(25): 21556–21564.

Sun, Wen, Jiangli Fan, Suzhen Wang, Yao Kang, Jianjun Du, and Xiaojun Peng. 2018. "Biodegradable drug-loaded hydroxyapatite nanotherapeutic agent for targeted drug release in tumors." *ACS Applied Materials & Interfaces* 10 (9): 7832–7840.

Sun, Yi, Yaying Chen, Xiaoyu Ma, Yuan Yuan, Changsheng Liu, Joachim Kohn, and Jiangchao Qian. 2016. "Mitochondria-targeted hydroxyapatite nanoparticles for selective growth inhibition of lung cancer in vitro and in vivo." *ACS Applied Materials & Interfaces* 8 (39): 25680–25690.

Svenskaya, Yulia, Bogdan Parakhonskiy, Albrecht Haase, Vsevolod Atkin, Evgeny Lukyanets, Dmitry Gorin, and Renzo Antolini. 2013. "Anticancer drug delivery system based on calcium carbonate particles loaded with a photosensitizer." *Biophysical Chemistry* 182: 11–15.

Tateiwa, Daisuke, Shinichi Nakagawa, Hiroyuki Tsukazaki, Rintaro Okada, Joe Kodama, Junichi Kushioka, Zeynep Bal, Yuichiro Ukon, Hiromasa Hirai, and Takashi Kaito. 2021. "A novel BMP-2–loaded hydroxyapatite/beta-tricalcium phosphate microsphere/hydrogel composite for bone regeneration." *Scientific Reports* 11(1): 1–13.

Trofimov, Alexey D., Anna A. Ivanova, Mikhail V. Zyuzin, and Alexander S. Timin. 2018. "Porous inorganic carriers based on silica, calcium carbonate and calcium phosphate for controlled/modulated drug delivery: Fresh outlook and future perspectives." *Pharmaceutics* 10(4): 167.

Trushina, Daria B., Tatiana V. Bukreeva, and Maria N. Antipina. 2016. "Size-controlled synthesis of vaterite calcium carbonate by the mixing method: Aiming for nanosized particles." *Crystal Growth & Design* 16(3): 1311–1319.

Trushina, Daria B., Tatiana V. Bukreeva, Mikhail V. Kovalchuk, and Maria N. Antipina. 2014. "$CaCO_3$ vaterite microparticles for biomedical and personal care applications." *Materials Science and Engineering: C* 45: 644–658.

Tsikourkitoudi, Vasiliki, Jens Karlsson, Padryk Merkl, Edmund Loh, Birgitta Henriques-Normark, and Georgios A. Sotiriou. 2020. "Flame-made calcium phosphate nanoparticles with high drug loading for delivery of biologics." *Molecules* 25(7): 1747.

Turner, T.M., R.M. Urban, R.M. Leven, M. Hawkins, E.H. Nichols, J.M. McPherson, and J.O. Galante. 2001. "Locally delivered rhTGF-β2 enhances bone ingrowth and bone regeneration at local and remote sites of skeletal injury." *Journal of Orthopaedic Research* 19 (1): 85–94.

Uskoković, Vuk, and Tejal A. Desai. 2013. "Phase composition control of calcium phosphate nanoparticles for tunable drug delivery kinetics and treatment of osteomyelitis. I. Preparation and drug release." *Journal of Biomedical Materials Research Part A* 101 (5): 1416–1426.

Uthappa, U.T., O.R. Arvind, G. Sriram, Dusan Losic, Madhuprasad Kigga, and Mahaveer D. Kurkuri. 2020. "Nanodiamonds and their surface modification strategies for drug delivery applications." *Journal of Drug Delivery Science and Technology* 60: 101993.

Uthappa, U.T., Varsha Brahmkhatri, G. Sriram, Ho-Young Jung, Jingxian Yu, Nikita Kurkuri, Tejraj M. Aminabhavi, Tariq Altalhi, Gururaj M. Neelgund, and Mahaveer D. Kurkuri. 2018. "Nature engineered diatom biosilica as drug delivery systems." *Journal of Controlled Release* 281: 70–83.

Uthappa, U.T., Mahaveer D. Kurkuri, and Madhuprasad Kigga. 2019. "Nanotechnology advances for the development of various drug carriers." In Prasad, R., Kumar, V., Kumar, M., Choudhary, D. (eds.) *Nanobiotechnology in Bioformulations*, 187–224. Springer, Cham.

Vallet-Regí, María, Francisco Balas, and Daniel Arcos. 2007. "Mesoporous materials for drug delivery." *Angewandte Chemie International Edition* 46 (40): 7548–7558.

Veljović, Dj., Eriks Palcevskis, Antonija Dindune, Slaviša Putić, Igor Balać, Rada Petrović, and Dj. Janaćković. 2010. "Microwave sintering improves the mechanical properties of biphasic calcium phosphates from hydroxyapatite microspheres produced from hydrothermal processing." *Journal of Materials Science* 45 (12): 3175–3183.

Vergaro, Viviana, Elisabetta Carata, Elisa Panzarini, Francesca Baldassare, Luciana Dini, and Giuseppe Ciccarella. 2015. "Synthesis of calcium carbonate nanocrystals and their potential application as vessels for drug delivery." *AIP Conference Proceedings.*

Verma, Ashwni, Shweta Sharma, Pramod Kumar Gupta, Awadhesh Singh, B Venkatesh Teja, Pankaj Dwivedi, Girish Kumar Gupta, Ritu Trivedi, and Prabhat Ranjan Mishra. 2016. "Vitamin B12 functionalized layer by layer calcium phosphate nanoparticles: A mucoadhesive and pH responsive carrier for improved oral delivery of insulin." *Acta Biomaterialia* 31: 288–300.

Verma, Ritu, Shubham Verma, and Sokindra Kumar. 2019. "Microsphere-A novel drug delivery system." *Research Chronicle in Health Sciences* 5 (1): 5–14.

Verron, Elise, Ibrahim Khairoun, Jerome Guicheux, and Jean-Michel Bouler. 2010. "Calcium phosphate biomaterials as bone drug delivery systems: A review." *Drug Discovery Today* 15 (13–14): 547–552.

Victor, Sunita Prem, and T.S. Sampath Kumar. 2008. "BCP ceramic microspheres as drug delivery carriers: Synthesis, characterisation and doxycycline release." *Journal of Materials Science: Materials in Medicine* 19 (1): 283–290.

Wang, Cheng, Shaoqing Chen, Lu Bao, Xuerong Liu, Fuqiang Hu, and Hong Yuan. 2020. "Size-controlled preparation and behavior study of phospholipid–calcium carbonate hybrid nanoparticles." *International Journal of Nanomedicine* 15: 4049.

Wang, Cheng, Min Han, Xuerong Liu, Shaoqing Chen, Fuqiang Hu, Jihong Sun, and Hong Yuan. 2019. "Mitoxantrone-preloaded water-responsive phospholipid-amorphous calcium carbonate hybrid nanoparticles for targeted and effective cancer therapy." *International Journal of Nanomedicine* 14: 1503.

Wang, Neng, Xuejun Cheng, Nan Li, Hong Wang, and Hongyu Chen. 2019. "Nanocarriers and their loading strategies." *Advanced Healthcare Materials* 8 (6): 1801002.

Wang, Shuang, Dezhi Ni, Hua Yue, Nana Luo, Xiaobo Xi, Yugang Wang, Min Shi, Wei Wei, and Guanghui Ma. 2018. "Exploration of antigen induced $CaCO_3$ nanoparticles for therapeutic vaccine." *Small* 14 (14): 1704272.

Wang, Xiaoqiang, Rui Kong, Xiaoxiao Pan, Hai Xu, Daohong Xia, Honghong Shan, and Jian R. Lu. 2009. "Role of ovalbumin in the stabilization of metastable vaterite in calcium carbonate biomineralization." *The Journal of Physical Chemistry B* 113(26): 8975–8982.

Wang, Yongsheng, Ying Xin Moo, Chunping Chen, Poernomo Gunawan, and Rong Xu. 2010. "Fast precipitation of uniform $CaCO_3$ nanospheres and their transformation to hollow hydroxyapatite nanospheres." *Journal of Colloid and Interface Science* 352(2): 393–400.

Wang, Zhaozhen, Xujie Liu, Vidmi Taolam Martin, Mohamed Abdullahi Abdi, Lijun Chen, Yong Gong, Yiran Yan, Liming Song, Zhongxun Liu, and Xianliao Zhang. 2020. "Sequential delivery of BMP2-derived peptide P24 by thiolated chitosan/calcium carbonate composite microspheres scaffolds for bone regeneration." *Journal of Nanomaterials* 2020. https://doi.org/10.1155/2020/4929151.

Wei, Yan, Ruize Sun, Hui Su, Hao Xu, Lichuang Zhang, Di Huang, Ziwei Liang, Yinchun Hu, Liqin Zhao, and Xiaojie Lian. 2021. "Synthesis and characterization of porous $CaCO_3$ microspheres templated by yeast cells and the application as pH value-sensitive anticancer drug carrier." *Colloids and Surfaces B: Biointerfaces* 199: 111545.

Westrøm, Sara, Marion Malenge, Ida Sofie Jorstad, Elisa Napoli, Øyvind S. Bruland, Tina B. Bønsdorff, and Roy H. Larsen. 2018. "Ra-224 labeling of calcium carbonate microparticles for internal α-therapy: Preparation, stability, and biodistribution in mice." *Journal of Labelled Compounds and Radiopharmaceuticals* 61 (6): 472–486.

Williams, David F. 2008. "On the mechanisms of biocompatibility." *Biomaterials* 29 (20): 2941–2953.

Won, Yu-Ho, Ho Seong Jang, Ding-Wen Chung, and Lia A. Stanciu. 2010. "Multifunctional calcium carbonate microparticles: Synthesis and biological applications." *Journal of Materials Chemistry* 20 (36): 7728–7733.

Wu, Hongfeng, Zhongtao Li, Jiaoqing Tang, Xiao Yang, Yong Zhou, Bo Guo, Lin Wang, Xiangdong Zhu, Chongqi Tu, and Xingdong Zhang. 2019. "The in vitro and in vivo anti-melanoma effects of hydroxyapatite nanoparticles: Influences of material factors." *International Journal of Nanomedicine* 14: 1177.

Wu, Shizhou, Lei Lei, Chongyun Bao, Jin Liu, Michael D. Weir, Ke Ren, Abraham Schneider, Thomas W. Oates, Jun Liu, and Hockin H.K. Xu. 2021. "An injectable and antibacterial calcium phosphate scaffold inhibiting Staphylococcus aureus and supporting stem cells for bone regeneration." *Materials Science and Engineering: C* 120: 111688.

Wu, Victoria M., Jarrett Mickens, and Vuk Uskoković. 2017. "Bisphosphonate-functionalized hydroxyapatite nanoparticles for the delivery of the bromodomain inhibitor JQ1 in the treatment of osteosarcoma." *ACS Applied Materials & Interfaces* 9 (31): 25887–25904.

Wu, Yan, Lisa Woodbine, Antony M. Carr, Amit R. Pillai, Ali Nokhodchi, and Mohammed Maniruzzaman. 2020. "3D printed calcium phosphate cement (CPC) scaffolds for anti-cancer drug delivery." *Pharmaceutics* 12(11): 1077.

Xiang, Yubin, Jie Han, Guilong Zhang, Furu Zhan, Dongqing Cai, and Zhengyan Wu. 2018. "Efficient synthesis of starch-regulated porous calcium carbonate microspheres as a carrier for slow-release herbicide." *ACS Sustainable Chemistry & Engineering* 6 (3): 3649–3658.

Xiao, Douxin, Jingli Cheng, Wenlong Liang, Lianli Sun, and Jinhao Zhao. 2021. "Metal-phenolic coated and prochloraz-loaded calcium carbonate carriers with pH responsiveness for environmentally-safe fungicide delivery." *Chemical Engineering Journal* 418: 129274.

Xiong, Long, Jianhua Zeng, Aihua Yao, Qiquan Tu, Jingtang Li, Liang Yan, and Zhiming Tang. 2015. "BMP2-loaded hollow hydroxyapatite microspheres exhibit enhanced osteoinduction and osteogenicity in large bone defects." *International Journal of Nanomedicine* 10: 517.

Xu, Renliang. 2008. "Progress in nanoparticles characterization: Sizing and zeta potential measurement." *Particuology* 6 (2): 112–115.

Yazdian-Robati, Rezvan, Atefeh Arab, Mohammad Ramezani, Houshang Rafatpanah, Amirhossein Bahreyni, Maryam Sadat Nabavinia, Khalil Abnous, and Seyed Mohammad Taghdisi. 2019. "Smart aptamer-modified calcium carbonate nanoparticles for controlled release and targeted delivery of epirubicin and melittin into cancer cells in vitro and in vivo." *Drug Development and Industrial Pharmacy* 45 (4): 603–610.

Yoo, Jihye, Changhee Park, Gawon Yi, Donghyun Lee, and Heebeom Koo. 2019. "Active targeting strategies using biological ligands for nanoparticle drug delivery systems." *Cancers* 11 (5): 640.

Yuan, Yuan, Changsheng Liu, Jiangchao Qian, Jing Wang, and Yuan Zhang. 2010. "Size-mediated cytotoxicity and apoptosis of hydroxyapatite nanoparticles in human hepatoma HepG2 cells." *Biomaterials* 31 (4): 730–740.

Zarkesh, Ibrahim, Mohammad Hossein Ghanian, Mahmoud Azami, Fatemeh Bagheri, Hossein Baharvand, Javad Mohammadi, and Mohamadreza Baghaban Eslaminejad. 2017. "Facile synthesis of biphasic calcium phosphate microspheres with engineered surface topography for controlled delivery of drugs and proteins." *Colloids and Surfaces B: Biointerfaces* 157: 223–232.

Zeng, Zhi, Han-bo Feng, Meng-en Hao, and Yi Zhang. 2021. "One-pot approach to form in situ colchicine-containing nano-hydroxyapatite within micro-emulsion composite system for sustained transdermal delivery." *Composites Communications* 25: 100698.

Zepp, Fred. 2010. "Principles of vaccine design—lessons from nature." *Vaccine* 28: C14–C24.

Zhang, Nan-nan, Ri-sheng Yu, Min Xu, Xing-yao Cheng, Chun-miao Chen, Xiao-ling Xu, Chen-ying Lu, Kong-jun Lu, Min-jiang Chen, and Meng-lu Zhu. 2018. "Visual targeted therapy of hepatic cancer using homing peptide modified calcium phosphate nanoparticles loading doxorubicin guided by T1 weighted MRI." *Nanomedicine: Nanotechnology, Biology and Medicine* 14 (7): 2167–2178.

Zhang, Yong, and Miqin Zhang. 2002. "Calcium phosphate/chitosan composite scaffolds for controlled in vitro antibiotic drug release." *Journal of Biomedical Materials Research: An Official Journal of The Society for Biomaterials, The Japanese Society for Biomaterials, and The Australian Society for Biomaterials and the Korean Society for Biomaterials* 62 (3): 378–386.

Zhao, Pengxuan, Minsi Li, Yan Chen, Chuanchuan He, Xiaojuan Zhang, Ting Fan, Tan Yang, Yao Lu, Robert J. Lee, and Xiang Ma. 2019. "Selenium-doped calcium carbonate nanoparticles loaded with cisplatin enhance efficiency and reduce side effects." *International Journal of Pharmaceutics* 570: 118638.

Zhao, Xinxin, SuXiu Ng, Boon Chin Heng, Jun Guo, LwinLwin Ma, Timothy Thatt Yang Tan, Kee Woei Ng, and Say Chye Joachim Loo. 2013. "Cytotoxicity of hydroxyapatite nanoparticles is shape and cell dependent." *Archives of Toxicology* 87(6): 1037–1052.

Zhao, Zongmin, Anvay Ukidve, Vinu Krishnan, and Samir Mitragotri. 2019. "Effect of physicochemical and surface properties on in vivo fate of drug nanocarriers." *Advanced Drug Delivery Reviews* 143: 3–21.

Zhou, Zi-Fei, Tuan-Wei Sun, Feng Chen, Dong-Qing Zuo, Hong-Sheng Wang, Ying-Qi Hua, Zheng-Dong Cai, and Jun Tan. 2017. "Calcium phosphate-phosphorylated adenosine hybrid microspheres for anti-osteosarcoma drug delivery and osteogenic differentiation." *Biomaterials* 121: 1–14.

Ziegler, J., U. Mayr-Wohlfart, S. Kessler, D. Breitig, and K.-P. Günther. 2002. "Adsorption and release properties of growth factors from biodegradable implants." *Journal of Biomedical Materials Research: An Official Journal of The Society for Biomaterials, The Japanese Society for Biomaterials, and The Australian Society for Biomaterials and the Korean Society for Biomaterials* 59(3): 422–428.

Part C

Synthetic Porous Materials

Chapter 7

Metal-Organic Frameworks (MOFs)-Based Carriers for Tumor Therapy

Mahesh P. Bhat and Kyeong-Hwan Lee
Chonnam National University

CONTENTS

7.1 INTRODUCTION

Metal-organic frameworks (MOFs) are a promising class of crystalline porous coordination polymers (PCPs) (Furukawa et al. 2013; Zhou, Long, and Yaghi 2012; Meek, Greathouse, and Allendorf 2011). They are a type of hybrid material created by the self-assembly of metallic clusters or ions with organic molecules acting as bridges, resulting in one-/two-/three-dimensional network known as MOFs. In 1995, Yaghi's group reported the first MOF and studied the selective binding and removal of guest molecules in a microporous MOF composed of 1,3,5-benzenetricarboxylate (BTC) and cobalt cation (Yaghi, Li, and Li 1995). Due to their high surface area and pore volume, as well as tunable pore size and chemical composition, MOFs have

DOI: 10.1201/9781003217114-10

been studied for a variety of applications over the last two decades, including chemical separation (Petit 2018), catalysis (Shen et al. 2016), sensing (Zhu et al. 2013), semiconductors (Subudhi, Tripathy, and Parida 2021), bioimaging (Gallis et al. 2017), and gas storage and separation (Bonneau et al. 2020). In recent years, there has been a lot of interest in the biomedical applications of MOFs for drug delivery (Uthappa, Sriram, et al. 2020; Uthappa, Brahmkhatri, et al. 2018; Uthappa et al. 2019). It is worthwhile to mention that when MOF are reduced to the nanoscale, they transform into effective nanocarriers for drug delivery in imaging, chemotherapy, photothermal therapy, and photodynamic therapy (Yang and Yang 2020). In addition, MOF composite materials are gaining interest for various applications (Bhat, Uthappa, and Kurkuri 2021; Uthappa et al. 2021).

Cancer/tumor is one of the most dangerous diseases to mankind, and its morbidity has been constantly increasing. Although cancer treatments have advanced and survival rates have increased in recent years, the heterogeneity of cancer required the development of more therapeutic options (DeSantis et al. 2019; Uthappa, Sriram, et al. 2018; Uthappa, Brahmkhatri, et al. 2018; Uthappa et al. 2019; Uthappa, Sriram, et al. 2020; Uthappa, Arvind, et al. 2020; Bhat, Uthappa, et al. 2021; Kurkuri and Aminabhavi 2004). Common cancer treatments involve chemotherapy, radiotherapy, and surgery, but they come with a handful of side effects caused by nonspecific anticancer agent tissue dispersion, insufficient drug concentrations at the tumor sites, and unmanageable toxicity. Immunotherapy, a new type of tumor therapy that has gained popularity in recent years, has a stronger anticancer effect, but it is riskier and only works for a limited number of patients (Meng et al. 2020). One of the most promising approach is tumor therapy to emerge in recent years is cancer targeting. Targeting anticancer drugs to tumor tissues has the potential to improve local drug concentration, increase therapeutic benefits, and decrease side effects (Gao et al. 2014).

As nanotechnology has progressed, multifunctional therapeutic agents have become more prominent. In the preclinical stage, a multifunctional therapeutic could aid in cancer diagnosis and treatment. Over the last few decades, a variety of nanomaterials have been created as drug carriers, including inorganic mesoporous silica (Watermann and Brieger 2017), quantum dots (McHugh et al. 2018), metal nanoparticles (Sharma, Goyal, and Rath 2018), organic micelles (Palazzolo et al. 2018), liposomes (Belfiore et al. 2018), polymersomes (Guan, Rizzello, and Battaglia 2015), and dendrimers (Yang 2016). However, such nanocarriers have a variety of limitations, including low biocompatibility, cytotoxicity, and restricted drug-loading capacity (Bendre et al. 2022). For safe and effective delivery of drugs, the designed carriers should be nontoxic, biocompatible, and biodegradable in nature (Mahapatro and Singh 2011; Liu et al. 2022). As a result, several efforts have been undertaken to develop multifunctional systems that may be used for both cancer diagnostic and treatment or theranostics purposes. In addition, nanotechnology is gaining importance in sensing applications, which could be an alternative to chemical biosensors (Madhuprasad et al. 2016; Sriram et al. 2016; Bhat et al. 2016; Patil et al. 2017; Patil et al. 2018; Bhat et al. 2019; Bhat et al. 2020; Bhat, Kurkuri, et al. 2021).

In this context, MOFs have been extensively studied as a multifunctional platform. They offer unique characteristics such a wide external surface area, porous architectures, tunable size, configurable frameworks, and biocompatibility (Falsafi et al. 2021; Tong et al. 2021). Because of their ideal features, such as enhanced drug-loading efficacy, porous frameworks, and flexible pore volume, they are promising materials for biomedical applications. The surface of MOFs can be easily modified as smart therapeutic agents to increase biodistribution, biodegradability, and biocompatibility, as well as provide intelligent drug release and prevent uncontrolled burst release (Guo et al. 2021; Nicks et al. 2021; Simon-Yarza et al. 2018; Rojas, Arenas-Vivo, and Horcajada 2019). In this chapter, we have discussed the development on MOF-based targeted drug delivery systems capable of releasing therapeutic agents once they reach diseased tissues and cells are reviewed. In addition, MOF synthesis methods and various stimuli-responsive MOFs platforms for tumor therapy such as pH, temperature, enzyme, photoresponsive systems, redox, and magnetic field–assisted drug delivery as well as their applications in tumor therapy are discussed in detail.

7.2 MOF SYNTHESIS

MOFs are produced by combining the inorganic and organic components in a high-end chemical reaction to produce a structural network. In order to determine the safety of MOF synthesis for biological applications, the chemistry of MOF synthesis must also be thoroughly explored. Figure 7.1 shows some of the most common procedures including rapid precipitation, hydro/solvothermal synthesis, surfactant-mediated thermal synthesis, microwave-assisted technique, mechanochemical technique, sonochemical technique, electrochemical synthesis, spray-drying technique, reverse microemulsion technique, modulated synthesis, post-synthesis, and one-pot synthesis. In terms of generating MOFs with various physiochemical properties, functionalization, and mass production capacity and each technique has its own set of advantages (González et al. 2021; Wu and Yang 2017; Wang et al. 2014; Zhou et al. 2018; Zheng, Zhang, and Su 2021; Rojas, Arenas-Vivo, and Horcajada 2019; Beg et al. 2017; Stock and Biswas 2012).

The solvothermal procedure, which is one of the earliest methods for producing MOFs, is frequently used to create MOFs. Yang et al. employed a

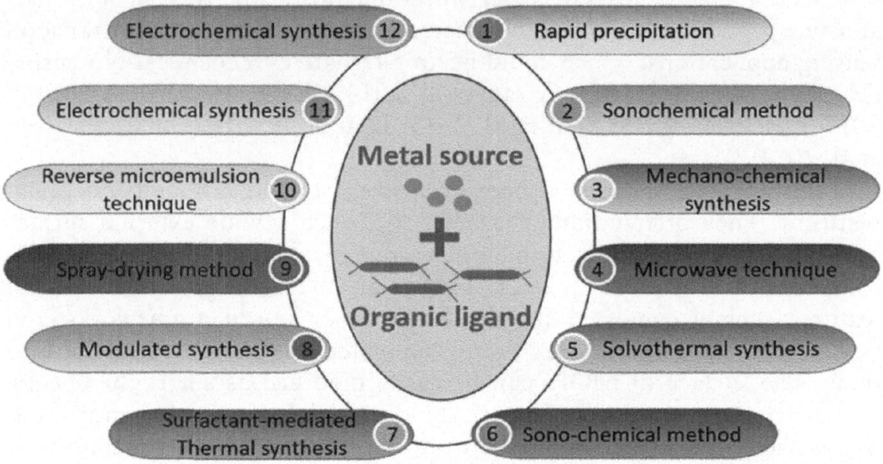

Figure 7.1 Various techniques involved in the MOF synthesis.

solvothermal technique to develop IRMOF-3 (Yang et al. 2017), where folic acid (FA) was used to make post-synthesis changes to IRMOF-3. Further, to create Fe_3O_4@IRMOF-3 (Fe_3O_4 nanoparticles into porous isoreticular MOFs), Angshuman et al. used a mixed solvent solvothermal method (Ray Chowdhuri, Bhattacharya, and Sahu 2016). The material was soaked in a mixture of dimethylformamide (DMF) and ethanol with polyvinylpyrrolidone (PVP), followed by heating at 100°C for 4 hours to produce dark-brown nanoparticles (NPs). The particle size of synthetic IRMOF-3 was <100 nm, while Fe_3O_4@IRMOF-3 was around 200 nm. Under physiological conditions for 4 days, the hydrophobic nanoplatform contained paclitaxel, which had a drug-loading capacity of 12.32% and was released at a rate of 65%. Nian et al. also used the solvothermal method to synthesize brown N_3-UiO-66-NH_2 MOF (Nian et al. 2017) (zirconium-based MOF). The size of these nanocrystals was consistent, and they had good drug-loading properties. However, solvothermal NPs can have large particle sizes, making them unsuitable for targeted administration via post-synthesis modification. To control particle size and promote functionalization of drug-loaded particles, the ratio of metal ions to organic ligands and their synthetic reaction process must be carefully adjusted. The rapid precipitation approach can produce NPs with smaller particle sizes, but the NPs produced by this process are typically in the form of cluster morphologies, lack a definite crystal shape, and random single crystals. Christopher et al. used several amines derivatives (trioctylamine, tributylamine, trimethylamine) to design ZIF-90 with varying particle sizes (60–90, 200–300, and 100–200 nm, respectively) (Jones et al. 2016). The particle size gradually increases as the reaction temperature rises. When amine is added, this method can quickly create MOF particles through precipitation.

In the production of MOFs, the one-pot synthesis approach is widely used and to make CQ@ZIF-8 (chloroquine diphosphate@ zeolitic imidazolate framework) with an 18% drug loading (Shi et al. 2018). The obtained MOFs are in regular octahedral structure with a particle size of ~250 nm. ZIF-8 is found to be stable under physiological environments; however, in acidic environment, the structure is disrupted. Song et al. used the similar process to produce ZnPc@ZIF-8/CTAB, which has a drug-loading capacity of 29.5% (Song et al. 2018). The intracellular reactive oxygen species increased when the photosensitizer ZnPc (zinc phthalocyanines) was released, resulting in an anticancer effect. Due to their one-step synthesis and ability to target weak acidic conditions, ZIF-8-derived nano-drug-loading systems have received a lot of attention as a carrier for delivering hydrophilic and hydrophobic drugs. Wang et al. also used a one-pot synthesis technique to produce pH and redox-responsive tumor targeting MOF (DOX@TTMOF) (Wang et al. 2015) (doxorubicin@ tumor targeting MOF). Shi et al. have created Ce-MOF (Cerium-MOF) using a one-pot synthesis method (Shi et al. 2017). The ATP (adenosine triphosphate) aptamer was then coupled with the Ce-MOF functionalized gold electrode. Electrochemical impedance spectroscopy was used to detect serum ATP in tumor patients using an ATP aptamer. Su et al. used for one-pot encapsulation approach to make UiO-66@AgNCs@Apt@DOX (zirconium MOF-embedded silver nanoclusters using AS1411 aptamer loaded with doxorubicin) with high loading efficiency (Su et al. 2019). Due to the ease of synthesis, most of the researchers use a one-pot approach for MOF synthesis.

However, in order to achieve high drug-loading capacity when employing a MOF for drug loading, the drugs must have a high affinity for the carrier. If the drugs being supplied contain an acidic group, for example, ZIF-8 can show high loading ability. However, not all tumor drugs contain acidic groups, thus ZIF-8's function as a drug carrier is limited. Zhang et al. loaded cytarabine (Ara) with ZIF-8, but significant drug-loading capacity was not achieved due to a lack of drug-acting group (Zhang et al. 2018). As a result, they combined cytarabine (Ara) with new indocyanine green (IR820) to create a ZIF-8-encapsulated prodrug. This strategy increased drug-loading capacity considerably, implying that structural change or other methods to increase MOF drug-loading capacity can be used to improve drug and carrier affinity.

MOFs can also be synthesized by other variety of methods, and Zhang et al. produced ZIF-90 by ultrasonication of precursors with strong stirring conditions (Zhang et al. 2017). The synthesized ZIF-90 has a particle size of <300 nm, making them suitable for drug carriers. They loaded fluorouracil (5-FU) and doxorubicin (DOX) into ZIF-90, which improved efficacy and eliminated drug resistance for pH-responsive drug delivery. Later, Jia et al. used a microwave-assisted approach to synthesis methylene blue@THA-NMOF-76@cRGD (THA: 4,4,4-trifluoro-1-(9-hexylcarbazol-3-yl)-1,3-butanedione, NMOF: nanoscale MOF, and cRGD: cyclic ArgGly-Asp peptide) (Jia et al. 2018). The synthesized MOF showed an average particle size of 89 nm and homogeneity, which are highly resistant to light and acid. Cai et al. presented a method for synthesizing Fe-soc-MOF for photothermal therapy using a liquid-solid-solution (LSS) process (Cai et al. 2019). The MOF particles are about 100 nm in size, which is substantially smaller than earlier approaches. Further, Yu et al. developed a template-directed synthesis technique, (Yu et al. 2015) by developing skeletal and interconnected ZIF-8 crystals with long and soft filamentous micelle, which is subsequently removed to yield ZIF-8 hollow nanotubes. The drug-loading efficiency of this nanotube was 350%, and it was successful in bypassing the reticuloendothelial system (RES), resulting in a prolonged drug delivery. In another report, Cao et al. used a surfactant to assist in the production of ZIF-8 hollow nanospheres encapsulating 10-hydroxycamptothecin (HCPT) for tumor therapy (Cao et al. 2015) and emerged as a novel concept for MOF synthesis.

Generally, in drug delivery field, low drug loading and burst release are common limitations involved in the development of single nanocarriers. Because some MOFs have a low biocompatibility, their clinical usage is limited. In this context, scientific communities have been striving to overcome these issues in recent years. The composite nanocarriers have been demonstrated to be more effective in the treatment of cancers. For example, MnCo-MOF (manganese substituted cobalt MOF) is extremely hazardous and should never be used in humans (Cai et al. 2020). Wang et al. developed polydopamine hybrid nanogels (Wang et al. 2018), which could significantly lower MOF toxicity while also increasing the photosensitizer's photothermal conversion efficiency. In vitro and in vivo tests revealed that these materials are biocompatible and have a good photothermal effect. From this study, it was observed that the same methodology can be applied to other MOFs which are used in therapeutic applications. Besides, Abhik et al. investigated the impact of Fe_3O_4 NPs and MOFs complexes on drug loading and releasing behaviors (Bhattacharjee, Gumma, and Purkait 2018). The drug loading of the composite was found to be greater than that of a single nanocarrier. DOX-loaded Fe_3O_4@MIL-100 did not exhibit any rapid release behavior; however, it showed release over a period of 25 days. All of these studies described as better examples for MOF-derived composite materials for tumor therapy. This shows that it is possible to continue and develop MOF-based multifunctional composite materials to conduct more advanced anticancer research/tumor therapies.

7.3 PROPERTIES OF MOFs AS A CARRIER

MOFs have a high surface area, a large pore diameter, and excellent biocompatibility; are nontoxic to humans; and are biodegradable. As a result,

MOFs can be used to deliver drugs. To maximize drug-loading capacity, control the drug release rate, and accurately deliver the drug to the target, we must strategically tune the pore size, particle size, stability, and other aspects of the MOFs. The fundamental properties of MOFs that must be considered as drug carriers are discussed briefly in this section. The effect of MOF pore size on drug-loading capabilities, controlling particle size to achieve desired functional transfer of MOF, biocompatibility, and stability are among the important properties. In general, larger pore sizes indicate greater drug-loading capability. As a result, hollow MOFs are regarded as efficient carriers for drug-loading and multifunctional targeted drug delivery. Recently, Gao et al. produced a hollow ZIF-8 bearing 51% drug-loading capacity (Gao et al. 2016). By modifying the pore size of MOFs and also by using different organic ligands could possible to improve drug-loading capacity. In recent years, few studies in this field, which gives future directions in this research, which will investigate the impact of MOF NPs with various pore diameters and drug-loading performances can be tuned.

Another important property of drug-loaded MOFs is particle size. The ability of the drug delivery system to target specific sites can be determined by particle size. When the particle size is around 100 nm, the drug-loading mechanism makes it relatively simple to passively target malignant tissues. MOF particle sizes should ideally be less than 100 nm to avoid clearance by the RES and hepatic macrophages in order to achieve active or multifunctional targeting, and thereby controlling the particle size of MOFs is one of the critical factors that need to be considered. In one such work, Duan et al. adjusted the particle size of AZIF-8 (amorphous zeolitic imidazolate framework-8), in addition to assessing the effect of particle size on tumor treatment (Duan et al. 2018). They used nontoxic poly-allylamine hydrochloride (PAH) to precisely control the particle size of the AZIF-8 in a one-pot synthesis procedure, breaking the tradition of being unable to control the particle size of MOFs and having to use harmful solvents for synthesis and modification. The addition of PAH altered the nucleation rate of AZIF-8, resulting in a variation in particle size. The more PAH produced by AZIF-8, the larger the particle size; however, no other physical or chemical characteristics were investigated. AZIF-8 MOF with 60 nm demonstrated the strongest therapeutic benefits in a series of in vitro and in vivo studies, with excellent biocompatibility and tumor absorption capacity. Furthermore, Gao et al. (2017) have studied the magnetic sensitization, light sensitivity, active targeting, and chemotherapeutic drug-loading properties of Fe-MIL-53-NH_2 MOF. They also investigated the variables that affect particle size. They discovered that the lower reactant concentration yield, the greater the particle size of Fe-MIL-53-NH_2. Furthermore, the impact of benzoic acid on the particle size of UIO-66-NH_2, which was made using the hydrothermal approach, was investigated (Gao et al. 2018). In contrast to the preceding, the smaller the MOF particle size, the lower the benzoic acid used in the reaction. Thus, the effect of reactant concentration on the particle size of MOFs was represented in these tests. These studies, on the other hand, merely confirmed the factors that determine particle size; however, there was no insight into particle size's effectiveness and safety. Few researches focused solely on drug-loading capacity, ignoring the impact of particle size on bodily circulation. Even with the maximum drug loading, the system is swiftly metabolized and also resulted in the death of the model animal upon entering the systemic circulation. As a result, therapeutic benefits are impossible to achieve. Such research is obviously of no consequence. MOF-based nanocarriers used in cancer treatment have a wide range of particle sizes, and there has been a lack of comprehensive particle size evaluation in their application. This also serves as a foundation for future research.

The most basic requirement for drug-loading systems is stability. Some intelligent drug-loaded nanosystems have attracted researchers' attention in order to improve the efficacy and reduce the toxicity of anticancer treatments. To ensure efficacy and safety, these NPs must be stable while stored in vitro. As a result, the drug-loaded nanosystems should be stable in vivo before reaching the tumor site and responsive to drug release at the tumor site. Rachel et al. developed Zn-MTX NCP and Zr-MTX NCP (MTX: methotrexate, NCP: nanoscale coordination polymers) materials, respectively, utilizing Zn^{2+} and Zr^{4+} as metal centers, and discovered that both were unstable (Huxford et al. 2012). In the water, the particles may polymerize, causing the surface liposome to rupture. Finally, they created Gd-MTX NCP via microwave heating. After that, the phospholipid bilayer was wrapped around the MOF. The drug-loading system was found to be stable. Thus, any drug-loading system should consider the impact of each component on the system's stability. Thus, more research on the impacts of stability on the body's efficacy and toxicity is needed.

7.3.1 MOFs in Tumor Therapy

The integrity of regulatory circuits that control cell proliferation and maintenance is critical for normal cells. In cancer cells, regulatory circuits are disrupted, and the type and behavior of the cancer cell vary depending on the type of damage to the regulatory circuits (Lim et al. 2015). This feature can be used to treat tumor cells in a variety of ways, including passive, active, physicochemical, and a combination of the aforementioned methods (Baeza, Colilla, and Vallet-Regí 2015). By selectively hosting, transporting, and directing therapeutic agents to the tumor, targeted MOFs can overcome the lack of selectivity of certain drugs. Thus, the dose required for conventional chemotherapy can be reduced, resulting in improved therapeutic efficacy while reducing unwanted side effects. By modifying the surface of nanomaterials with antibodies or appropriate ligands/linkers, specific cells

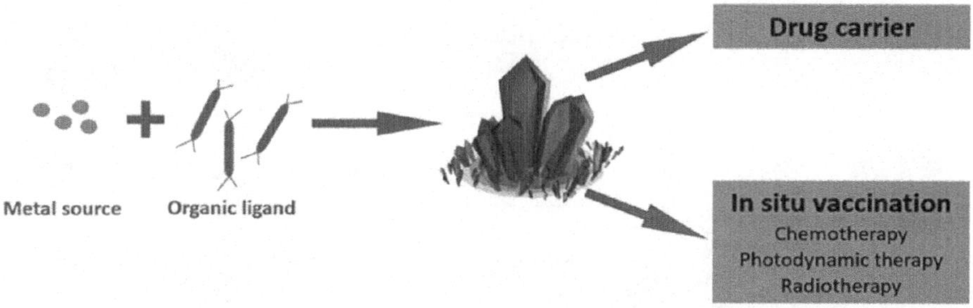

Figure 7.2 Schematic illustration of application of MOFs in tumor therapy.

and organs within the body can be targeted. Figure 7.2 shows the synthesis and applications of MOFs in various fields.

7.3.2 pH-Responsive MOFs

The pH of the tumor microenvironment is 5.7–7.8, the pH of lysosomes is 4.5–5.0, and the pH of endosomes is 5.5–6.0, all of which are lower than the pH of blood and normal tissues present in the human body. Using a pH-responsive method, encapsulated drug is transported and released in a controlled manner to many target sites, including gastrointestinal tract, tumor microenvironment, and cellular lysosomal/endosomal compartments. Aerobic glycolysis is the preferred energy source of cancer cells', irrespective of oxygen levels. As a result, lactate overproduction in the tumor microenvironment lowers the extracellular matrix's pH. The functional groups present in MOF such as pyridine group ($-C_5H_4N$), carboxyl group ($-COOH$), imidazolyl ($-C_3H_3N_2$), imino group ($-NH-$), phenolic hydroxyl group ($-C_6H_4OH$), daunosamine ($C_6H_{13}NO_3$), hydrazine (H_2N-NH_2), amide ($-CO$-$NH-$), amino group ($-NH_2$), benzoic imine bond, Schiff-base bond, and epoxy bond are pH responsive. In an acidic environment, the aforementioned functional groups protonate. Under certain pH conditions, the existing functional groups with side chains and the material backbone can be ionized, resulting in a conformational conversion of the complex resulting in dissolution or swelling. PH-responsive delivery systems have been developed using polyethylene glycol (PEG), polyethylene chitosan, polyacrylic acid (PAA), gelatine, and carboxymethyl cellulose. Wang et al. (2020) categorized pH-responsive MOF-based drug release mechanisms into the following: protonation-induced coordination bond breakage; pH-breakable bonds; pH-sensitive compounds; and host–guest interactions. Figure 7.3 represents the pH-simulative drug release mechanisms.

A few carboxylate-based MOFs, such as Fe-MIL-100, are protonated under acidic environments, enhancing electrostatic interactions and causing the cleavage of coordination between metal cluster and organic ligand.

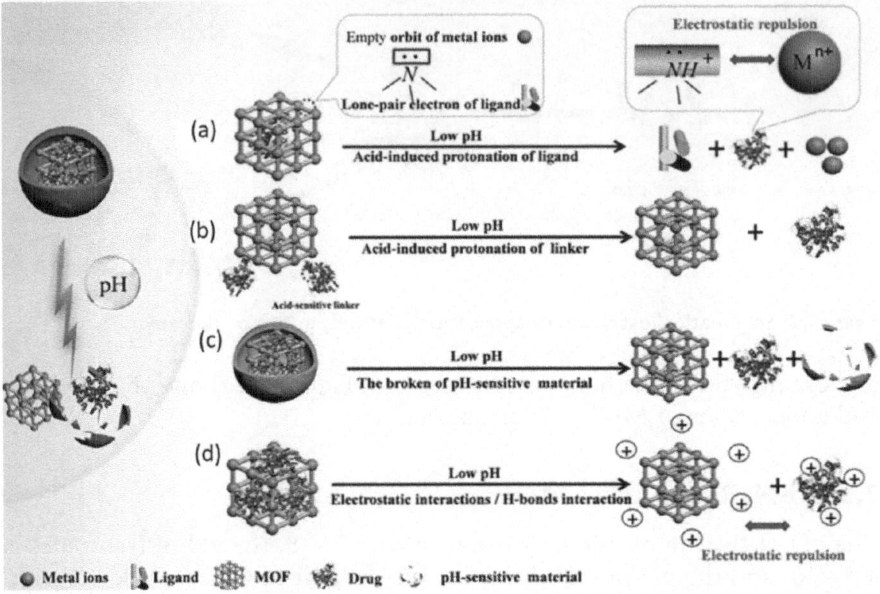

Figure 7.3 Mechanism of pH-responsive drug delivery in MOF. (a) Coordination bond breakage due to protonation. (b) pH-induced cleavage of linkers. (c) pH-sensitive molecules; and d) host–guest interaction. (Reproduced from reference Y. Wang et al. 2020 with permission from Elsevier.)

In this context, the magnetic nanomaterial Fe_3O_4@SiO_2@Fe-MIL-100 was developed to ensure the delivery of celecoxib, a common hydrophobic drug, into cancer cells. At physiological pH 7.4, a high adsorption ability was observed, but at acidic pH 5, a burst release was observed, making the produced nanocarrier suitable for cancer therapy (Lajevardi et al. 2020). With Fe-MIL-101 and NH_2-Fe-MIL-100, Cabrera-Garca et al. produced a novel drug delivery system that was covalently bonded to 20-(S)-camptothecin (CPT). CPT was esterified with various linker chains, and the resulting prodrugs were then attached to the amine groups of MOFs via amidation or click chemistry reactions. The obtained results revealed that the nanoplatform is extremely stable at physiological pH levels. Due to their potential and great response to the acidic condition, cell internalization of the CPT-loaded Fe-MIL-101 derivatives was improved. At pH 5, there was a 2- to 4-fold increase in drug release, which assisted intracellular discharge via endosomolytic effects (Cabrera-García et al. 2019). UiO-66 produced via solvothermal synthesis of $ZrCl_4$ (Zirconium(IV) chloride) with the ligand 1,4-dicarboxybenzene (BDC) is another example of porous and biocompatible MOFs. The protonation of carboxylate linker causes the framework to collapse in an acidic environment, allowing the cargo molecule to escape.

Gupta et al. developed UiO-66 MOF with a biocompatible PEG layer and loaded it with anticancer drug docetaxel (PEG@DTX@UiO-66). Their findings showed that low pH can shorten the time of drug release which can be attributed to faster disintegration of MOF particles at low pH compared to physiological pH (Gupta et al. 2019).

Cleavage of the coordination bond owing to protonation can be witnessed in ZIF-8 MOFs. The pH-responsive nanocomposites having a core-shell structure were developed by Lei et al. Here the ZIF-8 was produced in water by self-assembly of poly(-caprolactone)-block-poly (quaternized vinylbenzyl chloride/bipyridine) (PCL-b-q(PVBC/BPy), BCP) polymeric aggregates. The DOX is encapsulated in the micelle cores or vesicle inner cavities. To prevent the burst drug release in the physiological environment, ZIF-shell acts as a gatekeeper/barrier. The drug release from the core-shell structure (BCP@ZIF-8) was observed on demand in response to low pH, compared to bare polymeric aggregates loaded with DOX (Lei et al. 2020). Using a similar strategy, Ren et al. developed DOX-loaded pH and redox dual-responsive nanocarrier with a ZIF-8 nanostructure at the core and an organosilica shell using a one-pot synthesis technique (Ren et al. 2019). The core was encased in a biodegradable organosilica with multiple disulfide connections functioning as "gatekeepers" to create the core-shell structure. Because of the permeability and retention effect, the produced carrier was stable under normal conditions and has ability to quickly accumulate in tumor sites (enhanced permeability and retention). Also, flow cytometry and confocal imaging revealed that MOF can enter and completely release DOX in the cytosol of tumor cells when pH is low and glutathione levels are high, resulting in improved cytotoxicity against tumor cells.

The use of pH-sensitive systems using pH-responsive MOFs is another approach. Sivakumar et al. developed chitosan-capped Fe-MIL-88B-NH_2 as a pH-responsive DOX carrier. The chitosan capping layer prevents the Fe-MIL-88B-NH_2 MOFs structure from breaking by forming an insoluble gel-like structure at basic pH, whereas it promotes disintegration at acidic pH. The DOX was released into the tumor microenvironment using the physiochemical characteristics of chitosan (Sivakumar et al. 2017). Another method for synthesising pH-responsive MOFs is to use electrostatic, hydrogen-bonding and stacking are the interactions between the host and the guest (Zhao et al. 2019). To facilitate protonation, several functional groups must be coupled to drugs and ligands in order for electrostatic interactions to occur. Due to a pH change, electrostatic repulsion and charge reversal may occur, resulting in a higher rate of drug release. Few drugs with aromatic rings can form hydrogen bonds and interact with the MOF benzene rings, resulting in higher loading and better drug release control (Lin et al. 2017). The conjugated 1,3,6,8-tetrakis (p-benzoic acid) pyrene (H4TBAPy) linker was used to synthesize the Mg (H_2TBAPy) $(H_2O)_3C_4H_8O_2$ (TDL-Mg) MOF. Further, the loading content of 5-FU was

28.2 wt. % and achieved slow drug release. Because of the synergistic effect of polydirectional hydrogen-bonding interactions, multiple interactions, and limited channels, appropriate host–guest interactions were achieved, allowing the loading content of 76% for 5-FU drug to from the TDL-Mg carrier for 72 hours, which is a reasonable time for clinical applications (Hu et al. 2020). Thus, host–guest interactions were found to be good options to achieve controlled drug release.

7.3.3 Thermoresponsive MOFs

Temperature, as a major factor affecting materials on a nanoscale to atomic level, can be used as a variety of stimuli in porous materials such as MOF to control or activate the drug release process. Thermoresponsive materials can change phases at temperatures above or below a certain threshold. These phase shifts are known as the lower and upper critical solution temperatures (LCST or UCST).

Wu et al. produced a magnetic UiO-66 MOF (Fe_3O_4@UiO-66@WP6) coated with a water-soluble carboxylate pillararene (WP6). In this system, pillararene nanovalve-operated MOFs and core-shell nanocomposites were created to provide a theranostics platform for MRI-guided tumor therapy and multi-stimuli-responsive drug release. Figure 7.4 illustrates the synthesis and drug (5-Fu) release strategy of Fe_3O_4@UiO-66-NH_2, where Fe_3O_4 NPs and UiO-66 MOF were used as the core and shell, respectively (Wu, Gao, et al. 2018). Lin et al. investigated visual irradiation activated and regulated the release of small molecules from Zn-GA MOFs using L-glutamic acid and the nontoxic metal ion Zn^{2+}. The L-glutamic acid (GA) is a biocompatible amino acid with two carboxylic and one amine functional groups that can be used to coordinate metal centers. The antitumor drug methotrexate (MTX) was loaded onto Zn-GA using an in situ synthesis. The resulting drug carrier has several advantages, including dual temperature and pH responsiveness, adequate loading capability, low toxicity, and biocompatibility (Lin et al. 2018).

In its natural state, the polymer PNIPAM (poly(N-isopropyl acrylamide)) is not suitable for drug delivery. At 32°C and in physiologically relevant conditions, PNIPAM becomes hydrophobic. On the other hand, tailoring the transition temperature is possible by changing the side chain, molecular weight, structure, or copolymerization of the polymer with other hydrophobic or hydrophilic polymers. As a result, PNIPAM derivatives have become popular in thermosensitive drug delivery systems (Kokardekar, Shah, and Mody 2012). To address this, Nagata et al. recently covered UiO-66 MOF with PNIPAM copolymer, resulting in an MOF that can release a guest molecule in a regulated manner in response to changes in temperature and pH. When the globule conformation occurs at temperatures above 40°C and the pH is below 4.01, the guest molecule cannot be

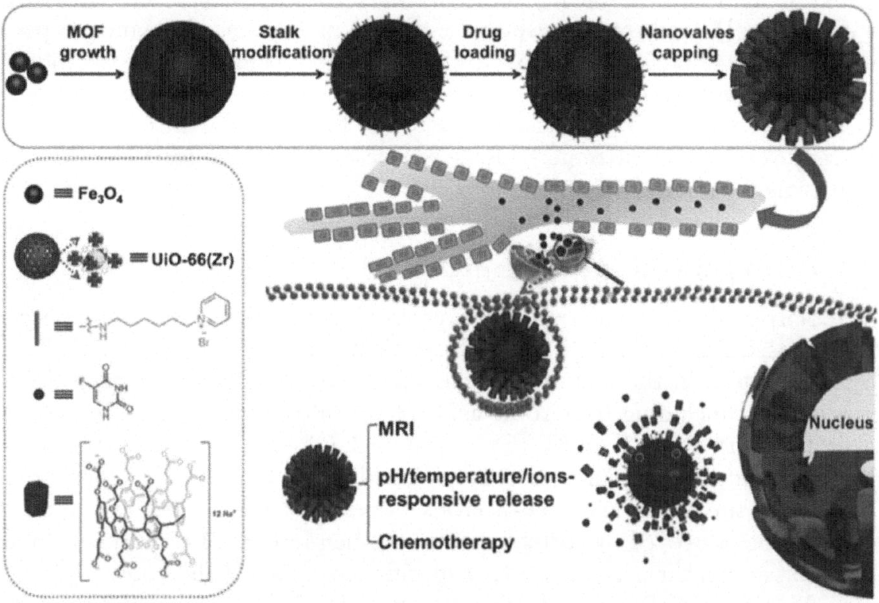

Figure 7.4 Schematic illustration of the synthesis and drug release stimuli of the Fe_3O_4@UiO-66@WP6 theranostics nanoplatform. (Reproduced from reference M.-X. Wu, Gao, et al. 2018 with permission from John Wiley and Sons.)

released; nevertheless, when the coil conformation happens at temperatures below 25°C and the pH is above 6.86, the guest molecule can be successfully released (Nagata, Kokado, and Sada 2020). Furthermore, H_2NPDA ((2E, 2′E)-3,3′-(naphthalene-1,4-diyl) diacrylic acid) was used as an organic linker in the production of the Zr-based MOF ZJU-801, which exhibited thermoresponsive properties (Jiang et al. 2017). To control the release of the drug at physiological temperatures, Silva et al. employed lanthanide ions (Eu^{3+} and/or Tb^{3+} ions) implanted in the ZIF-8 MOF structure as the shell and gold (Au) NPs as the core by functioning as sensitive nanothermometers and heaters, respectively. In this context, they developed (ZIF-8, Eu_xTb_y)@AuNP as a thermoresponsive material for controlled administration of model pharmacological compounds, caffeine and 5-FU. The system was also subjected to computational simulations. In this study, ZIF-8 was used and AuNPs as heaters and lanthanide ions as nanothermometers to control drug release in tumor cells at a physiological condition (Silva et al. 2019). A hybrid nanocomposite was produced that combines MOFs and a thermosensitive hydrogel to create an injectable implant. ($Zn_4O(C_8H_5NO_4)_3$, IRMOF-3) and poly(D, L-lactidecoglycolide)-poly(ethylene glycol)-poly(D, L-lactide-coglycolide) triblock copolymers (PLGA-PEG-PLGA) have been widely studied in terms of clinical applications. The proposed platform has a high drug-loading capacity, reduced toxicity in oral cancer cells in vitro, a constant pH, and thermoresponsive dual-drug release. The nanocomposite displayed remarkable tumor inhibition in vivo, tumor apoptosis induction, and tumor angiogenesis regression due to the synergistic effects of Cel (Celecoxib) and DOX. According to the findings, the anticipated local therapy resulted in extremely low systemic toxicity and no evident organ impairment (Tan et al. 2020).

7.3.4 Enzyme-Responsive MOFs

Materialswithhighenzymesensitivitywereemployedtocreateenzyme-responsive MOF-based drug delivery systems. Several enzyme-responsive materials have been employed in the majority of enzyme-responsive MOFs for drug delivery vehicles, including hyaluronic acid (HA)/hyaluronidase (HAase), pectin/pectinase, and Cy3-GRRGKC (Cy3: cyanine 3, GRRGKC: peptide)/cathepsin B (CaB). Some enzymes are overexpressed and can be found in high concentrations at the site of action or in cancerous tissues. Enzyme-responsive polymers can thus be destroyed by redox processes in the presence of certain enzymes, resulting in quicker drug release in a specific bio-milieu of the body.

Gold NPs functionalized with the cyanine 3 (Cy3)-labeled substrate peptide (Cy3-GRRGKC) (Au-Cy3P) and ZIF-8 (a pH-sensitive zeolitic imidazolate MOF) were used as the core and shell, respectively, to create the Au-Cy3P@ZIF-8 using the properties of both MOFs and NPs, as well as the CaB activity and acidic microenvironment. The nanoprobe's ZIF-8 shell might be disassembled in the acidic environment, allowing CaB to detect the exposed substrate peptide. The fluorescence was activated when the Cy3-labeled fragment left the AuNP surface after CaB cleavage of the Cy3-labeled peptides. As a result, a "signal on" method was used to produce a sensitive and precise CaB detection strategy. Because the lysosome microenvironment is more acidic than the cytoplasm (normal pH of 4.5–6.0), a precise targeted imaging technique to record the enzyme's activity in living cells was established. As a result, the imaging technique was able to detect lysosomal CaB, which is essential for cellular internalization. The prepared system aids in the understanding of how to build a dual-recognition nanoplatform. It also proves that stepwise-responsive imaging can be used in particular biomedical applications (Shen et al. 2018). In order to construct a combination of chemo- and photodynamic treatment, Kim et al. used a natural polysaccharide (hyaluronic acid) as a polymeric gatekeeper with sufficient biocompatibility over porphyrinic MOF containing Zr (PCN-224). One of the benefits of covering MOFs with the HA gatekeeper was the stable modification of the surface, which would protect the drug within the pore due to multiple coordination linkages between MOF and HA. Here the MOFs have excellent colloidal stability in water due to the hydrophilic HA on their surface; HA can be used as a cancer-targeting ligand in selective drug delivery due to its association with overexpressed CD44 (a cell surface glycoprotein antigen that serves as HA receptor) on the tumor cell surface; and HAdase degrades HA and speeds up drug release into the cancer cell (Liu et al. 2016). Because of its large surface area, MOF has a high capacity for DOX loading through physical adsorption. By blocking the pore's entrance and trapping drug molecules inside the MOF structure, HA prevented drug molecules from being released prematurely via polyvalent coordination bonds and electrostatic interactions. The HAdase enzyme initiated the drug release, and the HA-DOX-PCN system was created specifically to target cancer cells. In vitro studies combining chemotherapy and PDT (photodynamic treatment) revealed that light irradiation had a higher therapeutic efficacy. This nanocarrier has a wide range of applications in drug delivery to the site of action, cancer targeting, and PDT (Kim et al. 2019).

NANs (nucleic acid nanocapsule) enter cells via endocytosis when an enzyme-triggered breakdown occurs, resulting in the release of intracellular molecules. They showed that combining a triggerable release with the large storage capacity of NANs and MOFs enables the integration of a wide range of molecular cargos into a nanomaterial with programmable capabilities and controllable release profiles. The disintegration of MOF-NANs could be influenced by a number of factors, including pH variations and enzymes. Figure 7.5 represents the construction of selective release profiles for biological ecosystems that are more complex. Finally, the controllability of the release of tiny plasmids, proteins, and molecules was investigated using a combination of in vitro fluorescence assays and cytotoxicity experiments. MOF-NANs have the potential to be employed in diagnostic and therapeutic applications, according to the findings (Tolentino et al. 2020).

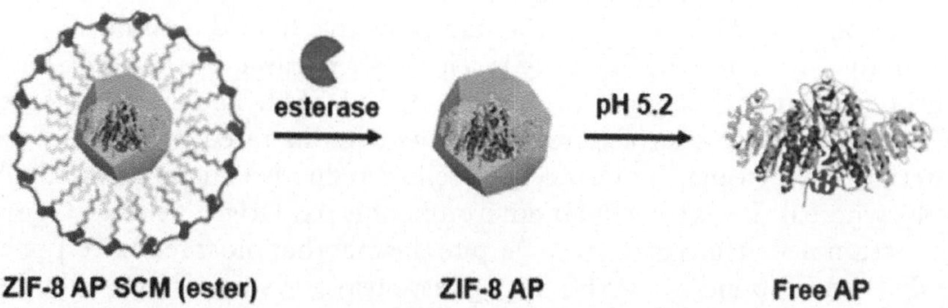

Figure 7.5 Schematic illustration of esterase and pH 5.2 triggered the release of alkaline phosphatase (AP) from the ZIF-8 SCM (surface-crosslinked micelle). (Reproduced from reference Tolentino et al. 2020 with permission from the Royal Society of Chemistry.)

7.3.5 Redox-Responsive MOFs

Redox-responsive MOFs release the drug when redox reaction occurs. Tumors have a redox potential that stimulates the production of redox-responsive carriers because they have both a reducing intracellular and an oxidizing extracellular environment. Glutathione concentrations in the nucleus and cytoplasm can cause redox-responsive carriers to lose structural integrity (Mura, Nicolas, and Couvreur 2013). In comparison to normal tissues, malignant tissues have exceptionally high GSH (glutathione) concentrations (2–10 mM in the cytoplasm) and are almost 100–1,000 times greater than the extracellular matrix and blood (2–20 μM) (Liu et al. 2017). GSH can be oxidized by oxidizing agents such as redox-active compounds and disulfide bonds since it is a potent reducing agent. The disulfide linkages can be found in a variety of compounds, including 4,4′-dithiobisbenzoic acid (4,4′-DTBA), 3,30-dithiobis (DTPC), and dithiodiglycolic acid. Several chemicals, such as 2,5-disulfanylterephthalic acid (BDC-$(SH)_2$), were employed to supply disulfide linkages in MOF structures in order to build glutathione-responsive MOFs. Furthermore, cations in some MOFs (such as redox-active ions Mn(IV) or Cu(II)) have a tendency to oxidize GSH, resulting in MOF degradation (Wang et al. 2020).

The copper ion was used to create 2D-MOFs of Cu-TCPP (tetrakis (4-carboxyphenyl)porphyrin) nanosheets that produce $^1O_2$ when they react with H_2O_2 in the tumor microenvironment, depleting GSH in the process. The produced Cu-TCPP can cause tumor cell death in vitro and in vivo with no adverse effects due to the production of $^1O_2$ and the blocking of $^1O_2$ scavenging by GSH. External light and oxygen stimulation, both of which are vital in PDT, are no longer required, paving the path for the development of cancer therapeutic methods (Tian et al. 2019). Further, Miao et al. developed a dual-sensitive hybrid MOF ($PMAA_{BACy}$@$(MOF)_{10}$@PDA) that was H_2O_2 (hydrogen peroxide) and GSH responsive. This MOF was made out of polymethylacrylic acid cores, a disulfide bond cross-linked structure, PDA coating, and a $PMAA_{BACy}/Fe^{3+}$-based MOF interlayer (Miao et al. 2019). In reaction to H_2O_2 and GSH, the dual-sensitive hybrid eliminated tumor cells in the site of action. The drug is selectively released by the DOX-loaded hybrid MOF at pathological levels of H_2O_2 and GSH. The precise release of DOX in the tumor microenvironment was demonstrated using this hybrid material. The cytoplasm of cancerous cells is reductive due to elevated GSH levels, whereas the extracellular environment is oxidative due to H_2O_2 overproduction in cancerous tissues. Despite the fact that most redox-responsive MOFs can respond to GSH, H_2O_2-responsive systems have only been described in a few cases in the context of cancer therapy. Gong et al. created a GSH-responsive MOF using zirconium (Zr^{4+}) ion, modulator benzoic acid (BA), and ligand 2,5-BDC-$(SH)_2$. By establishing disulfide connections between 6-mercaptopurine and BDC-SH_2, the thiol-containing anticancer drug 6-MP was efficiently loaded into the GSH-responsive MOF. In the

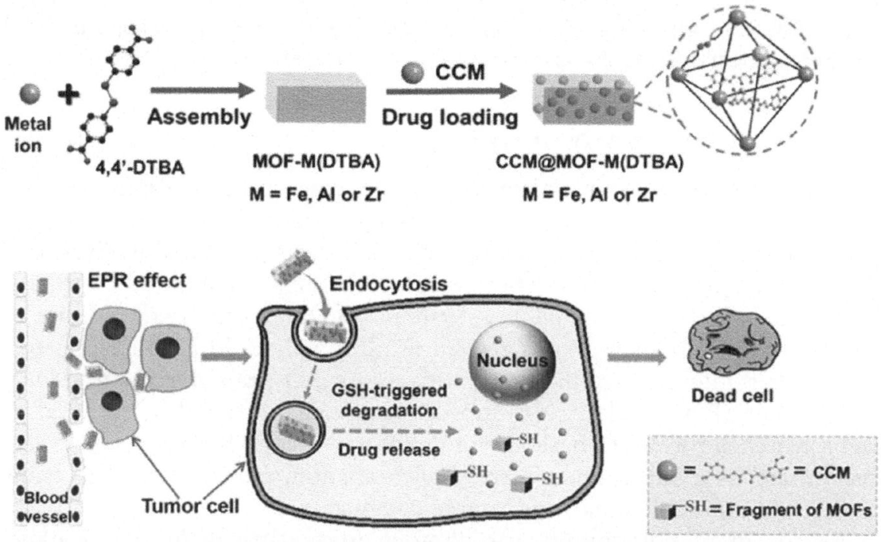

Figure 7.6 Schematic illustration of synthesis of curcumin (CCM) loaded Zr(DTBA) MOF and redox-responsive release of CCM in cancer cells. (Reproduced from reference B. Lei et al. 2018 with permission from American Chemical Society.)

presence of GSH, the disulfide bonds of MOFs were disrupted, resulting in the release of 6-MP. The drug-loaded MOF demonstrated a novel intracellular redox-responsive drug release ability. Cancer cells displayed higher cytotoxicity than normal cells, leading in tumor-selective chemotherapy that was more effective (Gong et al. 2020). Another GSH-responsive MOF, Zr(DTBA) MOF, containing organic ligand 4,4′-DTBA was loaded with curcumin. In vitro, studies revealed MOF-Zr(DTBA) showed a faster rate of drug release inside cancer cells, and preclinical testing showed that in vivo, the MOF-Zr(DTBA) had considerably stronger anticancer effect than free curcumin (Lei et al. 2018). Figure 7.6 shows the synthesis and release of curcumin from Zr(DTBA) MOF.

Redox-active elements (such as MnO_2 (manganese(IV) oxide) or cations like Cu(II)) also oxidize GSH, destroying redox-responsive molecules. Tian et al. developed a porphyrin-MOF (PCN-222) coated with MnO_2 (PCN@MnO_2) for MRI-guided drug-PDT dual therapy. To drain excess GSH in tumor tissue, MnO_2 was produced in situ on the surface of PAH-coated PCN-222. The PDT effect was increased as a result of GSH's inhibitory influence on$^1O_2$ production. The amount of GSH produced by the generated Mn^{2+} may be determined using T1-MRI. When Mn^{2+} was produced from MnO_2, the T1-MR shows brighter images, which can be attributed to a lower amount of GSH. Following the release of DOX, light irradiation effectively improved PDT, resulting in PDT/chemo dual therapy. The influence of GSH on $^1O_2$ formation was minimized as a result of the presence of MnO_2, allowing for better PDT efficiency and DOX release control for MRI-guided PDT chemotherapy (Tian et al. 2019).

7.3.6 Photoresponsive MOFs

Light is one of the most prevalent responses because it allows for fine control of intensity and depth of penetration. Here the photoactive chemicals such as anthracene, azobenzenedicarboxylate (AZB), porphyrin derivatives, and indocyanine green (ICG) have been employed as ligands in the MOF to produce light-responsive drug delivery systems. Further, altering the surface of certain photoresponsive materials can result in enhanced photoresponsiveness. The photosensitive materials such as Ag_3PO_4, polydopamine (PDA), polypyrrole (PPy), and UCNPs (up conversion nanoparticles) are used as light switches for MOF-based drug delivery systems. Because it is widely recognized as a naturally occurring phenomenon, photo-related cis–trans isomerization is called nature-inspired chemistry.

Among many compounds, the photochemistry of azobenzene is likely the most researched cis–trans isomerization. Trans–cis photo-isomerization causes major changes in molecular size, structure, and polarity, which opens up a lot of possibilities for making smart materials. Stefaniak et al. employed the photoresponsive linker AZB in UiO MOF (UiO-AZB). They discovered photo-isomerization of AZB linker led UiO-AZB nanocarriers to break down when exposed to light. Further, UiO-AZB was used to release the drugs in a photo-controllable strategy by concurrently cleaving the carrier. The anticancer drug 5-FU was used in photoresponsive architecture. To improve biocompatibility, stability, and half-life of MOF-containing 5-FU, PEG-NH_2 was coated on the MOF surface. In the absence of light, these drug delivery systems remained stable and only deteriorated when exposed to 340 nm light (Falsafi et al. 2021).

Photodynamic therapy (PDT) is a versatile tumor treatment that can be used in a variety of ways. PDT, unlike other tumor treatments, is less intrusive, has less cumulative toxicity, and has a higher rate of responsiveness. Additionally, some excited electrons in photosensitizers may be able to use the radiation pathway to return to the system's zero-point energy, and PDT allows for fluorescence imaging (Khdair et al. 2010). The MOF nanostructures with porphyrin have been proven as adaptable photosensitizers for PDT with excellent efficiency due to their biodegradability, practical functionality, and structural flexibility. For instance, smart PDT NPs that evolved O_2 for homologous tumor cell targeting and dual-mode cancer cell imaging (fluorescence/MRI) were developed. Porphyrin MOFs formed the basis of the core composition. The porphyrin MOFs core was then functionalized with a thin MnO_2 nanosheet (MMNPs) layer. This hybrid nanostructure responds to H_2O_2 with sensitivity under acidic environments. This feature increased O_2 production, which improved the efficiency of the O_2-mediated PDT. Furthermore, Mn^{2+} ions released into the solution allowed for MRI imaging, which was confirmed by T1-weighted MRI. The cancer cell membrane was viewed as a covering shell of MMNPs in order to achieve the ability to target cancer cells (CM-MMNPs). The microscopic images demonstrated that CM-MMNPs remained stable in a biological buffer while targeting homogenous cancer cells with remarkable efficiency. Due to the effective etching of the MnO_2 coating during endocytosis, the synthesized structure emitted red fluorescence after laser irradiation. The formation of singlet oxygen and Mn^{2+} appears to be favored by PDT and dual-mode imaging of cancer cells (Zhang et al. 2019).

PDT is largely cantered on the second type of oxygen-dependent process, which includes transferring energy from the excited state of photosensitizers (PS) to the molecular form of oxygen (O_2) to produce singlet oxygen or $^1O_2$, despite its potential in tumor therapy. Type II PDT's therapeutic efficacy is demonstrated in a hypoxic environment to resemble tumor environment. Type I PDT, on the other hand, has a greater tolerance to hypoxia because the ET (electron transfer) from the excited PS state to the O_2 molecules and organic molecules produces harmful radicals. As a result, Lan et al. created a TiTBP MOF made up of Ti-oxo chain secondary building units (SBUs) and photosensitizers 5,10,15,20-tetra(*p*-benzoato)porphyrin (TBP) ligands. This produced hydroxyl radicals ($^{\cdot}OH$), H_2O_2, and superoxide (O_2) in type I PDT. $TBP^{\bullet+}$ ligands and a Ti^{3+} core were created by transitioning electrons from heated TBP* species to SBUs based on Ti^{4+}. With a regression rate of >98% and a cure rate of 60%, the administration of four different ROSs resulted in significant tumor inhibitory activity (Lan et al. 2019).

The incorporation of photo-switchable compounds into drug carriers allows for their remote control of chemical and physical properties. MOFs are one type of smart, light-responsive material. By integrating photo-switchable molecules into MOFs, new functionality can be added, potentially leading to remotely controlled crystalline structures (Fan et al. 2021). Lin et al. created a photoresponsive nanoswitch MOF that could stimulate quick endo/lysosomal breach and oligonucleotide (siRNA (small-interfering ribonucleic acid) and RNAi (ribonucleic acid interference)) release. ZIF-8 with internal photothermal agent ICG carried siRNAs via electrostatic adsorption in the nanoswitch MOF. To facilitate the "off-to-on" switching, ICG absorbed light and generated local heat, resulting in rapid release of a high number of siRNAs and the dissociation of ZIF-8. The endo/lysosomal rupture occurred in this system as a result of mild UV irradiation and the pH sensitivity of Zn^{2+} and 2-methylimidazolate (MI) in endo/lysosomes in an acidic environment. This form of switching offers RNAi delivery for cancer therapy and a lot of spatiotemporal control. By recapturing, the fluorescence signals of ICG might be used to observe the transfer of siRNA at the same time by switching it "off-to-on." In addition, other therapeutic substances including DNA, protein, and anticancer drugs can also be transported using the nanoswitch (Lin et al. 2020).

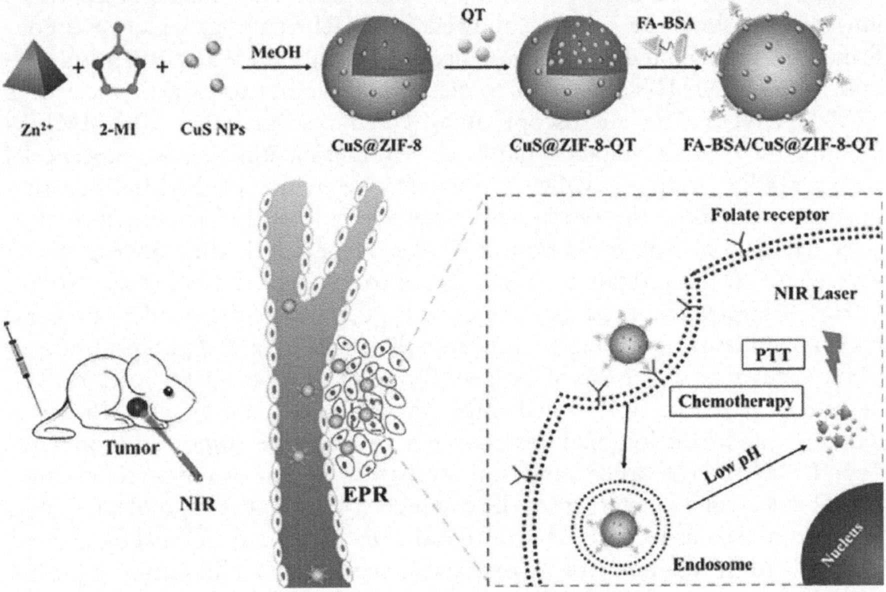

Figure 7.7 Schematic illustration of production of FA–BSA modified ZIF-8 (FA–BSA/CuS@ZIF-8-QT) and external stimuli-responsive release of drug in tumor microenvironment. (Reproduced from reference W. Jiang et al. 2018 with permission from American Chemical Society.)

A multifunctional chemo-photothermal system has recently gained popularity. This approach employs a nanomaterial system for drug administration and efficient photothermal conversion (Jiang et al. 2018). Figure 7.7 represents the photothermal-responsive release of drugs in tumor microenvironment. Photothermal therapy is the use of materials that attract and convert energy from near-infrared (NIR) light into thermal energy, resulting in localized hyperthermia (PTT). To combat tumor growth, the aforementioned approach can be applied. NIR irradiation has the ability to enter tissues with pinpoint accuracy and intensity. In the range of 700 – 1100 nm, blood and soft tissues are fairly transparent. PTT is favorable because it is just mildly aggressive and has a low risk of harming healthy tissues (Cai et al. 2018). As photothermal agents, a variety of materials, including metals and polymers, have been employed. Jiang et al. used Cu as a PTT therapeutic agent in ZIF-8 MOF and constructed a nanoplatform with numerous functions for the codelivery of CuS NPs and quercetin (QT) to synergistically combine chemotherapy and PTT. A coating of bovine serum albumin-folic acid (BSA-FA) was also employed to maintain the stability of CuS@ZIF-8-QT and increase QT bioavailability while allowing for tailored dosing. NIR fluorescence imaging demonstrated aggregation of BSA-FA/CuS@ZIF-8-QT in cancer cells via FA receptor-mediated endocytosis. NIR irradiation boosted synergistic efficacy of QT and CuS in vivo and in vitro anticancer assessments (Jiang et al. 2018). Li et al. successfully coated a single gold nanorod (AuNR) with ZIF-8 MOF to provide NIR-responsive photothermal and chemotherapeutic effects. Here the Au nanorods, compared to spherical AuNPs, have exceptionally robust LSPR (longitude surface plasmon resonance) adsorption characteristics in the near-infrared. The AuNR@ZIF-8 core-shell nanostructures demonstrated a high capacity for loading and releasing DOX in response to the two triggers of pH and NIR light at 808 nm and were successful as synergic chemo-photothermal treatment (Li et al. 2018).

Further, PTT is commonly achieved using coating MOFs with polymers such as PDA, PPy, and polyaniline (PANI). Polyaniline-coated ZIF-8 MOFs (nPANI@nZIF-8) were produced and employed as a 5-FU distribution system. Most of the encapsulated 5-FU (up to 68%) was released at pH 5.2 because the ZIF-8 network is pH responsive. The inclusion of nPANI drastically boosted NIR absorbance. In addition, local hyperthermia evolved as a result of the absorbed NIR, which enhanced drug diffusion from carrier at the site of action. This function facilitates on-demand 5-FU release by using an NIR laser (980 nm) and raising the hyperthermia to around 70°C (80%) (Silva et al. 2018).

Furthermore, PDA drastically improved the biocompatibility of ZIF-8 MOF as a pH-responsive platform. In addition, MOF's reactivity to NIR irradiation resulted in hyperthermia, which caused tetradecanol (phase change material) to phase change on the carriers surface, leading to drug release and synergistic thermo-chemotherapy (Wu et al. 2018). Figure 7.8 illustrates the synthesis of ZIF-8 MOF and NIR irradiation drug release mechanisms. Another MOF that is used in PTT is the Fe-soc-MOF carrier. It was made up of 3,3,5,5-azo benzenetetracarboxylic acid ligand and building blocks of iron carboxylate trimer molecules with oxygen at their center. After that, PPy was added to Fe-soc-MOF that had been treated with PEG. The MOF nanocomposites were highly effective in the detection and treatment of cancer in vitro and in vivo, according to the results of utilizing Fe-soc-MOF@PPy as a PTT agent (Cai et al. 2019).

7.3.7 Magnetic Field-Responsive MOFs

Magnetic NPs, superparamagnetic iron oxide NPs (SPIONs), can be used as built therapies and are incorporated with other materials (MOF) to give them magnetic qualities. Drug delivery using MOFs has unique structures that use external magnetic fields as a stimulus to release their payload. These systems are employed as an external magnetic field to transport drug-loaded magnetic NPs to the site of action and release them on demand, therefore increasing therapeutic efficiency. Magnetic MOFs are nontoxic and have a high drug-loading capacity as well as a high transverse relativity for MR imaging (Xie et al. 2011).

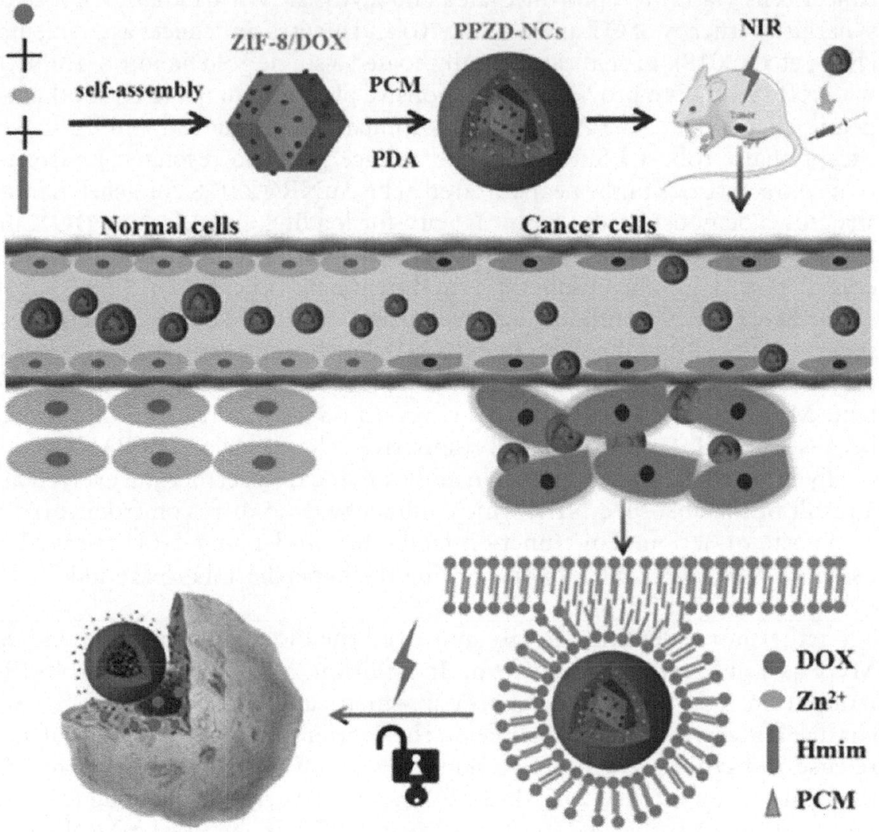

Figure 7.8 Schematic illustration of the synthesis of PDA-PCM@ZIF-8/DOX and controlled release through thermo-chemotherapy. (Reproduced from reference Wu et al. 2018 with permission from Elsevier.)

Zhao et al. produced a theranostics Fe_3O_4@UiO-66 core-shell composite on UiO-66 MOF functioning as the shell and being generated in situ on the Fe_3O_4 core to transport drugs while allowing for MR imaging. The shell of UiO-66 was merely used to encapsulate the drug in these composites, while the core of Fe_3O_4 served as an MR (magnetic resonance) imaging contrast agent. The Fe_3O_4@UiO-66 core-shell was biocompatible, had a high drug-loading efficiency, and could be employed for magnetic resonance imaging (Zhao et al. 2016). Sene et al. created Fe_2O_3/MIL-100(Fe) composites with minimal toxicity and a potent anticancer platform. They employed the system in vivo as an useful agent for MRI imaging due to its outstanding relaxivity properties (Sene et al. 2017). The role of Fe-MIL-100 MOF and its composite, Fe_3O_4@MIL-100 in delivering the anticancer drug DOX was investigated. The Fe_3O_4@MIL-100, which contained around 16 wt.% Fe_3O_4 NPs, exhibited the highest DOX-loading capacity (19 wt.%). The DOX release profiles from prepared systems in PBS (phosphate-buffered saline) with pH 7.4 at 37°C revealed that the kinetics become slower after the Fe_3O_4 NPs were incorporated (Bhattacharjee, Gumma, and Purkait 2018). Shi et al. employed a similar method to study Fe_3O_4-NH_2@MIL101-NH_2 MOF with a 36.02% DOX-loading capacity (Li et al. 2017). Later, Wang et al. have developed core-shell -Fe_2O_3/La-MOFs@SiO_2 NPs that may transport drugs in a multifunctional manner. The outcome of this study revealed that such systems are extremely biocompatible, have a large efficiency for drug loading, and can deliver pH-responsive release on demand. Due to its magnetic nature and bright blue fluorescence, the system has significant potential to be termed a magneto-responsive platform and magnetic resonance or fluorescence dual-mode imaging system (Sun et al. 2018).

7.4 CONCLUSION AND FUTURE PROSPECTIVE

MOF-based porous materials for drug delivery to a specific target for tumor therapy and diagnosis have shown great potential. MOF-based systems have adjustable pore size, biocompatible, efficient, and stable for a variety of drug delivery strategies against tumor. This chapter summarizes the most recent developments and advancements in MOF-based systems for tumor therapy and diagnosis.

Generally, MOFs-based drug-loaded granules rarely achieve long-term circulation in the body, generally are being metabolized prematurely by the body or cleared by the immune system, which result in reduced efficacy. As the drug-loaded particles circulate, the premature release of the chemotherapeutic drugs renders these drugs toxic to normal tissues. This issue can be overcome by surface modifying the MOFs surface for targeted drug delivery applications. Targeting strategies can maximize efficacy while minimizing negative consequences. The evolution of multifunctional MOFs may be able to compensate for the drawbacks of single targeting approaches. On the other hand, MOF-based NPs with multitargeted responses have become the most often employed technique. The development of these intelligent systems could lead to better drug release control, precise drug transportation, accurate tumor imaging, high tumor penetration, and enhanced tumor therapies.

ACKNOWLEDGMENTS

Prof. Kyeong-Hwan Lee thanks Korea Institute of Planning and Evaluation for Technology in Food, Agriculture and Forestry (IPET) and Korea Smart Farm R&D Foundation (KosFarm) through the Smart Farm

Innovation Technology Development Program, funded by the Ministry of Agriculture, Food and Rural Affairs (MAFRA), Ministry of Science and ICT (MSIT), Rural Development Administration (RDA) (grant no. 42103204).

REFERENCES

Baeza, Alejandro, Montserrat Colilla, and María Vallet-Regí. 2015. "Advances in mesoporous silica nanoparticles for targeted stimuli-responsive drug delivery." *Expert Opinion on Drug Delivery* 12 (2): 319–337.

Beg, Sarwar, Mahfoozur Rahman, Atul Jain, Sumant Saini, Patrick Midoux, Chantal Pichon, Farhan Jalees Ahmad, and Sohail Akhter. 2017. "Nanoporous metal organic frameworks as hybrid polymer–metal composites for drug delivery and biomedical applications." *Drug Discovery Today* 22 (4): 625–637.

Belfiore, Lisa, Darren N. Saunders, Marie Ranson, Kristofer J. Thurecht, Gert Storm, and Kara L. Vine. 2018. "Towards clinical translation of ligand-functionalized liposomes in targeted cancer therapy: Challenges and opportunities." *Journal of Controlled Release* 277: 1–13.

Bendre, Akhilesh, Mahesh P. Bhat, Kyeong-Hwan Lee, Tariq Altalhi, Mohammed Ayad Alruqi, and Mahaveer Kurkuri. 2022. "Recent developments in microfluidic technology for synthesis and toxicity-efficiency studies of biomedical nanomaterials." *Materials Today Advances* 13: 100205.

Bhat, Mahesh P., Madhuprasad Kigga, Harshith Govindappa, Pravin Patil, Ho-Young Jung, Jingxian Yu, and Mahaveer Kurkuri. 2019. "A reversible fluoride chemosensor for the development of multi-input molecular logic gates." *New Journal of Chemistry* 43 (32): 12734–12743.

Bhat, Mahesh P., Mahaveer Kurkuri, Dusan Losic, Madhuprasad Kigga, and Tariq Altalhi. 2021. "New optofluidic based lab-on-a-chip device for the real-time fluoride analysis." *Analytica Chimica Acta* 1159: 338439.

Bhat, Mahesh P., Madhuprasad, Pravin Patil, S. K. Nataraj, Tariq Altalhi, Ho-Young Jung, Dusan Losic, and Mahaveer D. Kurkuri. 2016. "Turmeric, naturally available colorimetric receptor for quantitative detection of fluoride and iron." *Chemical Engineering Journal* 303: 14–21.

Bhat, Mahesh P., U. T. Uthappa, and Mahaveer D. Kurkuri. 2021. "Surface-functionalized diatom silica as a bio-absorbent for the removal of toxins from water." In Thangadurai, D., Sangeetha, J., Prasad, R. (eds.) *Bioprospecting Algae for Nanosized Materials*, 383–402. Springer, Cham.

Bhat, Mahesh P., Shraddha Vinayak, Jingxian Yu, Ho-Young Jung, and Mahaveer Kurkuri. 2020. "Colorimetric receptors for the detection of biologically important anions and their application in designing molecular logic gate." *ChemistrySelect* 5 (42): 13135–13143.

Bhat, Shrinath, U. T. Uthappa, Tariq Altalhi, Ho-Young Jung, and Mahaveer D. Kurkuri. 2021. "Functionalized porous hydroxyapatite scaffolds for tissue engineering applications: A focused review." *ACS Biomaterials Science & Engineering*. doi: 10.1021/acsbiomaterials.1c00438.

Bhattacharjee, Abhik, Sasidhar Gumma, and Mihir Kumar Purkait. 2018. "Fe_3O_4 promoted metal organic framework MIL-100 (Fe) for the controlled release of doxorubicin hydrochloride." *Microporous and Mesoporous Materials* 259: 203–210.

Bonneau, Mickaele, Christophe Lavenn, Patrick Ginet, Ken-ichi Otake, and Susumu Kitagawa. 2020. "Upscale synthesis of a binary pillared layered MOF for hydrocarbon gas storage and separation." *Green Chemistry* 22 (3): 718–724.

Cabrera-García, Alejandro, Elisa Checa-Chavarria, Eva Rivero-Buceta, Victoria Moreno, Eduardo Fernández, and Pablo Botella. 2019. "Amino modified metal-organic frameworks as pH-responsive nanoplatforms for safe delivery of camptothecin." *Journal of Colloid and Interface Science* 541: 163–174.

Cai, Mengru, Gongsen Chen, Liuying Qin, Changhai Qu, Xiaoxv Dong, Jian Ni, and Xingbin Yin. 2020. "Metal organic frameworks as drug targeting delivery vehicles in the treatment of cancer." *Pharmaceutics* 12 (3): 232.

Cai, Xuechao, Xiaoran Deng, Zhongxi Xie, Yanshu Shi, Maolin Pang, and Jun Lin. 2019. "Controllable synthesis of highly monodispersed nanoscale Fe-soc-MOF and the construction of Fe-soc-MOF@ polypyrrole core-shell nanohybrids for cancer therapy." *Chemical Engineering Journal* 358: 369–378.

Cai, Xuechao, Bei Liu, Maolin Pang, and Jun Lin. 2018. "Interfacially synthesized Fe-soc-MOF nanoparticles combined with ICG for photothermal/photodynamic therapy." *Dalton Transactions* 47 (45): 16329–16336.

Cao, Xin, Lin Dai, Luying Wang, Jing Liu, and Jiandu Lei. 2015. "A surfactant template-assisted strategy for synthesis of ZIF-8 hollow nanospheres." *Materials Letters* 161: 682–685.

DeSantis, Carol E., Kimberly D. Miller, Ann Goding Sauer, Ahmedin Jemal, and Rebecca L. Siegel. 2019. "Cancer statistics for african americans, 2019." *CA: A Cancer Journal for Clinicians* 69 (3): 211–233.

Duan, Dongban, Hui Liu, Mengxin Xu, Mengqi Chen, Yuxiang Han, Yaxin Shi, and Zhibo Liu. 2018. "Size-controlled synthesis of drug-loaded zeolitic imidazolate framework in aqueous solution and size effect on their cancer theranostics in vivo." *ACS Applied Materials & Interfaces* 10 (49): 42165–42174.

Falsafi, Monireh, Amir Sh Saljooghi, Khalil Abnous, Seyed Mohammad Taghdisi, Mohammad Ramezani, and Mona Alibolandi. 2021. "Smart metal organic frameworks: Focus on cancer treatment." *Biomaterials Science* 9 (5): 1503–1529.

Fan, Shuaikang, Shilin Wang, Xiaobin Wang, Zhuoyi Li, Xu Ma, Xinyi Wan, Shabab Hussain, and Xinsheng Peng. 2021. "Photogated proton conductivity of ZIF-8 membranes co-modified with graphene quantum dots and polystyrene sulfonate." *Science China Materials* 64 (8): 1997–2007.

Furukawa, Hiroyasu, Kyle E. Cordova, Michael O'Keeffe, and Omar M. Yaghi. 2013. "The chemistry and applications of metal-organic frameworks." *Science* 341 (6149): 1230444.

Gallis, Dorina F Sava, Lauren E. S. Rohwer, Mark A. Rodriguez, Meghan C. Barnhart-Dailey, Kimberly S. Butler, Ting S. Luk, Jerilyn A. Timlin, and Karena W. Chapman. 2017. "Multifunctional, tunable metal-organic framework materials platform for bioimaging applications." *ACS Applied Materials & Interfaces* 9 (27): 22268–22277.

Gao, Xuechuan, Ruixue Cui, Guanfeng Ji, and Zhiliang Liu. 2018. "Size and surface controllable metal–organic frameworks (MOFs) for fluorescence imaging and cancer therapy." *Nanoscale* 10 (13): 6205–6211.

Gao, Xuechuan, Xiao Hai, Huricha Baigude, Weihua Guan, and Zhiliang Liu. 2016. "Fabrication of functional hollow microspheres constructed from MOF shells: Promising drug delivery systems with high loading capacity and targeted transport." *Scientific Reports* 6 (1): 1–10.

Gao, Xuechuan, Manjue Zhai, Weihua Guan, Jingjuan Liu, Zhiliang Liu, and Alatangaole Damirin. 2017. "Controllable synthesis of a smart multifunctional nanoscale metal–organic framework for magnetic resonance/optical imaging and targeted drug delivery." *ACS Applied Materials & Interfaces* 9 (4): 3455–3462.

Gao, Yu, Jingjing Xie, Haijun Chen, Songen Gu, Rongli Zhao, Jingwei Shao, and Lee Jia. 2014. "Nanotechnology-based intelligent drug design for cancer metastasis treatment." *Biotechnology Advances* 32 (4): 761–777.

Gong, Ming, Jian Yang, Yongsheng Li, and Jinlou Gu. 2020. "Glutathione-responsive nanoscale MOFs for effective intracellular delivery of the anticancer drug 6-mercaptopurine." *Chemical Communications* 56 (47): 6448–6451.

González, Cesar M. Oliva, Boris I. Kharisov, Oxana V. Kharissova, and Thelma E. Serrano Quezada. 2021. "Synthesis and applications of MOF-derived nanohybrids: A review." *Materials Today: Proceedings* 46 (8): 3018–3029.

Guan, Lijuan, Loris Rizzello, and Giuseppe Battaglia. 2015. "Polymersomes and their applications in cancer delivery and therapy." *Nanomedicine* 10 (17): 2757–2780.

Guo, Yan, Yantao Li, Sijie Zhou, Qingsong Ye, Xingjie Zan, and Yan He. 2021. "Metal–organic framework-based composites for protein delivery and therapeutics." *ACS Biomaterials Science & Engineering*. doi: 10.1021/acsbiomaterials.0c01600.

Gupta, Vandana, Shanid Mohiyuddin, Abhay Sachdev, P. K. Soni, P. Gopinath, and Sachin Tyagi. 2019. "PEG functionalized zirconium dicarboxylate MOFs for docetaxel drug delivery in vitro." *Journal of Drug Delivery Science and Technology* 52: 846–855.

Hu, Zengchi, Chengfang Qiao, Zhengqiang Xia, Feng Li, Jing Han, Qing Wei, Qi Yang, Gang Xie, Sanping Chen, and Shengli Gao. 2020. "A luminescent mg-metal–organic framework for sustained release of 5-fluorouracil: Appropriate host–guest interaction and satisfied acid–base resistance." *ACS Applied Materials & Interfaces* 12 (13): 14914–14923.

Huxford, Rachel C., Kathryn E. deKrafft, William S. Boyle, Demin Liu, and Wenbin Lin. 2012. "Lipid-coated nanoscale coordination polymers for targeted delivery of antifolates to cancer cells." *Chemical Science* 3 (1): 198–204.

Jia, Jianguo, Yang Zhang, Min Zheng, Changfu Shan, Huicheng Yan, Wenyu Wu, Xuan Gao, Bo Cheng, Weisheng Liu, and Yu Tang. 2018. "Functionalized Eu(III)-based nanoscale metal–organic framework to achieve near-IR-triggered and-targeted two-photon absorption photodynamic therapy." *Inorganic Chemistry* 57 (1): 300–310.

Jiang, Ke, Ling Zhang, Quan Hu, Qi Zhang, Wenxin Lin, Yuanjing Cui, Yu Yang, and Guodong Qian. 2017. "Thermal stimuli-triggered drug release from a biocompatible porous metal–organic framework." *Chemistry–A European Journal* 23 (42): 10215–10221.

Jiang, Wei, Huiyuan Zhang, Jilian Wu, Guangxi Zhai, Zhonghao Li, Yuxia Luan, and Sanjay Garg. 2018. "CuS@ MOF-based well-designed quercetin delivery system for chemo–photothermal therapy." *ACS Applied Materials & Interfaces* 10 (40): 34513–34523.

Jones, Christopher G., Vitalie Stavila, Marissa A. Conroy, Patrick Feng, Brandon V. Slaughter, Carlee E. Ashley, and Mark D. Allendorf. 2016. "Versatile synthesis and fluorescent labeling of ZIF-90 nanoparticles for biomedical applications." *ACS Applied Materials & Interfaces* 8 (12): 7623–7630.

Khdair, Ayman, Di Chen, Yogesh Patil, Linan Ma, Q. Ping Dou, Malathy P. V. Shekhar, and Jayanth Panyam. 2010. "Nanoparticle-mediated combination chemotherapy and photodynamic therapy overcomes tumor drug resistance." *Journal of Controlled Release* 141 (2): 137–144.

Kim, Kibeom, Sungmin Lee, Eunji Jin, L. Palanikumar, Jeong Hyeon Lee, Jin Chul Kim, Jung Seung Nam, Batakrishna Jana, Tae-Hyuk Kwon, and Sang Kyu Kwak. 2019. "MOF× biopolymer: Collaborative combination of metal–organic framework and biopolymer for advanced anticancer therapy." *ACS Applied Materials & Interfaces* 11 (31): 27512–27520.

Kokardekar, Rashmi R., Vaibhav K. Shah, and Hardik R. Mody. 2012. "PNIPAM Poly (N-isopropylacrylamide): A thermoresponsive "smart" polymer in novel drug delivery systems." *Internet Journal of Medical Update-EJOURNAL* 7 (2): 60–63.

Kurkuri, Mahaveer D., and Tejraj M. Aminabhavi. 2004. "Poly(vinyl alcohol) and poly(acrylic acid) sequential interpenetrating network pH-sensitive microspheres for the delivery of diclofenac sodium to the intestine." *Journal of Controlled Release* 96 (1): 9–20.

Lajevardi, Aseman, Moayad Hossaini Sadr, Alireza Badiei, and Mahsa Armaghan. 2020. "Synthesis and characterization of Fe_3O_4@SiO_2@MIL-100(Fe) nanocomposite: A nanocarrier for loading and release of celecoxib." *Journal of Molecular Liquids* 307: 112996.

Lan, Guangxu, Kaiyuan Ni, Samuel S. Veroneau, Xuanyu Feng, Geoffrey T. Nash, Taokun Luo, Ziwan Xu, and Wenbin Lin. 2019. "Titanium-based nanoscale metal–organic framework for type I photodynamic therapy." *Journal of the American Chemical Society* 141 (10): 4204–4208.

Lei, Bingqian, Mengfan Wang, Zelei Jiang, Wei Qi, Rongxin Su, and Zhimin He. 2018. "Constructing redox-responsive metal–organic framework nanocarriers for anticancer drug delivery." *ACS Applied Materials & Interfaces* 10 (19): 16698–16706.

Lei, Zhentao, Qiuju Tang, Yanshan Ju, Yonghui Lin, Xiaowen Bai, Haipeng Luo, and Zaizai Tong. 2020. "Block copolymer@ZIF-8 nanocomposites as a pH-responsive multi-steps release system for controlled drug delivery." *Journal of Biomaterials Science, Polymer Edition* 31 (6): 695–711.

Li, Sheng, Ke Bi, Ling Xiao, and Xiaowen Shi. 2017. "Facile preparation of magnetic metal organic frameworks core–shell nanoparticles for stimuli-responsive drug carrier." *Nanotechnology* 28 (49): 495601.

Li, Yantao, Jun Jin, Dawei Wang, Jiawei Lv, Ke Hou, Yaling Liu, Chunying Chen, and Zhiyong Tang. 2018. "Coordination-responsive drug release inside gold nanorod@ metal-organic framework core–shell nanostructures for near-infrared-induced synergistic chemo-photothermal therapy." *Nano Research* 11 (6): 3294–3305.

Lim, Eun-Kyung, Taekhoon Kim, Soonmyung Paik, Seungjoo Haam, Yong-Min Huh, and Kwangyeol Lee. 2015. "Nanomaterials for theranostics: Recent advances and future challenges." *Chemical Reviews* 115 (1): 327–394.

Lin, Gan, Yang Zhang, Long Zhang, Junqing Wang, Ye Tian, Wen Cai, Shangui Tang, Chengchao Chu, JiaJing Zhou, and Peng Mi. 2020. "Metal-organic frameworks nanoswitch: Toward photo-controllable endo/lysosomal rupture and release for enhanced cancer RNA interference." *Nano Research* 13 (1): 238–245.

Lin, Wenxin, Yuanjing Cui, Yu Yang, Quan Hu, and Guodong Qian. 2018. "A biocompatible metal–organic framework as a pH and temperature dual-responsive drug carrier." *Dalton Transactions* 47 (44): 15882–15887.

Lin, Wenxin, Quan Hu, Ke Jiang, Yuanjing Cui, Yu Yang, and Guodong Qian. 2017. "A porous Zn-based metal-organic framework for pH and temperature dual-responsive controlled drug release." *Microporous and Mesoporous Materials* 249: 55–60.

Liu, Chaoqun, Zhaowei Chen, Zhenzhen Wang, Wei Li, Enguo Ju, Zhengqing Yan, Zhen Liu, Jinsong Ren, and Xiaogang Qu. 2016. "A graphitic hollow carbon nitride nanosphere as a novel photochemical internalization agent for targeted and stimuli-responsive cancer therapy." *Nanoscale* 8 (25): 12570–12578.

Liu, Gaoshuang, Mahesh P. Bhat, Cheol Soo Kim, Jangho Kim, and Kyeong-Hwan Lee. 2022. "Improved 3D-printability of cellulose acetate to mimic water absorption in plant roots through nanoporous networks." *Macromolecules* 55: 1855–1865.

Liu, Mengrui, Hongliang Du, Wenjia Zhang, and Guangxi Zhai. 2017. "Internal stimuli-responsive nanocarriers for drug delivery: Design strategies and applications." *Materials Science and Engineering: C* 71: 1267–1280.

Madhuprasad, Mahesh P. Bhat, Ho-Young Jung, Dusan Losic, and Mahaveer D. Kurkuri. 2016. "Anion sensors as logic gates: A close encounter?" *Chemistry – A European Journal* 22 (18): 6148–6178.

Mahapatro, Anil, and Dinesh K. Singh. 2011. "Biodegradable nanoparticles are excellent vehicle for site directed in-vivo delivery of drugs and vaccines." *Journal of Nanobiotechnology* 9 (1): 1–11.

McHugh, Kevin J., Lihong Jing, Adam M. Behrens, Surangi Jayawardena, Wen Tang, Mingyuan Gao, Robert Langer, and Ana Jaklenec. 2018. "Biocompatible semiconductor quantum dots as cancer imaging agents." *Advanced Materials* 30 (18): 1706356.

Meek, Scott T., Jeffery A. Greathouse, and Mark D. Allendorf. 2011. "Metal-organic frameworks: A rapidly growing class of versatile nanoporous materials." *Advanced Materials* 23 (2): 249–267.

Meng, Yiming, Jing Sun, Na Qv, Guirong Zhang, Tao Yu, and Haozhe Piao. 2020. "Application of molecular imaging technology in tumor immunotherapy." *Cellular Immunology* 348: 104039.

Miao, Yalei, Xubo Zhao, Yudian Qiu, Zhongyi Liu, Wenjing Yang, and Xu Jia. 2019. "Metal–organic framework-assisted nanoplatform with hydrogen peroxide/glutathione dual-sensitive on-demand drug release for targeting tumors and their microenvironment." *ACS Applied Bio Materials* 2 (2): 895–905.

Mura, Simona, Julien Nicolas, and Patrick Couvreur. 2013. “Stimuli-responsive nanocarriers for drug delivery.” *Nature Materials* 12 (11): 991–1003.

Nagata, Shunjiro, Kenta Kokado, and Kazuki Sada. 2020. “Metal–organic framework tethering pH-and thermo-responsive polymer for ON–OFF controlled release of guest molecules.” *CrystEngComm* 22 (6): 1106–1111.

Nian, Fuyu, Yafan Huang, Meiru Song, Juan-Juan Chen, and Jinping Xue. 2017. “A novel fabricated material with divergent chemical handles based on UiO-66 and used for targeted photodynamic therapy.” *Journal of Materials Chemistry B* 5 (31): 6227–6232.

Nicks, Joshua, Kezia Sasitharan, Ram R. R. Prasad, David J. Ashworth, and Jonathan A. Foster. 2021. “Metal-organic framework nanosheets: Programmable 2D materials for catalysis, sensing, electronics, and separation applications.” *Advanced Functional Materials* 31: 2103723.

Palazzolo, Stefano, Samer Bayda, Mohamad Hadla, Isabella Caligiuri, Giuseppe Corona, Giuseppe Toffoli, and Flavio Rizzolio. 2018. “The clinical translation of organic nanomaterials for cancer therapy: A focus on polymeric nanoparticles, micelles, liposomes and exosomes.” *Current Medicinal Chemistry* 25 (34): 4224–4268.

Patil, Pravin, Kanalli V. Ajeya, Mahesh P. Bhat, Ganesan Sriram, Jingxian Yu, Ho-Young Jung, Tariq Altalhi, Madhuprasad Kigga, and Mahaveer D. Kurkuri. 2018. “Real-time probe for the efficient sensing of inorganic fluoride and copper ions in aqueous media.” *ChemistrySelect* 3 (41): 11593–11600.

Patil, Pravin, Madhuprasad, Mahesh P. Bhat, Manasa G. Gatti, Shervin Kabiri, Tariq Altalhi, Ho-Young Jung, Dusan Losic, and Mahaveer Kurkuri. 2017. “Chemodosimeter functionalized diatomaceous earth particles for visual detection and removal of trace mercury ions from water.” *Chemical Engineering Journal* 327: 725–733.

Petit, Camille. 2018. “Present and future of MOF research in the field of adsorption and molecular separation.” *Current Opinion in Chemical Engineering* 20: 132–142.

Ray Chowdhuri, Angshuman, Dipsikha Bhattacharya, and Sumanta Kumar Sahu. 2016. “Magnetic nanoscale metal organic frameworks for potential targeted anticancer drug delivery, imaging and as an MRI contrast agent.” *Dalton Transactions* 45 (7): 2963–2973.

Ren, Shen-Zhen, Dan Zhu, Xiao-Hua Zhu, Bin Wang, Yu-Shun Yang, Wen-Xue Sun, Xiao-Ming Wang, Peng-Cheng Lv, Zhong-Chang Wang, and Hai-Liang Zhu. 2019. “Nanoscale metal–organic-frameworks coated by biodegradable organosilica for pH and redox dual responsive drug release and high-performance anticancer therapy.” *ACS Applied Materials & Interfaces* 11 (23): 20678–20688.

Rojas, Sara, Ana Arenas-Vivo, and Patricia Horcajada. 2019. “Metal-organic frameworks: A novel platform for combined advanced therapies.” *Coordination Chemistry Reviews* 388: 202–226.

Sene, Saad, M. Teresa Marcos-Almaraz, Nicolas Menguy, Joseph Scola, Jeanne Volatron, Richard Rouland, Jean-Marc Greneche, Sylvain Miraux, Clotilde Menet, and Nathalie Guillou. 2017. “Maghemite-nanoMIL-100 (Fe) bimodal nanovector as a platform for image-guided therapy.” *Chem* 3 (2): 303–322.

Sharma, Ankush, Amit K. Goyal, and Goutam Rath. 2018. "Recent advances in metal nanoparticles in cancer therapy." *Journal of Drug Targeting* 26 (8): 617–632.

Shen, Hong, Jintong Liu, Jianping Lei, and Huangxian Ju. 2018. "A core–shell nanoparticle–peptide@ metal–organic framework as pH and enzyme dual-recognition switch for stepwise-responsive imaging in living cells." *Chemical Communications* 54 (66): 9155–9158.

Shen, Kui, Xiaodong Chen, Junying Chen, and Yingwei Li. 2016. "Development of MOF-derived carbon-based nanomaterials for efficient catalysis." *Acs Catalysis* 6 (9): 5887–5903.

Shi, Pengfei, Yuanchao Zhang, Zhaopeng Yu, and Shusheng Zhang. 2017. "Label-free electrochemical detection of ATP based on amino-functionalized metal-organic framework." *Scientific Reports* 7 (1): 6500.

Shi, Zheqi, Xuerui Chen, Li Zhang, Shiping Ding, Xu Wang, Qunfang Lei, and Wenjun Fang. 2018. "FA-PEG decorated MOF nanoparticles as a targeted drug delivery system for controlled release of an autophagy inhibitor." *Biomaterials Science* 6 (10): 2582–2590.

Silva, Janine S. F., José Y. R. Silva, Gilberto F. de Sá, Silvany S. Araújo, Manoel A. Gomes Filho, Célia M. Ronconi, Thiago C. Santos, and Severino A. Júnior. 2018. "Multifunctional system polyaniline-decorated ZIF-8 nanoparticles as a new chemo-photothermal platform for cancer therapy." *ACS Omega* 3 (9): 12147–12157.

Silva, José Yago R., Yaicel G. Proenza, Leonis L. da Luz, Silvany de Sousa Araújo, Manoel Adrião Gomes Filho, Severino Alves Junior, Thereza A. Soares, and Ricardo L. Longo. 2019. "A thermo-responsive adsorbent-heater-thermometer nanomaterial for controlled drug release:(ZIF-8, EuxTby)@ AuNP core-shell." *Materials Science and Engineering: C* 102: 578–588.

Simon-Yarza, Teresa, Angelika Mielcarek, Patrick Couvreur, and Christian Serre. 2018. "Nanoparticles of metal-organic frameworks: On the road to in vivo efficacy in biomedicine." *Advanced Materials* 30 (37): 1707365.

Sivakumar, Palanisamy, Subramani Priyatharshni, K. B. Nagashanmugam, A. Thanigaivelan, and K. Kumar. 2017. "Chitosan capped nanoscale Fe-MIL-88B-NH2 metal-organic framework as drug carrier material for the pH responsive delivery of doxorubicin." *Materials Research Express* 4 (8): 085023.

Song, Mei-Ru, Dong-Yao Li, Fu-Yu Nian, Jin-Ping Xue, and Juan-Juan Chen. 2018. "Zeolitic imidazolate metal organic framework-8 as an efficient pH-controlled delivery vehicle for zinc phthalocyanine in photodynamic therapy." *Journal of Materials Science* 53 (4): 2351–2361.

Sriram, Ganesan, Pravin Patil, Mahesh P. Bhat, Raveendra M. Hegde, Kanalli V. Ajeya, Iranna Udachyan, M. B. Bhavya, Manasa G. Gatti, U. T. Uthappa, Gururaj M. Neelgund, Ho-Young Jung, Tariq Altalhi, Madhuprasad, and Mahaveer D. Kurkuri. 2016. "Current trends in nanoporous anodized alumina platforms for biosensing applications." *Journal of Nanomaterials* 2016: 1753574.

Stock, Norbert, and Shyam Biswas. 2012. "Synthesis of metal-organic frameworks (MOFs): Routes to various MOF topologies, morphologies, and composites." *Chemical Reviews* 112 (2): 933–969.

Su, Fangfang, Qiaojuan Jia, Zhenzhen Li, Minghua Wang, Linghao He, Donglai Peng, Yingpan Song, Zhihong Zhang, and Shaoming Fang. 2019. "Aptamer-templated silver nanoclusters embedded in zirconium metal–organic framework for targeted antitumor drug delivery." *Microporous and Mesoporous Materials* 275: 152–162.

Subudhi, Satyabrata, Suraj Prakash Tripathy, and Kulamani Parida. 2021. "Highlights of the characterization techniques on inorganic, organic (COF) and hybrid (MOF) photocatalytic semiconductors." *Catalysis Science & Technology* 11 (2): 392–415.

Sun, Keke, Chen Xu, Tianke Hu, Caixue Lin, Yifeng Wang, Yulin Li, Ling Li, and Yingxi Wang. 2018. "γ-Fe_2O_3/La-MOFs@ SiO_2 for magnetic resonance/fluorescence dual mode imaging and pH-drug delivery." *Materials Letters* 228: 216–219.

Tan, Guozhu, Yingtao Zhong, Linlin Yang, Yaodong Jiang, Jianqiang Liu, and Fei Ren. 2020. "A multifunctional MOF-based nanohybrid as injectable implant platform for drug synergistic oral cancer therapy." *Chemical Engineering Journal* 390: 124446.

Tian, Xue-Tao, Pei-Pei Cao, Hui Zhang, Yu-Hao Li, and Xue-Bo Yin. 2019. "GSH-activated MRI-guided enhanced photodynamic-and chemo-combination therapy with a MnO 2-coated porphyrin metal organic framework." *Chemical Communications* 55 (44): 6241–6244.

Tolentino, Mark Q., Alyssa K. Hartmann, David T. Loe, and Jessica L. Rouge. 2020. "Controlled release of small molecules and proteins from DNA-surfactant stabilized metal organic frameworks." *Journal of Materials Chemistry B* 8 (26): 5627–5635.

Tong, Pei-Hong, Ling Zhu, Yi Zang, Jia Li, Xiao-Peng He, and Tony D. James. 2021. "Metal-Organic Frameworks (MOFs) as host materials for the enhanced delivery of biomacromolecular therapeutics." *Chemical Communications* 57: 12098–12110.

Uthappa, U. T., O. R. Arvind, G. Sriram, Dusan Losic, Jung Ho Young, Madhuprasad Kigga, and Mahaveer D. Kurkuri. 2020. "Nanodiamonds and their surface modification strategies for drug delivery applications." *Journal of Drug Delivery Science and Technology* 60: 101993.

Uthappa, U. T., Mahesh P. Bhat, Ho-Young Jung, and Mahaveer D. Kurkuri. 2021. "Surface-functionalized diatoms for drug delivery and tissue engineering applications." In Thangadurai, D., Sangeetha, J., Prasad, R. (eds.) *Bioprospecting Algae for Nanosized Materials*, 275–289. Springer, Cham.

Uthappa, U. T., Varsha Brahmkhatri, G. Sriram, Ho-Young Jung, Jingxian Yu, Nikita Kurkuri, Tejraj M. Aminabhavi, Tariq Altalhi, Gururaj M. Neelgund, and Mahaveer D. Kurkuri. 2018. "Nature engineered diatom biosilica as drug delivery systems." *Journal of Controlled Release* 281: 70–83.

Uthappa, U. T., Madhuprasad Kigga, G. Sriram, Kanalli V. Ajeya, Ho-Young Jung, Gururaj M. Neelgund, and Mahaveer D. Kurkuri. 2019. "Facile green synthetic approach of bio inspired polydopamine coated diatoms as a drug vehicle for controlled drug release and active catalyst for dye degradation." *Microporous and Mesoporous Materials* 288: 109572.

Uthappa, U. T., G. Sriram, O. R. Arvind, Sandeep Kumar, Jung Ho Young, Gururaj M. Neelgund, Dusan Losic, and Mahaveer D. Kurkuri. 2020. "Engineering

MIL-100(Fe) on 3D porous natural diatoms as a versatile high performing platform for controlled isoniazid drug release, Fenton's catalysis for malachite green dye degradation and environmental adsorbents for Pb^{2+} removal and dyes." *Applied Surface Science* 528: 146974.

Uthappa, U. T., G. Sriram, Varsha Brahmkhatri, Madhuprasad Kigga, Ho-Young Jung, Tariq Altalhi, Gururaj M. Neelgund, and Mahaveer D. Kurkuri. 2018. "Xerogel modified diatomaceous earth microparticles for controlled drug release studies." *New Journal of Chemistry* 42 (14): 11964–11971.

Wang, Dongdong, Huihui Wu, Jiajia Zhou, Pengping Xu, Changlai Wang, Ruohong Shi, Haibao Wang, Hui Wang, Zhen Guo, and Qianwang Chen. 2018. "In situ one-pot synthesis of MOF–polydopamine hybrid nanogels with enhanced photothermal effect for targeted cancer therapy." *Advanced Science* 5 (6): 1800287.

Wang, Lisa J., Hexiang Deng, Hiroyasu Furukawa, Felipe Gándara, Kyle E. Cordova, Dani Peri, and Omar M. Yaghi. 2014. "Synthesis and characterization of metal–organic framework-74 containing 2, 4, 6, 8, and 10 different metals." *Inorganic Chemistry* 53 (12): 5881–5883.

Wang, Xiao-Gang, Zhi-Yue Dong, Hong Cheng, Shuang-Shuang Wan, Wei-Hai Chen, Mei-Zhen Zou, Jia-Wei Huo, He-Xiang Deng, and Xian-Zheng Zhang. 2015. "A multifunctional metal–organic framework based tumor targeting drug delivery system for cancer therapy." *Nanoscale* 7 (38): 16061–16070.

Wang, Ying, Jianhua Yan, Nachuan Wen, Hongjie Xiong, Shundong Cai, Qunye He, Yaqin Hu, Dongming Peng, Zhenbao Liu, and Yanfei Liu. 2020. "Metal-organic frameworks for stimuli-responsive drug delivery." *Biomaterials* 230: 119619.

Watermann, Anna, and Juergen Brieger. 2017. "Mesoporous silica nanoparticles as drug delivery vehicles in cancer." *Nanomaterials* 7 (7): 189.

Wu, Ming-Xue, Jia Gao, Fang Wang, Jie Yang, Nan Song, Xiaoyu Jin, Peng Mi, Jian Tian, Jiayan Luo, Feng Liang, and Ying-Wei Yang. 2018. "Multistimuli Responsive Core–Shell Nanoplatform Constructed from Fe_3O_4@MOF Equipped with Pillar[6]arene Nanovalves." *Small* 14 (17): 1704440.

Wu, Ming-Xue, and Ying-Wei Yang. 2017. "Metal–organic framework (MOF)-based drug/cargo delivery and cancer therapy." *Advanced Materials* 29 (23): 1606134.

Wu, Qiong, Meng Niu, Xiaowei Chen, Longfei Tan, Changhui Fu, Xiangling Ren, Jun Ren, Laifeng Li, Ke Xu, Hongshan Zhong, and Xianwei Meng. 2018. "Biocompatible and biodegradable zeolitic imidazolate framework/polydopamine nanocarriers for dual stimulus triggered tumor thermo-chemotherapy." *Biomaterials* 162: 132–143.

Xie, Jin, Gang Liu, Henry S. Eden, Hua Ai, and Xiaoyuan Chen. 2011. "Surface-engineered magnetic nanoparticle platforms for cancer imaging and therapy." *Accounts of Chemical Research* 44 (10): 883–892.

Yaghi, Omar M., Guangming Li, and Hailian Li. 1995. "Selective binding and removal of guests in a microporous metal–organic framework." *Nature* 378 (6558): 703–706.

Yang, Baochun, Mei Shen, Jianqiang Liu, and Fei Ren. 2017. "Post-synthetic modification nanoscale metal-organic frameworks for targeted drug delivery in cancer cells." *Pharmaceutical Research* 34 (11): 2440–2450.

Yang, Hu. 2016. "Targeted nanosystems: Advances in targeted dendrimers for cancer therapy." *Nanomedicine: Nanotechnology, Biology and Medicine* 12 (2): 309–316.

Yang, Jie, and Ying-Wei Yang. 2020. "Metal–organic frameworks for biomedical applications." *Small* 16 (10): 1906846.

Yu, Haizhou, Xiaoyan Qiu, Pradeep Neelakanda, Lin Deng, Niveen M. Khashab, Suzana P. Nunes, and Klaus-Viktor Peinemann. 2015. "Hollow ZIF-8 nanoworms from block copolymer templates." *Scientific Reports* 5 (1): 15275.

Zhang, Di, Zhongju Ye, Lin Wei, Haibin Luo, and Lehui Xiao. 2019. "Cell membrane-coated porphyrin metal–organic frameworks for cancer cell targeting and o2-evolving photodynamic therapy." *ACS Applied Materials & Interfaces* 11 (43): 39594–39602.

Zhang, Feng-Ming, Hong Dong, Xin Zhang, Xiao-Jun Sun, Ming Liu, Dou-Dou Yang, Xin Liu, and Jin-Zhi Wei. 2017. "Postsynthetic modification of ZIF-90 for potential targeted codelivery of two anticancer drugs." *ACS Applied Materials & Interfaces* 9 (32): 27332–27337.

Zhang, Huiyuan, Qian Li, Ruiling Liu, Xinke Zhang, Zhonghao Li, and Yuxia Luan. 2018. "A versatile prodrug strategy to in situ encapsulate drugs in MOF nanocarriers: A case of cytarabine-IR820 prodrug encapsulated ZIF-8 toward chemo-photothermal therapy." *Advanced Functional Materials* 28 (35): 1802830.

Zhao, Huai-Xin, Quan Zou, Shao-Kai Sun, Chunshui Yu, Xuejun Zhang, Rui-Jun Li, and Yan-Yan Fu. 2016. "Theranostic metal–organic framework core–shell composites for magnetic resonance imaging and drug delivery." *Chemical Science* 7 (8): 5294–5301.

Zhao, Huifang, Shijie Hou, Xudong Zhao, and Dahuan Liu. 2019. "Adsorption and pH-responsive release of tinidazole on metal–organic framework CAU-1." *Journal of Chemical & Engineering Data* 64 (4): 1851–1858.

Zheng, Yadan, Xiaoyuan Zhang, and Zhiqiang Su. 2021. "Design of metal-organic frameworks composites in anti-cancer therapies." *Nanoscale* 13: 12102–12118.

Zhou, Hong-Cai, Jeffrey R. Long, and Omar M. Yaghi. 2012. "Introduction to metal–organic frameworks." *Chemical Reviews* 112 (2): 673–674.

Zhou, Jingrong, Gan Tian, Lijuan Zeng, Xueer Song, and Xiu-wu Bian. 2018. "Nanoscaled metal-organic frameworks for biosensing, imaging, and cancer therapy." *Advanced Healthcare Materials* 7 (10): 1800022.

Zhu, Xi, Hanye Zheng, Xiaofeng Wei, Zhenyu Lin, Longhua Guo, Bin Qiu, and Guonan Chen. 2013. "Metal–organic framework (MOF): A novel sensing platform for biomolecules." *Chemical Communications* 49 (13): 1276–1278.

Chapter 8

Covalent Organic Frameworks (COFs) for Drug Delivery Applications

Arvind Raj, Richelle M. Rego, Mahaveer Kurkuri, and Madhuprasad Kigga
JAIN (Deemed-to-be-University)

CONTENTS

8.1 INTRODUCTION

An aging population along with a change in societal behaviors contributing to a gentle increase in health problems and thus depleting physical health is considered as one of the primary issues in recent times (Lancet 2020). To

DOI: 10.1201/9781003217114-11

address these issues, medication is being implemented, where precision medicine has the ability to use specific information about a person's disease and giving the correct treatment at the appropriate time. Nevertheless, there is limited evidence to show that precision medicine could overall improve cost-effectiveness, enhance clinical outcomes, and enhance the quality of care across populations and thereby creating a serious barrier for its adoption (Dzau and Ginsburg 2016). One of the main reasons for precision medicine to exhibit limitations is the poor delivery of drug to the targeted site (Tibbitt, Dahlman, and Langer 2016). To overcome these limitations, an advanced medicinal technique known as the drug delivery system (DDS) is used. The DDS plays a vital role in transporting the drug into the desired tissues, cells, and subcellular elements for targeted drug release and thereby increasing its efficiency through a variety of drug carriers (Li et al. 2019). Similarly, to improve the therapeutic effect of a drug and control the related side effects, active drug molecules need to selectively accumulate within the diseased area for a protracted period with high controllability (D. Liu et al. 2016).

It is a crucial challenge to find suitable nontoxic carriers which are effective in delivering the drugs to the desired targeted sites (Davis, Chen, and Shin 2010). Though various materials such as organic and inorganic porous polymers are studied for drug delivery (Shivanand and Sprockel 1998). The applications of these polymers are limited either by minimum drug-loading capacity or due to the uncontrolled release. To overcome these problems, metal-organic frameworks (MOFs) are used as a carrier for bio-applications and drug delivery (C.-Y. Sun et al. 2013). MOFs are well known for their porous coordinated structures constructed using metal ions and organic linkers (Rego, Sriram, et al. 2021; Kitagawa 2014). Due to their structural and functional tunability, they are utilized in many applications such as gas storage and separation, heterogeneous catalysis, chemical sensing, proton conductivity, and drug delivery (Jiao et al. 2019). Besides the outstanding features of MOF, they are also known for their nano-size structures owing to nano properties (Rego, Kuriya, et al. 2021). These properties make MOFs promising nanocarriers for theragnostic agent delivery (L. Wang, Zheng, and Xie 2018). MOFs have a massive potential, which allows the development of new structures and topologies altered for specific drug molecular structures and medicating requirements. Also, their biodegradability additionally corroborates the employment of nano-MOFs as drug carriers. The metal-to-ligand bonds establishing the network are comparatively labile, letting the framework break down into smaller byproducts, and thereby, this property prevents the irreversible growth of MOFs inside the body (Y. Sun et al. 2020). Additionally, by observing the character of the network, major framework degradation produces a space for constant, burst, or stimuli-dependent release kinetics of the drug. Even though their application as a drug carrier is notable, they have stability issues in drug delivery, and MOFs extend the problem of unwanted cytotoxicity due to the presence of inorganic metal nodes along with organic linkers. For instance, though certain metals such as zinc and iron are found in remarkable quantities inside the body, their prolonged accumulation can be toxic (Scicluna and Vella-Zarb 2020).

On the other hand, covalent organic frameworks (COFs) are potential contenders because of their stability and lack of metal centers, and thus they are intended for drug delivery applications. COFs are a recently established class of crystalline porous materials, which are mainly constructed from lightweight elements like boron, nitrogen, carbon, and oxygen (Wu and Yang 2017). These organic linkers/units connected by covalent bonds have attracted many researchers in recent years. COFs are obtained by the gathering of symmetric and rigid organic building blocks. These building blocks are observed to sustain their geometry throughout the reversible reactions. The structure of COFs is significantly tunable by the choice of linkers and building blocks combined for the development of porous 2D or 3D networks (Chen et al. 2019). COFs as nanocarriers have a spread of properties similar to MOFs such as highly tuneable porosity, ordered networks, optional building blocks, predicable areas, and good thermal and chemical stability (Cote et al. 2005), as shown in Figure 8.1.

COFs are constructed using organic linkers through a condensation reaction, and the covalent bonds developed in the frameworks allow high thermal stability. The properties of COFs are employed in many applications such as gas storage and separation, catalysis, optoelectronics, sensing organic molecules, and drug delivery (Díaz and Corma 2016).

According to the existing reports, many researchers have used polymer nanoparticles (PNPs) as the most operative drug carriers. In general, PNPs consist of better biodegradable properties having a higher drug-loading capacity and flow time as compared to other nanocarrier systems, which make PNPs as one of the better candidates in drug delivery applications. On the the hand, COFs having similar properties like PNPs can also be used for drug delivery systems (Butterfield et al. 2017). Additionally, the non-existence of metal ions in COFs also reduces the degree of unwanted cytotoxicity which makes COFs a better carrier for drug delivery (Zhou et al. 2010).

8.2 LINKERS FOR THE SYNTHESIS OF COFs

The linkage of organic precursors is an important parameter that decides the 2D or 3D nature of COFs. Therefore, by categorizing the linkage used in COFs, one can get to know essential information regarding the structural formation of COFs. Figure 8.2 shows the different types of 2D and

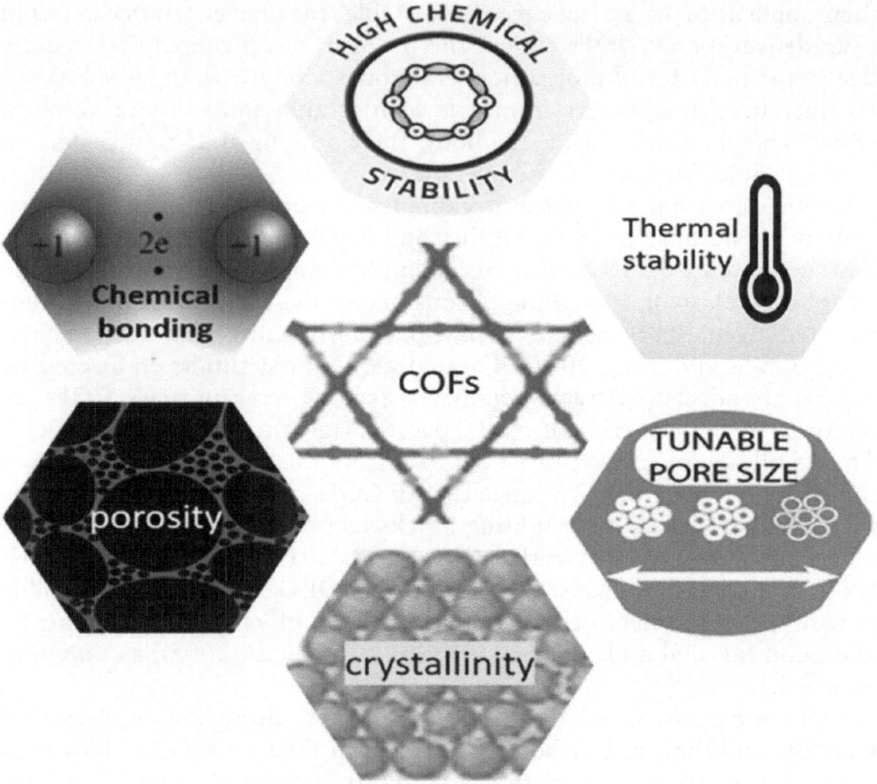

Figure 8.1 Schematic representation showing various properties of COFs.

3D COFs. In the following section, we are briefly discussing the diverse linkages and their properties for the formation of COFs.

8.2.1 Boron-Oxygen Linkage

The initial structures of COFs were designed utilizing boron-oxygen (B-O) linkage. The Yaghi group was the first one to report the B-O-linked 2D COF (Cote et al. 2005). The boroxine-based COF network (COF-1) was synthesized by condensation of diboronic acid at 120°C. Furthermore, diboronic acid reacts with hexahydroxytriphenylene to form hexagonal framework with B-O linkages. COFs with B-O linkages have good thermal stability with an orderly arranged structure (Smith et al. 2015). The first 3D COF was obtained using catechol and was synthesized by the condensation method giving boronated ester rings. Owing to its highly porous structure, the COF-103 showed a high surface area of 4,210 m^2/g and low-density crystals (COF-108, 0.17 g/cm^3) (El-Kaderi et al. 2007).

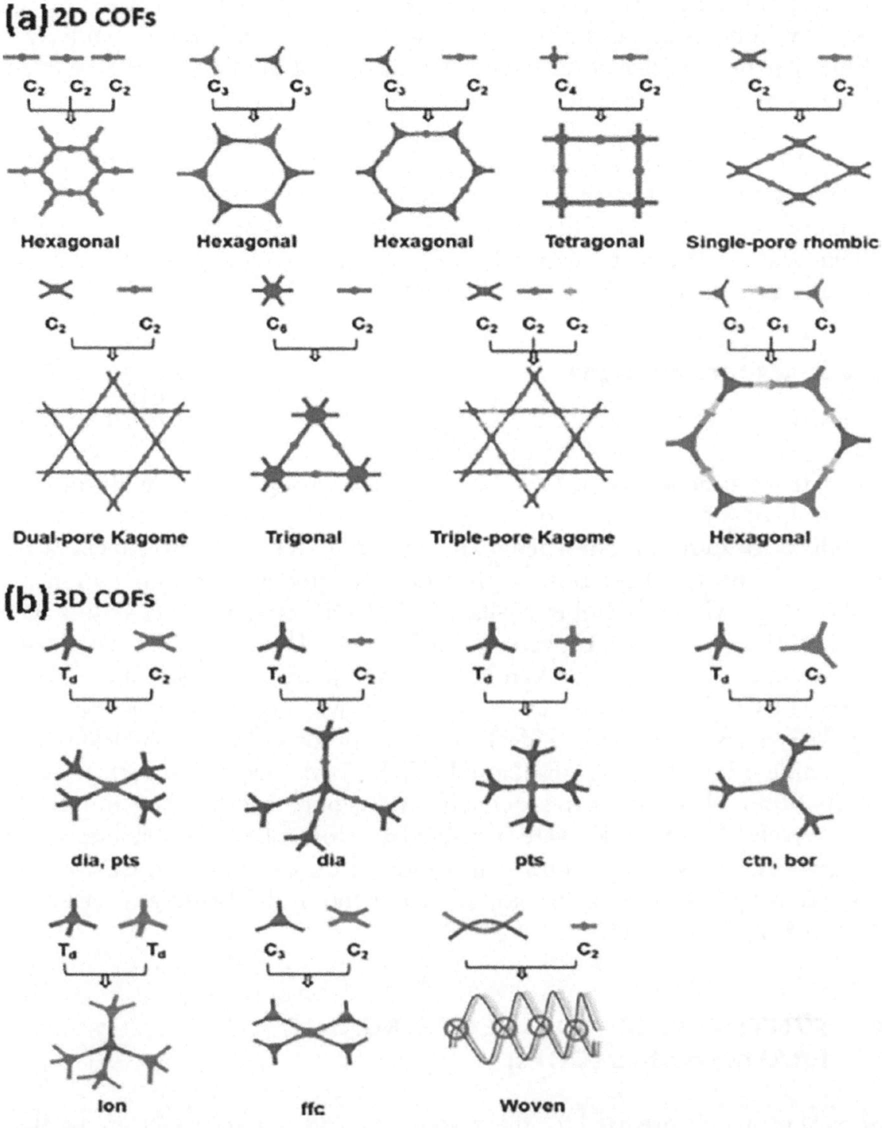

Figure 8.2 Topological diagrams for (a) 2D and (b) 3D COFs. (Reproduced with approval from (Abuzeid, EL-Mahdy, and Kuo 2021).)

8.2.2 Carbon-Nitrogen Linkage

Compared to the B-O bond, the C=N bond has higher stability due to the presence of π-conjugations throughout the framework. Such imine-based COFs offer better chemical stability and also give scope to various applications such as drug delivery and other biomedical applications. Yaghi's group was the first to report an imine-based 2D COF which was synthesized by condensing tetra (*p*-aminophenyl) porphyrin (TAPP) and terephthaldehyde. Furthermore, the layered sheet-like 2D COF with extended planar symmetry of π-conjugation among the porphyrin moieties enables charge carrier mobility (Wan et al. 2011). The first imine-based 3D COF (COF-300) reported by Yaghi's group was synthesized from terephthaladehyde and tetrakis-(4-aminophenyl)methane (TAPM). The COF-300 has a diamond structure with a five-fold interpenetration with high stability up to a temperature of 490°C, which is insoluble in water and common organic solvents as well (Uribe-Romo et al. 2009).

8.2.3 Other Linkages

Apart from B-O and C-N linkages, there are a few other linkages that were used for the development of COFs with C-C linkages and C-O linkages. The nitriles attached to the C=C bond showed strong electron-withdrawing effects giving reversibility to the C=C linkage by affecting the chemical stability. In addition, the chemically oxidized 2D COF linked via C=C linkage shows excellent results for semiconductor applications (Jin et al. 2017). Polyaryl-based and ether-based 2D COFs containing C-O linkages such as JUC-506 (Jilin University China) and JUC-505 COFs have been studied (Guan et al. 2019). Yan et al. came up with two polyimide-based COFs, PI-COF-4, and PI-COF-5. The COF was synthesized by condensing TAPM and thioacetic acid (TAA) with pyromellitic dianhydride. The polyimide (PI) COF, PI-COF-4, and PI-COF-5 possessed high surface areas of 2,430 and 1,876 m^2/g, respectively, and a pore width of 13 and 10 Å, respectively. These COFs were inspected for controlled drug delivery, and the two PI-COFs loaded with drugs showed an excellent release control, obtaining 95% of the cancer antigen from the initial loading after about 6 days (Fang et al. 2015).

8.3 SYNTHESIS OF COVALENT ORGANIC FRAMEWORKS (COFs)

Several protocols are used for the synthesis of COFs. In this section, we discuss the general approaches followed for the synthesis of COFs, as shown in Figure 8.3.

8.3.1 Solvothermal Synthesis

The COF synthesis was first achieved through the solvothermal method reported by (Cote et al. 2005), and this method still remains a popular method to synthesize COFs. The organic linkers are placed in a reaction

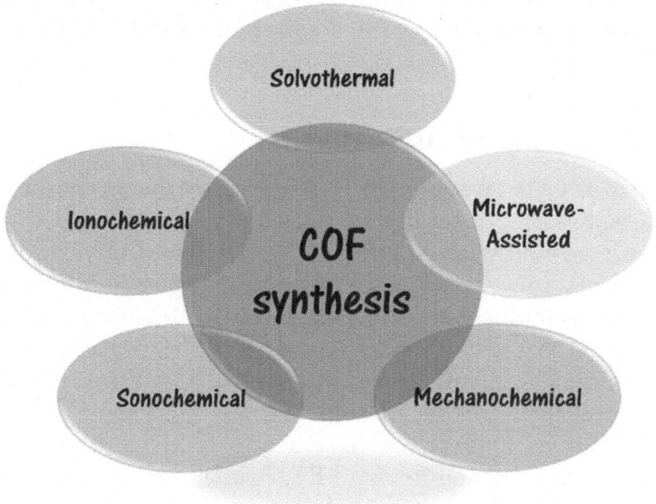

Figure 8.3 Schematic representation showing different methods involved in the synthesis of COFs.

vessel with the suitable solvent/solvent mixture and catalysts if required. The reactor vessel is placed in a sealed container or Teflon-lined steel autoclave. The reaction vessel is kept in a furnace for heating under a constant temperature higher than the boiling point of the solvent. Such conditions increase the solubility of the organic linkers and thus improve the reaction kinetics. The morphologies obtained by this method are common agglomerates in various forms such as flake, flower, rod, spherical, or particles being irregular in the nanometer range. Peng et al. testified the room temperature batch synthesis of azine, imine, and enamine-linked COFs (Peng et al. 2016).

8.3.2 Microwave-Assisted Synthesis

For many decades, microwave synthesis has been implemented in organic chemistry. Microwave reaction occurs in the region between radio and infrared frequencies producing electromagnetic radiation. The heating depends on the ability of the matter to absorb microwaves and convert them into heat. Among different reactions done through solvothermal synthesis, an early approach for the synthesis of COFs was carried out with the irradiation of microwaves. Campbell et al. established the synthesis of COF-5 through the microwave-assisted synthesis in just 20 minutes. Additionally, these COF also exhibited a high surface area of 2,000 m^2/g (Campbell et al. 2009), which was better than the surface areas reported in the solvothermal method. Additionally, other components such as mode stirrers and turntables can also be present to ensure homogeneity inside the cavity (Diaz de Grenu et al. 2021).

8.3.3 Mechanochemical Synthesis

The synthesis of COFs was also been achieved by the mechanical grinding of the organic linkers. Generally, in a mechanochemical synthesis, the two precursors are ground with a motor and pestle. The COF synthesis via the mechanochemical route provides the same yield as the solvothermal method. Nevertheless, mechanochemically synthesized COFs were not much crystalline compared to a solvothermal method and showed a very low surface area of 100 m^2/g. The chemical stability of mechanochemically synthesized COFs was equivalent to that of solvothermal synthesized COFs (Biswal et al. 2013). However, there has been a drastic increase in the degree of structural order in solid and in turn BET (Brunauer-Emmett-Teller) surface area by using the liquid-assisted grinding method (LAG). In the LAG-based synthesis, a catalytic amount of liquid was added to the COF linkers, which increase the rate of the reaction. This method was successfully applied for the synthesis of imine, hydrazine, and β-ketoenamine-based COFs (Biswal et al. 2013).

8.3.4 Sonochemical Synthesis

In this method, the ultrasound is used to form bubbles in the solvent which grow and collapse in a process called cavitation, which is responsible for the formation of COFs. This process leads to very high pressures and temperatures in the solution which accelerates the chemical reaction. Yang's group examined this method for the construction of COF-1 and COF-5. This technique showed promising results in a short period of time (0. 5–2 hours). Additionally, this method yielded COF with a high surface area of 2,122 m^2/g, and the reaction could be increased up to a 0.5 L batch size (Yang et al. 2012). This method can be used to synthesize highly porous COFs in a short period of time.

8.3.5 Ionothermal Synthesis

In this technique, ionic liquids are used to facilitate the synthesis of COFs, where the lattice is formed due to the solvent and the structural directing components or template for the formation of COFs. The first report on ionothermally synthesized COF was triazine linkage-based COF, namely covalent triazine-based frameworks (CTFs) (Kuhn, Antonietti, and Thomas 2008). At a high temperature (400°C), cyclotrimerization of aromatic nitrile linker was heated with $ZnCl_2$. Also, $ZnCl_2$ acts as a catalyst for cyclotrimerization. CTFs have high thermal stabilities, and due to their amorphous nature, they are used in catalysis applications. However, due to the harsh reaction conditions, the crystallinity of these materials is limited. Nevertheless, recently there are many improvements progressed using the ionothermal method for the synthesis of COFs. Recently, a polyimide-linked COF (PI-COF) was synthesized (Maschita et al. 2020) in $ZnCl_2$ solution and the eutectic salt mixture by heating at 300°C for 48 hours. These COFs possess a high surface area and also present high thermal stability. Therefore, the PI-COFs show a great prospect for drug delivery applications.

8.4 DRUG DELIVERY APPLICATION

Drug delivery systems are used to transport drugs effectively to the targeted site (Uthappa, Kurkuri, and Kigga 2019). Many materials have been developed for these applications such as diatoms (Uthappa, Brahmkhatri, et al. 2018; Uthappa et al. 2020), xerogels (Uthappa, Sriram, et al. 2018), MOFs (Abánades Lázaro and Forgan 2019), etc. However, COFs are emerging materials in this application due to their organic structure. The COFs displayed better results in drug delivery applications. COFs being a representative class of porous material have been used for the loading and release of drugs in an aqueous medium. The biocompatibility and stability of COFs for drug delivery were studied based on three major aspects: (i) poor dispersion of COFs in water in comparison with other common porous materials; (ii) reversible bonding that is highly sensitive to the surrounding environment; and (iii) drug-loading capacity and controllable release efficacy as the drug loading depends on the surface energy to enclose drugs. Figure 8.4 depicts the general schematic representation, where anticancer drugs are delivered to the targeted site. Keeping these main factors, the following sections discuss the use of COFs in drug delivery applications.

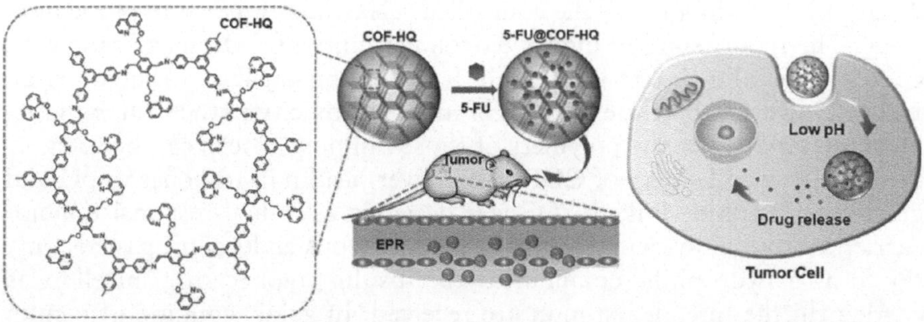

Figure 8.4 Schematic representation of drug (5-FU) loading in COF (COF-HQ) and drug releasing on the targeted site. (Reproduced with approval from (Jia et al. 2020).)

8.4.1 2D COFs

2D COFs are gaining special attention as the organic sheets are extended in two dimensions, which make a unique structure, and they can be synthesized easily. These 2D sheets will be in layers one above the other due to the π-π interactions. This results in a porous space that is functional and thus giving a large surface area, high crystallinity, low density, and biodegradability. These properties crafted them as a potential material for various applications from energy to biomedical sciences (Bhunia, Deo, and Gaharwar 2020). Zhao et al. have studied an imine-based 2D COF, namely, PI-3-COF and PI-2-COF. These COFs were analyzed for their efficiency to transport the drug by inspecting their loading, biocompatibility, dispersibility, in vitro cytotoxicity, and drug release patterns (Bai et al. 2016). The spherical 2D COFs (size ≈ 50 nm) exhibited good biocompatibility. The loading and release of the drug were studied using 5-fluorouracil (5-FU), captopril, and ibuprofen. These kinds of drugs were loaded into dried COF samples in hexane solution with continuous stirring for about 6 hours. The COFs loaded with drugs were further made distinctive using powered X-ray diffraction (PXRD), Fourier Transform Infrared Spectroscopy (FTIR), and thermogravimetric analysis (TGA). The drug-loading capability was also analyzed by TGA. The drug efficiency and the pore size of 2D COF are directly correlated to the loading and releasing of the specific drugs. It was noticed that the loading capacity of PI-2-COF was high (up to ≈ 30%) with 5-FU showing high cytotoxicity in MCF7 (Michigan cancer foundation-7) tumor cells. Similarly, another imine-based 2D COF (TTI-COF) was examined by (Vyas et al. 2016). The COF was synthesized using triazinetriphenyl aldehyde and triazinetriphenyl amine as precursors. TTI-COF was used as a drug carrier for quercetin which is an anticancer drug. The drug is released on MDA-MB-231 (i.e., human mammary carcinoma) to test the activity of the drug-loaded COF. In another study, an imine-derived COF drug reservoir is used between porous PCL (polycaprolactone) films for drug delivery applications. They used a dye (methylene blue) and a model drug (oxytocin) to analyze the controlled release and hindrance of the molecule. The report showed higher biocompatibility of COF membrane with good cell viability (>80%) and high drug-loading capacity (Alanagh et al. 2020). However, there are chances of inherent toxicity in the COF building block materials, but the polymers of those building blocks can be used for the efficiency and safety of COFs. To deliver insulin in response to pH and glucose, a boroxine-linked COF was designed as a dual-responsive nanocarrier. Additionally, with the use of percutaneous endoscopic gastrostomy (PEG) as a hydrophilic component, the insulin trapped in a micelle was carried till the intended stimuli are received. In acidic conditions, insulin was released due to the increase in pH and glucose. This was performed on A549 cells (i.e., lung carcinoma epithelial cells), and it was degraded into biocompatible products in mice (Zhang, Ji, et al. 2020). This is a promising discovery for COFs to be used in protein-based drug delivery systems and a major breakthrough for COFs as a drug carrier. A one-pot synthesized 2D COF (TAPB-DMTP-COF) with doxorubicin (DOX) was tested for chemotherapeutic efficiency. This 2D COF showed a high loading capacity (32.1 wt.%) and release of the drug in response to the pH (Sainan Liu et al. 2019). Therefore, the 2D COF (TAPB-DMTP-COF) can be used to treat tumor cells with reduced side effects.

8.5 3D COFs

3D COFs are very rarely studied compared to 2D COFs due to the limited choice of organic linkers which can offer many reactive sites in polyhedral geometry. To date, the majority of COFs reported are 2D layered with 1D pore channels where the interlayer packing is modulated by strong non-covalent bonding. Even though 3D COFs are rarely explored, their interconnected pore channels may provide a better opportunity with superior properties such as molecular diffusivity enhancement [48]. Additionally, due to the structure and porosity, there are many other functions such as placing rotatable dipolar linkers in the framework which gives a net response of electric field to the COFs are possible (Dürholt, Jahromi, and Schmid 2019). A 3D-polyimide-COF (PI-COF) was synthesized by selecting tetrahedral building units of various sizes to feature the interpenetrated or non-interpenetrated structures as shown in Figure 8.5. Also, the PI-COFs had a very high thermal stability and also a good surface area of 2,403 m^2/g. This 3D-polyimide-COF (PI-COF) was the first 3D COF used for drug delivery applications. Additionally, it can be noted that the loading and releasing of the drug molecule were highly controlled (Fang et al. 2015). Therefore, the 3D-PI-COFs can also demonstrate immense prospects in pharmaceutical applications.

Zhu et al. synthesized an organic 3D-Cage COF-1 (cage-6-NH_2) for drug delivery applications. This 3D-Cage COF had a unique feature to switch between the small pore and the large pore having a surface area of 1,040 and 1,336 m^2/g, respectively. These features can be used for the loading of drugs in two different sizes (Zhu et al. 2020). Recently, Zhang et al. synthesized a type of disulfide and hydrazide bond having a building unit, 4,4'-dihydrazide diphenyldisulfide (DHDS). These building blocks were used to develop PEGylated, pH, and redox dual-sensitive CONs (denoted HY/SS-CONs) for higher loading and release of DOX. The HY/SS-CONs can attain very low premature leakage and very high loading of the drug at physiological conditions (C. Wang et al. 2020). These COFs are a promising solution in drug delivery and can also be tested for other pharmaceutical applications. Table 8.1 briefly summarizes various COFs used in drug delivery applications.

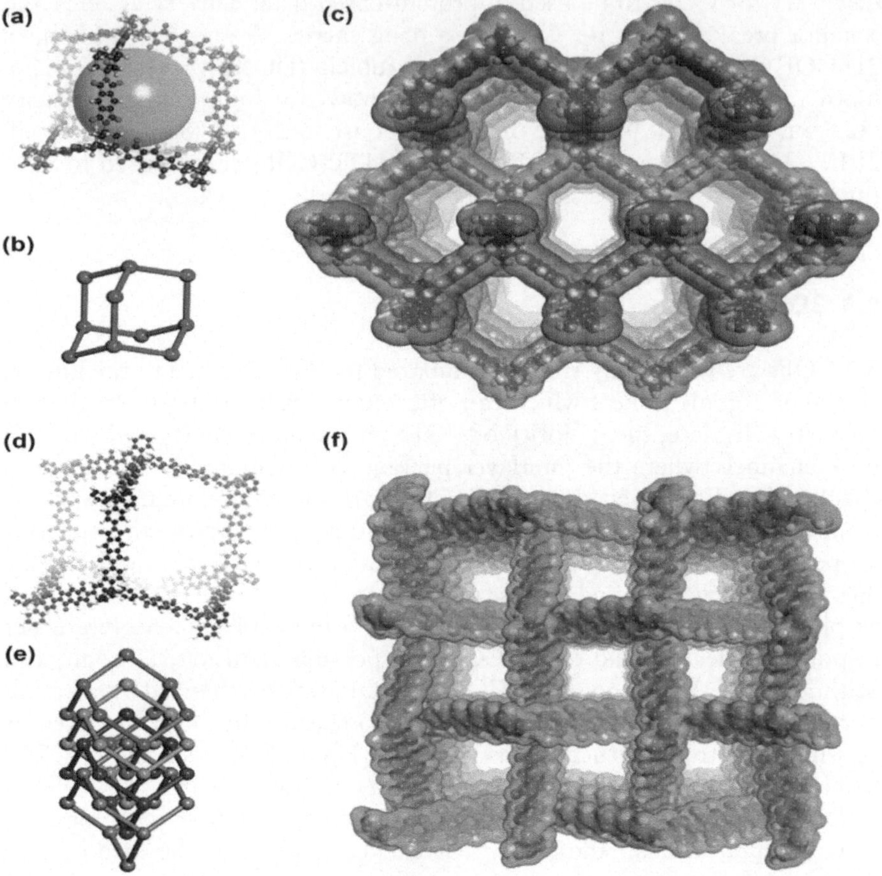

Figure 8.5 (a–c) Structures of 3D-Pi-COF-4. (d–f) Structures of Pi-COF-5. (Reproduced with approval from (Fang et al. 2015).)

8.6 COF COMPOSITES

Even though COFs are used widely in various fields, it is observed that there is a limitation for COF-based materials due to their intrinsic drawbacks. For example, the poor dispersion and porosity of microcrystalline COF powders in many solvents restrict their processability toward practical applications. Therefore, it is crucial to understand innovative methods to obtain COFs with additional functionalities and properties to meet the current demands. To overcome these issues, significant efforts have been taken to combine different functional materials with COFs. Additionally, they can also exhibit different physical and chemical properties depending upon the composite materials used.

Table 8.1 Representative COFs and Their Use in Drug Delivery Applications

Year	*COFs*	*Linkage*	*Drugs*	*Biological Activity Studies*
2016	PI-3-COF, PI-2-COF	Imine	5-FU	MCF-7 (Bai et al. 2016)
2016	TTI-COF	Imine	Drug delivery of quercetin	MDA-MB-231, MCF-10A (Vyas et al. 2016)
2019	TAPB-DMTP-COF	Imine	DOX	HeLa, L929 (Sainan Liu et al. 2019)
2017	TpASH-FA	Hydrazone and β-ketoenamine	5-FU	MDA-MB-231 (Mitra et al. 2017)
2018	PEG_x-CCM@APTES-COF-1	Boroxine	DOX	HeLa (Zhang et al. 2018)
2020	PEG_{350}-CCM@APTES-COF-1	Boroxine	Pazopanib	Renca, bEnd.3, 786-O, HK-2 (Zhang, Jiang, et al. 2020)
2020	F68@SS-COF	Imine	DOX	HepG2 (Shuai Liu et al. 2020)
2019	COF@IR783@CAD	Boronate ester	Cis-aconityldoxorubicin	4T1 (K. Wang et al. 2019)
2020	PFD@$COF_{TTA-DHTA}$@PLGA-PEG, NM-PPIX	Imine	Pirfenidone	CT26 (S.-B. Wang et al. 2020)
2020	COF-HQ	Imine	5-FU	B16F10 tumor-bearing mice with PBS (1) (Jia et al. 2020).
2020	PcS@COF-1	Boroxine	(Porphyrin photosensitizer phthalocyanines) PcS@COF-1 as a photodynamic therapy agent	CT26 colorectal tumor-bearing mice (Tong et al. 2020).

The magnetic COF composite was expected to show good prospects in drug delivery and many other applications. A COF thin film composite (TpASH COF) was synthesized by Banerjee and coworkers for drug delivery applications (Mitra et al. 2017). The amine was used to anchor the targeting ligands to the specific site for drug delivery. TpASH COF was loaded with the targeted 5-fluorouracil drug to enable the release of the drug to specific tumor cells. The COF was also expected to reduce the side effects by eliminating nonspecific targeting. Additionally, the COF showed good antitumor activity, and with a dosage of 50 μg/mL, 14% of the cells were viable. Besides, the TpASH COF was used for the delivery of drugs to breast cancer cells by receptor-mediated endocytosis.

Zhang's group synthesized a COF nanocarrier that is redox responsive and used for the transport of drugs (Shuai Liu et al. 2020). This COF consists of disulfide (SS-COF) and pluronic F68 surfactant synthesized by the self-assembly approach. The F68@SS-COF was spherical in nature with an approximate size of 140 nm and could enclose DOX by π-π and hydrophobic interactions. Additionally, the F68@SS-COF structure collapsed after the uptake of tumor cells as it was brought by glutathione (GSH) in tumor cells releasing the pre-loaded DOX drug. Thereby, the nanocarrier was responsive to the intercellular GHS for a controlled drug release to the targeted site. A new series of water-dispersible polymer-COF nanocomposite was developed by the self-assembly of amine-factionalized COF (APTES-COF-1) and polyethylene-glycol-modified monofunctional curcumin derivative (PEG-CCM). This COF composite acts on the cancer cells emitting fluorescence light as a response. This fluorescent light can enable the tracking of the COF-based material and the anticancer drug (DOX) release performance to the targeted site as shown in Figure 8.6. Additionally, the composite COF also represents high thermal stability (≈300°C), and a good loading capacity (9.71 ± 0.13wt.%) of DOX drug (Zhang et al. 2018).

Liu and coworkers have reported a multifunctional COFs-based core-shell nanocomposite for drug delivery. However, the surface area of the COF composite was less (51.79 m^2/g) compared to 2D COFs. Nevertheless, the COF composite had a good dispersity, excellent magnetic and photothermal performance in various media, and was highly efficient in targeted drug delivery systems. Also, the composite COF significantly quenched the fluorescence of DOX. Therefore, visual detection of the drug loading was possible by fluorescence "turn-off" (Zhao et al. 2021). Several attempts were made to combine COFs with metal ions that can be used for drug delivery applications. For instance, a porphyrin-based covalent triazine framework with manganese metal was developed for the in vitro delivery of IBU drugs (Luo et al. 2017). It is noteworthy to mention that the porphyrins combine with the COF in good coordination, and thus, the composite had good porosity and thermal stability. These features allow the high intake and release of drugs intended for targeted drug delivery applications.

8.7 CONCLUSION AND FUTURE ASPECTS

The current chapter evaluates various improvements made in the field of COFs for drug delivery applications. COFs are an emerging field that finds immense use in drug delivery applications because of their engrossing features. As there are no transition/heavy metals present in COFs, they are a remarkable and nontoxic tool for drug delivery applications. COFs offer high thermal stability, large porosity, and porous structures. Such fascinating properties of COFs provide high drug-loading capacity with improved stability to carry the various drugs to the targeted site without any structural

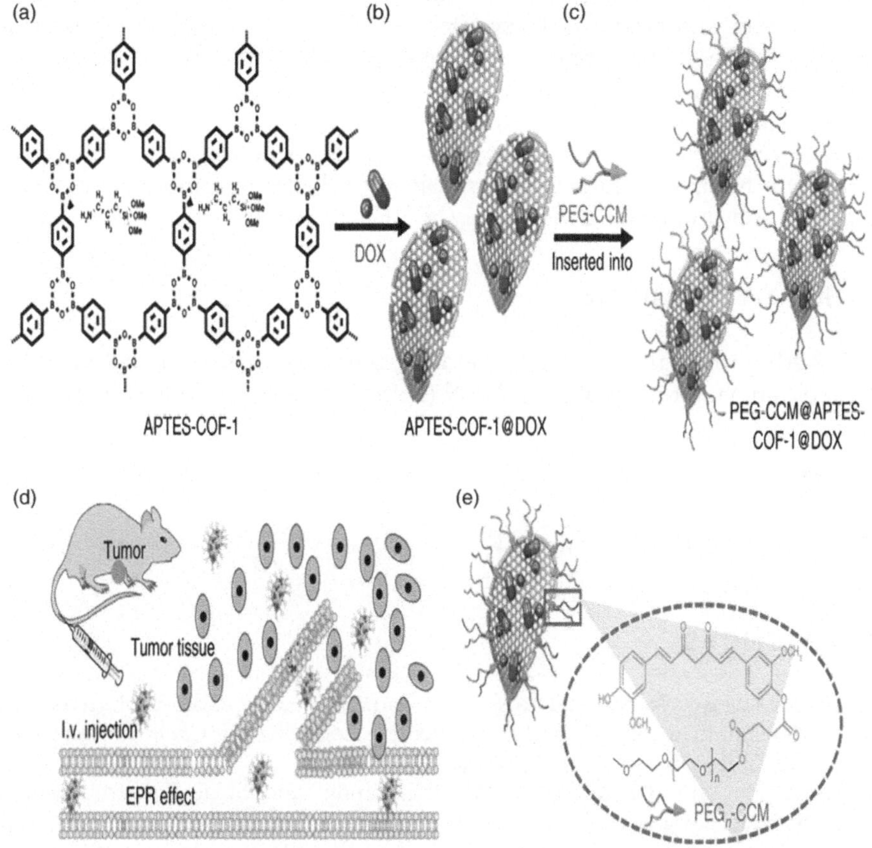

Figure 8.6 (a–d) Schematic representation of DOX loaded in APTES-COF-1 undergoing various interactions to release the drug at targeted site emitting fluorescence light as a response. (e) PEG-CCM blocking the pores of APTES-COF. (Reproduced with approval from (Zhang et al. 2018).)

disintegration and good dispersity in various media. 2D COFs were studied extensively for drug delivery applications due to various advantages such as biodegradability, large pores, high surface area, well-ordered structure, and tunable surface features. However, there are some drawbacks in 2D COFs which need to be resolved such as poor physiological stability and scalability. On the other hand, 3D COFs are very rarely explored for drug delivery applications, but they have a unique structure with two different pore sizes. These features aided 3D COFs to load two different sizes of drugs. Additionally, due to the intrinsic drawbacks, scientists have developed composites of COFs with pluronic F68 surfactant, metal oxides, thin films, and water-dispersible polymers. These composites can be a good tool for drug delivery applications by overcoming some of the existing drawbacks. Additionally, COFs combined with other nanocarriers could display superior results in the drug delivery field. Additionally, the synthesis of COFs has also been improvised, and new methods have been discovered for rapid synthesis. Therefore, the future perspective demands stable, high drug-loading capacities, and a targeted drug delivery approach. Nonetheless, the research field of COF is still an emerging area that could show promising results in drug delivery applications, can be used as targeted drug delivery vehicles in a more appropriate manner, and could emerge as one of the efficient porous carriers near future.

ACKNOWLEDGMENT

The authors recognize the provision delivered by Centre for Research in Functional Materials (CRFM), JAIN (Deemed-to-be University), India.

NOTE

There are no conflicts of interests.

REFERENCES

Abánades Lázaro, Isabel, and Ross S. Forgan. 2019. "Application of zirconium MOFs in drug delivery and biomedicine." *Coordination Chemistry Reviews* 380: 230–259. doi: 10.1016/j.ccr.2018.09.009.

Abuzeid, Hesham R., Ahmed F. M. EL-Mahdy, and Shiao-Wei Kuo. 2021. "Covalent organic frameworks: Design principles, synthetic strategies, and diverse applications." *Giant* 6: 100054. doi: 10.1016/j.giant.2021.100054.

Alanagh, Hamideh Rezvani, Iman Rostami, Mohammad Taleb, Xiaoqing Gao, Yadong Zhang, Abdul Muqsit Khattak, Xiao He, Lianshan Li, and Zhiyong Tang. 2020. "Covalent organic framework membrane for size selective release of small molecules and peptide in vitro." *Journal of Materials Chemistry B* 8 (35): 7899–7903.

Bai, Linyi, Soo Zeng Fiona Phua, Wei Qi Lim, Avijit Jana, Zhong Luo, Huijun Phoebe Tham, Lingzhi Zhao, Qiang Gao, and Yanli Zhao. 2016. "nanoscale covalent organic frameworks as smart carriers for drug delivery." *Chemical Communications* 52 (22): 4128–4131.

Bhunia, Sukanya, Kaivalya A. Deo, and Akhilesh K. Gaharwar. 2020. "2D covalent organic frameworks for biomedical applications." *Advanced Functional Materials* 30 (27): 2002046.

Biswal, Bishnu P., Suman Chandra, Sharath Kandambeth, Binit Lukose, Thomas Heine, and Rahul Banerjee. 2013. "Mechanochemical synthesis of chemically stable isoreticular covalent organic frameworks." *Journal of the American Chemical Society* 135 (14): 5328–5331.

Butterfield, John T., Hidong Kim, Daniel J. Knauer, Wendy K. Nevala, and Svetomir N. Markovic. 2017. "Identification of a peptide-peptide binding motif in the coating of nab-paclitaxel nanoparticles with clinical antibodies: Bevacizumab, rituximab, and trastuzumab." *Scientific Reports* 7 (1): 1–9.

Campbell, Neil L, Rob Clowes, Lyndsey K. Ritchie, and Andrew I. Cooper. 2009. "Rapid microwave synthesis and purification of porous covalent organic frameworks." *Chemistry of Materials* 21 (2): 204–206.

Chen, Lixiao, Qi Wu, Jie Gao, Hui Li, Shuqing Dong, Xiaofeng Shi, and Liang Zhao. 2019. "Applications of covalent organic frameworks in analytical chemistry." *TrAC Trends in Analytical Chemistry* 113: 182–193.

Cote, Adrien P., Annabelle I. Benin, Nathan W. Ockwig, Michael O'Keeffe, Adam J. Matzger, and Omar M. Yaghi. 2005. "Porous, crystalline, covalent organic frameworks." *Science* 310 (5751): 1166–1170.

Davis, Mark E., Zhuo Chen, and Dong M. Shin. 2010. "Nanoparticle therapeutics: An emerging treatment modality for cancer." *Nanoscience and Technology: A Collection of Reviews from Nature Journals*, 7: 239–250.

Diaz de Grenu, Borja, Juan Torres, Javier García-González, Sara Muñoz-Pina, Ruth de Los Reyes, Ana M. Costero, Pedro Amorós, and Jose V. Ros-Lis. 2021. "Microwave-assisted synthesis of covalent organic frameworks: A review." *ChemSusChem* 14 (1): 208–233.

Díaz, Urbano, and Avelino Corma. 2016. "Ordered covalent organic frameworks, COFs and PAFs. From preparation to application." *Coordination Chemistry Reviews* 311: 85–124.

Dürholt, Johannes P., Babak Farhadi Jahromi, and Rochus Schmid. 2019. "Tuning the electric field response of MOFs by rotatable dipolar linkers." *ACS Central Science* 5 (8): 1440–1448.

Dzau, Victor J., and Geoffrey S. Ginsburg. 2016. "Realizing the full potential of precision medicine in health and health care." *Jama* 316 (16): 1659–1660.

El-Kaderi, Hani M., Joseph R. Hunt, José L. Mendoza-Cortés, Adrien P. Côté, Robert E. Taylor, Michael O'Keeffe, and Omar M. Yaghi. 2007. "Designed synthesis of 3D covalent organic frameworks." *Science* 316 (5822): 268–272.

Fang, Qianrong, Junhua Wang, Shuang Gu, Robert B. Kaspar, Zhongbin Zhuang, Jie Zheng, Hongxia Guo, Shilun Qiu, and Yushan Yan. 2015. "3D porous crystalline polyimide covalent organic frameworks for drug delivery." *Journal of the American Chemical Society* 137 (26): 8352–8355.

Guan, Xinyu, Hui Li, Yunchao Ma, Ming Xue, Qianrong Fang, Yushan Yan, Valentin Valtchev, and Shilun Qiu. 2019. "Chemically stable polyarylether-based covalent organic frameworks." *Nature Chemistry* 11 (6): 587–594.

Jia, Yutao, Lina Zhang, Binnan He, Yulong Lin, Jing Wang, and Meng Li. 2020. "8-hydroxyquinoline functionalized covalent organic framework as a PH sensitive carrier for drug delivery." *Materials Science and Engineering: C* 117: 111243.

Jiao, Long, Joanne Yen Ru Seow, William Scott Skinner, Zhiyong U. Wang, and Hai-Long Jiang. 2019. "Metal–organic frameworks: Structures and functional applications." *Materials Today* 27: 43–68. doi: 10.1016/j.mattod.2018.10.038.

Jin, Enquan, Mizue Asada, Qing Xu, Sasanka Dalapati, Matthew A. Addicoat, Michael A. Brady, Hong Xu, Toshikazu Nakamura, Thomas Heine, and Qiuhong Chen. 2017. "Two-dimensional Sp2 carbon–conjugated covalent organic frameworks." *Science* 357 (6352): 673–676.

Kitagawa, Susumu. 2014. "Metal–organic frameworks (MOFs)." *Chemical Society Reviews* 43 (16): 5415–5418.

Kuhn, Pierre, Markus Antonietti, and Arne Thomas. 2008. "Porous, covalent triazine-based frameworks prepared by ionothermal synthesis." *Angewandte Chemie International Edition* 47 (18): 3450–3453. doi: 10.1002/anie.200705710.

Lancet, The. 2020. "COVID-19: Protecting health-care workers." *Lancet (London, England)* 395 (10228): 922.

Li, Chong, Jiancheng Wang, Yiguang Wang, Huile Gao, Gang Wei, Yongzhuo Huang, Haijun Yu, et al. 2019. "Recent progress in drug delivery." *Acta Pharmaceutica Sinica B* 9 (6): 1145–1162. doi: 10.1016/j.apsb.2019.08.003.

Liu, Dong, Fang Yang, Fei Xiong, and Ning Gu. 2016. "The smart drug delivery system and its clinical potential." *Theranostics* 6 (9): 1306.

Liu, Sainan, Chunling Hu, Ying Liu, Xueyan Zhao, Maolin Pang, and Jun Lin. 2019. "One-pot synthesis of DOX@ covalent organic framework with enhanced chemotherapeutic efficacy." *Chemistry–A European Journal* 25 (17): 4315–4319.

Liu, Shuai, Jumin Yang, Ruiwei Guo, Liandong Deng, Anjie Dong, and Jianhua Zhang. 2020. "Facile fabrication of redox-responsive covalent organic framework nanocarriers for efficiently loading and delivering doxorubicin." *Macromolecular Rapid Communications* 41 (4): 1900570.

Luo, Yali, Jun Liu, Yunfei Liu, and Yinong Lyu. 2017. "Porphyrin-based covalent triazine frameworks: Porosity, adsorption performance, and drug delivery." *Journal of Polymer Science Part A: Polymer Chemistry* 55 (16): 2594–2600.

Maschita, Johannes, Tanmay Banerjee, Gökcen Savasci, Frederik Haase, Christian Ochsenfeld, and Bettina V. Lotsch. 2020. "Ionothermal synthesis of imide-linked covalent organic frameworks." *Angewandte Chemie International Edition* 59 (36): 15750–15758. doi: 10.1002/anie.202007372.

Mitra, Shouvik, Himadri Sekhar Sasmal, Tanay Kundu, Sharath Kandambeth, Kavya Illath, David Díaz Díaz, and Rahul Banerjee. 2017. "Targeted drug delivery in covalent organic nanosheets (CONs) via sequential postsynthetic modification." *Journal of the American Chemical Society* 139 (12): 4513–4520. doi:10.1021/jacs.7b00925.

Peng, Yongwu, Wai Kuan Wong, Zhigang Hu, Youdong Cheng, Daqiang Yuan, Saif A. Khan, and Dan Zhao. 2016. "Room temperature batch and continuous flow synthesis of water-stable covalent organic frameworks (COFs)." *Chemistry of Materials* 28 (14): 5095–5101.

Rego, Richelle M., Gangalakshmi Kuriya, Mahaveer D. Kurkuri, and Madhuprasad Kigga. 2021. "MOF based engineered materials in water remediation: Recent trends." *Journal of Hazardous Materials* 403: 123605.

Rego, Richelle M., Ganesan Sriram, Kanalli V. Ajeya, Ho-Young Jung, Mahaveer D. Kurkuri, and Madhuprasad Kigga. 2021. "Cerium based UiO-66 MOF as a multipollutant adsorbent for universal water purification." *Journal of Hazardous Materials* 416: 125941. doi: 10.1016/j.jhazmat.2021.125941.

Scicluna, Marie Christine, and Liana Vella-Zarb. 2020. "Evolution of nanocarrier drug-delivery systems and recent advancements in covalent organic framework–drug systems." *ACS Applied Nano Materials* 3 (4): 3097–3115.

Shivanand, Padmaja, and Omar L. Sprockel. 1998. "A controlled porosity drug delivery system." *International Journal of Pharmaceutics* 167 (1–2): 83–96.

Smith, Brian J., Nicky Hwang, Anton D. Chavez, Jennifer L. Novotney, and William R. Dichtel. 2015. "Growth rates and water stability of 2D boronate

ester covalent organic frameworks." *Chemical Communications* 51 (35): 7532–7535.
Sun, Chun-Yi, Chao Qin, Xin-Long Wang, and Zhong-Min Su. 2013. "Metal-organic frameworks as potential drug delivery systems." *Expert Opinion on Drug Delivery* 10 (1): 89–101.
Sun, Yujia, Liwei Zheng, Yu Yang, Xu Qian, Ting Fu, Xiaowei Li, Zunyi Yang, He Yan, Cheng Cui, and Weihong Tan. 2020. "Metal–organic framework nanocarriers for drug delivery in biomedical applications." *Nano-Micro Letters* 12 (1): 1–29.
Tibbitt, Mark W., James E. Dahlman, and Robert Langer. 2016. "Emerging frontiers in drug delivery." *Journal of the American Chemical Society* 138 (3): 704–717. doi:10.1021/jacs.5b09974.
Tong, Xiaoning, Shaoju Gan, Jinhui Wu, Yiqiao Hu, and Ahu Yuan. 2020. "A nano-photosensitizer based on covalent organic framework nanosheets with high loading and therapeutic efficacy." *Nanoscale* 12 (13): 7376–7382.
Uribe-Romo, Fernando J., Joseph R. Hunt, Hiroyasu Furukawa, Cornelius Klock, Michael O'Keeffe, and Omar M. Yaghi. 2009. "A crystalline imine-linked 3-D porous covalent organic framework." *Journal of the American Chemical Society* 131 (13): 4570–4571.
Uthappa, U. T., Varsha Brahmkhatri, G. Sriram, Ho-Young Jung, Jingxian Yu, Nikita Kurkuri, Tejraj M. Aminabhavi, Tariq Altalhi, Gururaj M. Neelgund, and Mahaveer D. Kurkuri. 2018. "Nature engineered diatom biosilica as drug delivery systems." *Journal of Controlled Release* 281: 70–83.
Uthappa, U. T., Mahaveer D. Kurkuri, and Madhuprasad Kigga. 2019. "Nanotechnology advances for the development of various drug carriers." In Prasad, R., Kumar, V., Kumar, M., Choudhary, D. (eds.) *Nanobiotechnology in Bioformulations*, 187–224. Springer, Cham.
Uthappa, U. T., G. Sriram, O. R. Arvind, Sandeep Kumar, Gururaj M. Neelgund, Dusan Losic, and Mahaveer D. Kurkuri. 2020. "Engineering MIL-100 (Fe) on 3D porous natural diatoms as a versatile high performing platform for controlled isoniazid drug release, Fenton's catalysis for malachite green dye degradation and environmental adsorbents for Pb^{2+} removal and dyes." *Applied Surface Science* 528: 146974.
Uthappa, U. T., G. Sriram, Varsha Brahmkhatri, Madhuprasad Kigga, Ho-Young Jung, Tariq Altalhi, Gururaj M. Neelgund, and Mahaveer D. Kurkuri. 2018. "Xerogel modified diatomaceous earth microparticles for controlled drug release studies." *New Journal of Chemistry* 42 (14): 11964–11971.
Vyas, Vijay S., Medhavi Vishwakarma, Igor Moudrakovski, Frederik Haase, Gökcen Savasci, Christian Ochsenfeld, Joachim P. Spatz, and Bettina V. Lotsch. 2016. "Exploiting noncovalent interactions in an imine-based covalent organic framework for quercetin delivery." *Advanced Materials* 28 (39): 8749–8754.
Wan, Shun, Felipe Gándara, Atsushi Asano, Hiroyasu Furukawa, Akinori Saeki, Sanjeev K. Dey, Lei Liao, Michael W. Ambrogio, Youssry Y. Botros, and Xiangfeng Duan. 2011. "Covalent organic frameworks with high charge carrier mobility." *Chemistry of Materials* 23 (18): 4094–4097.
Wang, Chaoyu, Huiming Liu, Shuai Liu, Zhijun Wang, and Jianhua Zhang. 2020. "PH and redox dual-sensitive covalent organic framework nanocarriers to

resolve the dilemma between extracellular drug loading and intracellular drug release." *Frontiers in Chemistry* 8: 488.

Wang, Kui, Zhe Zhang, Lin Lin, Kai Hao, Jie Chen, Huayu Tian, and Xuesi Chen. 2019. "Cyanine-assisted exfoliation of covalent organic frameworks in nanocomposites for highly efficient chemo-photothermal tumor therapy." *ACS Applied Materials & Interfaces* 11 (43): 39503–39512.

Wang, Lei, Min Zheng, and Zhigang Xie. 2018. "Nanoscale metal–organic frameworks for drug delivery: A conventional platform with new promise." *Journal of Materials Chemistry B* 6 (5): 707–717.

Wang, Shi-Bo, Zhao-Xia Chen, Fan Gao, Cheng Zhang, Mei-Zhen Zou, Jing-Jie Ye, Xuan Zeng, and Xian-Zheng Zhang. 2020. "Remodeling extracellular matrix based on functional covalent organic framework to enhance tumor photodynamic therapy." *Biomaterials* 234: 119772.

Wu, Ming-Xue, and Ying-Wei Yang. 2017. "Applications of covalent organic frameworks (COFs): From gas storage and separation to drug delivery." *Chinese Chemical Letters* 28 (6): 1135–1143. doi: 10.1016/j.cclet.2017.03.026.

Yang, Seung-Tae, Jun Kim, Hye-Young Cho, Sangho Kim, and Wha-Seung Ahn. 2012. "Facile synthesis of covalent organic frameworks COF-1 and COF-5 by sonochemical method." *RSC Advances* 2 (27): 10179–10181.

Zhang, Guiyang, Yan Ji, Xinle Li, Xiaoyun Wang, Mengmeng Song, Huilin Gou, Shan Gao, and Xudong Jia. 2020. "Polymer–covalent organic frameworks composites for glucose and PH dual-responsive insulin delivery in mice." *Advanced Healthcare Materials* 9 (June). doi:10.1002/adhm.202000221.

Zhang, Guiyang, Bo Jiang, Chunyong Wu, Yanfeng Liu, Yidan He, Xin Huang, Wei Chen, Kai Xi, Hongqian Guo, and Xiaozhi Zhao. 2020. "Thin platelet-like COF nanocomposites for blood brain barrier transport and inhibition of brain metastasis from renal cancer." *Journal of Materials Chemistry B* 8 (20): 4475–4488.

Zhang, Guiyang, Xinle Li, Qiaobo Liao, Yanfeng Liu, Kai Xi, Wenyu Huang, and Xudong Jia. 2018. "Water-dispersible PEG-curcumin/amine-functionalized covalent organic framework nanocomposites as smart carriers for in vivo drug delivery." *Nature Communications* 9 (1): 2785. doi:10.1038/s41467-018-04910-5.

Zhao, Kai, Peiwei Gong, Jie Huang, Yan Huang, Dandan Wang, Jingyi Peng, Duyi Shen, Xiaofeng Zheng, Jinmao You, and Zhe Liu. 2021. "Fluorescence turn-off magnetic COF composite as a novel nanocarrier for drug loading and targeted delivery." *Microporous and Mesoporous Materials* 311: 110713.

Zhou, Zhihua, Qingfeng Yi, Yongyi Gao, Qingquan Liu, Lihua Liu, Wennan Zeng, and Xiaoping Liu. 2010. "Evaluation of the potential cytotoxicity of metals associated with implanted biomaterials (II)." *Journal of Medical Engineering & Technology* 34 (7–8): 455–461. doi:10.3109/03091902.2010.519813.

Zhu, Qiang, Xue Wang, Rob Clowes, Peng Cui, Linjiang Chen, Marc A. Little, and Andrew I. Cooper. 2020. "3D cage COFs: A dynamic three-dimensional covalent organic framework with high-connectivity organic cage nodes." *Journal of the American Chemical Society* 142 (39): 16842–16848.

Chapter 9

Nanoporous Anodic Alumina (NAA) for Drug Delivery Applications

Dusan Losic
The University of Adelaide

Shaheer Maher
The University of Adelaide
and
Assiut University

CONTENTS

9.1 INTRODUCTION

To address long-standing limitations of conventional drug delivery based on injections, oral (e.g., pills, tablets, and capsules), or topical formulations (e.g., creams and ointments) because of limited drug solubility, poor

DOI: 10.1201/9781003217114-12

biodistribution, lack of selectivity, and side effects, considerable research has been directed in the last decades toward the development of new and more efficient drug delivery systems [1–3]. In particular, bioactive therapeutic agents such as proteins, nucleic acids, enzymes, and genes administered through oral or intravenous routes can be degraded prematurely by metabolism or by enzymatic conditions existing in gastrointestinal tracts [3,4]. These challenges have contributed to drive the exploration of new drug delivery concepts where the application of nanotechnology and new nanomaterials was regarded as the most promising specifically for their applications in addressing life-threatening conditions such as cancer, heart disease, diabetes, and mental illness etc. [4]. A range of new nanoscale materials in different forms, dimensions, and chemical compositions have been explored in the past two decades as nanocarriers for drug delivery applications such as nanoparticles, nanofibers, dendrimers, liposomes, polymer micelles, carbon nanotubes, fullerenes, graphene sheets, nanocrystals, viral vectors, and virus-like particles (VLP) [5,6]. They are shown to provide a number of advantages such as excellent protection of sensitive active ingredients, sustainable and controllable drug release, delivery of multiple doses, elimination of frequent injection, and flexibility to be used for conventional, targeting, and localized drug delivery systems. Several nanoparticles-based therapeutics delivery systems have been clinically approved and used for real applications with many in the last stage of clinical evaluation and approval. Among them, nanocarriers porous and tubular one-dimensional (1D) morphologies and their 2D surfaces (e.g., nanoporous anodic alumina (NAA), porous silicon (pSi), and nanotubular titania (TiO_2)), have been very attractive and widely explored for delivery of a broad range of therapeutics. This is due to their unique features such as tailorable pore/nanotube structure, surface chemistry, high surface area, high loading capability, low-cost fabrication, and biocompatibility [5,7–11]. They have offered new avenues toward the development of new smart drug delivery systems with improved therapeutic efficiency that includes a wide range of delivery routes such as localized, sustainable, controllable, targeting, and triggered [10–14]. In particular, localized drug delivery using drug-releasing implants, capsules, platforms, stents, etc. can offer many advantages providing locally optimal concentrations of often expensive drugs without diluting them across the entire body while optimizing their bioavailability by avoiding rapid breakdown and serious side effects.

This chapter aims to provide an update and overview on the recent advancements in the field of NAA drug delivery systems and their applications. In the first section, the fundamental fabrication process, their properties, and biocompatibility of NAA associated with their biomedical applications are briefly introduced. The following section describes the engineering of different NAA nanostructures and their modifications that were recently reported for drug delivery applications showing their advantages and limitations. More details and demonstration of concepts for their application for localized, targeted, and triggered drug delivery systems as well as biocapsules and stents have been elaborated showing the most important examples of in vitro and in vivo studies. Finally, a general overview on recent trends in this field presenting key challenges and future perspectives has been concluded.

9.2 NANOPOROUS ANODIC ALUMINA (NAA): STRUCTURE, PREPARATION, AND PROPERTIES

Nanoporous anodic alumina (NAA) can be described as a thin oxide film created by electrochemical anodization process that is composed of alumina (aluminum oxide—Al_2O_3) hexagonal arrays of vertically aligned cylindrical nanopore structures with closed hemispherical bottom (Figure 9.1) [7,15,16]. They have remarkable properties such as unique ordered porous structures, chemical and thermal stability, hardness, and high surface area [14]. The pore structures of NAA are characterized by several key parameters such as pore organization (hexagonal), pore diameter, interpore distance (cell diameter), wall thickness, pore length, and barrier layer thickness (Figure 9.1b). By controlling anodization conditions, these parameters can be precisely tuned in the range of about 10–400 nm for pore diameter, 50–600 nm for interpore distance, pore aspect ratio from 10 to 5,000, a thickness of the porous layer from 10 to 150 nm, a pore density from 109 to 1,011 cm^2, and porosity from 5% to 50% [7,14,15,17,18].

NAA is prepared by the anodization of aluminum (Al) which is scalable and a prime example of the self-ordered electrochemical anodization process. Over the past decade, we have witnessed the emergence of various applications based on NNA membranes such as template synthesis of nanomaterials, molecular separation, nanofluidics, microfluidics, sensing, photonics, catalysis, supercapacitors, energy storage, drug delivery, tissue engineering, etc. with more than 5,000 published papers [14,16]. Numerous studies over the last decades have explored the anodization conditions of Al metal, such as the applied potential, current, pH, electrolyte type, electrolyte composition and concentration, temperature, and pre-patterning of the surface (Figure 9.1c–e) in order to achieve improved control of the self-ordering process and fabricate NAA with highly ordered pore structures with controllable pore diameters, internal geometries, and interpore spacing [14,16]. Three electrolytes including sulfuric, oxalic, and phosphoric acids are commonly used for preparation of NAA by anodization processes at constant voltage (potentiostatic mode), which is also called "mild" anodization (MA). Using these acids and conditions, three typical sizes of pre-diameters of NAA can be obtained: with sulfuric at 25 V for an interpore distance (Dint) = 63 nm, with oxalic acid at 40 V for Dint = 100 nm,

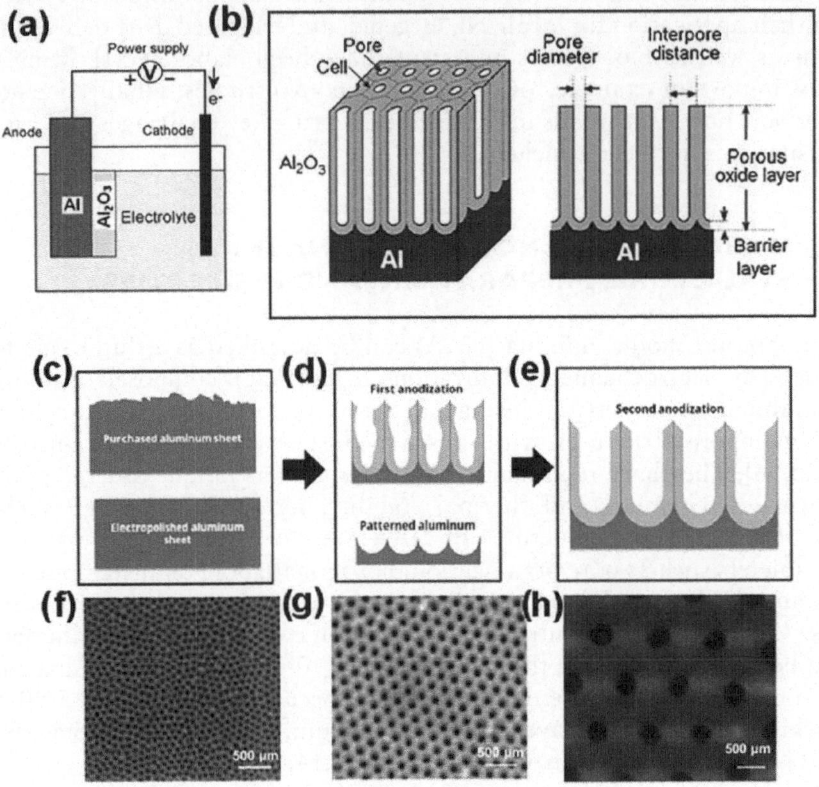

Figure 9.1 (a) Schematic of electrochemical cell for preparation of nanoporous anodic alumina (NAA) on Al substrate using electrochemical anodization. (b) The scheme of NAA structure showing typical pore structures and structural features. (c–e) The schematic of the two-step anodization process starting from aluminum sheet followed by electropolishing treatment to decrease surface roughness: the first anodization step is further chemically treated to remove the sacrificial oxide layer followed by the second step anodization to obtain desired oxide thickness. (f–h) SEM images of typical NAA structures (top view) obtained in (f) sulfuric, (g) oxalic, and (h) phosphoric acids, respectively. (c–e: Reprinted with permission from ref. [19]. Copyright 2016, Springer.)

and with phosphoric acid at 195 V for Dint = 500 nm (Figure 9.2f–h) [14,16]. Several studies have shown that other acids such as chromic, boric, citric, and tartaric acid can also be used for preparation of NAA, at different voltages providing specific pore diameters [14,16]. The most significant progress toward the fabrication of NAA with a high degree of pore order has been made by Masuda and Fukuda by introducing a two-step anodization

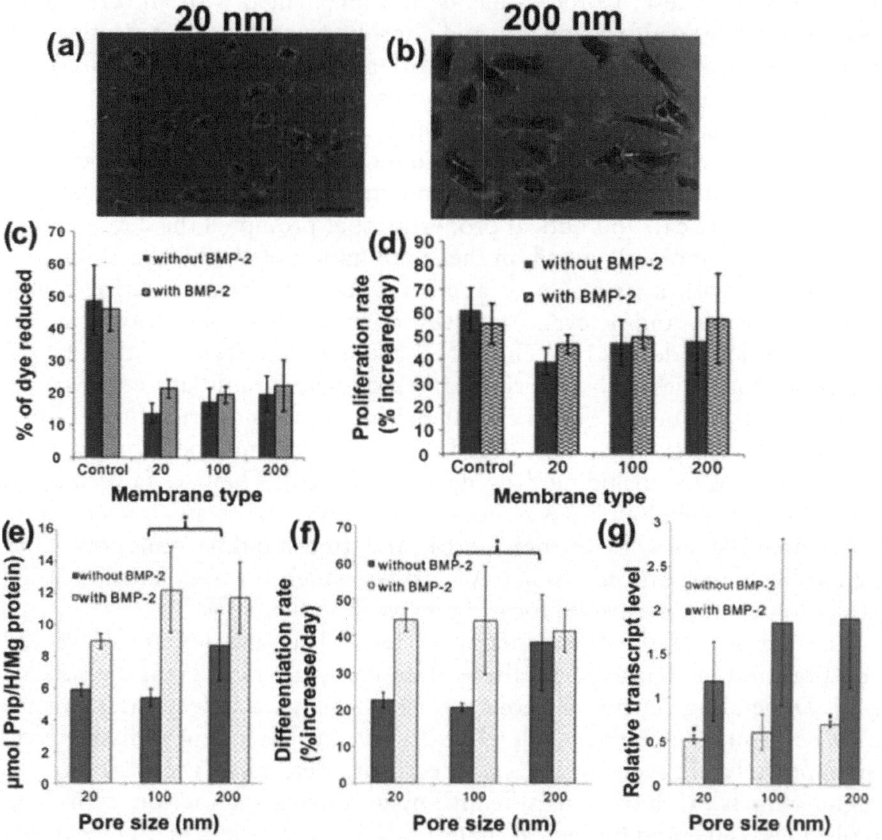

Figure 9.2 W20-17 cell morphology after cell culturing for 2 days on (a) 20 nm and (b) 200 nm. (c) Alamar blue assay profile of proliferated cells after 7 days. (d) Day-wise analysis of increase in cell number from 2 to 7 days. (e) Alkaline phosphatase (ALP) activity after 14 days of cell culture, with polystyrene as a control, and NAA (20, 100, and 200 nm), with and without the addition of BMP-2. (f) Measurement of cell differentiation rate by analyzing increase in ALP activity by time (12 days) from days 2 to 14. (g) OC gene expression with and without BMP-2 was analyzed at 14 days. (Adapted with permission from ref. [48]. Copyright 2014, Scientific Research Publishing.)

approach [17]. They generated a porous layer after removal of the first anodization step and used the pre-structuring of Al to facilitate the propagation of pores with long-range order over the entire surface in a subsequent second anodization step. The main disadvantage of this process is the slow fabrication speed (1–2 nm/hour), which requires a very long time (2 days) to prepare an NAA membrane. To address this problem, a new method called hard (HA) or high-field anodization has been introduced by the Gösele group that provides higher anodization and fabrication speeds of 50–100 nm/hour [18]. The HA process has been implemented with all three common electrolytes (sulfuric, oxalic, and phosphoric acid) using potentiostatic and galvanostatic mode and provides more options for controlling pore diameters and interpore distance compared to mild anodization.

NAA with structured internal geometries of pores raised considerable promise in the development of advanced molecular separation strategies or as a template for the fabrication of nanowires and nanotubes with unique magnetic, electrical, and optical properties that prompted the development of several new methods based on the combination of chemical etching and anodization with a variation of applied voltage or current during anodization, pulsing, and/or cyclic anodization using both potentiostatic and galvanostatic mode [14,16]. The NNA could be fabricated with a broad range of geometries such as periodically modulated, multilayered, tree-like branched, three-tiered branched, hierarchical, asymmetric (funnel-like), ratchet-type, bottle-neck, perforated, etc. providing unique properties for many applications including drug delivery [19–24]. They are fabricated in several forms including NAA structured film on Al substrate, free-standing NAA membranes with opened pores, and free-standing nanopores and nanotubes de-assembled from NAA arrays which are very attractive for designing 1D nano capsules for drug delivery applications.

The surface of NAA is inherently charged as a consequence of the equilibration of charged crystalline alumina lattice defects on the surface [25]. Depending on the net concentration of lattice defects, the surface may be positively or negatively charged with an attendant redistribution of oppositely charged lattice and electronic defects in the near-surface region which can have a significant impact during interaction with drug molecules, cells, and biological material [25]. Hence, it is highly desirable to modify the surface of NAA to improve biocompatibility for applications that involve interaction with biomolecules and cells such as protein separation, immunoisolations, cell adsorption/growth, and tissue engineering. In the case of drug delivery applications, the surface modifications and functionalization of NAA are very important to improve their drug-loading and drug-releasing performance for tailoring desired drug-release kinetics (burst or slow with zero order), designing stimulated drug-release concepts, combining with sensing functions, etc. Various solid and soft surface modification techniques of NAA have been explored in the past, including atomic layer deposition (ALD), chemical vapor deposition (CVD), thermal vapor metal deposition, chemical, electrochemical deposition, sol–gel layer-by-layer deposition, and plasma polymerization [14,24,26,27]. The soft surface functionalizations were performed using organic molecules such as silanes, polythiols, n-alkanoic acids, polyelectrolyte layers, poly(ethylene glycol) (PEG), chitosan, poly(sodium styrenesulfonate) (PSS), proteins, lipid bilayers, plasma polymers, carbon, and graphene [7,14,28–37].

9.3 BIOCOMPATIBILITY

Biocompatibility, a general term describing the property of a material being compatible with living tissue, is the prerequisite for the application of new biomaterials to be used for real-life clinical applications [38]. This safety evaluation is defined in terms of cellular response and tissue integration of implantable biomaterials and their ability when exposed to the body or bodily fluids to function without eliciting detrimental local or systemic immunological responses. Alumina (Al_2O_3) or bioceramic alumina is proven as nontoxic and biocompatible biomaterial, which is widely used clinically in dentistry and orthopedics as dental and orthopedic implants [39,40]. Alumina is a bioinert material, highly insoluble, with excellent chemical stability and resistance, which are key properties defining their biocompatibility and safe biomedical applications. In recent years, considerable in vitro and in vivo studies have been performed to confirm the biocompatibility of NAA biomaterials and NAA-based devices such as implants and stents and to better understand its behavior with different cell lines and tissues including bone, epithelial, muscular, and blood cells as well as neuronal tissues [38–44].

9.4 IN VITRO BIOCOMPATIBILITY STUDIES

It is well established that surface composition, surface energy, surface roughness, and surface topography of nanoporous alumina (and biomaterials in general) affect their biocompatibility (i.e., cellular response and tissue integration) [39,40]. Understanding the mechanisms behind cell adhesion, behavior, and differentiation in response to NAA surfaces is critical for the development of new methods for enhanced cell culture processes and their translations into implantable devices and drug delivery systems. However, the influence of surface micro and nano-topography on cells' behavior and interaction is still not well understood or even controversial. A major challenge in the case of biomedical implant research is to understand these key parameters in order to design optimized implant surfaces that are capable to promote in vitro and in vivo bio-integration. Pioneering studies by Desai et al. have demonstrated that the nanoporous and nanotubular titania surface is a favorable template for bone cell growth and differentiation and provides clear evidence that osteoblasts activity can be significantly enhanced using controlled nano-topographies [30,40,41]. These surfaces supported higher cell adhesion, proliferation, and viability for up to 7 days of culture when compared to plain surfaces. Studies on osteoblast response to NNA indicated that pore diameters of ~100 nm are optimal for bone in-growth assuming it will maintain blood supply in the connective tissues [40]. However, later studies on NAA have revealed that smaller pores of

AAO are more favorable for bone cells' growth [43,44]. Thus, this debate about influence of the NAA pore diameters on cells' adhesion, differentiation, and proliferation is still not closed [39–43].

Studies using NAA with smaller pores (diameters of 30–80 nm) on osteoblast confirm extending the growth of osteoblasts into the nanopores which produced an active matrix in the form of fibrous extensions that contain calcium and phosphorus (the typical elements of the bone matrix) [44–46]. SEM images showed that the osteoblasts were extending growth processes into the nanopores while cells showed a spherical morphology after 1 day, and after 2 days, spherical morphology was lost. By day 4, osteoblasts showed active matrix production in the form of fibrous extensions, i.e., normal phenotype and morphology. The lengths of these bundles were many times greater than the cell diameters. Similar conclusion was reached by Popat et al. who reported that NAA membranes showed significantly improved osteoblast adhesion and proliferation in comparison with amorphous alumina, aluminum, and glass [40,41,47], revealing that NAA can work as a framework in which osteoblasts can generate new bone. Cells cultured on NAA membranes showed higher protein content and more extracellular matrix, indicating significantly improved performance. In another study by Popat et al. [41], which aimed to investigate osteogenic differentiation, the marrow stromal cell viability and the cytotoxicity on NAA surfaces (pore size 79 nm) are shown to increase ~45% in cell adhesion, proliferation, and viability; 35% increase in enzyme activity; and 50% increase in matrix production in comparison with the amorphous alumina surface. It is postulated that these nanoporous structures which are not able to allow cellular in-growth due to their size will instead be filled with collagen and bone matrix. Further improved osteoblast adhesion and growth on NAA with the pore diameters (30–80 nm) were reported with modified surfaces by physically adsorbing vitronectin or covalently immobilizing a cellular adhesive peptide of arginine–glycine–aspartic acid–cysteine (RGDC) [37]. The rationale for protein attachment is explained because protein and peptide modifications influence cell adhesion. Moreover, to analyze the dissolution rate, NAA material was placed in cell culture medium along with growing cells. It was found that after 9 days of incubation, membrane lost only 0.03% of its weight which is far below the toxic level [40]. These encouraging studies show the potential of porous NAA to be used as a biocompatible platform for bone growth and orthopedic implant applications; however, more studies are needed in the future.

A recent pore-size dependence study by Pujari-Palmer et al. also confirmed that the nano-topography of the surface of NAA has a significant impact on bone cells' behavior [48]. The bone marrow stromal cell growth study using NAA membranes, with different pore diameters (20, 100, and 200 nm) monitored by alkaline phosphatase (ALP) expressions, showed that the cells on NAA membranes with a pore diameter of 20 nm were flat and round shape while being elongated on 200 nm pores (Figure 9.2). The rate of cell proliferation was found to be higher on the control surfaces compared to NAA surfaces when analyzed with Alamar blue assay with no significant differences considering the proliferation rate among different pore diameters. The higher ALP activity in cells was observed on 200 nm pores as compared to 20 and 100 nm NAA pores after 14 days culture. This trend was observed in the cells differentiation rate, showing that the differentiation rate was higher on the 200 nm pores as compared to 100 nm pores without the addition of bone morphogenic protein-2 (BMP-2) and showing no significant difference for all surfaces with the BMP-2 addition (Figure 9.2).

The study by Hoess and coworkers [49] found that by cultivating hepatocytes cell line HepG2 on NAA membranes pore diameters of 70 and 260 nm showed good cell growth conditions with excellent proliferation and adhesion for up to 4 days with normal morphology and no signs of toxicity. It was observed that filopodia structures were created by penetrating inside the larger pores with a diameter of more than 200 nm indicating the importance of pore dimensions [50]. In another study by Ni et al. to assess the proliferation and attachment of preosteoblast (MC3T3-E1) cell lines, fabricated NAA with pore diameters between 25 and 70 nm were used [51]. Results showed moderate differences in preosteoblast attachment, but the proliferation rate was found to be dramatically increased at the larger pore sizes, i.e., 50 and 75 nm. The influence of the NAA pore depth (50–2,000 nm) is studied by Thakur et al. using vascular endothelial cells (ECV 304) showing that for shallow pores (50 and 200 nm pore depth), the cells were found to be round with the presence of actin in an amorphous form throughout the cytosol distribution with no major differences [52]. However, on higher deep pores (+2,000 nm), the cells' morphology and their arrangement in its cytosol compartment depend mainly on the pore diameters with no influence on the pore depth [52].

The interactions between NAA with different pore diameters (20 and 200 nm) and whole blood and platelet-rich plasma were investigated by Karlsson and coworkers [43–45]. The blood-implant contact leads to a series of interlinked events such as protein adsorption, complement activation, platelet and leucocytes adhesion/activation, and activation of the coagulation cascade leading to the surface covered with plasma proteins and platelets particles. Immunocytochemical staining and SEM analysis indicated different behavior of NAA with different pore sizes (20–200 nm) in contact with whole blood. NAA with 200 nm pore diameters caused lower complement activation, high platelet, and nonsignificant platelet microparticle adsorption. On the contrary, NAA with 20 nm pore diameters caused higher complement activation, negligible platelet, and significant microparticle adsorption [45–47]. It is postulated that different protein adsorption and patterning are created on the surface of NAA depending on the pore size, affecting the availability of receptors and binding sites, and also platelet activation. In another study by Karlsson and coworkers, NAA membranes were coated with collagen I, serum, fibrinogen, IgG, and albumin to determine in vitro cell viability of osteoblastic cells (MG63) and the pore size-dependent responses. The strongest response in the cell numbers was noticed when NAA membranes (20 and 200 nm pore size) were incubated with collagen I. Cells cultivated on fibrinogen-coated membrane were found to be more viable on 20 nm as compared to 200 nm structure. The reason for observed results can be attributed to the physical characteristics, i.e., size and shape of fibrinogen. It was also reported that albumin has more binding affinity to this substrate than IgG [46].

To test the biocompatibility of NAA tubular structures with different lengths and aspect ratios which are considered carriers for drug delivery application, our team fabricated NAA nanotubes (NAANTs) with different lengths (500–5,800 nm) through pulse anodization and performed the systematic cytotoxicity evaluation to determine the influence of their lengths, the aspect ratio, concentration, and time [53–55]. Results from these toxicity studies are summarized in Figures 9.3 and 9.4 [54]. Systematic cytotoxicity evaluations were conducted using RAW 264.7 mouse macrophage cells and MDA-MB 231-TXSA human breast cancer cells through several toxicity parameters, including cell viability and morphology, pro-inflammatory response, mitochondrial depolarization, lysosomal membrane permeabilization (LMP), induction of autophagy, and endoplasmic reticulum (ER) stress. The results confirmed that toxicity patterns of NAA nanotubes with different aspect ratios were cell-type dependent and strongly related to NAANTs dose, time, and importantly their aspect ratio. Long NAANTs triggered enhanced cell death, morphological changes, tumor necrosis factor α (TNF- α) release, LMP, and ER stress than short NAANTs. The toxic aspect ratio of NAANTs was determined to be 7.8, which is shorter than that of other previously reported high aspect ratio nanomaterials. The determination of this toxic aspect ratio window provides an important information to control the toxicity of this type of nanomaterials and their application as nanocarriers for their advanced drug delivery application.

In an additional study of the concentration dependence of NNA nanotubes on toxicity, NAA nanotubes with concentrations from 1.56 to 100 μg/mL were used for toxicity experiments for 1–5 days on breast cancer cells (MDA-MB231-TXSA) and macrophage cells (RAW264.7) and characterized by Alamar blue and crystal violet bioassays (Figure 9.4a–d). It was demonstrated that even after 5 days, no toxicity patterns were observed in both cell lines indicating that NAA nanotubes did not have any negative impact on cell growth and morphology (Figure 9.4e). To evaluate the interaction between NAAs nanotubes and cell lines, transmission electron microscopy (TEM) examination was carried out as depicted in Figure 9.4f–j, confirming NAA tubes were inside and taken by the RAW264.7 cells with

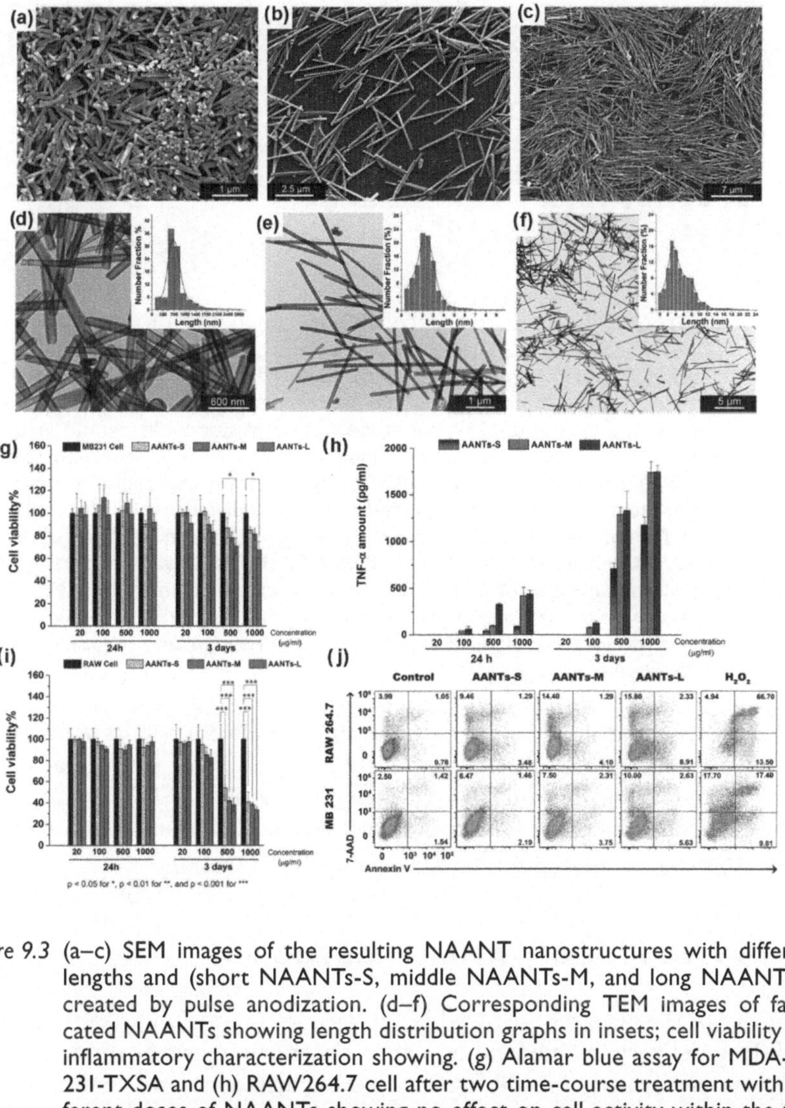

Figure 9.3 (a–c) SEM images of the resulting NAANT nanostructures with different lengths and (short NAANTs-S, middle NAANTs-M, and long NAANTs-L) created by pulse anodization. (d–f) Corresponding TEM images of fabricated NAANTs showing length distribution graphs in insets; cell viability and inflammatory characterization showing. (g) Alamar blue assay for MDA-MB 231-TXSA and (h) RAW264.7 cell after two time-course treatment with different doses of NAANTs showing no effect on cell activity within the first 24 h but impact the cell viability after 3 days in a dose- and length-dependent pattern. (h) RAW 264.7 TNF-α production respond to NAANTs detected by ELISA showing cells produced a significant amount of TNF-α after 3 days of treatment at high doses in all three types of NAANTs. However, short NAANTs-S did not induce TNF-α generation at a concentration of 100 mg/mL after 3 days of treatment. No TNF-α production was found at the lowest dose treatment. (j) Representative scatter plot of Annexin-V assay and (e) statistics analysis for MDA-MB 231-TXSA cell and RAW 264.7 cell lines after 100 mg/mL NAANTs treatment for 3 days. NAANTs-S and NAANTs-M induced necrosis but did not trigger apoptosis; NAANTs-L triggered stronger necrosis and apoptosis as compared to shorter ones, although they did not induce significant cell death (late apoptosis). The level of significance was set to a probability of $p<0.05$ for *, $p<0.01$ for **, and $p<0.001$ for ***. (Adapted with permission from ref. [54]. Copyright 2014, Elsevier.)

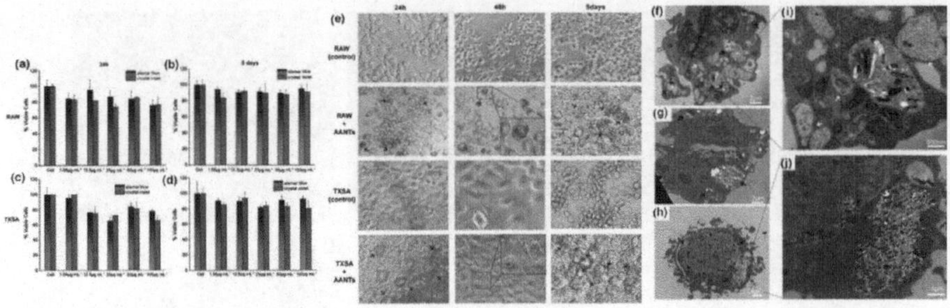

Figure 9.4 (a–d) Cell toxicity studies of NAA nanotubes on RAW264.7 and MDA-MB231-TXSA cell lines within 24 hours and 5 days to confirm the concentration and the time dependence. Cells have more than 80% viability in both cell lines, demonstrating the biocompatibility of NAANTs. (e) Light microscope images of NAA nanotubes (concentration 100 mg/mL) incubated with two cell lines. Black arrows indicate that cells are closely surrounded by NNA nanotubes, but no cell viability inhibition was found during 5-day experiment. Insets show magnified views of individual cells after 48 hours. (f–j) TEM images of NAA nanotubes (100 mg/mL) internalized by RAW264.7 macrophage cells (f, g, and i) and MDA-MB231-TXSA cell (h and j); (i) and (j) are magnified views of (f) and (i). The black arrows identify NAANTs inside cells; white arrows indicate the fusion of autophagic vacuoles, in which cellular debris was located inside. (Adapted with permission from ref. [55]. Copyright 2015, Elsevier.)

the bonding of autophagosome with autophage. These results successfully demonstrate the uptake of NAA nanotubes inside the cell without any toxic effects. Comparing the influence of different sizes on NAA nanotubes, it was again confirmed that nanotubes with smaller length (700 nm) have the lowest toxicity compared with longer nanotubes [55].

9.5 IN VIVO BIOCOMPATIBILITY STUDIES

Majority of the research involved NAA used as a model platform for localized drug delivery, biomedical implants, coronary stents, or immune isolation was performed considering in vitro experiments, with only a few in vivo studies. It is worth noting that, even NAA substrates show promising in vitro results for their real-life applications, it is critical to have more in vivo investigations to confirm their performance before moving into clinical studies.

One of the pioneering in vivo biocompatibility studies of NAA was performed for coronary stents applications using the rabbit restenosis model, which proved biocompatibility and absence of inflammation [56]. However, the following study by other groups on in vivo biocompatibility of stents alumina porous coatings investigated using the pig restenosis model indicates an inflammatory response which can be explained by differences in substrates [57,58]. The studies on immunoisolation using capsules with NAA membranes with 75 nm pore diameter showed that they are nontoxic with no significant complement activation in vitro [42]. However, in vivo implantation of these capsules into the peritoneal cavity of rats induces a transient inflammatory response. To address this problem, NAA membrane was modified by polyethylene glycol (PEG) for minimizing this inflammatory response. Blood vessels are seen in the tissue treated with PEG-modified capsules, which suggests that the major amount of inflammation is due to the procedure itself, whereas surrounding tissues are relatively undisturbed. Considering that the inflammatory response of NAA can be minimized by PEG surface functionalization, further investigations are required to establish whether surface modifications can eliminate or minimize observed inflammatory/restenosis effects.

A novel method to study the ex vivo drug release in bones was introduced by our group using the Zetos bioreactor able to keep bones in live conditions over 5–6 days (Figure 9.5) [59–61]. For this study, Al wires with an NAA layer were fabricated and used as a model of bone drug-releasing implants (NAA-Al) and their ex vivo biocompatibility study [59–61]. These NAA-Al implants with pore diameter (30–35 nm) and depth of 10–60 μm were fabricated by electrochemical anodization. The NAA nanopores of the implants were loaded with rhodamine B (RB) dye as a model drug and placed directly into bovine trabecular bone cores using the needle puncture procedure, and drug elution kinetics was measured in the bone culture chamber by live fluorescence imaging as presented in Figure 9.5. To evaluate the stability of inserted NAA-Al implants as well as interaction within the bone, the entire ex vivo–treated implants were taken out of the bone chamber to evaluate the stability of NAA structures. The digital photograph as well as the SEM image presented in Figure 9.5f–i confirmed that inserted implants retained their surface texture and the pore structure after 11 days of media perfusion inside the bone. Biocompatibility study of these Al wire implants was performed using human osteoblast cells, which responded with strong growth and adhesion to the NAA surface with no visible cell death after 3 days. Histology examination of implants reveals the presence of live osteocyte cells along with an insertion area demonstrating the harmlessness of the implant device to adjacent areas, which makes the system suitable for clinical practice (Figure 9.5j–l).

9.6 DRUG DELIVERY APPLICATIONS OF NAA

Owing to its unique porous structure for loading and release of therapeutic molecules as well as its biocompatibility, NAA biomaterial had attracted considerable attention in the past two decades to be explored for

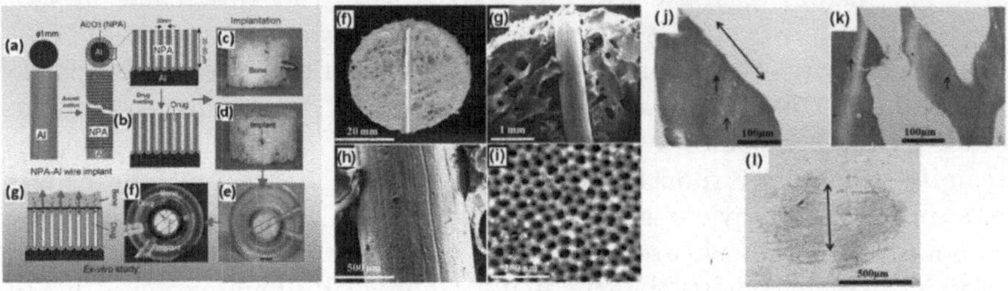

Figure 9.5 (a) Scheme of Al wire implant preparation, drilling-guided drug-loaded implant insertion into the ex vivo bone model and in situ release measurements. (f–i) Stability of the NAA-Al wire implant inserted into marrow-less bone. Digital image of the implant in the cross section of bone collected and prepared at the end of the ex vivo study using decalcification, cross-sectioning, and platinum coating (f). SEM images showing porous bone structure with placement of the implant (g), stable and unchanged surface morphology (h–i) and clear nanopores of the inserted implant; (j–k) Stained histology of bone core implanted with NAA-Al wires. Light microscopic images showing the presence of viable osteocytes along the drilled areas as well as adjacent to the implant position (j) and in distant areas of the bone core (k). Digital image of hematoxylin–eosin stained a representative histology sample (l) prepared from the decalcified bone core at the end of the ex vivo study, with a double-headed black arrow indicating the location of the implant. (Adapted with permission from ref. [59]. Copyright 2015, Royal Society of Chemistry.)

biomedical applications including drug delivery. The use of NAA for drug delivery applications has been explored across several domains including in vitro studies to demonstrate the delivery of different drugs, engineering of sustainable and controllable drug-releasing systems, development of therapeutic devices for bone and dental tissue engineering, coronary stent implants, carriers for transplanted cells, and immunoisolation with some in vivo studies, which are presented in the following sections.

9.6.1 In Vitro Studies of NAA as Carriers for Drug Delivery

The NAA as potential drug-releasing implants for localized drug delivery has been less explored in comparison to TNTs based on the fact that titanium materials are commonly used as orthopedic and dental implants. Most of these drug delivery application studies were in vitro based and focused to explore the influence of NAA structures and their structural and surface chemistry modification on drug-release kinetics using different types of drug molecules demonstrating new concepts for controllable, targeting, and triggered drug-release [8–11,16].

When the NAA platform, with drugs loaded inside nanopores, comes into contact with the physiological solution inside the host body, the drug release from nanopores is governed by a diffusion and process of the mass transfer of drug molecules from the nanopores [10]. This is controlled by a number of factors such as the solubility of drug molecules, their diffusion coefficient, molecular size, charge and surface chemistry, the dimensions of nanopores (diameter and length), their charge and surface chemistry, interfacial interaction between drug molecules, and so on. Thus all these aspects should be considered for NAA applications as carriers for designing drug delivery systems [10,11]. The ultimate aim of employing NAA was to provide a sustainable and controllable release of drug molecules from NAA pores with favorable release kinetics (optimized drug-release rate and time of release) for a broad range of clinical therapies [8,10]. In particular, the focus of these studies was to eliminate the undesired burst release of drug and to establish strategies capable of providing sustained and long-term release with zero-order kinetics [8]. To achieve these goals and design NAA platforms with optimized drug delivery performances, several approaches to improve drug-loading and drug-release performance of NAA implants were explored considering the structural modification of NAA (pore diameters, length, and shapes), chemical modifications (by means of altering the internal surface chemistry) and by combining with other materials (biopolymer coating, nanoparticles (NP), polymeric micelles, graphene, external triggering agents, etc.) [8–11,16].

Surface functionalization of NAA by introducing different functional groups is recognized as one of the simplest and most efficient strategies not only to alter and tailor slow drug-release kinetics but also to improve the overall physicochemical properties and biocompatibility [14,62]. Many surface modification approaches for the functionalization of NAA structures have been explored to improve drug-release performances that include: chemical modification by silanization using different types of silanes (3-aminopropyl trimethoxysilane (APTES), octadecyltrimethoxysilane (ODS), etc.), phosponic compounds, dopamine, polymer grafting using polyacrylic acid (PAA), poly(N-isopropylacrylamide) (PNIPAM), polystyrene sulfonate/poly-allylamine hydrochloride(PSS/PAH), plasma polymerization, atomic layer deposition (ALD), modification with nanoparticles (Ag, Se, etc.), and carbon materials (CNT, carbon nanodots, graphene, etc.) [14,16,19,28,30,32–36,62].

In a pioneering study, Kapoor et al. [63] explored the effect of NAA pore size and functionalization with hydrophilic and hydrophobic surface chemical groups on the loading and release of ibuprofen (IBU). Surface functionalization with hydrophobic groups resulted in low drug loading (approximately 20%) and fast release (85% over a period of 5 hours), whereas hydrophilic groups resulted in significantly higher drug loadings (21%–45%) and slower rate of release (12%–40% over a period of 5 hours). Based on the results, the authors suggested surfaces modified with both hydrophobic and hydrophilic groups such as “Janus particles.” In a similar study, Das et al. [64] investigated the influence of surface density of the OH group on ibuprofen loading and release. It was found that the density variation of OH does not affect the morphological parameters such as surface area, pore size, and distribution. A high degree of ibuprofen loading was possible as high as 26%. It was shown that in vitro ibuprofen release kinetics was influenced by the OH surface groups. When the concentration of the OH group increased, the resulting interaction of ibuprofen molecules was stronger which lead to slower drug release from the NAA structure.

In terms of improving drug-releasing performances of NAA, our group conducted several studies to show that the release of drugs from NAA platforms can be controlled not only by manipulating its pore geometries but also by other approaches using surface modification such as NAA coating with polymers and loading with nanoparticle carriers and micellar nanocarrier with encapsulating drug molecules [8,10,16,60–62,65–68]. Our results from these studies showed that drug molecules were eluted more rapidly from nanopores with bigger diameters, which is in good agreement with previous studies. Furthermore, we demonstrated that the initial burst release of indomethacin could be drastically reduced from 50% to around 25% by functionalizing the NAA surface with amine- or penta-fluoro-terminated silanes. The study by Marsal and coworkers reported the impact of pore geometries on the release of drug from 3D-NAA nanostructures [69]. They fabricated different 3D structures (multilayered nanofunnels (NFs) and inverted funnels (IFs), consisting of cylindrical pores with varied pore diameter) which were loaded with doxorubicin (1 mg/mL). Results of their release profiles modeled by Higuchi (short-term) and Korsmeyer–Peppas (long-term) equations confirmed sustained drug elution profile for more than 60 days without an initial burst release. It was shown that pore geometry impacted the release kinetics including the total amount of drug loaded inside the pores. Regarding the short-term release, the release rates from inverted funnels were lower than straight pores (SPs) despite having the same pore diameter [69].

Important advancement has been recently reported by our group for developing a new and facile method to control drug release from NAA which combines both structural and chemical modification of pores in one step [67,68]. The concept presented in Figure 9.6a is based on applying a thin plasma polymer film on the top of NAA after drug loading into the nanopores. It was hypothesized that applying a plasma polymer layer of a different thickness would allow control over pore diameter at the surface and hence, control the rate of drug release which was successfully demonstrated using several different drug molecules such as anti-inflammatory, antibiotics, proteins, growth factors, antibodies, and anticancer drugs [67,68,70]. Plasma polymerization is attractive because it is a one-step drying technique which prevents elution of the loaded drug by solvents while excluding any contamination. The release profiles of loaded drug, vancomycin, with

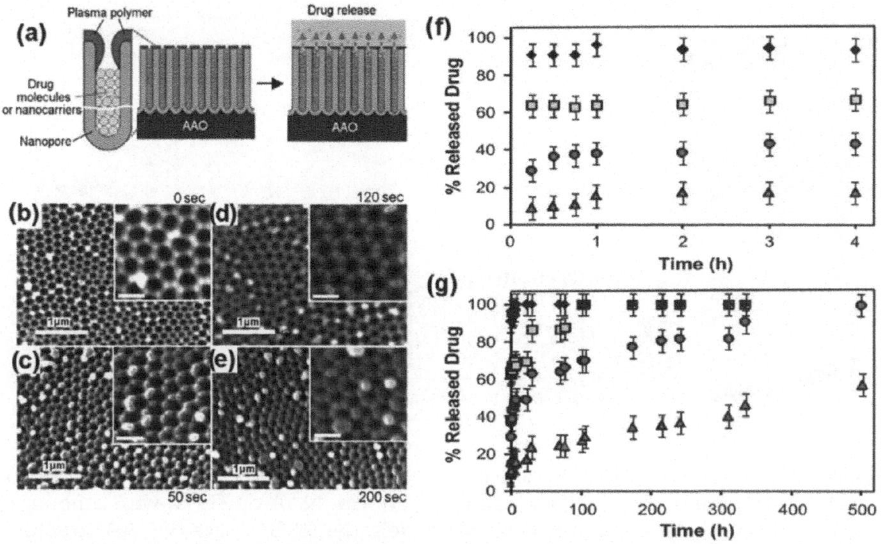

Figure 9.6 (a) The schematic representation of plasma modification of NAA platform for controlled drug release (drug loading with loaded drug (vancomycin) inside of the pores. (b–e) SEM images of the top surface of the NAA layer modified with allylamine plasma polymer using deposition times of (b) 0 (i.e., control), (c) 50 s, (d) 120 s, and (e) 200 s. Scale bars in insets are 200 nm and (f–g) controlled release of drug vancomycin from plasma-modified NAA during (f) 4 hours (burst release) and (b) 500 hours (sustained release). Plasma deposition times were 50 seconds (squares), 120 seconds (circles), 200 seconds (triangles), and control (no plasma deposition, diamonds). Adapted with permission from ref. [67]. Copyright 2010, Royal Society of Chemistry.)

and without plasma polymer film on top deposited for times of 50, 120, and 200 seconds showed construable and significantly lower release without significant burst with only half of the drug was released after 500 hours (Figure 9.6b–g). By controlling a plasma polymer layer with different thickness, it was possible to control over pore diameter and hence the rate of drug releases to achieve favorable zero-order release kinetics from the NAA platform over several weeks. This concept of plasma-modified NAA is successfully demonstrated for slow and extended release of other bioactive macromolecules, such as monoclonal antibodies (rituximab) used to treat cell malignancies of chronic lymphocytic leukemia and non-Hodgkin lymphoma [70]. This study showed that long-term zero-order release of rituximab could be achieved in a biologically active form for several weeks [67].

Another promising strategy showing that NAA platforms can be used as therapeutic implants for loading and releasing drug nanocarriers such as polymer micelles loaded with drugs is demonstrated by our group aiming not only to extend their sustained drug release but also to provide new

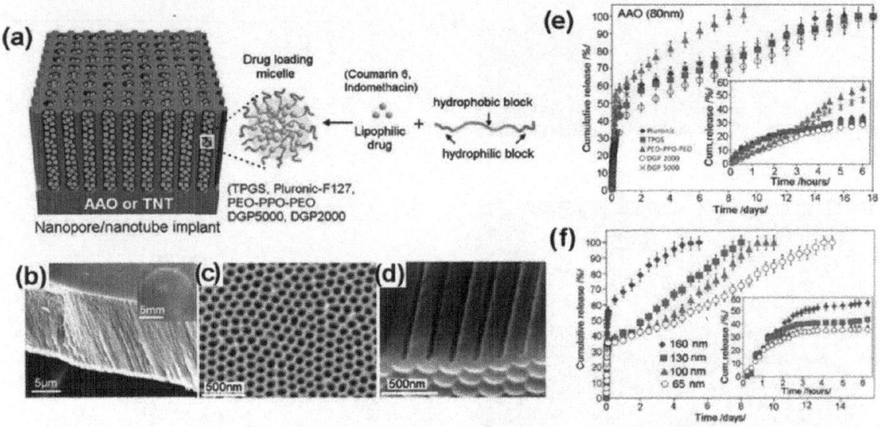

Figure 9.7 (a) Scheme of the therapeutic device that integrates polymer micelles as drug nanocarrier and nanoporous platform (NAA or TNTs) with nanopore/nanotube structures as implants models. (b–c) SEM image of NAA structure showing (b) cross section (whole NAA is shown in inset). (c) The top surface and (d) the bottom of pore structure with closed ends. (e) Comparative release of several drugs unloaded micelles (Pluronic F127, TPGS, PEO–PPO–PEO, DGP 2000, and DGP 5000) from NAA with the pore diameters of 80 nm. (f) Release profiles of TPGS polymeric micelles (unloaded) from NAA with different pore diameters of 65, 100, 130, and 160 nm. The inset shows the burst release for the first 6 hours. (Adapted with permission from ref. [66]. Copyright 2015, Royal Society of Chemistry.)

functionality as multiple drug release of several drugs for combined therapies [9,10,65,66]. The concept is summarized in Figure 9.7. Five types of polymeric micelles:

(TPGS), Pluronic F127, PEO(260)–PPO(400)–PEO(260), (DGP 5000), and (DGP 2000) unloaded and drug loaded with a size of 10–25 nm were loaded into NAA with pore diameters from 65 to 180 nm to confirm their release pattern and influence of the pore dimensions. The release kinetics of drug-loaded polymeric micelles from NAA was confirmed to be two phased with a burst release of 31%–55% in the first 6–8 hours, followed by a slow release phase over 8–22 days (Figure 9.7e–f). This release pattern is especially useful in bone implant therapies that require a large initial dose followed by a prolonged dose over a few weeks. Additionally, by applying plasma polymer film on the top of NAA, the release could be extended considerably to several months, the burst release almost suppressed, and zero-order drug-release kinetics over a period of more than 4 weeks could be achieved. This concept for multiple and sequential drug delivery and combination therapy using two different polymer micelles loaded with two to three different drugs (e.g., antibiotics and inflammatory) was successfully demonstrated using TNTs platforms but applicable for NAA as well [65,66,71–74].

Most of the previous drug delivery studies were performed using NAA in 2D forms such as free-standing membranes, films, or NAA layers on other surfaces that are very relevant for potential implant or device applications. Apart from these forms, our team explored other NAA forms created on Al wire as potential implants inside bone and free-standing NAA nanotubes that can be applied as drug nanocarriers [59–61].Figure 9.8a–d demonstrates the design of a suitable platforms for bone insertion that can be used for a wide variety of bone implant functions, including localized drug delivery to treat bone infection and bone inflammation and promote osseo-integration and localized cancer therapy that is not possible with conventional implants forms (e.g., plates). In vitro drug release from three types of NAA-Al wire implants with variable layer thickness (20.4, 40.8, and 61.2 μm) is presented in Figure. 9.8e–f. The drug-release graphs showed a two-phase pattern with an initial sharp increase or burst release in the

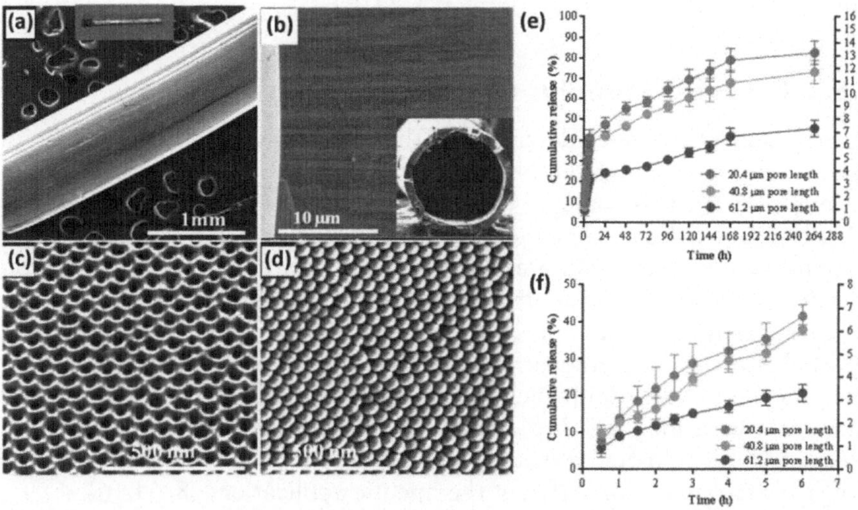

Figure 9.8 (a) Scanning electron microscopy (SEM) images of prepared NAA-Al wire implants showing (a) a low-resolution image of a portion of wire (the whole implant in the inset, length: 10 mm), (b) a cross-section view of the NAA layer showing nanopore length growth and a cross-sectional view of wire after removal of Al showing the cylindrical NAA layer around the wire, (c) the top surface of NAA showing nanopore structures, and (d) the bottom surfaces of closed ends of the nanopores (Al is removed for imaging purpose). (e–f) In vitro drug release of model drug (RB) from NAA-Al wire implants with an average pore diameter of 33 nm and pore layer thicknesses of 20.4 μm, 40.8 μm, and 61.2 μm into phosphate buffer saline for 11 days. Data represent mean st. dev. from at least 3 or 4 samples. (Adapted with permission from ref. [60]. Copyright 2015, Royal Society of Chemistry.)

first 6 hours with the release of 20%–40%, followed by the second one with a slow and steady release until 11 days of measurements. After 11 days, 61.2 μm also showed the lowest total release of only 42%, while 40.8 μm and 20.4 μm released about 70% and 80% of loaded drug, respectively.

A new type of nanocarriers based on NAA called NAA nanotubes (NAANT) electrochemically engineered by a unique pulse anodization process, which enables precise control of the nanotube geometry, was introduced by our group and demonstrated to be used for potential cancer therapy [53–55]. The concept is shown in Figure 9.9. The NAANTs with a length of about 600 nm showed exceptional loading capacity (104 ± 14.4 μg/mg) with tumor necrosis factor-related apoptosis-inducing ligand (Apo2L/TRAIL). The ability of these biocompatible NAANTs loaded with Apo2L/TRAIL for successful killing of cancer cells is demonstrated by in vitro cell study showing a significant decrease in viability of MDA-MB231-TXSA cancer cells due to apoptosis induction. Interestingly, we found that NAANTs tend to compact on cancer cell surfaces, which may be beneficial for Apo2L/-TRAIL-receptor binding through localized drug release surrounding the cell.

9.6.2 External Stimulus and Triggered Drug Release

In drug delivery systems described in the previous sections, the release of loaded drug molecules from NAA pore structures follows a release mechanism in which kinetics can be expressed in terms of diffusion of loaded or adsorbed molecules inside nanopores. This diffusion process and release of drug molecules from nanopores can be altered in different ways by controlling pore dimensions, pores surface chemistry, applying degradable polymer coatings, or incorporating the drugs in polymer micelles, etc. However, it is desirable for certain therapeutics applications to control release by environmental or external stimuli such as pH, temperature, light, electrical, electromagnetic, or magnetic field. Many of these concepts were explored and successfully demonstrated using NAA carriers loaded with real or model drugs and proposed for different therapeutic applications [8–11,16].

An electrically responsive drug delivery system based on the NAA membrane was developed by Jeon et al. using the electropolymerization of NAA with polypyrrole doped with dodecyl benzenesulfonate anion (PPy/DBS) [75]. The main idea of this concept was to actuate NAA pore size electrically, by utilizing the volume change in volume of PPy/DBS layer depending on the electrochemical state which is confirmed with fluorescence measurements of fluorescently labeled BSA used as a drug model (Figure 9.10). Apart from the fast-switching time (<10 seconds) of the opening and closing stage of pores, it was demonstrated that pores in the open state could provide a high flux of drugs from the NAA platform, which makes this carrier system suitable for emergency treatment of diseases where urgent

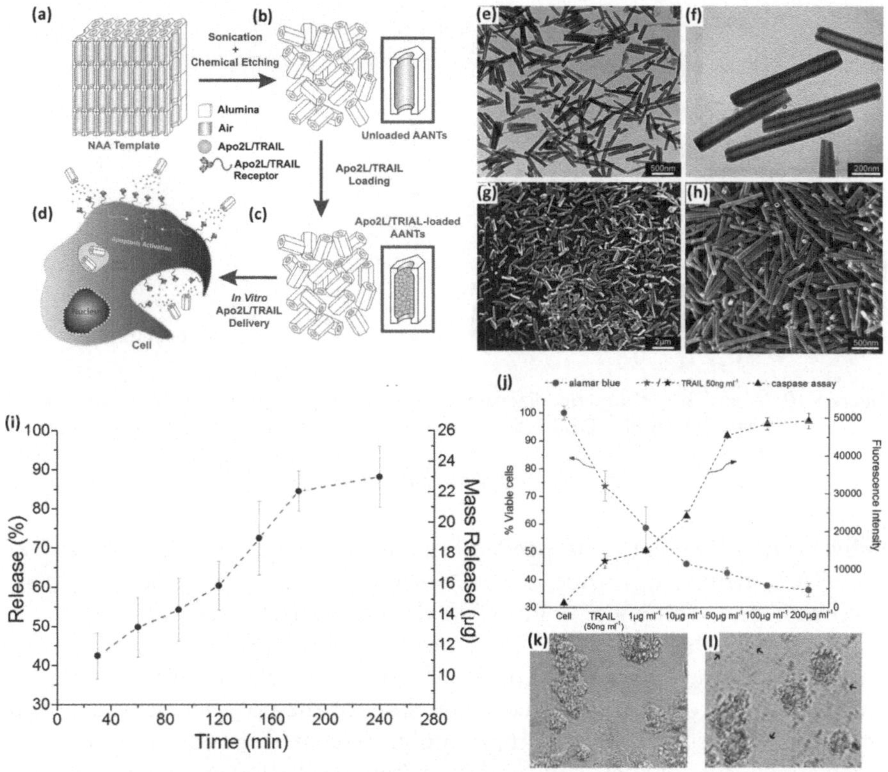

Figure 9.9 (a–d) Schematic illustration showing fabrication of NAANTs and in vitro drug delivery from them for cancer therapy. (a) Resulting nanoporous anodic alumina structure obtained after pulse anodization of aluminum foil. (b) Free-standing A NAANTs obtained after wet chemical etching and sonication. (c) Apo2L/TRAIL loading inside NAANTs. (d) In vitro Apo2L/ TRAIL release from NAANTs and apoptosis mechanism killing breast cancer cells (MDA-MB231-TXSA). (e–h) SEM images of NAA nanotubes (NAANT) fabricated by pulse anodization with the length of NAANTs around 600 nm; the inner and outer diameters of 50 and 100 nm, respectively, with 25 nm at the nanotube mouth; (i) In vitro drug-release profile of NAANTs loaded with Apo2L/TRAIL in PBS solution at 37°C. (j–l) In vitro Apo2L/TRAIL delivery by NAANTs showing (e) Alamar blue and caspase assays after 165 minutes of NAANT-Apo2L/TRAIL treatment. (f–g) Cell apoptosis images induced by 50 ng/mL of Apo2L/TRAIL and 100 mg/mL of NAANTs-Apo2L/TRAIL after 120 minutes treatment. Black arrows denote NAANTs in the media surrounding cells. (Adapted with permission from ref. [54]. Copyright 2014, Elsevier.)

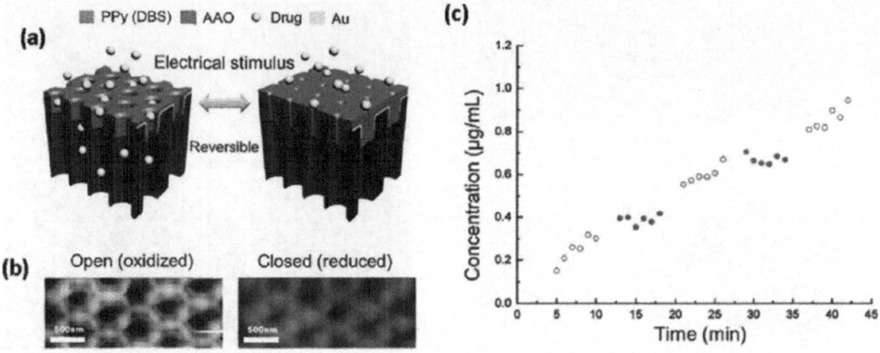

Figure 9.10 (a and b) Schematic diagram of electrically responsive NAA membrane coated with PPy-DBS indicating reversible cycle of pore opening reduction (drug release) between oxidation and reduction states. (Reprinted with permission from ref. [74]. Copyright 2011, American Chemical Society.)

delivery of therapeutics is needed. In another study by Abelow et al., the NAA membranes were coated with polypyrrole (PPy) and poly(3,-4-ethylenedioxythiophone) (PEDOT) doped with chloride and p-toluene sulfonate (Tosylate) through vapor-phase polymerization technique [76]. Molecular diffusion rates of tannic acid used as a model drug were measured based on oxidation or reduction state of the polymer. It was shown that the diffusion through these polymer-coated nanostructures was faster when the polymer is in oxidation state while slower in the reduction state which is shown to provide different drug release. This behavior was explained by swelling/deswelling of confined polymer coatings inside the porous structure that is causing the changes of the pore diameters and subsequently impacting the drug release.

The concept of light-switchable NAA drug delivery system was demonstrated by our team (Kumeria et al.) showing controlled photoresponsive molecular transport of Rose Bengal (RosB) dye used as a model drug across the NAA membrane modified with photo-switchable peptide (PSP) [77]. In this study, an azobenzene-derived peptide was immobilized along the internal part of 3-aminopropyl trimethoxysilane (APTES)-modified nanopore channels for a change in effective pore diameter of the structure and subsequently, tracking the movement of dye molecules using a change in cis/trans configuration of the peptide. The NAA/PSP membrane was first treated with light of a wavelength of 400 nm for a duration of 60 minute, which resulted in low molecular transport; however, when the exposure was changed to 364 nm, an increasing trend was observed in the dye concentration due to change in the isomeric property. It was shown that exposing the structure to 364 nm wavelength leads to reversible switching in azobenzene structure from trans to cis isomer showing the ability of this system to provide light stimulus triggered release of active molecules from NAA nanopores.

Recently, Porta-i-Batalla et al. reported stimuli-driven drug delivery system using pH-responsive polyelectrolytes modified NAA substrates [69]. The NAA structures were modified by subsequent dipping in solutions of negative poly(styrene sulfonate) (PAS) and positive poly(allylamine hydrochloride) (PAH) to get two, five, and eight layers, respectively, followed by loading of doxorubicin (DOX) used as a model drug. Polyelectrolyte-coated samples were placed in 1 mg/mL of DOX solution, and the pH was adjusted to 2.0 to increase the permeability of polyelectrolyte layers and for the diffusion of DOX molecules inside PSS/PAH layers. Drug-release kinetics were evaluated using photoluminescence spectroscopy in two different pH mediums 5.2 and 7.4 for over 5 days based on a change in pH and the number of polyelectrolyte layers. When pH was changed to 8.0, the contraction of the polyelectrolyte multilayers occurred, which results in the entrapment of drug molecules inside the films. It was demonstrated that at acidic pH, DOX was released at a faster rate and was found to be in correlation with the number of polyelectrolyte bilayers. On the other hand, at alkaline pH, the drug-release kinetics were not linear with the number of polyelectrolytes bilayers, which suggest that only the drug located near the release medium was released. To test the pH responsiveness of the system, a sudden change of pH was performed during the release which led to another burst release confirming the same concept. In a study by Zhao et al., a dual stimuli (pH and temperature) NAA membrane was demonstrated for controlled drug release of dexamethasone [78]. The NAA membranes were fabricated by two-step anodization in which the first part was coated with biocompatible colloid and the remaining part was used for drug loading. The pH and temperature-responsive drug release of prepared NAA membranes was characterized by combination of the voltammetry technique and UV–vis spectrophotometry under different pH conditions (5.2, 6.4, and 7.4) and different temperatures (25°C, 35°C, 40°C, and 50°C). Results showed that there was an increase in drug-release rate four to six times at acidic pH and high temperature (50°C). To investigate the versatility of this system, another anticancer drug (DOX) was used showing a similar drug-release pattern with higher release efficiency at pH 5.2 as compared to neutral pH (7.4).

9.6.3 Coronary Stents Implants

Percutaneous transluminal coronary angioplasty (PTCA) was introduced in clinical practice in 1977 followed by the development of endovascular prostheses (stents), which were clinically applied for the first time in 1987 and are regularly used until the present time [79]. The coronary stent implantation was shown to be superior to conventional angioplasty in the treatment of coronary artery disease. However, still there are some limitations in the use of PTCA due to vessel closure and restenosis in 30%–50% of patients [80]. Despite advances, restenosis remains one of the most crucial challenges in interventional cardiology. Experimental evidence suggests five major restenosis mechanisms after stent implantation: (i) elastic retraction, (ii) thrombus formation at the injured area, (iii) inflammation, (iv) proliferation of smooth muscle cells, and (v) extensive formation of extracellular matrix which are causing problems such as thrombocytes aggregates and inflammation signs with lymphocytes and eosinophils surrounding the stents [80–82]. To overcome these disadvantages, the concept of drug-eluting stents has been recently introduced, where drugs were trapped in polymer films coated on stents which allow a controlled drug release [82]. Several active coatings of stents that suppress neointima proliferation by releasing anti-inflammatory or antiproliferative therapeutics, e.g., immunosupressive drugs (tacrolimus, sirolimus) and cytostatic drugs (paclitaxel) were reported [81–85]. Although the clinical use of polymer-coated stents has been clinically approved, their inflammatory problems are still not resolved and need further improvement where several other possibilities such as metal, carbons, ceramic, and porous oxide layers as NAA were also explored [80].

A promising approach to address these problems was reported by designing stainless steel coronary stents coated with an NAA layer which was filled with anti-inflammatory drugs [86]. The design of these types of active stents is one of the most important examples of drug-releasing NAA devices explored by Wieneke et al. using 316 L stainless steel stents with NAA coatings loaded with immunosuppressive drug tacrolimus (60 and 120 µg) [86] shown in Figure 9.11. SEM image of these stents with NAA layer fabricated by electrochemical anodization on an aluminum film deposited on stainless steel stent surface is shown in Figure 9.11a and b. Bare stents, coated stents, and drug-loaded coated stents were fabricated and implanted in the carotid artery of New Zealand white rabbits. Drug release was monitored by extracting whole blood at different time intervals and measuring with HPLC (Figure 9.11c and d). It was shown that NAA-coated stents served as an excellent platform for loading and releasing drugs within therapeutic range followed by a significant reduction in neointima thickness. The effect of NAA pore diameter and depth on the drug release was also tested. Results showed sustained release up to 40 hours with pore diameters ~20 nm, and further delay was achieved by changing pore depth from 1 to 4.4 µm. Similarly, Kang et al. used NAA-coated stents for controlled drug release fabricated through anodization of Al on stents [87]. In this study, the effect of different pore sizes and depth of NAA on drug release was studied showing that an increase in pore diameter leads to an increase in drug-release rate, whereas the

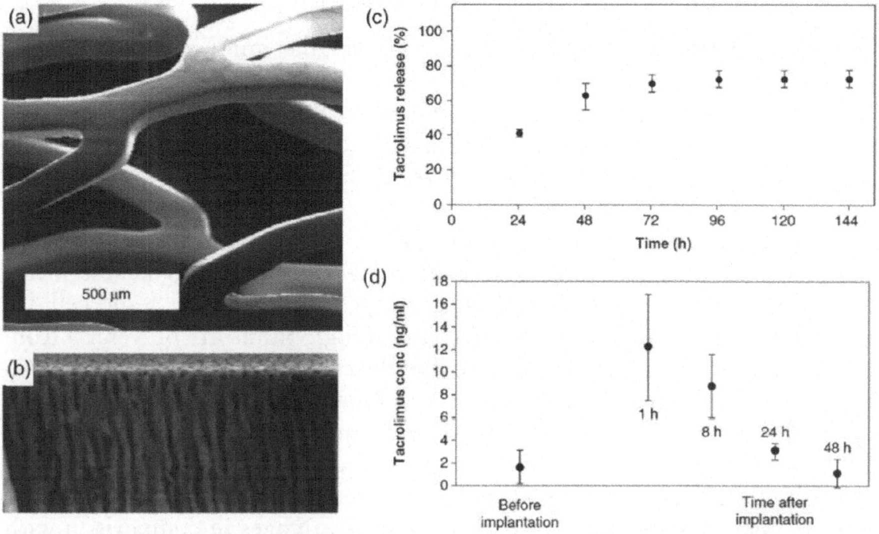

Figure 9.11 (a) SEM image of coronary stents with NAA layer on the surface with (b) cross-section image of NAA layer with pore size between 5 and 15 nm and pore density $10^{12}/cm^2$ allowing sufficient drug loading with tacrolimus. (c) In vitro drug release showing cumulative tacrolimus release within the first 144 h with ~75% of the loaded 60 mg tacrolimus has been eluted that after 72 hours and (d) In vivo drug release with the time course of whole blood tacrolimus concentration after stent implantation in the carotid arteries of rabbits. (Adapted with permission from ref. [86].)

increase in pore depth decreases the amount of drug being released from the pores. An early animal study indicated a good vascular compatibility of the stent with regard to loading and releasing tacrolimus from the porous structure. However, disappointing results were reported from a subsequent animal study using NAA-modified stents, with evidence of particle debris shed from the NAA contributing to increased neointimal hyperplasia [88]. Due to the unsatisfactory clinical performance, further development of this concept and technology has been abandoned. These results can be explained by unsatisfactory deposition of Al film on stainless steel and its delamination which is a problem that is required to be solved.

Despite these disappointing results caused by lack of fabrication of robust NAA layer on stent surface, previous studies using porous NAA stents are very encouraging performance. There is a huge room for further improvements of these types of stents by improving robustness to avoid debris formation through designing optimized pore structure and surface modification to increase their compatibility and loading capacity including controlled and sustained release.

9.6.4 Biocapsules for Immunoissolation

The encapsulation of living cells such as the cellular immunoisolation using microfabricated capsules with semipermeable barriers has been investigated over the past several decades as a potential treatment for a number of diseases such as diabetes mellitus, Parkinson's, and Alzheimer's [31,89]. The encapsulation of living cells is recognized as a promising therapy since it is proven that immunoprotected cells such as pancreatic islets or hepatocytes can respond physiologically both in vitro and in vivo to appropriate stimuli [89]. Therapeutic cells can be encapsulated within a semipermeable membrane that provides the exchange of insulin, oxygen, nutrients, and cellular waste; however, larger entities such as immunoglobulins are prevented from penetrating the membrane and destroying the cells. Typical immunoisolation devices such as polymeric membrane and biocapsules were used, but there are several issues associated with their performances, including poor chemical resistance, inadequate mechanical strength, and broad pore size distributions [89–91]. NAA membranes are recognized as an alternative to address many of these disadvantages offering many advantages in comparison with polymer membranes to design more advanced implantable biocapsules. Key advantages are better mechanical and chemical stability, adjustable pore size and surface chemistry, and easy incorporation into microfabricated devices.

Pioneering research to explore NAA for cellular encapsulation was performed by Desai and coworkers to demonstrate NAA's capability to release immunoglobulin (IgG), glucose, and insulin [89–93]. They designed a special device consisting of NAA layers on aluminum tubes and demonstrated their applications as implantable biocapsules as an alternative treatment for type 1 diabetes. The NAA with average pore sizes of 46, 58, and 75 nm fabricated by two-step anodization processes were filled with insulin-secreting MIN6 insulinoma cells and placed within a collagen matrix. Results indicated that the release of insulin from these NAA biocapsules continued for up to 3 hours suggesting that the encapsulated cells were able to produce new insulin. Gong et al. showed the use of NAA platform as therapeutic biocapsules for immunoisolation to demonstrate their controlled drug release [94]. Figure 9.12a shows photos of these biocapsules fabricated by electrochemical anodization, consisting of an NAA porous layer with pore diameters of 25–55 nm. To prove their controlled release ability, the study used several model molecules such as fluorescein (Mw 400 Da), fluorescein isotiocyanate, and dextran conjugates (with molecular weight (Mw) 4, 20, 70, and 150 kDa). The results from this study showed that it is possible to control the diffusion of small molecular weight proteins (~3.5 nm diameter) with no limitation, while transport of larger molecules (>30 nm diameter) was prevented. The later work by this team demonstrated the feasibility of using NAA capsules for the encapsulation of cells [92–94]. These NAA capsules (pore diameter 46–75 nm) incorporated with insulin-secreting MIN6 cells showed that they could act as effective semipermeable devices allowing

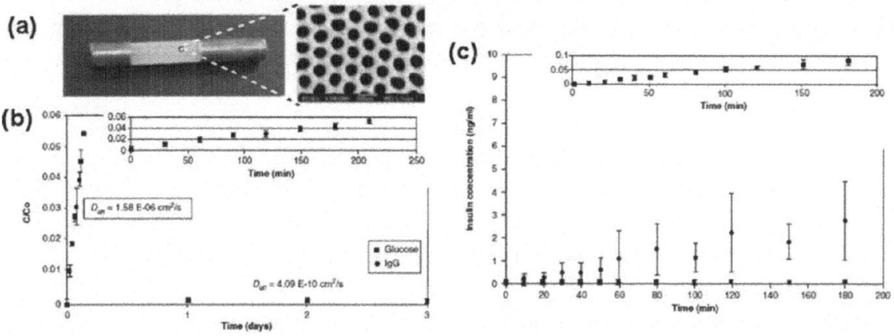

Figure 9.12 (a) Photos of completed NAA capsule (b) Normalized release of glucose (squares, Deff= $1.58\ 10^{-6} cm^2/s$) and IgG (diamonds, Deff= $4.09\ 10^{-10} cm^2/s$) through a NAA membrane with a nominal pore size of 75 nm. Inset: glucose release on a 210-minute timescale. (c) Insulin release from encapsulated (experimental, squares) and unencapsulated (control, diamonds) MIN6 cells following a step increase in glucose. The nominal pore size used for the encapsulated cells was 75 nm. Inset: enlarged graph of experimental data. (Reproduced with permission from ref. [94].)

the transport of glucose and insulin while impeding the transport of larger proteins such as immunoglobulin G. Figure 9.12b shows fast release of glucose and hindered the release of IgG over 4 days from fabricated NAA capsules. The release profile of insulin through the NNA membrane from encapsulated MIN6 cells in response to an increase in glucose level is shown in Figure 9.12c. This experiment suggests that the encapsulated cells not only could release insulin in response to glucose but were also able to produce new insulin. Furthermore, it is important to emphasize that cells retained their viability in the close proximity of NAA membrane showing future promises of this approach for clinical immunoisolation.

9.7 CONCLUSION AND FUTURE PERSPECTIVES

This chapter presents the recent progress in using NAA materials prepared by electrochemical anodization for drug delivery applications. The NAA biomaterials, fabricated in different forms because of their many favorable properties including high surface area, low-cost production, biocompatibility, and unique pore structure which can be used as a perfect reservoir for loading and releasing therapeutic molecules, had attracted considerable attention in last two decades to be explored for biomedical applications including drug delivery. The attractiveness of NAA is also based on their versatility to control pore and nanotube dimensions, geometries, and their surface chemistry that provide a massive opportunity to design tailorable drug-releasing platforms that can be adjusted and optimized for broad therapeutic applications required for addressing many health problems in cancer treatment, orthopedics, diabetes, infections, heart diseases, etc.

Also, this chapter presents the summary of key concepts for advancing NAA using a broad range of structural or chemical modifications for drug delivery applications showing most promising approaches to achieve favorable drug-releasing kinetics with sustained, controllable, and triggered drug-release capabilities important for specific therapies. These examples have proven that there is still plenty of room for further advance in the applications of NAA material.

The future research potentially has multiple directions which include: (i) increasing the biocompatibility by covalent immobilization of therapeutic molecules on the implant surfaces, e.g., anti-bacterial and anti-inflammatory drugs; (ii) achieving controlled and sustained drug elution over long period of the time using specific surface modification and structural design of pores and combining with biocompatible polymers; (iii) further development of stimuli-responsive systems such as external magnetic field, NIR light, temperature, and ultrasound; (iv) the implementation of NAA into microfabrication devices for creating chip-based drug delivery platforms which is also one of the future directions; (v further studies are necessary to understand how these small systems pass through different barriers in the body and to examine other long-term behaviors, including failure modes and component clearance; and (vi) more in vivo studies which are still missing to translate NAA platforms to be acceptable for clinical applications and translation for real applications.

Recent progress in this field is only the beginning of a long journey of further research in terms of correlating NAA surface chemistry with tissue responses along with new clinical approaches are expected, not only in orthopedics implants but also for the treatment of several other diseases (heart, cancer, diabetes, Parkinson's, Alzheimer's, etc.). In addition, the combination of the NAA platforms with existing technologies such as MEMS, NEMS, lab on a chip, wireless communication, and Internet of Thing (IOT) technologies is proposed to drive the designing of a new generation of integrated therapeutic drug delivery systems that have the potential to revolutionize this field with significant impact.

ACKNOWLEDGMENTS

The authors acknowledge the support of Australian Research Council (IH 15000003) and the School of Chemical Engineering at the University of Adelaide. SM thanks for the support from the Australian Government Training Program Scholarship and Forrest George and Sandra Lynne Young Supplementary Scholarship.

REFERENCES

1. Drews J. Drug discovery: A historical perspective. *Science.* 2000 Mar 17;287(5460):1960–4.
2. Mainardes R.M., Silva L.P. Drug delivery systems: Past, present, and future. *Curr Drug Targets.* 2004 Jul;5(5):449–55.
3. Ranade V.V., Cannon J.B. *Drug Delivery Systems.* 3rd ed.: CRC Press, Boca Raton, FL; 2011.
4. Fahr A., Liu X. Drug delivery strategies for poorly water-soluble drugs. *Expert Opin Drug Deliv.* 2007 Jul;4(4):403–16.
5. de Villiers M.M., Aramwit P., Kwon G.S., (eds.) *Nanotechnology in Drug Delivery.* 1 ed.: Springer, New York; 2009.
6. Hughes G.A. Nanostructure-mediated drug delivery. *Nanomedicine.* 2005 Mar;1(1):22–30.
7. Losic D., Santos A., (eds.) *Electrochemically Engineered Nanoporous Materials: Methods, Properties and Applications.* Springer International Publishing AG, Germany; 2015.
8. Losic D., Simovic S. Self-ordered nanopore and nanotube platforms for drug delivery applications. *Expert Opin Drug Deliv* 2009 Dec;6(12):1363–81.
9. Losic D., Aw M.S., Santos A., et al. Titania nanotube arrays for local drug delivery: Recent advances and perspectives. *Expert Opin Drug Deliv.* 2015;12(1):103–27.
10. Sinn Aw M., Kurian M., Losic D. Non-eroding drug-releasing implants with ordered nanoporous and nanotubular structures: Concepts for controlling drug release. *Biomater Sci.* 2014;2(1):10–34. doi: 10.1039/C3BM60196J.
11. Kapruwan P., Ferré-Borrull J., Marsal L.F. Nanoporous anodic alumina platforms for drug delivery applications: Recent advances and perspective. *Adv Mater Interfaces.* 2020;7(22):2001133.
12. Zhao Y., Tavares A.C., Gauthier M.A. Nano-engineered electro-responsive drug delivery systems. *J Mater Chem B.* 2016;4(18):3019–30. doi: 10.1039/C6TB00049E.
13. Gultepe E., Nagesha D., Casse B.D.F., et al. Sustained drug release from non-eroding nanoporous templates. *Small.* 2010;6(2):213–16.
14. Md Jani A.M., Losic D., Voelcker N.H. Nanoporous anodic aluminium oxide: Advances in surface engineering and emerging applications. *Prog Mater Sci.* 2013;58(5):636–704.
15. Ghicov A., Schmuki P. Self-ordering electrochemistry: A review on growth and functionality of TiO_2 nanotubes and other self-aligned MOx structures. *Chem Commun.* 2009:2009(20):2791–808. doi: 10.1039/B822726H.
16. Losic D., Santos A., (eds.) *Nanoporous Alumina: Fabrication, Structure, Properties and Applications.* 1 ed.: Springer International Publishing AG, Germany; 2015.
17. Masuda H., Fukuda K. Ordered metal nanohole arrays made by a two-step replication of honeycomb structures of anodic alumina. *Science.* 1995;268(5216):1466–8.
18. Lee W., Ji R., Gösele U., et al. Fast fabrication of long-range ordered porous alumina membranes by hard anodization. *Nat Mater.* 2006;5(9):741–7.

19. Porta-i-Batalla M., Eckstein C., Xifré-Pérez E., et al. Sustained, controlled and stimuli-responsive drug release systems based on nanoporous anodic alumina with layer-by-layer polyelectrolyte. *Nanoscale Res Lett.* 2016;11(1):372.
20. Meng G., Jung Y.J., Cao A., et al. Controlled fabrication of hierarchically branched nanopores, nanotubes, and nanowires. *Proc Natl Acad Sci USA.* 2005;102(20):7074–8.
21. Ho A.Y.Y., Gao H., Lam Y.C., et al. Controlled fabrication of multitiered three-dimensional nanostructures in porous alumina. *Adv Funct Mater.* 2008;18(14):2057–63.
22. Losic D., Lillo M., Losic Jr. D. Porous alumina with shaped pore geometries and complex pore architectures fabricated by cyclic anodization. *Small.* 2009;5(12):1392–7.
23. Losic D., Losic D. Preparation of porous anodic alumina with periodically perforated pores. *Langmuir.* 2009;25(10):5426–31.
24. Losic D., Velleman L., Kant K., et al. Self-ordering electrochemistry: A simple approach for engineering nanopore and nanotube arrays for emerging applications*. *Aust J Chem.* 2011;64:294–301.
25. Kipke S., Schmid G. Nanoporous alumina membranes as diffusion controlling systems. *Adv Funct Mater.* 2004;14:1184–8.
26. Lee W., Scholz R., Nielsch K., et al. A template-based electrochemical method for the synthesis of multisegmented metallic nanotubes. *Angew Chem Int Ed.* 2005;44(37):6050–4.
27. Altalhi T., Ginic-Markovic M., Han N., et al. Synthesis of carbon nanotube (CNT) composite membranes. *Membranes.* 2010;1(1):37–47.
28. Losic D., Cole M.A., Dollmann B., et al. Surface modification of nanoporous alumina membranes by plasma polymerization. *Nanotechnology.* 2008;19(24):245704.
29. Yu Y., Kant K., Shapter J.G., et al. Gold nanotube membranes have catalytic properties. *Microporous Mesoporous Mater.* 2012;153:131–6.
30. Velleman L., Triani G., Evans P.J., et al. Structural and chemical modification of porous alumina membranes. *Microporous Mesoporous Mater.* 2009;126(1):87–94.
31. Schmitt E.K., Nurnabi M., Bushby R.J., et al. Electrically insulating pore-suspending membranes on highly ordered porous alumina obtained from vesicle spreading. *Soft Matter.* 2008;4(2):250–3. doi: 10.1039/B716723G.
32. Szczepanski V., Vlassiouk I., Smirnov S. Stability of silane modifiers on alumina nanoporous membranes. *J Membr Sci.* 2006;281(1):587–91.
33. Popat K.C., Mor G., Grimes C.A., et al. Surface modification of nanoporous alumina surfaces with poly(ethylene glycol). *Langmuir.* 2004;20(19):8035–41.
34. Mutalib Md Jani A., Anglin E.J., McInnes S.J.P., et al. Nanoporous anodic aluminium oxide membranes with layered surface chemistry. *Chem Commun.* 2009;2009 (21):3062–4. doi:10.1039/B901745C.
35. Mutalib Md Jani A., Kempson I.M., Losic D., et al. Dressing in layers: Layering surface functionalities in nanoporous aluminum oxide membranes. *Angew Chem Int Ed Engl.* 2010 Oct 18;49(43):7933–7.
36. Chang C.-S., Suen S.-Y. Modification of porous alumina membranes with n-alkanoic acids and their application in protein adsorption. *J Membr Sci.* 2006;275(1):70–81.

37. Leary Swan E.E., Popat K.C., Desai T.A. Peptide-immobilized nanoporous alumina membranes for enhanced osteoblast adhesion. *Biomaterials.* 2005;26(14):1969–76.
38. Ratner B.D. Chapter 3- The biocompatibility of implant materials. In: Badylak S.F., (ed.) *Host Response to Biomaterials.* Oxford: Academic Press; 2015. pp. 37–51.
39. Sedel L. Evolution of alumina-on-alumina implants: A review. *Clin Orthop Relat Res.* 2000;379:48–54.
40. Popat K.C., Leary Swan E.E., Mukhatyar V., et al. Influence of nanoporous alumina membranes on long-term osteoblast response. *Biomaterials.* 2005;26(22):4516–22.
41. Popat K.C., Chatvanichkul K.I., Barnes G.L., et al. Osteogenic differentiation of marrow stromal cells cultured on nanoporous alumina surfaces. *J Biomed Mater Res A.* 2007 Mar 15;80(4):955–64.
42. La Flamme K.E., Popat K.C., Leoni L., et al. Biocompatibility of nanoporous alumina membranes for immunoisolation. *Biomaterials.* 2007;28(16):2638–45.
43. Karlsson M., Johansson A., Tang L., et al. Nanoporous aluminum oxide affects neutrophil behaviour. *Microsc Res Tech.* 2004;63(5):259–65.
44. Karlsson M., Pålsgård E., Wilshaw P.R., et al. Initial in vitro interaction of osteoblasts with nano-porous alumina. *Biomaterials.* 2003 Aug;24(18):3039–46.
45. Ferraz N., Carlsson J., Hong J., et al. Influence of nanoporesize on platelet adhesion and activation. *J Mater Sci Mater Med.* 2008 Sep;19(9):3115–21.
46. Karlsson M., Tang L. Surface morphology and adsorbed proteins affect phagocyte responses to nano-porous alumina. *J Mater Sci Mater Med.* 2006;17(11):1101–11.
47. Popat K.C., Daniels R.H., Dubrow R.S., et al. Nanostructured surfaces for bone biotemplating applications. *J Orthop Res.* 2006 Apr;24(4):619–27.
48. Pujari-Palmer S., Lind T., Xia W., et al. Controlling osteogenic differentiation through nanoporous alumina. *J Biomater Nanobiotechnol.* 2014;5(2): 7.
49. Friedmann A., Hoess A., Cismak A., et al. Investigation of cell–substrate interactions by focused ion beam preparation and scanning electron microscopy. *Acta Biomater.* 2011;7(6):2499–507.
50. Poinern G.E., Le X.T., O'Dea M., et al. Chemical synthesis, characterisation, and biocompatibility of nanometre scale porous anodic aluminium oxide membranes for use as a cell culture substrate for the vero cell line: A preliminary study. *Biomed Res Int.* 2014;2014:238762.
51. Ni S., Li C., Ni S., et al. Understanding improved osteoblast behavior on select nanoporous anodic alumina. *Int J Nanomed.* 2014;9(1):3325–34.
52. Thakur S., Massou S., Benoliel A.M., et al. Depth matters: Cells grown on nano-porous anodic alumina respond to pore depth. *Nanotechnology.* 2012;23(25):255101.
53. Wang Y., Santos A., Evdokiou A., et al. Rational design of ultra-short anodic alumina nanotubes by short-time pulse anodization. *Electrochim Acta.* 2015;154:379–86.
54. Wang Y., Santos A., Kaur G., et al. Structurally engineered anodic alumina nanotubes as nano-carriers for delivery of anticancer therapeutics. *Biomaterials.* 2014 Jul;35(21):5517–26.

55. Wang Y., Kaur G., Zysk A., et al. Systematic in vitro nanotoxicity study on anodic alumina nanotubes with engineered aspect ratio: Understanding nanotoxicity by a nanomaterial model. *Biomaterials*. 2015 Apr;46:117–30.
56. Gunn J., Cumberland D. Stent coatings and local drug delivery; state of the art. *Eur Heart J*. 1999 Dec;20(23):1693–700.
57. Kollum M., Farb A., Schreiber R., et al. Particle debris from a nanoporous stent coating obscures potential antiproliferative effects of tacrolimus-eluting stents in a porcine model of restenosis. *Catheter Cardiovasc Interv*. 2005 Jan;64(1):85–90.
58. Sigler M., Paul T., Grabitz R.G. Biocompatibility screening in cardiovascular implants. *Z Kardiol*. 2005 Jun;94(6):383–91.
59. Rahman S, Atkins G.J, Findlay D.M., et al. Nanoengineered drug releasing aluminium wire implants: A model study for localized bone therapy. *J Mater Chem B*. 2015;3(16):3288–96. doi: 10.1039/C5TB00150A.
60. Rahman S., Ormsby R., Santos A., et al. Nanoengineered drug-releasing aluminium wire implants: Comparative investigation of nanopore geometry, drug release and osteoblast cell adhesion. *RSC Adv*. 2015;5(92):75004–14. doi: 10.1039/C5RA10418A.
61. Rahman S., Gulati K., Kogawa M., et al. Drug diffusion, integration, and stability of nanoengineered drug-releasing implants in bone ex-vivo. *J Biomed Mater Res A*. 2016 Mar;104(3):714–25.
62. Saji V.S., Kumeria T., Gulati K., et al. Localized drug delivery of selenium (Se) using nanoporous anodic aluminium oxide for bone implants. *J Mater Chem B*. 2015;3(35):7090–8. doi: 10.1039/C5TB00125K.
63. Kapoor S., Hegde R., Bhattacharyya A.J. Influence of surface chemistry of mesoporous alumina with wide pore distribution on controlled drug release. *J Control Release*. 2009;140(1):34–39.
64. Das S.K., Kapoor S., Yamada H., et al. Effects of surface acidity and pore size of mesoporous alumina on degree of loading and controlled release of ibuprofen. *Microporous Mesoporous Mater*. 2009;118(1):267–72.
65. Aw M.S., Kurian M., Losic D. Polymeric micelles for multidrug delivery and combination therapy. *Chemistry (Easton)*. 2013 Sep 16;19(38):12586–601.
66. Aw M.S., Simovic S., Addai-Mensah J., et al. Polymeric micelles in porous and nanotubular implants as a new system for extended delivery of poorly soluble drugs. *J Mater Chem*. 2011;21(20):7082–9. doi: 10.1039/C0JM04307A.
67. Simovic S., Losic D., Vasilev K. Controlled drug release from porous materials by plasma polymer deposition. *Chem Commun*. 2010;46(8):1317–9. doi: 10.1039/B919840G.
68. Simovic S., Losic D., Vasilev K. Controlled release from porous platforms. *Pharm Technol*. 2011;35:68–71.
69. Porta-i-Batalla M., Xifré-Pérez E., Eckstein C., et al. 3D nanoporous anodic alumina structures for sustained drug release. *Nanomaterials*. 2017;7(8):227.
70. Simovic S., Diener K.R., Bachhuka A., et al. Controlled release and bioactivity of the monoclonal antibody rituximab from a porous matrix: A potential in situ therapeutic device. *Mater Lett*. 2014;130:210–4.
71. Aw M.S., Addai-Mensah J., Losic D. A multi-drug delivery system with sequential release using titania nanotube arrays. *Chem Commun*. 2012;48(27):3348–50. doi: 10.1039/C2CC17690D.

72. Aw M.S., Addai-Mensah J., Losic D. Magnetic-responsive delivery of drug-carriers using titania nanotube arrays. *J Mater Chem.* 2012;22(14):6561–3. doi: 10.1039/C2JM16819G.
73. Sinn Aw M., Addai-Mensah J., Losic D. Polymer micelles for delayed release of therapeutics from drug-releasing surfaces with nanotubular structures. *Macromol Biosci.* 2012 Aug;12(8):1048–52.
74. Santos A., Sinn Aw M., Bariana M., et al. Drug-releasing implants: Current progress, challenges and perspectives. *J Mater Chem B.* 2014;2(37):6157–82. doi: 10.1039/C4TB00548A.
75. Jeon G., Yang S.Y., Byun J., et al. Electrically actuatable smart nanoporous membrane for pulsatile drug release. *Nano Lett.* 2011 Mar 9;11(3):1284–8.
76. Abelow A.E., Persson K.M., Jager E.W.H., et al. Electroresponsive nanoporous membranes by coating anodized alumina with poly(-3,4-ethylenedioxythiophene) and polypyrrole. *Macromol Mater Eng.* 2014;299(2):190–7.
77. Kumeria T., Yu J., Alsawat M., et al. Photoswitchable membranes based on peptide-modified nanoporous anodic alumina: Toward smart membranes for on-demand molecular transport. *Adv Mater.* 2015;27(19):3019–24.
78. Zhao X.-P., Wang S.-S., Younis M.R., et al. Thermo and pH dual – actuating smart porous anodic aluminum for controllable drug release. *Adv Mater Interfaces.* 2018;5(13):1800185.
79. Cherian A.M., Nair S.V., Maniyal V., et al. Surface engineering at the nanoscale: A way forward to improve coronary stent efficacy. *APL Bioeng.* 2021;5(2):021508.
80. Borhani S., Hassanajili S., Ahmadi Tafti S.H., et al. Cardiovascular stents: Overview, evolution, and next generation. *Prog Biomater.* 2018 Sep;7(3):175–205.
81. Buccheri D., Piraino D., Andolina G., et al. Understanding and managing in-stent restenosis: A review of clinical data, from pathogenesis to treatment. *J Thorac Dis.* 2016 Oct;8(10):E1150–62.
82. Camenzind E., Scheerder ID, (eds.) *Local Drug Delivery for Coronary Artery Disease.* CRC Press, Boca Raton, FL, 2005.
83. Chatterjee S., Pandey A. Drug eluting stents: Friend or foe? A review of cellular mechanisms behind the effects of Paclitaxel and sirolimus eluting stents. *Curr Drug Metab.* 2008 Jul;9(6):554–66.
84. Wieneke H., Dirsch O., Sawitowski T., et al. Synergistic effects of a novel nanoporous stent coating and tacrolimus on intima proliferation in rabbits. *Catheter Cardiovasc Interv.* 2003 Nov;60(3):399–407.
85. Wieneke H., Sawitowski T., Wnendt S., et al. Stent coating: A new approach in interventional cardiology. *Herz.* 2002 Sep;27(6):518–26.
86. Karoussos I.A., Wieneke H., Sawitowski T., et al. Inorganic materials as drug delivery systems in coronary artery stenting. *Materialwiss Werkstofftech.* 2002;33(12):738–46.
87. Kang H.-J., Kim D.J., Park S.-J., et al. Controlled drug release using nanoporous anodic aluminum oxide on stent. *Thin Solid Films.* 2007;515(12):5184–7.
88. Tsujino I., Ako J., Honda Y., et al. Drug delivery via nano-, micro and macroporous coronary stent surfaces. *Expert Opin Drug Deliv.* 2007 May;4(3):287–95.

89. Tao S.L., Desai T.A. Microfabricated drug delivery systems: From particles to pores. *Adv Drug Deliv Rev.* 2003 Feb 24;55(3):315–28.
90. Ferrari M., Desai T., Bhatia S., (eds.) *Therapeutic Micro/Nanotechnology*, Vol. III. Springer, New York; 2007. (BioMEMS and Biomedical Nanotechnology).
91. Desai T.A., West T., Cohen M., et al. Nanoporous microsystems for islet cell replacement. *Adv Drug Deliv Rev.* 2004 Sep 22;56(11):1661–73.
92. La Flamme K.E., LaTempa T.J., Grimes C.A., et al. The effects of cell density and device arrangement on the behavior of macroencapsulated beta-cells. *Cell Transplant.* 2007;16(8):765–74.
93. La Flamme K.E., Mor G., Gong D., et al. Nanoporous alumina capsules for cellular macroencapsulation: Transport and biocompatibility. *Diabetes Technol Ther.* 2005 Oct;7(5):684–94.
94. Gong D., Yadavalli V., Paulose M., et al. Controlled molecular release using nanoporous alumina capsules. *Biomed Microdev.* 2003;5(1):75–80.

Chapter 10

Electrochemically Nano-engineered Titanium Implants towards Local Drug Delivery Applications

Karan Gulati
The University of Queensland

CONTENTS

DOI: 10.1201/9781003217114-13

ABBREVIATIONS

AMPs:	antimicrobial peptides
BMP-2:	bone morphogenetic protein-2
BMSCs:	bone marrow stromal cells
EA:	electrochemical anodization
EST:	electrical stimulation therapy
HAP:	hydroxyapatite
IBR:	initial burst release
KRSR:	lysine–arginine–serine–arginine
MRSA:	methicillin-resistant *Staphylococcus aureus*
MWCNTs:	multi-walled carbon nanotubes
NPs:	nanoparticles
NSAIDs:	nonsteroidal anti-inflammatory drugs
PLGA:	poly(lactic-co-glycolic acid)
PTH:	parathyroid hormone
RGDC:	arginine–glycine–aspartic acid–cysteine
ROS:	reactive oxygen species
STI:	soft-tissue integration
TNPs:	titania nanopores
TNTs:	titania nanotubes

10.1 INTRODUCTION

Owing to their excellent biocompatibility, mechanical and corrosion resistance characteristics, titanium and its alloys have been widely used in orthopaedic and dental implant settings for decades (Guo, Gulati, et al. 2021a; Chopra, Gulati, and Ivanovski 2021d). Ti-based implants have become primary choice to correct/replace diseased/damaged tissues like bones and teeth. Formation of a few nms thick TiO_2 layer on Ti upon exposure to air attributes to the biocompatibility of Ti (Guo, Gulati, et al. 2021b). However, Ti is bio-inert, and early establishment and long-term maintenance of implant-tissue integration may be challenged, especially in compromised patient conditions (poor bone quality or quantity) (Gulati and Ivanovski 2017). The success of Ti implants is dependent on the management of the *3Is*: integration, immunomodulation and infection (Guo, Gulati, et al. 2021a; Chopra et al. 2022). Since the surface of the implant is the first site of contact for the surrounding cells, appropriate surface characteristics including topographical, chemical and biological functionalities are needed to enhance implant-tissue integration, reduce inflammation and prevent infection. As a result, most attempts at optimizing implant bioactivity have been focussed on increasing surface roughness, which has significantly reduced implant failures clinically. Catering to the need for enhanced bioactivity, surface modification of Ti-based implants has been performed in the macro, micro and nanoscales, as reviewed elsewhere (Guo, Gulati, et al. 2021a).

Nanoscale modification or nano-engineering of Ti implants has outperformed the micro-scale modifications, as established in various in vitro and in vivo investigations (Martinez-Marquez et al. 2020; Zhang, Gulati, et al. 2021). Various techniques employed to impart nanotopography on Ti implants can be categorized into physical, chemical, mechanical, electrochemical and biomolecule modification (Gulati, Kogawa, et al. 2015; Chopra, Gulati, and Ivanovski 2021a). Thermal, ion implantation, plasma and physical vapour deposition treatments (physical modification) involve the use of electric, kinetic or thermal energy to enable the deposition of specific particles onto the implant surface. These techniques have been commonly employed to modify Ti implants with alumina, zirconia, titania and hydroxyapatite. Further, a simple immersion of implant in acidic or alkaline solutions can enable chemical modification, whereby altered surface chemistry or incorporation of chemical moieties can improve corrosion resistance, enhance bioactivity and decontaminate the surface (Guo, Gulati, et al. 2021a). Chemical vapour deposition and sol-gel methods are also used to enhance implant bioactivity. Machining, grinding, blasting and polishing constitute the mechanical techniques that involve shaping/removal of material and has been used to achieve improved mechanical and wettability properties (Guo, Gulati, et al. 2021b). Besides, the use of abrasive particles to roughen the implant surface can augment surface reactivity. Electrochemical modification involves anodization, whereby a growth of 10 nm to 40 μm of TiO_2 on Ti implants allows for ion incorporation from electrolyte and fabrication of controlled topographies, which offer corrosion protection and enhanced bioactivity. Under optimized conditions, when the implant is immersed in the electrolyte containing F and water, self-ordering of TiO_2 nanotopographies can be achieved upon supply of constant voltage and current, as detailed in further sections (Gulati and Ivanovski 2017). Ti implants have also been modified with biomolecules including peptides or proteins, which has shown promising outcomes towards enhancing bone-implant contact (Chopra, Gulati, and Ivanovski 2021e; Guo, Gulati, et al. 2021b). Further, the use of bioactive polymers like chitosan or incorporation of CaP via immersion in simulated body fluid have also enhanced implant bioactivity (Gulati, Zhang, et al. 2021).

Among the various nano-engineering strategies employed, electrochemical anodization (EA) stands out as it permits the fabrication of controlled TiO_2-based nanotopographies including nanotubes and nanopores, which not only augment the bioactivity of conventional implants but also enable loading and local release of potent therapeutics. Local drug delivery bypasses the limitations associated with oral/systemic administration and allows for customized therapies, which can be tailored for specific therapeutic needs.

This chapter focusses on the next generation of nano-engineered Ti implants modified using anodization to fabricate nanotubes towards local therapy applications. This will inform the readers of the latest developments with respect to Ti implants modified with nanostructures for various therapies including integration, infection and inflammation, providing an improved understanding of the efficacy of each therapy and the possible clinical translation challenges.

10.2 ELECTROCHEMICALLY NANO-ENGINEERED TI IMPLANTS

Of the various strategies employed to nano-engineer Ti implants, electrochemical anodization (EA) stands out attributed to:

- Easy, cost-effective and scalable fabrication
- Fabrication of self-ordered TiO_2 nanostructures (nanotubes and nanopores)
- Control over nanostructure dimensions
- Modification of Ti and its alloys of various shapes and geometries
- Applicable to modify wide-variety of metal-based surfaces

Briefly, as presented in Figure 10.1, EA involves immersion of anode (target Ti) and cathode (Ti or Pt) in appropriate electrolyte (often organic electrolyte containing fluoride and water) and supply of constant voltage and current (Gulati, Aw, et al. 2012). Dependent on various influencing factors (electrolyte composition, pH, voltage, current, time, etc.) and attainment of an equilibrium between metal oxidation and dissolution, self-ordering of nanotubular or nanoporous TiO_2 structures is obtained on the target Ti (anode) (Gulati, Zhang, et al. 2021). These structures include titania nanotubes (TNTs), nanopores (TNPs), nanograss, nanotemplate, etc. (Li et al. 2018a). The most popular anodization-based Ti implant modification are TNTs. TNTs are like test tubes, open at top and closed at bottom (diameter: 10–300 nm, length: 0.5–300 μm), and hence suitable to accommodate drugs/proteins for their local elution post implantation (Gulati, Aw, et al. 2012). Recent advances with respect to EA of Ti-based implants include: fabrication of dual micro-nano structures (Gulati et al. 2017; Gulati et al. 2018), fabrication of stable nanopores on micro-machined implants (Gulati, Li, and Ivanovski 2018) and modification of clinical implants with controlled nanotopography (Gulati, Aw, and Losic 2011; Li et al. 2018a). Further, more recently, the concept of electrolyte ageing (repeated use of electrolyte to anodize non-target Ti prior to EA of target Ti) to fabricate controlled and stable TNTs and TNPs has emerged (Guo, Oztug, et al. 2021b; Gulati, Santos, et al. 2015). It is noteworthy that EA is a versatile

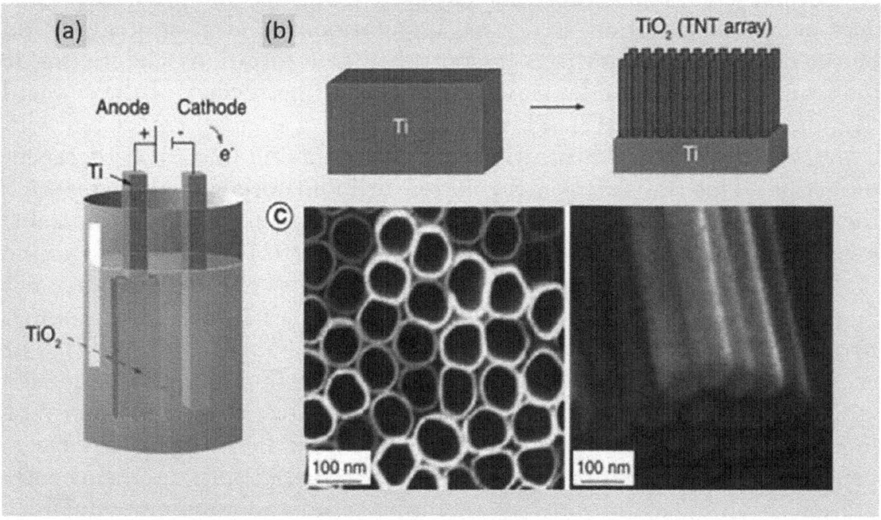

Figure 10.1 Electrochemical anodization of titanium to fabricate TNTs. Scheme showing (a) electrochemical setup and (b) self-ordering of TNTs. SEM images (c) show top and bottom views of TNTs. (Adapted with permission from Gulati, Aw, et al. 2012.)

technique and has been used to modify various metals including Al, Zr, Zn, Cu, Fe, etc. for applications ranging from solar cells, purification, photocatalysis to biomedical implants (Chopra, Gulati, and Ivanovski 2021b, c; Saji et al. 2015; Alsawat et al. 2015; Roy, Berger, and Schmuki 2011; Roy et al. 2010; Chopra et al. 2022).

10.3 DRUG DELIVERY FROM NANO-ENGINEERED TI IMPLANTS

TNTs by themselves offer enhanced bioactivity attributed to nanoscale roughness, as reviewed previously (Gulati, Kogawa, et al. 2015). However, severe complications like the onset of infection or inflammation, or compromised patient conditions (poor bone quality/quantity), demand therapeutic intervention (Chen et al. 2021). Reduced healing around implants presents a significant health and economic challenges, especially in patients with ongoing conditions and aged patients (Trajkovski et al. 2012). Commonly used oral or systemic administration faces limitations including poor local availability of drugs (attributed to traumatized tissue post implantation and poor blood supply), repeated drug administration polluting the entire body and reduced patient compliance. Further, unattended local conditions such as infection and inflammation or poor bone-implant integration can result in severe complications including need for decontamination, resurgery and reimplantation, and even amputation. An ideal strategy would be the release of potent drugs in controlled concentrations directly inside the traumatized bone microenvironment from the surface of the implant (Caplin and García 2019). This would bypass challenges associated with conventional drug administration and ensure maximized local therapeutic action. This has led to a revolution in biomaterials/implant research focussed on the fabrication of drug-eluting implants with customizable local therapy (Quarterman, Geary, and Salem 2021). It is worth noting that local therapy has the potential to not only improve implant outcomes but can also enable effective therapies towards conditions like tumours, bone infections (osteomyelitis) and osteoporosis (Gulati et al. 2013). The vacant volume of the nanotubes in anodized Ti implants can be loaded with any therapeutic for its local elution via diffusion, once the modified implant is placed. From bare drugs/proteins to micelle-encapsulated drugs, peptides and metal nanoparticles, various local therapies including integration (both bone and soft-tissue), antibacterial and immunomodulatory functions can be achieved from the TNTs-modified implants, as described schematically in Figure 10.2 (Gulati, Zhang, et al. 2021). Next, we take a close look at various therapies that can be achieved from TNTs/Ti implants towards long-term implant success.

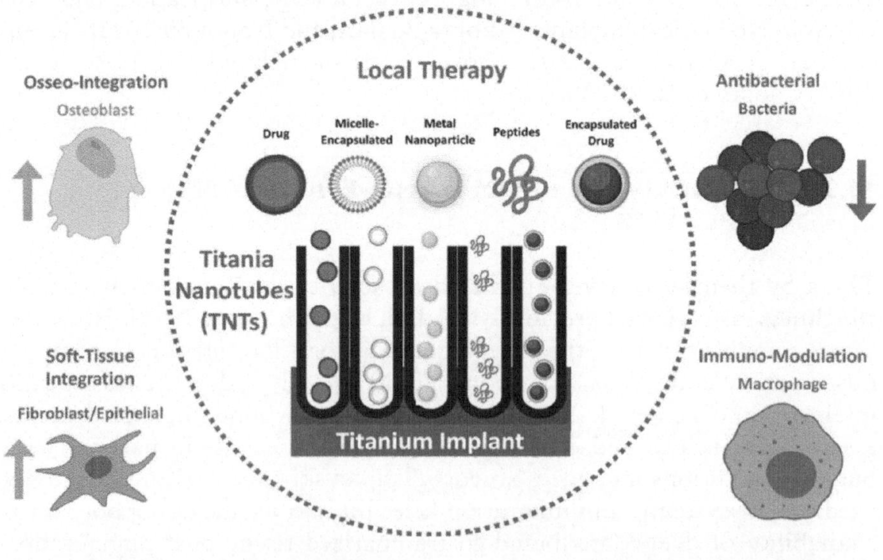

Figure 10.2 Schematic representation of local drug delivery from TNTs modified Ti implants towards various therapies. (Adapted with permission from Gulati, Zhang, et al. 2021. Copyright 2021 American Chemical Society.)

10.3.1 Antibacterial Therapy

Immediately after implant placement, the cells 'race to invade' the compromised site, which dictates the implant outcome (Guo, Gulati, et al. 2021b). The adhesion of bacteria is influenced by the implant surface characteristics including topography and chemistry, and by environmental conditions (temperature, pH and host proteins) and the type of pathogen (gram positive or negative, species, shape, etc.). Upon contact of bacteria to the implant surface, as cascade of events takes place, starting with physiochemical interaction, molecular/cellular interaction to bacterial biofilm formation/maturation and bacterial proliferation (Filipović et al. 2020). It is worth noting that for orthopaedic implants, the presence of bacteria on patient's body and on the operating surfaces may be the source for pathogenesis (Chevalier and Gremillard 2009). While for dental implants, oral microbes are constantly present in the oral microenvironment, and their ingress can happen via the physiological barrier (trans-mucosal integration) (Guo, Gulati, et al. 2021a). Additional details on bacterial adhesion on implants and the surface science behind bacterial invasion can be found elsewhere (Zhang, Zhao, et al. 2021). Various investigations on fabricating the next generation of implants have been focussed on finding appropriate bacteriostatic and bactericidal responses, across micro- and nanoscales (Lee et al. 2020). While TNTs may be an ideal candidate to locally elute potent antibiotics, bare TNTs can enhance bacterial adhesion via incorporated F ions (from anodization electrolyte), dead bacteria on surface and amorphous nature of TNTs. Hence, the bioactive TNTs with synergistic antibiotic therapy may provide an optimum solution. A recent review by Chopra et al. described the influence of TNTs topography and chemistry (diameter, hydrophilicity, and crystallinity) on bacterial adhesion (Chopra, Gulati, and Ivanovski 2021e). Current section will shine light on the use of TNTs towards local elution of antibacterial agents or antibiotics towards maximum therapeutic effect.

10.3.1.1 Release of Antibiotics

Clinically utilized and commonly prescribed antibiotics such as gentamicin, vancomycin and amoxicillin have been loaded inside TNTs towards their local elution (Pawlik et al. 2017; Park et al. 2014). In a pioneering attempt, Popat et al. loaded gentamicin inside TNTs towards its local release and observed a reduction in the adhesion of *S. epidermidis*, while maintaining favourable bioactivity towards osteoblasts (Popat et al. 2007). While common antibiotics may work against various bacteria, they are ineffective against resistant bacteria like methicillin-resistant *Staphylococcus aureus* (MRSA). To address this challenge, Ma et al. utilized antimicrobial peptides (AMPs) loaded inside TNTs and reported almost 99.9% bactericidal effect against MRSA (Ma et al. 2012).

10.3.1.2 Controlled Release Using Biopolymers

Inherently antibacterial and bioactive polymers like chitosan hold great promise to cover open ends of drug-loaded TNTs to control initial burst release (IBR, which can be around 40%–70% of the payloads) (Gulati, Johnson, et al. 2016; Gulati, Ramakrishnan, et al. 2012). It is noteworthy that a very high IBR can result in local cytotoxicity and early consumption of antibiotics. As a result, various attempts have been made using biopolymers like chitosan, silk, polydopamine and PLGA [poly(lactic-co-glycolic acid)] to cover the drug-loaded TNTs towards achieving long-term sustained release patterns (Ungureanu et al. 2016; Ding et al. 2018; Mokhtari et al. 2018). For example, polydopamine-assisted loading of torularhodin (Ungureanu et al. 2016), Ag NPs (Jia et al. 2016) and Zn-Ag NPs (Ding et al. 2018) inside TNTs enabled growth inhibition of various bacteria [*E. coli*: 60%, *S. aureus*: 66%, *E. faecalis*: 60%, *B. subtilis*: 40%, *P. aeruginosa*: 66%], trap-killing antimicrobial potency and high antibacterial with better cytocompatibility, respectively. Chitosan has been used to incorporate 58S bioactive glass (Mokhtari et al. 2018) and indomethacin (Aw, Gulati, and Losic 2011a) to achieve superior antibacterial activity (*E. coli* and *S. aureus*) and increased cell adhesion ability, respectively. Further, chitosan-coated gentamicin-loaded TNTs exhibited superior antibacterial and antibiofilm capabilities while augmenting osteoblast adhesion in vitro (Kumeria et al. 2015). Additionally, electrospun silk fibroin nanofibres on vancomycin-loaded TNTs demonstrated superior antibacterial activity against *S. aureus*, as compared to controls (Fathi, Akbari, and Taheriazam 2019).

10.3.1.3 Release of Metal Ions/Nanoparticles

Metal ions or nanoparticles (NPs), especially Ag, have been widely used to dope TNTs towards achieving efficient bactericidal functions, often striking a balance between bioactivity and cytotoxicity (Chen, Cai, Fang, Lai, Li, et al. 2013;Das et al. 2008;Gunputh et al. 2018). Besides Ag, Au (Xu et al. 2019), Cu (Zhang et al. 2018;Zong et al. 2017), B, P and Ca (Sopchenski et al. 2018) have also been immobilized inside/on TNTs to achieve bactericidal efficacy using various strategies including sputtering, micro-arc oxidation and chemical reduction. Au NPs–loaded TNTs demonstrated antibacterial efficacy against *P. gingivalis* and *F. nucleatum* upon UV irradiation, while maintaining immunomodulatory functions (Xu et al. 2019). Similarly, magnetically sputtered Au NPs in TNTs showed antibacterial action against *S. aureus*, and no ROS were produced from the Au NPs in dark (Wang, Feng, et al. 2016). To dope TNTs with Ag, micro-arc oxidation (Jia et al. 2016), magnetron sputtering (Gao et al. 2014), electrophoresis (Mirzaee, Vaezi, and Palizdar 2016), photo-reduction (Hajjaji et al. 2018), immersion/anodization in $AgNO_3$ solution (Das et al. 2008), chemical reduction (Gunputh et al. 2018) and spin-coating (Chen, Cai, Fang, Lai, Li, et al. 2013) have been utilized to enable release of Ag ions or NPs towards high antibacterial efficacy, while maintaining biocompatibility. Further, dual antibacterial and antifungal actions against *Candida albicans*, *Candida parapsilosis* and *Streptococcus mutans* were achieved for Ag and Zn NPs doped TNTs (achieved via direct current magnetron sputtering) (Roguska et al. 2018). The local elution of Ag-Zn eliminated the microbes within 3 hours (bacteria) or 24 hours (fungus) contact. Similarly, folic acid–conjugated ZnO quantum dots (with vancomycin) (Xiang et al. 2018) and (poly-DL-lactic acid) with Ga (Dong et al. 2019) have also been used in conjunction with TNTs to reduce bacterial adhesion, while maintaining favourable cytocompatibility.

10.3.2 Immunomodulatory

Understanding how an implant surface influences the balance between pro- and anti-inflammatory macrophages is crucial in designing the next generation of immunomodulatory implants, rather than inert implants (Gulati, Hamlet, and Ivanovski 2018). If the implant surface illicit unfavourable immune response, excessive inflammation, fibrosis and scarring can happen, which can result in implant rejection and fibrous capsule formation, leading to implant failure. It has also been shown that nanoscale surface topography enhances protein adsorption and reduces immune activation (Gulati, Kogawa, et al. 2015). The influence of TNTs characteristics including topography, chemistry and local elution of anti-inflammatory drugs have been reported, as reviewed elsewhere (Gulati, Hamlet, and Ivanovski 2018). TNTs diameter influences the activity of immune cells (macrophages, leukocytes, neutrophils or monocytes) with conflicting in vitro results reported with respect to finding the most appropriate diameter range. This may be attributed to the influence of chemistry or topography of the TNTs (Guo, Oztug, et al. 2021c) or the use of varied surface sterilization techniques (Guo, Oztug, et al. 2021a), which are often not appropriately described or explored in bioactivity evaluation focussed studies. However, it is noteworthy that 60–70 nm TNTs diameter is considered appropriate towards reducing macrophage functions.

Further details on the influence of surface topography and chemistry of TNTs on immunomodulatory functions in vitro can be found elsewhere (Gulati, Hamlet, and Ivanovski 2018). TNTs have been utilized to locally elute potent immunomodulatory drugs including nonsteroidal anti-inflammatory drugs (NSAIDs). It is noteworthy that conventional therapy using NSAIDs via oral/intravenous delivery has been associated with delayed bone healing and gastrointestinal/renal toxicity, and their local controlled elution may be the most optimum therapy strategy (Goodman et al. 2002). Ibuprofen, a potent NSAID, has been loaded in TNTs, and controlled release has been obtained based on varying dimensions (Doadrio et al. 2015), with interaction between the drugs and TNTs being electrostatic bonding. Further, ibuprofen was loaded inside PLGA/TNTs composite, which delayed the release in vitro and augmented mechanical stability (Jia and Kerr 2013). Additionally, to increase the loading of ibuprofen and delay its release, TNTs were hydrothermally treated with antimicrobial TiO_2 nanoparticles (Wang et al. 2015). Another drug commonly used to optimize drug delivery from TNTs is NSAID indomethacin. The attempts optimizing indomethacin release (reduced IBR and delayed release) from TNTs can be summarized as (i) periodically tailored TNTs (sustained release up to 17 days) (Gulati, Kant, et al. 2015); (ii) coating of chitosan and PLGA onto drug-loaded TNTs (release delayed to weeks, with favourable osteoblast responses) (Gulati, Ramakrishnan, et al. 2012; Gulati, Kogawa, et al. 2016); and (iii) drug encapsulation inside pluronic F127 polymeric micelle prior to loading inside TNTs (suitable for other sensitive drugs/proteins) (Aw, Gulati, and Losic 2011b). Indomethacin has also been loaded with antibiotics and other drugs to enable synergistic, sequential and triggered therapies (Jayasree, Ivanovski, and Gulati 2021), which will be discussed in further sections.

10.3.3 Osseointegration

TNTs have been widely explored to study the functions of osteoblasts in an attempt to promote osteogenesis via their nanoscale topography and mechanical stimulation (Gulati, Maher, Findlay, et al. 2016; Gulati, Aw, et al. 2012). It has been reported that controlled and local elution of bone-forming proteins or growth factors (orthobiologics) from the implant surface directly inside the bone microenvironment may be more appropriate as compared to systemic administration (Vo, Kasper, and Mikos 2012). Potent growth factors like bone morphogenetic protein-2 (BMP-2) (Balasundaram, Yao, and Webster 2008), alendronate (Shen et al. 2016), ibandronate (Lee et al. 2011) and parathyroid hormone (PTH) (Gulati, Kogawa, et al. 2016) have been incorporated inside TNTs towards augmenting osteoblast functions for osseointegration.

10.3.3.1 Release of Growth Factors

In 2008, in a pioneering attempt, Balasundaram et al. chemically immobilized 'knuckle epitope' [CKIPKASSVPTELSAISTLYL] of BMP-2 onto TNTs followed by culturing human osteoblasts (Balasundaram, Yao, and Webster 2008). The study revealed maximum cellular adhesion for BMP-2 modified TNTs, as compared to the controls. In 2013, Lee et al. utilized anodized dental screws (mimicking dental implants) with TNTs modified with N-acetyl cysteine (NAC, drug with anti-inflammatory and osteogenic properties) and implanted in rad mandible in vivo and observed time-dependent new bone formation (Lee et al. 2013). Additionally, bone-forming abilities of Ti implants have also been enhanced using TNTs incorporated with growth factors like pamidronic acid (nitrogen-containing bisphosphonate) (Koo et al. 2013) and parathyroid hormone (Gulati, Kogawa, et al. 2016); and peptide sequences arginine–glycine–aspartic acid–cysteine (RGDC) (Cao et al. 2012) and lysine–arginine–serine–arginine (KRSR) (Sun et al. 2013). TNTs modified with KRSR upregulated osteoblast adhesion and differentiation (Sun et al. 2013), while RGDC modification enhanced adhesion and osteogenic differentiation of rat bone marrow stromal cells (BMSCs) (Cao et al. 2012). Since osseointegration may be further challenged in compromised conditions with poor bone quality/quantity like osteoporosis and diabetes, it is crucial to study the performance of modified implants in such conditions. In 2011, Xiao et al. reported TNTs on dental implant screws towards augmented osteogenesis in osteoporotic model in vivo (Xiao et al. 2011). Briefly, dual micro-nano TNTs structures on HF-modified machined implant screws significantly increased bone-implant contact, bone volume ratio and maximal pull-out force for TNTs modification, post implantation for 12 weeks in ovariectomized sheep.

10.3.3.2 Release of Metal Nanoparticles

Metal ions or nanoparticles have also been used as therapeutics inside TNTs to orchestrate osteogenesis. For instance, immunosuppressive Au NPs (gelatin stabilized or electrochemically deposited) were loaded inside TNTs, which enhanced osteoblast attachment and proliferation (Wang, Bai, et al. 2016;Neupane et al. 2011). Zhao et al. reported loading of varied amounts of Sr ions inside TNTs of varied diameters and achieved delayed release (over 30 days) and enhanced cellular adhesion of rat MSCs (at 1 hour) (Zhao et al. 2013). The authors also reported that Sr release from TNTs promoted osteogenic differentiation of MSCs and did not cause any cytotoxicity. Further, in separate studies, Sr-Ca (Zhang, Wang, et al. 2020) and Sr-Ag (Pan, Liu, et al. 2020) co-doping have also been utilized to enable enhanced osteogenic activity.

Additionally, Ta was vacuum deposited on annealed TNTs, which augmented ALP activity and osteoblast mineralization and bone nodule formation (Frandsen et al. 2014). Another study used rare earth element La to enhance osteogenic potential of Sr-doped TNTs, and the data revealed enhanced hydrophilicity, protein adsorption and upregulated expression of osteogenic genes (Zhang, Zhang, et al. 2020). Many studies have also established the use of Zn doping on TNTs to stimulate osteoblast functions (Pan et al. 2021;Pan, Hu, et al. 2020;Chen et al. 2020).

10.3.3.3 Bioactive Polymers

Bioactive polymers like chitosan and PLGA can not only cover the open ends of drug-loaded TNTs, but also simultaneously enhance osteoblast functions, as demonstrated in a pioneering study in 2012 (Gulati, Ramakrishnan, et al. 2012). Further, to induce osteogenic differentiation of stem cells, BMP-2 incorporated inside TNTs using polydopamine-assisted chemical conjugation or gelatin/chitosan multi-layering enabled a sustained release (Hu et al. 2012;Lai et al. 2011). Alternatively, polydopamine-Ag/CaP (Li et al. 2015), Se-chitosan (Chen, Cai, Fang, Lai, Hou, et al. 2013), and chitosan/gelatin-icariin (Zhang et al. 2016) have also been used to modify TNTs towards enhancing bone cell activity.

10.3.4 Soft-Tissue Integration

Formation of a barrier towards ingress of oral microbes via the establishment of soft-tissue integration (STI) at the transmucosal region of dental implant is crucial for implant success (Guo, Gulati, et al. 2021b). To augment STI at the dental implant, various topographical, chemical and bioactive modifications have been performed, aimed at upregulating the functions of gingival fibroblasts and oral epithelial cells, as reviewed recently (Guo, Gulati, et al. 2021a). Anodized nanostructures including TNTs and TNPs have been used towards enhancing STI. In vitro studies have reported enhanced functions for human dermal fibroblasts on TNTs (Tan et al. 2017) and increased proliferation and alignment parallel to TNPs for human gingival fibroblasts (Gulati et al. 2018, 2020). Additionally, application of hydrothermal treatment on anodized dual micro-nano topography (TNPs) augmented the proliferation of gingival epithelial (GE1) cells as compared to untreated TNPs (Miyata and Takebe 2013).

Interestingly, only a few studies have utilized the drug loading/release ability of TNTs towards augmenting STI. In 2011, Ma et al. loaded various concentrations (250, 500 and 1,000 ng/mL) of FGF-2 (fibroblast growth factor-2) immobilized on Ag NPs inside TNTs and obtained significantly enhanced activity of human gingival fibroblasts (proliferation, adhesion and extracellular matrix formation) (Ma et al. 2011). Of the various loaded TNTs, 500 ng/mL concentration was most optimum towards upregulation of fibroblast functions and VEGF and LAMA1 gene expression in vitro. Proteins like BSA (bovine serum albumin) have also been utilized to enhance STI. Briefly, 80 nm diameter TNTs were modified with BSA followed by culture of human gingival fibroblasts for 1 hour to 14 days (Liu et al. 2014). BSA-TNTs and bare TNTs both enhanced the initial cell adhesion (1–3 hours), while bare TNTs showed enhanced cell proliferation at day 14. Further, hydroxyapatite (HAP) precipitated TNPs have been used to achieve enhanced STI ability using gingival epithelial cells (Takebe et al. 2014) and fibroblasts (Miura and Takebe 2012).

10.3.5 Synergistic Therapies

Combining *3Is*: integration, infection and inflammation therapies into a single implant surface may be the most appropriate implant surface modification strategy, catering to most encountered conditions directly inside the bone microenvironment. More recently, titania nanopores (nanotubes fused together) have been used to achieve tailored bioactivity, whereby the bioactivity of osteoblasts and fibroblast was enhanced with mechanical stimulation, while macrophage proliferation was reduced with the morphology representing an inactivated state (Gulati et al. 2018). Other attempts at enabling multiple synergistic therapies include the use of biopolymers which enhance bioactivity while restricting the release of antibiotics for sustained release, whereby both osteogenic and antibacterial functions can be achieved simultaneously (Kumeria et al. 2015). It is worth noting that biopolymers like chitosan are inherently antibacterial and osteogenic, and their coating can easily enable synergistic actions, as shown in previous sections (Gulati, Johnson, et al. 2016).

In one such attempt, Huo et al. loaded Zn inside TNTs using hydrothermal treatment (varying TNTs dimensions and treatment times) and investigated the antibacterial (against *Staphylococcus aureus*) and osteogenic performances (using rat bone MSCs) (Huo et al. 2013). Zn loading enabled a dose-dependent bactericidal effect, while enhancing the adhesion, mineralization and osteogenic differentiation of MSCs. Similarly, dual antibacterial and enhanced bioactivity functions have also been reported from Ag-incorporated TNTs (Gao et al. 2014; Mei et al. 2014). Cheng et al. reported dual loading of Sr and Ag (via simple treatment with $Sr(OH)_2$ and $AgNO_3$ solutions) and reported osteoinductive and antimicrobial efficacy, respectively (Cheng et al. 2016). Upon implantation in male rat tibia in vivo for 6 weeks, Sr/Ag-TNTs enabled a complete healing of bone defect, and implantation in ovariectomized rats revealed enhanced trabecular bone and enhanced osseointegration. Further, Chen et al. enabled combined anticancer, osteogenic and antibacterial functions from Se-chitosan doped TNTs (as described in the next section) (Chen, Cai, Fang, Lai, Hou, et al. 2013).

Next, dual Sm/Sr-doped TNTs, achieved via combined anodization, hydrothermal treatment and dopamine self-assembly, enabled slow release of Sm and Sr ions which showed improved antibacterial (Sm) and osteogenic (Sr) functions (Zhang, Huang, et al. 2020). Additionally, combined multiple therapies were achieved from TNTs doped with Ca/P (promoters of osteogenesis) and Zn (antibacterial), including wear resistance and improved stability (electrochemical and mechanical) (Alves, Rossi, Ribeiro, Werckmann, et al. 2017;Alves, Rossi, Ribeiro, Toptan, et al. 2017). It is noteworthy that while metallic ions or NPs can enable potent therapeutic functions, such modified implants are a *double-edged sword*, and therapeutic efficacy and toxicity evaluations must be thoroughly investigated to enable clinical translation (Gulati, Scimeca, et al. 2021).

10.3.6 Anticancer

Tumours and cancers can be effectively treated via local elution from the implant surface as compared to chemotherapy which is often associated with adverse side effects. In one of the pioneering studies, potent chemotherapeutic doxorubicin (1,200 μg) was loaded inside TNTs (diameter 170nm, length 70μm) fabricated on Ti wires, and the in vitro release confirmed only 25% IBR and 100% release in 8days (Gulati, Aw, and Losic 2012; Karan et al. 2013). Additionally, antineoplastic drug cisplatin has also been loaded and locally eluted from TNTs (Xiao et al. 2009). In 2013, Chen et al. reported the use of selenium-chitosan modified TNTs towards dual anticancer and antibacterial functions (Chen, Cai, Fang, Lai, Hou, et al. 2013). TNTs were electrodeposited with Se and then coated with chitosan. Modified TNTs inhibited the growth of cancerous osteoblasts while maintaining and enhancing the proliferation of healthy osteoblasts in vitro. Attributed to the chitosan coating, a sustained release for 3weeks was obtained and long-term antibacterial activity against *E. coli* was reported. Similarly, nanoporous alumina implants modified with Se-chitosan enabled controlled local release, dependent on chitosan coating and the type of Se modification used (Saji et al. 2015).

In 2016, Kaur et al. reported the use of TNTs/Ti wires loaded with TRAIL (TNF-related apoptosis-inducing ligand) towards localized cancer treatment. Both 2D in vitro and 3D ex vivo breast cancer cell models showed a significant reduction in cell viability when incubated with TRAIL-TNTs. Further, testing in in vivo tumour model revealed significantly reduced tumour burden, which makes such drug-eluting implants suitable towards tumour chemotherapy, especially in conditions where surgical removal of tumour is not possible.

10.4 TRIGGERED LOCAL THERAPY

Local release from TNTs implants may not be a long-term solution as the consumption of drugs can retrigger bacterial adhesion, and the therapeutic dosage cannot be changed once implanted. As a result, the development of trigger-based drug delivery, whereby the drug release can be turned *on or off*, via an internal or external stimuli, can minimize drug wastage and can be a more cost-effective and patient compliant option (Jayasree, Ivanovski, and Gulati 2021). Briefly, these triggers can be internal (pH changes) or external (magnetic field, ultrasound, electrical stimulation, etc.) as schematically presented in Figure 10.3 (Jayasree, Ivanovski, and Gulati 2021).

10.4.1 Internal Triggers

Defroxamine was loaded in 70nm diameter TNTs followed by layer-by-layer (LBL) coating of chitosan and HA-gentamicin and around

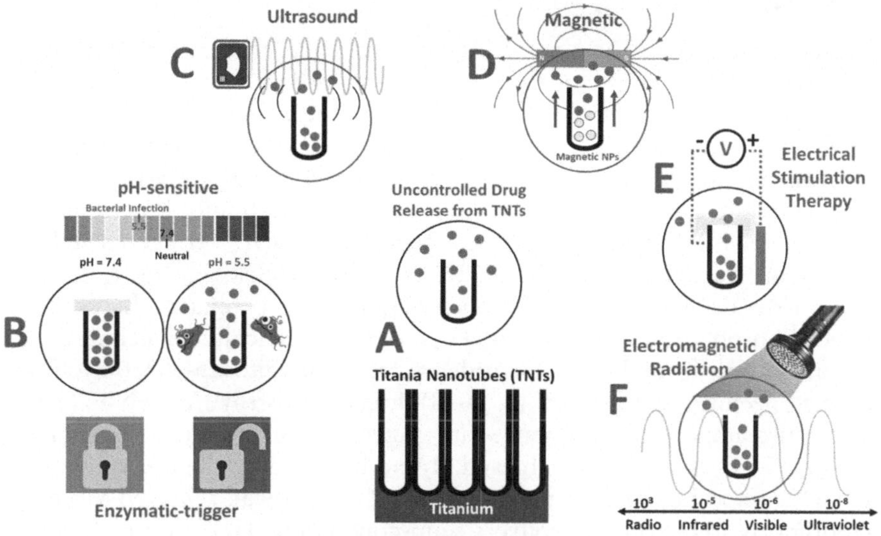

Figure 10.3 Triggered therapies from TNT-modified implants. (Reprinted from Jayasree, Ivanovski, and Gulati 2021, with permission from Elsevier.)

30% of the drug was released within 12 hours and 70% within 72 hours (Yu et al. 2020). Upon enzymatic trigger, 60% of the drug was released within 12hours, while osteogenic differentiation of MSCs and reduced adhesion of *S. aureus* and *E. coli* was observed in vitro. Similarly, upon application of trigger, IBR of vancomycin from TNTs LBL-coated with catechol modified HA and chitosan increased from <10% (4 hours) to ~44% (4 hours), with enhanced antibacterial and osseointegration abilities as demonstrated in infected rat femur model in vivo (Yuan et al. 2018). It is noteworthy that bacterial infection can change local physiological pH from 7.4 to 5.5, which can be utilized as another internal trigger to release potent antibiotics as the bacterial infection starts (Dong et al. 2017). As a result, various antibacterial agents including Ag NPs and vancomycin have been released via pH trigger from TNTs (Dong et al. 2017). In 2017, Dong et al. immobilized Ag NPs onto TNTs using pH liable acetal linker (AL) and achieved only 0.25 ppm IBR within 2 hours, which was accelerated to 0.75 ppm upon change of pH to 5.5, showing appropriate bactericidal efficacy against *S. aureus* and *E. coli* at 2 hours. Further, vancomycin bound to TNTs modified with folic acid–conjugated ZnO quantum dots, triggered IBR from 125 μg/mL within 5 hours to 280 μg/mL, with potent antibacterial efficacy against *S. aureus* (Xiang et al. 2018). While internal triggers can have drug release controlled by microbial load, it is noteworthy that once triggered, entire payloads can get released within a short time.

10.4.2 External Triggers

Triggers external to the site of implantation like electric/magnetic field, radiofrequency or light can enable a dose-dependent release, allowing for further therapeutic customization (Gulati, Maher, Chandrasekaran, et al. 2016). In the pioneering attempt, Sirivisoot et al. incorporated penicillin/streptomycin inside TNTs (with multi-walled carbon nanotubes/MWCNTs grown within TNTs) and electrodeposited PPy and finally functionalized with PLGA-NHS towards demonstrating electrically triggered release (Sirivisoot, Pareta, and Webster 2011). With electrical trigger, around 80% of the drug was released, which augmented osteoblast adhesion and reduced fibroblast adhesion in vitro. Similarly, electrically triggered release of vancomycin from TNTs electrodeposited with chitosan-vancomycin gel has also been reported (Shi et al. 2013). It is noteworthy that TNTs (TiO_2) are semi-conducting, and hence full potential for electrical stimulation therapy (EST) may not be achieved. To address this challenge, conversion of TiO_2 nanotubes into Ti nanotubes on Ti wires was achieved via magnesiothermic reduction to convert semi-conducting TiO_2 into conducting Ti, towards enhancing the EST performance of implants (Gulati, Maher, Chandrasekaran, et al. 2016).

Further, on-demand release of micelle-encapsulated NSAID indomethacin from TNTs pre-loaded with Fe_3O_4 and Au NPs (with up-conversion NPs) was achieved via magnetic (Aw, Addai-Mensah, and Losic 2012) and radiofrequency (Bariana et al. 2014) triggers, respectively. However, these triggers may be associated with accidental triggers upon magnetic field exposure and controversies with respect to RF exposure on cells. Light or radiation can also be used to enable turning the release of payloads *on or off*. For instance, visible light was used to release tetracycline-chlorhexidine and ampicillin from N_2-doped TNTs (Oh et al. 2013) and functionalized heat-treated TNTs with Au NPs (Xu et al. 2016), respectively. Further, UV irradiated 7-methoxycoumarin-3-carboxylic acid incorporated TNTs (with Fe_3O_4 NPs and dye attached with silane linker) enabled photo-induced killing of tumour cells in vitro (Shrestha et al. 2009); however, UV can stimulate photocatalysis on TNTs which can cause cell cytotoxicity. Ultrasound waves have also been utilized to enable the release of potent therapeutics (indomethacin (Aw and Losic 2013) and tetracyclin (Zhou et al. 2018)) from modified TNTs. It is worth noting that while ultrasound waves can enhance drug permeation into the tissues and disrupt biofilms, they may damage sensitive drugs/proteins due to high cavitation force.

10.5 CYTOTOXICITY CONCERNS

Numerous in vivo investigations have established the safety and biocompatibility of TNTs (bare or with drugs), and the absence of fibrous capsule formation and inflammation around the TNTs/Ti implants is strong evidence that such nano-engineered implants are non-toxic. However, most in vivo investigations are short term and without mechanical loading. Further, it is crucial to have fabrication of reproducible and stable nanotubes, which are well adherent onto the underlying substrate, thereby minimizing any leaching of ions or breakage under loading conditions (Li et al. 2018b). It is worth noting that the release of Ti NPs from Ti implants has been reported to cause aseptic loosening of the implant (Bijukumar et al. 2018). And the release of ions can also have a detrimental effect on the osteo-immunomodulation. Further, implant degradation and release of nanoparticulates can accumulate in various organs and cause complications. Interestingly, only few studies have investigated the cytotoxicity from TNTs.

It is also known that Ti ions can damage RNA, DNA and phopsholipids and can cause osteolysis and implant failure (Vasconcelos et al. 2016). Ion release from TNTs-based implants can be intentional (for therapeutic purposes) or unintentional (chemical breakdown or physical destruction) (Gulati, Scimeca, et al. 2021). If an unintentional release of TiO_2 in the form of nanoparticles happens, it may induce a dose-dependent pro-inflammatory response, as demonstrated for human gingival fibroblasts in vivo (Garcia-Contreras et al. 2014). Another toxicity concern for TNTs is the chemical moieties incorporated from the anodization electrolyte rich in F and TiF_6 ions (Guo, Oztug, et al. 2021b). It is noteworthy that complete removal of F and organic electrolyte components may not be possible, even after thorough sterilization (Guo, Oztug, et al. 2021a), which can influence the chemistry of the TNTs (Guo, Asli Kocak Oztug, et al. 2021); however, this remains largely underexplored. The release of such ions over time needs further investigations.

Besides, the intentional use of therapeutic and trigger-enabling metal NPs or ions (Zn, Au, Ag, etc.) can also leach out from TNTs and interact with cells. These NPs can form protein corona and can enter cells, where NPs can produce toxic cations disrupting mitochondrial functions and generating reactive oxygen species (ROS) (Sabella et al. 2014). A recent review focusses on understanding and optimizing therapy from metal-doped Ti implants with appropriate bioactivity and controlled/minimal cytotoxicity (Gulati, Scimeca, et al. 2021).

TNTs modified implants also pose cytotoxicity risks due to high local release of potent therapeutics, mechanical failure under loading conditions, corrosion (both chemical and electrochemical) and use of external triggers for on-demand release. It is worth noting that high IBR of antibiotics like vancomycin and gentamicin can alter cell signalling pathways which can inhibit cellular functions (Chang, Goldberg, and Caplan 2006). Additionally, there is always a risk of development of antibiotic resistance in microbes if the release is not regulated or controlled. Ideally, the local release should be within the safe therapeutic window and should not cause cytotoxicity.

10.6 RESEARCH CHALLENGES AND FUTURE DIRECTIONS

TNTs are a promising bioactive surface modification for Ti-based implants that can enable controlled, tailored and triggered local elution of potent drugs. TNTs dimensions, pre-encapsulation of drugs, biopolymer coating of drug-loaded TNTs and use of NPs to enable triggers show promising outcomes in vitro and short-term in vivo; however, for their clinical translation, long-term testing under loading conditions in vivo is needed. Hence, testing under loading and with varied pH and physiological conditions (both healthy and compromised conditions, inflammation or infection) must be performed.

Further, predicting the concentration of drugs that will be needed in vivo in traumatized tissue conditions is cumbersome. Hence, quantification of drugs inside the bone microenvironment and its successful uptake by the cells are important considerations. Tools like in vitro 3D cell culture models (Gulati, Kogawa, et al. 2016) and ex vivo 3D tissue models (Aw et al. 2012; Daish et al. 2017; Rahman et al. 2016; Kaur et al. 2016) can be used to quantify release in real traumatized 3D tissue, which is more physiologically relevant than a conventional in vitro PBS release media (which maintains a very high diffusion gradient). Under implantation trauma, blood coagulation and compromised tissue porosity can significantly impede drug release from TNTs, as diffusion gradient is compromised (Kaur et al. 2016). The in vitro optimized release does not translate into real implant conditions and only showcases the 'proof of concept', which may be very distant from clinical translation. Further, increased protein adhesion onto drug-loaded TNTs can block the pores, thereby restricting its release.

Overall, to ensure successful clinical translation, the TNTs/Ti implants must survive packaging, implantation surgery and long-term (>10–15 years) operation under mechanical loading (Gulati, Zhang, et al. 2021). Further, such modified implants should successfully enable synergistic therapies (*3Is*: integration, infection and inflammation management) without initiating any immunotoxicity. The next generation of nano-engineered Ti implants would allow for multiple tailored therapies and triggered functionality. Such 'smart' implants may be custom 3D printed (matching patients' tissue defect), followed by anodization to fabricate controlled nanostructures, and loading of drugs and functionalization to control/trigger its release, which caters to the specific therapeutic needs of the patient.

10.7 CONCLUSIONS

Anodized nano-engineered Ti-based implants with TNTs are a promising strategy to achieve augmented bioactivity and local release of potent drugs/proteins for maximized local therapeutic action, bypassing systemic/oral therapeutic administration. Numerous therapies including osseo- and soft-tissue integration, antibacterial activity and immunomodulation can be achieved from TNTs via loading and controlled release of specific drugs or proteins. Additionally, anticancer and trigger-enabled therapies (based on internal or external stimuli) can also be achieved from TNTs modification, attributed to the ease of TNTs' functionalization. While such local drug-eluting implants hold great promise to advance conventional Ti-based orthopaedic and dental implants, several challenges including long-term in vivo testing in compromised conditions under loading and in-depth cytotoxicity evaluation of intentional or unintentional release of ions or nanoparticles remain underexplored.

ACKNOWLEDGEMENTS

Karan Gulati is supported by the National Health and Medical Research Council (NHMRC) Early Career Fellowship (APP1140699).

REFERENCES

Alsawat, Mohammed, Tariq Altalhi, Karan Gulati, Abel Santos, and Dusan Losic. 2015. "Synthesis of carbon nanotube–nanotubular titania composites by catalyst-free CVD process: Insights into the formation mechanism and photocatalytic properties." *ACS Applied Materials & Interfaces* 7 (51):28361–28368. doi: 10.1021/acsami.5b08956.

Alves, Sofia A., André L. Rossi, Ana R. Ribeiro, Fatih Toptan, Ana M. Pinto, Jean-Pierre Celis, Tolou Shokuhfar, and Luís A. Rocha. 2017. "Tribo-electrochemical behavior of bio-functionalized TiO_2 nanotubes in artificial saliva: Understanding of degradation mechanisms." *Wear* 384: 28–42.

Alves, Sofia A., Andre L. Rossi, Ana R. Ribeiro, Jacques Werckmann, Jean-Pierre Celis, Luis A. Rocha, and Tolou Shokuhfar. 2017. "A first insight on the biofunctionalization mechanisms of TiO_2 nanotubes with calcium, phosphorous and zinc by reverse polarization anodization." *Surface and Coatings Technology* 324: 153–166.

Aw, Moom Sinn, Jonas Addai-Mensah, and Dusan Losic. 2012. "Magnetic-responsive delivery of drug-carriers using titania nanotube arrays." *Journal of Materials Chemistry* 22 (14):6561–6563.

Aw, Moom Sinn, Karan Gulati, and Dusan Losic. 2011a. "Controlling drug release from titania nanotube arrays using polymer nanocarriers and biopolymer coating." *Journal of Biomaterials and Nanobiotechnology* 2 (5):477.

Aw, Moom Sinn, Karan Gulati, and Dusan Losic. 2011b. "Controlling drug release from titania nanotube arrays using polymer nanocarriers and biopolymer coating." *Journal of Biomaterials and Nanobiotechnology* 2(5):8. doi: 10.4236/jbnb.2011.225058.

Aw, Moom Sinn, Kamarul A. Khalid, Karan Gulati, Gerald J. Atkins, Peter Pivonka, David M. Findlay, and Dusan Losic. 2012. "Characterization of drug-release kinetics in trabecular bone from titania nanotube implants." *International Journal of Nanomedicine* 7:4883–4892 doi: 10.2147/IJN.S33655.

Aw, Moom Sinn, and Dusan Losic. 2013. "Ultrasound enhanced release of therapeutics from drug-releasing implants based on titania nanotube arrays." *International Journal of Pharmaceutics* 443 (1–2):154–162.

Balasundaram, Ganesan, Chang Yao, and Thomas J Webster. 2008. "TiO_2 nanotubes functionalized with regions of bone morphogenetic protein-2 increases osteoblast adhesion." *Journal of Biomedical Materials Research Part A* 84 (2):447–453.

Bariana, Manpreet, Moom Sinn Aw, Eli Moore, Nicolas H. Voelcker, and Dusan Losic. 2014. "Radiofrequency-triggered release for on-demand delivery of therapeutics from titania nanotube drug-eluting implants." *Nanomedicine* 9 (8):1263–1275.

Bijukumar, Divya Rani, Abhijith Segu, Júlio C.M. Souza, XueJun Li, Mark Barba, Louis G. Mercuri, Joshua J. Jacobs, and Mathew Thoppil Mathew. 2018. "Systemic and local toxicity of metal debris released from hip prostheses: A review of experimental approaches." *Nanomedicine: Nanotechnology, Biology and Medicine* 14 (3):951–963.

Cao, Xin, Wei-qiang Yu, Jing Qiu, Yan-fang Zhao, Yi-lin Zhang, and Fu-qiang Zhang. 2012. "RGD peptide immobilized on TiO_2 nanotubes for increased bone marrow stromal cells adhesion and osteogenic gene expression." *Journal of Materials Science: Materials in Medicine* 23 (2):527–536.

Caplin, Jeremy D., and Andrés J. García. 2019. "Implantable antimicrobial biomaterials for local drug delivery in bone infection models." *Acta Biomaterialia* 93:2–11. doi: 10.1016/j.actbio.2019.01.015.

Chang, Yuhan, Victor M. Goldberg, and Arnold I. Caplan. 2006. "Toxic effects of gentamicin on marrow-derived human mesenchymal stem cells." *Clinical Orthopaedics and Related Research (1976–2007)* 452: 242–249.

Chen, Bo, Yapeng You, Aobo Ma, Yunjia Song, Jian Jiao, Liting Song, Enyu Shi, Xue Zhong, Ying Li, and Changyi Li. 2020. "Zn-incorporated TiO_2 nanotube surface improves osteogenesis ability through influencing immunomodulatory function of macrophages." *International Journal of Nanomedicine* 15: 2095.

Chen, Xiuyong, Kaiyong Cai, Jiajia Fang, Min Lai, Yanhua Hou, Jinghua Li, Zhong Luo, Yan Hu, and Liling Tang. 2013. "Fabrication of selenium-deposited and chitosan-coated titania nanotubes with anticancer and antibacterial properties." *Colloids and Surfaces B: Biointerfaces* 103:149–157.

Chen, Xiuyong, Kaiyong Cai, Jiajia Fang, Min Lai, Jinghua Li, Yanhua Hou, Zhong Luo, Yan Hu, and Liling Tang. 2013. "Dual action antibacterial TiO_2 nanotubes incorporated with silver nanoparticles and coated with a quaternary ammonium salt (QAS)." *Surface and Coatings Technology* 216:158–165.

Chen, Yun-Chu, Sheryhan F. Gad, Dhawal Chobisa, Yongzhe Li, and Yoon Yeo. 2021. "Local drug delivery systems for inflammatory diseases: Status quo, challenges, and opportunities." *Journal of Controlled Release* 330:438–460. doi: 10.1016/j.jconrel.2020.12.025.

Cheng, Hao, Wei Xiong, Zhong Fang, Hanfeng Guan, Wei Wu, Yong Li, Yong Zhang, Mario Moisés Alvarez, Biao Gao, and Kaifu Huo. 2016. "Strontium

(Sr) and silver (Ag) loaded nanotubular structures with combined osteoinductive and antimicrobial activities." *Acta Biomaterialia* 31: 388–400.

Chevalier, Jerome, and Laurent Gremillard. 2009. "Ceramics for medical applications: A picture for the next 20 years." *Journal of the European Ceramic Society* 29 (7):1245–1255.

Chopra, Divya, Karan Gulati, and Sašo Ivanovski. 2021a. "Bed of nails: Bioinspired nano-texturing towards antibacterial and bioactivity functions." *Materials Today Advances* 12:100176. doi: 10.1016/j.mtadv.2021.100176.

Chopra, Divya, Karan Gulati, and Sašo Ivanovski. 2021b. "Micro+nano: Conserving the gold standard microroughness to nanoengineer zirconium dental implants." *ACS Biomaterials Science & Engineering* 7 (7):3069–3074. doi: 10.1021/acsbiomaterials.1c00356.

Chopra, Divya, Karan Gulati, and Sašo Ivanovski. 2021c. "Towards clinical translation: Optimized fabrication of controlled nanostructures on implant-relevant curved zirconium surfaces." *Nanomaterials* 11 (4):868.

Chopra, Divya, Karan Gulati, and Sašo Ivanovski. 2021d. "Understanding and optimizing the antibacterial functions of anodized nano-engineered titanium implants." *Acta Biomaterialia* 127:80–101. doi: 10.1016/j.actbio.2021.03.027.

Chopra, Divya, Anjana Jayasree, Tianqi Guo, Karan Gulati, and Sašo Ivanovski. 2022. "Advancing dental implants: Bioactive and therapeutic modifications of zirconia." *Bioactive Materials* 13:161–178. doi: 10.1016/j.bioactmat.2021.10.010.

Daish, C., R. Blanchard, K. Gulati, D. Losic, D. Findlay, D. J. E. Harvie, and P. Pivonka. 2017. "Estimation of anisotropic permeability in trabecular bone based on microCT imaging and pore-scale fluid dynamics simulations." *Bone Reports* 6:129–139. doi: 10.1016/j.bonr.2016.12.002.

Das, Kakoli, Susmita Bose, Amit Bandyopadhyay, Balu Karandikar, and Bruce L. Gibbins. 2008. "Surface coatings for improvement of bone cell materials and antimicrobial activities of Ti implants." *Journal of Biomedical Materials Research Part B: Applied Biomaterials* 87 (2):455–460.

Ding, Xiyu, Yanmei Zhang, Jinyan Ling, and Changjian Lin. 2018. "Rapid mussel-inspired synthesis of PDA-Zn-Ag nanofilms on TiO_2 nanotubes for optimizing the antibacterial activity and biocompatibility by doping polydopamine with zinc at a higher temperature." *Colloids and Surfaces B: Biointerfaces* 171:101–109.

Doadrio, Antonio L., A. Conde, M. A. Arenas, J. M. Hernández-López, J. J. de Damborenea, Concepción Pérez-Jorge, Jaime Esteban, and Maria Vallet-Regí. 2015. "Use of anodized titanium alloy as drug carrier: Ibuprofen as model of drug releasing." *International Journal of Pharmaceutics* 492 (1):207–212. doi: 10.1016/j.ijpharm.2015.07.046.

Dong, Junjie, Dong Fang, Lei Zhang, Quan Shan, and Yunchao Huang. 2019. "Gallium-doped titania nanotubes elicit anti-bacterial efficacy in vivo against Escherichia coli and Staphylococcus aureus biofilm." *Materialia* 5:100209.

Dong, Yiwen, Hui Ye, Yi Liu, Lihua Xu, Zuosu Wu, Xiaohui Hu, Jianfeng Ma, Janak L Pathak, Jinsong Liu, and Gang Wu. 2017. "pH dependent silver nanoparticles releasing titanium implant: A novel therapeutic approach to control peri-implant infection." *Colloids and Surfaces B: Biointerfaces* 158: 127–136.

Fathi, Mehdi, Babak Akbari, and Afshin Taheriazam. 2019. "Antibiotics drug release controlling and osteoblast adhesion from Titania nanotubes arrays using silk fibroin coating." *Materials Science and Engineering: C* 103:109743.

Filipović, Urška, Raja Gošnak Dahmane, Slaheddine Ghannouchi, Anamarija Zore, and Klemen Bohinc. 2020. "Bacterial adhesion on orthopedic implants." *Advances in Colloid and Interface Science* 283:102228.

Frandsen, Christine J., Karla S. Brammer, Kunbae Noh, Gary Johnston, and Sungho Jin. 2014. "Tantalum coating on TiO_2 nanotubes induces superior rate of matrix mineralization and osteofunctionality in human osteoblasts." *Materials Science and Engineering: C* 37: 332–341.

Gao, Ang, Ruiqiang Hang, Xiaobo Huang, Lingzhou Zhao, Xiangyu Zhang, Lin Wang, Bin Tang, Shengli Ma, and Paul K. Chu. 2014. "The effects of titania nanotubes with embedded silver oxide nanoparticles on bacteria and osteoblasts." *Biomaterials* 35 (13):4223–4235.

Garcia-Contreras, Rene, Rogelio J. Scougall-Vilchis, Rosalia Contreras-Bulnes, Yumiko Kanda, Hiroshi Nakajima, and Hiroshi Sakagami. 2014. "Induction of prostaglandin E2 production by TiO_2 nanoparticles in human gingival fibroblast." *In vivo* 28 (2):217–222.

Goodman, Stuart, Ting Ma, Michael Trindade, Takashi Ikenoue, Ippe Matsuura, Neal Wong, Nora Fox, Mark Genovese, Don Regula, and R. Lane Smith. 2002. "COX-2 selective NSAID decreases bone ingrowth in vivo." *Journal of Orthopaedic Research* 20 (6):1164–1169. doi: 10.1016/S0736-0266(02)00079-7.

Gulati, Karan, Gerald Atkins, David Findlay, and Dusan Losic. 2013. *Nano-Engineered Titanium for Enhanced Bone Therapy*, Vol. 8812, SPIE NanoScience+Engineering: SPIE, San Diego, CA.

Gulati, Karan, Moom Sinn Aw, David Findlay, and Dusan Losic. 2012. "Local drug delivery to the bone by drug-releasing implants: Perspectives of nano-engineered titania nanotube arrays." *Therapeutic Delivery* 3 (7):857–873. doi: 10.4155/tde.12.66.

Gulati, Karan, Moom Sinn Aw, and Dusan Losic. 2011. "Drug-eluting Ti wires with titania nanotube arrays for bone fixation and reduced bone infection." *Nanoscale Research Letters* 6 (1):571. doi: 10.1186/1556-276X-6-571.

Gulati, Karan, Moom Sinn Aw, and Dusan Losic. 2012. "Nanoengineered drug-releasing Ti wires as an alternative for local delivery of chemotherapeutics in the brain." *International Journal of Nanomedicine* 7:2069–2076. doi: 10.2147/IJN.S29917.

Gulati, Karan, Stephen M. Hamlet, and Sašo Ivanovski. 2018. "Tailoring the immuno-responsiveness of anodized nano-engineered titanium implants." *Journal of Materials Chemistry B* 6 (18):2677–2689. doi: 10.1039/C8TB00450A.

Gulati, Karan, and Sašo Ivanovski. 2017. "Dental implants modified with drug releasing titania nanotubes: Therapeutic potential and developmental challenges." *Expert Opinion on Drug Delivery* 14 (8):1009–1024. doi: 10.1080/17425247.2017.1266332.

Gulati, Karan, Lucas Johnson, Ramesh Karunagaran, David Findlay, and Dusan Losic. 2016. "In situ transformation of chitosan films into micro-tubular structures on the surface of nanoengineered titanium implants." *Biomacromolecules* 17 (4):1261–1271. doi: 10.1021/acs.biomac.5b01037.

Gulati, Karan, Krishna Kant, David Findlay, and Dusan Losic. 2015. "Periodically tailored titania nanotubes for enhanced drug loading and releasing performances." *Journal of Materials Chemistry B* 3 (12):2553–2559. doi: 10.1039/C4TB01882F.

Gulati, Karan, Masakazu Kogawa, Shaheer Maher, Gerald Atkins, David Findlay, and Dusan Losic. 2015. "Titania nanotubes for local drug delivery from implant surfaces." In Losic, D., Santos, A. (eds.) *Electrochemically Engineered Nanoporous Materials*, 307–355. Springer, Cham.

Gulati, Karan, Masakazu Kogawa, Matthew Prideaux, David M. Findlay, Gerald J. Atkins, and Dusan Losic. 2016. "Drug-releasing nano-engineered titanium implants: Therapeutic efficacy in 3D cell culture model, controlled release and stability." *Materials Science and Engineering: C* 69:831–840. doi: 10.1016/j.msec.2016.07.047.

Gulati, Karan, Tao Li, and Sašo Ivanovski. 2018. "Consume or conserve: Microroughness of titanium implants toward fabrication of dual micro–nanotopography." *ACS Biomaterials Science & Engineering* 4 (9):3125–3131. doi: 10.1021/acsbiomaterials.8b00829.

Gulati, Karan, Shaheer Maher, Soundarrajan Chandrasekaran, David M. Findlay, and Dusan Losic. 2016. "Conversion of titania (TiO_2) into conductive titanium (Ti) nanotube arrays for combined drug-delivery and electrical stimulation therapy." *Journal of Materials Chemistry B* 4 (3):371–375. doi: 10.1039/C5TB02108A.

Gulati, Karan, Shaheer Maher, David M. Findlay, and Dusan Losic. 2016. "Titania nanotubes for orchestrating osteogenesis at the bone–implant interface." *Nanomedicine* 11 (14):1847–1864. doi: 10.2217/nnm-2016-0169.

Gulati, Karan, Ho-Jin Moon, P. T. Sudheesh Kumar, Pingping Han, and Sašo Ivanovski. 2020. "Anodized anisotropic titanium surfaces for enhanced guidance of gingival fibroblasts." *Materials Science and Engineering: C* 112:110860. doi: 10.1016/j.msec.2020.110860.

Gulati, Karan, Ho-Jin Moon, Tao Li, P. T. Sudheesh Kumar, and Sašo Ivanovski. 2018. "Titania nanopores with dual micro-/nano-topography for selective cellular bioactivity." *Materials Science and Engineering: C* 91:624–630. doi: 10.1016/j.msec.2018.05.075.

Gulati, Karan, Matthew Prideaux, Masakazu Kogawa, Luis Lima-Marques, Gerald J. Atkins, David M. Findlay, and Dusan Losic. 2017. "Anodized 3D–printed titanium implants with dual micro- and nano-scale topography promote interaction with human osteoblasts and osteocyte-like cells." *Journal of Tissue Engineering and Regenerative Medicine* 11 (12):3313–3325. doi: 10.1002/term.2239.

Gulati, Karan, Saminathan Ramakrishnan, Moom Sinn Aw, Gerald J. Atkins, David M. Findlay, and Dusan Losic. 2012. "Biocompatible polymer coating of titania nanotube arrays for improved drug elution and osteoblast adhesion." *Acta Biomaterialia* 8 (1):449–456. doi: 10.1016/j.actbio.2011.09.004.

Gulati, Karan, Abel Santos, David Findlay, and Dusan Losic. 2015. "Optimizing anodization conditions for the growth of titania nanotubes on curved surfaces." *The Journal of Physical Chemistry C* 119 (28):16033–16045. doi: 10.1021/acs.jpcc.5b03383.

Gulati, Karan, Jean-Claude Scimeca, Sašo Ivanovski, and Elise Verron. 2021. "Double-edged sword: Therapeutic efficacy versus toxicity evaluations of doped titanium implants." *Drug Discovery Today* 26 (11):2734–2742. doi: 10.1016/j.drudis.2021.07.004.

Gulati, Karan, Yifan Zhang, Ping Di, Yan Liu, and Sašo Ivanovski. 2021. "Research to clinics: Clinical translation considerations for anodized nano-engineered titanium implants." *ACS Biomaterials Science & Engineering*. doi: 10.1021/acsbiomaterials.1c00529.

Gunputh, Urvashi Fowdar, Huirong Le, Richard D. Handy, and Christopher Tredwin. 2018. "Anodised TiO_2 nanotubes as a scaffold for antibacterial silver nanoparticles on titanium implants." *Materials Science and Engineering: C* 91:638–644.

Guo, Tianqi, Karan Gulati, Himanshu Arora, Pingping Han, Benjamin Fournier, and Sašo Ivanovski. 2021a. "Orchestrating soft tissue integration at the transmucosal region of titanium implants." *Acta Biomaterialia* 124:33–49. doi: 10.1016/j.actbio.2021.01.001.

Guo, Tianqi, Karan Gulati, Himanshu Arora, Pingping Han, Benjamin Fournier, and Sašo Ivanovski. 2021b. "Race to invade: Understanding soft tissue integration at the transmucosal region of titanium dental implants." *Dental Materials* 37 (5):816–831. doi: 10.1016/j.dental.2021.02.005.

Guo, Tianqi, Necla Asli Kocak Oztug, Pingping Han, Sašo Ivanovski, and Karan Gulati. 2021a. "Influence of sterilization on the performance of anodized nanoporous titanium implants." *Materials Science and Engineering: C* 130:112429. doi: 10.1016/j.msec.2021.112429.

Guo, Tianqi, Necla Asli Kocak Oztug, Pingping Han, Sašo Ivanovski, and Karan Gulati. 2021b. "Old is gold: Electrolyte aging influences the topography, chemistry, and bioactivity of anodized TiO_2 nanopores." *ACS Applied Materials & Interfaces* 13 (7):7897–7912. doi: 10.1021/acsami.0c19569.

Guo, Tianqi, Necla Asli Kocak Oztug, Pingping Han, Sašo Ivanovski, and Karan Gulati. 2021c. "Untwining the topography-chemistry interdependence to optimize the bioactivity of nano-engineered titanium implants." *Applied Surface Science* 570:151083. doi: 10.1016/j.apsusc.2021.151083.

Hajjaji, A., M. Elabidi, K. Trabelsi, A.A. Assadi, B. Bessais, and S. Rtimi. 2018. "Bacterial adhesion and inactivation on Ag decorated TiO_2-nanotubes under visible light: Effect of the nanotubes geometry on the photocatalytic activity." *Colloids and Surfaces B: Biointerfaces* 170:92–98.

Hu, Yan, Kaiyong Cai, Zhong Luo, Dawei Xu, Daichao Xie, Yuran Huang, Weihu Yang, and Peng Liu. 2012. "TiO_2 nanotubes as drug nanoreservoirs for the regulation of mobility and differentiation of mesenchymal stem cells." *Acta Biomaterialia* 8 (1):439–448.

Huo, Kaifu, Xuming Zhang, Hairong Wang, Lingzhou Zhao, Xuanyong Liu, and Paul K Chu. 2013. "Osteogenic activity and antibacterial effects on titanium surfaces modified with Zn-incorporated nanotube arrays." *Biomaterials* 34 (13):3467–3478.

Jayasree, Anjana, Sašo Ivanovski, and Karan Gulati. 2021. "ON or OFF: Triggered therapies from anodized nano-engineered titanium implants." *Journal of Controlled Release* 333:521–535. doi: 10.1016/j.jconrel.2021.03.020.

Jia, Huiying, and Lei L. Kerr. 2013. "Sustained ibuprofen release using composite poly(lactic-co-glycolic Acid)/titanium dioxide nanotubes from Ti implant surface." *Journal of Pharmaceutical Sciences* 102 (7):2341–2348. doi: 10.1002/jps.23580.

Jia, Zhaojun, Peng Xiu, Ming Li, Xuchen Xu, Yuying Shi, Yan Cheng, Shicheng Wei, Yufeng Zheng, Tingfei Xi, and Hong Cai. 2016. "Bioinspired anchoring AgNPs onto micro-nanoporous TiO_2 orthopedic coatings: Trap-killing of bacteria, surface-regulated osteoblast functions and host responses." *Biomaterials* 75:203–222.

Karan, Gulati, J. Atkins Gerald, M. Findlay David, and Losic Dusan. 2013. "Nano-engineered titanium for enhanced bone therapy." *Proceedings of the SPIE*. doi: 10.1117/12.2027151.

Kaur, Gagandeep, Tamsyn Willsmore, Karan Gulati, Irene Zinonos, Ye Wang, Mima Kurian, Shelley Hay, Dusan Losic, and Andreas Evdokiou. 2016. "Titanium wire implants with nanotube arrays: A study model for localized cancer treatment." *Biomaterials* 101:176–188. doi: 10.1016/j.biomaterials.2016.05.048.

Koo, Tae-Hyung, Jyoti S. Borah, Zhi-Cai Xing, Sung-Mo Moon, Yongsoo Jeong, and Inn-Kyu Kang. 2013. "Immobilization of pamidronic acids on the nanotube surface of titanium discs and their interaction with bone cells." *Nanoscale Research Letters* 8 (1):1–9.

Kumeria, Tushar, Htwe Mon, Moom Sinn Aw, Karan Gulati, Abel Santos, Hans J. Griesser, and Dusan Losic. 2015. "Advanced biopolymer-coated drug-releasing titania nanotubes (TNTs) implants with simultaneously enhanced osteoblast adhesion and antibacterial properties." *Colloids and Surfaces B: Biointerfaces* 130:255–263 doi: 10.1016/j.colsurfb.2015.04.021.

Lai, Min, Kaiyong Cai, Li Zhao, Xiuyong Chen, Yanhua Hou, and Zaixiang Yang. 2011. "Surface functionalization of TiO2 nanotubes with bone morphogenetic protein 2 and its synergistic effect on the differentiation of mesenchymal stem cells." *Biomacromolecules* 12 (4):1097–1105.

Lee, Sang Won, K. Scott Phillips, Huan Gu, Mehdi Kazemzadeh-Narbat, and Dacheng Ren. 2020. "How microbes read the map: Effects of implant topography on bacterial adhesion and biofilm formation." *Biomaterials* 268:120595.

Lee, Seung-Jae, Tae-Ju Oh, Tae-Sung Bae, Min-Ho Lee, Yunjo Soh, Byung-Il Kim, and Hyung Seop Kim. 2011. "Effect of bisphosphonates on anodized and heat-treated titanium surfaces: An animal experimental study." *Journal of Periodontology* 82 (7):1035–1042.

Lee, Young-Hee, Govinda Bhattarai, Il-Song Park, Ga-Ram Kim, Go-Eun Kim, Min-Ho Lee, and Ho-Keun Yi. 2013. "Bone regeneration around N-acetyl cysteine-loaded nanotube titanium dental implant in rat mandible." *Biomaterials* 34 (38):10199–10208.

Li, Ming, Qian Liu, Zhaojun Jia, Xuchen Xu, Yuying Shi, Yan Cheng, and Yufeng Zheng. 2015. "Polydopamine-induced nanocomposite Ag/CaP coatings on the surface of titania nanotubes for antibacterial and osteointegration functions." *Journal of Materials Chemistry B* 3 (45):8796–8805.

Li, Tao, Karan Gulati, Na Wang, Zhenting Zhang, and Sašo Ivanovski. 2018a. "Bridging the gap: Optimized fabrication of robust titania nanostructures on complex implant geometries towards clinical translation." *Journal of Colloid and Interface Science* 529:452–463 doi: 10.1016/j.jcis.2018.06.004.

Li, Tao, Karan Gulati, Na Wang, Zhenting Zhang, and Sašo Ivanovski. 2018b. "Understanding and augmenting the stability of therapeutic nanotubes on anodized titanium implants." *Materials Science and Engineering: C* 88:182–195 doi: 10.1016/j.msec.2018.03.007.

Liu, Xiangning, Xiaosong Zhou, Shaobing Li, Renfa Lai, Zhiying Zhou, Ye Zhang, and Lei Zhou. 2014. "Effects of titania nanotubes with or without bovine serum albumin loaded on human gingival fibroblasts." *International Journal of Nanomedicine* 9:1185.

Ma, Menghan, Mehdi Kazemzadeh-Narbat, Yu Hui, Shanshan Lu, Chuanfan Ding, David D.Y. Chen, Robert E.W. Hancock, and Rizhi Wang. 2012. "Local delivery of antimicrobial peptides using self-organized TiO_2 nanotube arrays for peri-implant infections." *Journal of Biomedical Materials Research Part A* 100 (2):278–285.

Ma, Qianli, Shenglin Mei, Kun Ji, Yumei Zhang, and Paul K Chu. 2011. "Immobilization of Ag nanoparticles/FGF-2 on a modified titanium implant surface and improved human gingival fibroblasts behavior." *Journal of Biomedical Materials Research Part A* 98 (2):274–286.

Martinez-Marquez, Daniel, Karan Gulati, Christopher P. Carty, Rodney A. Stewart, and Sašo Ivanovski. 2020. "Determining the relative importance of titania nanotubes characteristics on bone implant surface performance: A quality by design study with a fuzzy approach." *Materials Science and Engineering:* C 114:110995. doi: 10.1016/j.msec.2020.110995.

Mei, Shenglin, Huaiyu Wang, Wei Wang, Liping Tong, Haobo Pan, Changshun Ruan, Qianli Ma, Mengyuan Liu, Huiling Yang, and Liang Zhang. 2014. "Antibacterial effects and biocompatibility of titanium surfaces with graded silver incorporation in titania nanotubes." *Biomaterials* 35 (14):4255–4265.

Mirzaee, Majid, Mohammadreza Vaezi, and Yahya Palizdar. 2016. "Synthesis and characterization of silver doped hydroxyapatite nanocomposite coatings and evaluation of their antibacterial and corrosion resistance properties in simulated body fluid." *Materials Science and Engineering: C* 69:675–684.

Miura, Shingo, and Jun Takebe. 2012. "Biological behavior of fibroblast-like cells cultured on anodized-hydrothermally treated titanium with a nanotopographic surface structure." *Journal of Prosthodontic Research* 56 (3):178–186.

Miyata, Kyohei, and Jun Takebe. 2013. "Anodized-hydrothermally treated titanium with a nanotopographic surface structure regulates integrin-$\alpha6\beta4$ and laminin-5 gene expression in adherent murine gingival epithelial cells." *Journal of Prosthodontic Research* 57 (2):99–108.

Mokhtari, Hamidreza, Zahra Ghasemi, Mahshid Kharaziha, Fathollah Karimzadeh, and Farzaneh Alihosseini. 2018. "Chitosan-58S bioactive glass nanocomposite coatings on TiO_2 nanotube: Structural and biological properties." *Applied Surface Science* 441:138–149.

Neupane, Madhav Prasad, Il Song Park, Tae Sung Bae, Ho Keun Yi, Motohiro Uo, Fumio Watari, and Min Ho Lee. 2011. "Titania nanotubes supported gelatin stabilized gold nanoparticles for medical implants." *Journal of Materials Chemistry* 21 (32):12078–12082.

Oh, Seunghan, Kyung-Suk Moon, Joo-Hee Moon, Ji-Myung Bae, and Sungho Jin. 2013. "Visible light irradiation-mediated drug elution activity of nitrogen-doped TiO_2 nanotubes." *Journal of Nanomaterials* 2013. doi: 10.1155/2013/802318.

Pan, Changjiang, Youdong Hu, Zhihao Gong, Ya Yang, Sen Liu, Li Quan, Zhongmei Yang, Yanchun Wei, and Wei Ye. 2020. "Improved blood compatibility and endothelialization of titanium oxide nanotube arrays on titanium surface by zinc doping." *ACS Biomaterials Science & Engineering* 6 (4):2072–2083.

Pan, Changjiang, Tingting Liu, Ya Yang, Tao Liu, Zhihao Gong, Yanchun Wei, Li Quan, Zhongmei Yang, and Sen Liu. 2020. "Incorporation of Sr^{2+} and Ag nanoparticles into TiO_2 nanotubes to synergistically enhance osteogenic and antibacterial activities for bone repair." *Materials & Design* 196: 109086.

Pan, Changjiang, Tingting Liu, Ziqin Zhang, Xiaolei Zhang, Xinglong Qiao, Youdong Hu, Qiuyang Zhang, and Zhongmei Yang. 2021. "Preparation of chitosan-Zn^{2+} complex coating on polydopamine-modified TiO_2 nanotubes to enhance osteoblast behaviors." *Materials Letters* 282: 128665.

Park, Se Woong, Donghyun Lee, Yong Suk Choi, Hoon Bong Jeon, Chang-Hoon Lee, Ji-Hoi Moon, and Il Keun Kwon. 2014. "Mesoporous TiO_2 implants for loading high dosage of antibacterial agent." *Applied surface science* 303:140–146.

Pawlik, Anna, Magdalena Jarosz, Karolina Syrek, and Grzegorz D. Sulka. 2017. "Co-delivery of ibuprofen and gentamicin from nanoporous anodic titanium dioxide layers." *Colloids and Surfaces B: Biointerfaces* 152: 95–102.

Popat, Ketul C, Matthew Eltgroth, Thomas J. LaTempa, Craig A. Grimes, and Tejal A. Desai. 2007. "Decreased Staphylococcus epidermis adhesion and increased osteoblast functionality on antibiotic-loaded titania nanotubes." *Biomaterials* 28 (32):4880–4888.

Quarterman, Juliana C., Sean M. Geary, and Aliasger K. Salem. 2021. "Evolution of drug-eluting biomedical implants for sustained drug delivery." *European Journal of Pharmaceutics and Biopharmaceutics* 159:21–35. doi: 10.1016/j.ejpb.2020.12.005.

Rahman, Shafiur, Karan Gulati, Masakazu Kogawa, Gerald J. Atkins, Peter Pivonka, David M. Findlay, and Dusan Losic. 2016. "Drug diffusion, integration, and stability of nanoengineered drug-releasing implants in bone ex-vivo." *Journal of Biomedical Materials Research Part A* 104 (3):714–725. doi: 10.1002/jbm.a.35595.

Roguska, Agata, Anna Belcarz, Justyna Zalewska, Marcin Hołdyński, Mariusz Andrzejczuk, Marcin Pisarek, and Grazyna Ginalska. 2018. "Metal TiO_2 nanotube layers for the treatment of dental implant infections." *ACS Applied Materials & Interfaces* 10 (20):17089–17099.

Roy, Poulomi, Steffen Berger, and Patrik Schmuki. 2011. "TiO_2 nanotubes: Synthesis and applications." *Angewandte Chemie International Edition* 50 (13):2904–2939.

Roy, Poulomi, Doohun Kim, Kiyoung Lee, Erdmann Spiecker, and Patrik Schmuki. 2010. "TiO_2 nanotubes and their application in dye-sensitized solar cells." *Nanoscale* 2 (1):45–59.

Sabella, Stefania, Randy P. Carney, Virgilio Brunetti, Maria Ada Malvindi, Noura Al-Juffali, Giuseppe Vecchio, Sam M. Janes, Osman M. Bakr, Roberto Cingolani, and Francesco Stellacci. 2014. "A general mechanism for intracellular toxicity of metal-containing nanoparticles." *Nanoscale* 6 (12):7052–7061.

Saji, Viswanathan S., Tushar Kumeria, Karan Gulati, Matthew Prideaux, Shafiur Rahman, Mohammed Alsawat, Abel Santos, Gerald J. Atkins, and Dusan Losic. 2015. "Localized drug delivery of selenium (Se) using nanoporous anodic aluminium oxide for bone implants." *Journal of Materials Chemistry B* 3 (35):7090–7098. doi: 10.1039/C5TB00125K.

Shen, Xinkun, Pingping Ma, Yan Hu, Gaoqiang Xu, Kui Xu, Weizhen Chen, Qichun Ran, Liangliang Dai, Yonglin Yu, and Caiyun Mu. 2016. "Alendronate-loaded hydroxyapatite-TiO 2 nanotubes for improved bone formation in osteoporotic rabbits." *Journal of Materials Chemistry B* 4 (8):1423–1436.

Shi, Xiaowen, Huiping Wu, Yuanyuan Li, Xiaoquan Wei, and Yumin Du. 2013. "Electrical signals guided entrapment and controlled release of antibiotics on titanium surface." *Journal of Biomedical Materials Research Part A* 101 (5):1373–1378.

Shrestha, Nabeen K., Jan M. Macak, Felix Schmidt-Stein, Robert Hahn, Claudia T. Mierke, Ben Fabry, and Patrik Schmuki. 2009. "Magnetically guided titania nanotubes for site-selective photocatalysis and drug release." *Angewandte Chemie International Edition* 48 (5):969–972.

Sirivisoot, Sirinrath, Rajesh Pareta, and Thomas J. Webster. 2011. "Electrically controlled drug release from nanostructured polypyrrole coated on titanium." *Nanotechnology* 22 (8):085101.

Sopchenski, L., S. Cogo, M.F. Dias-Ntipanyj, S. Elifio-Espósito, K.C. Popat, and P. Soares. 2018. "Bioactive and antibacterial boron doped TiO_2 coating obtained by PEO." *Applied Surface Science* 458:49–58.

Sun, Shengjun, Weiqiang Yu, Yilin Zhang, and Fuqiang Zhang. 2013. "Increased preosteoblast adhesion and osteogenic gene expression on TiO_2 nanotubes modified with KRSR." *Journal of Materials Science: Materials in Medicine* 24 (4):1079–1091.

Takebe, J., K. Miyata, S. Miura, and S. Ito. 2014. "Effects of the nanotopographic surface structure of commercially pure titanium following anodization–hydrothermal treatment on gene expression and adhesion in gingival epithelial cells." *Materials Science and Engineering: C* 42:273–279.

Tan, Jing, Chanjuan Zhao, Jie Zhou, Ke Duan, Jianxin Wang, Xiong Lu, Jie Weng, and Bo Feng. 2017. "Co-culturing epidermal keratinocytes and dermal fibroblasts on nano-structured titanium surfaces." *Materials Science and Engineering: C* 78:288–295.

Trajkovski, Branko, Ansgar Petersen, Patrick Strube, Manav Mehta, and Georg N. Duda. 2012. "Intra-operatively customized implant coating strategies for local and controlled drug delivery to bone." *Advanced Drug Delivery Reviews* 64 (12):1142–1151. doi: 10.1016/j.addr.2012.05.016.

Ungureanu, Camelia, Cristina Dumitriu, Simona Popescu, Monica Enculescu, Vlad Tofan, Marian Popescu, and Cristian Pirvu. 2016. "Enhancing antimicrobial activity of TiO_2/Ti by torularhodin bioinspired surface modification." *Bioelectrochemistry* 107:14–24.

Vasconcelos, Daniel M., Susana G. Santos, Meriem Lamghari, and Mário A. Barbosa. 2016. "The two faces of metal ions: From implants rejection to tissue repair/regeneration." *Biomaterials* 84: 262–275.

Vo, Tiffany N., F. Kurtis Kasper, and Antonios G. Mikos. 2012. "Strategies for controlled delivery of growth factors and cells for bone regeneration." *Advanced Drug Delivery Reviews* 64 (12):1292–1309.

Wang, Cunyang, Yu Bai, Yulong Bai, Jingjun Gao, and Wen Ma. 2016. "Enhancement of corrosion resistance and bioactivity of titanium by Au nanoparticle-loaded TiO_2 nanotube layer." *Surface and Coatings Technology* 286:327–334.

Wang, Guomin, Hongqing Feng, Ang Gao, Qi Hao, Weihong Jin, Xiang Peng, Wan Li, Guosong Wu, and Paul K. Chu. 2016. "Extracellular electron transfer from aerobic bacteria to Au-loaded TiO_2 semiconductor without light: A new bacteria-killing mechanism other than localized surface plasmon resonance or microbial fuel cells." *ACS Applied Materials & Interfaces* 8 (37):24509–24516.

Wang, Zhang, Chunlin Xie, Fei Luo, Ping Li, and Xiufeng Xiao. 2015. "P25 nanoparticles decorated on titania nanotubes arrays as effective drug delivery system for ibuprofen." *Applied Surface Science* 324:621–626. doi: 10.1016/j.apsusc.2014.10.147.

Xiang, Yiming, Xinmei Liu, Congyang Mao, Xiangmei Liu, Zhenduo Cui, Xianjin Yang, Kelvin W.K. Yeung, Yufeng Zheng, and Shuilin Wu. 2018. "Infection-prevention on Ti implants by controlled drug release from folic acid/ZnO quantum dots sealed titania nanotubes." *Materials Science and Engineering: C* 85: 214–224.

Xiao, J., H. Zhou, L. Zhao, Y. Sun, S. Guan, B. Liu, and L. Kong. 2011. "The effect of hierarchical micro/nanosurface titanium implant on osseointegration in ovariectomized sheep." *Osteoporosis International* 22 (6):1907–1913.

Xiao, XiLin, LiXia Yang, ManLi Guo, ChunFeng Pan, QingYun Cai, and ShouZhuo Yao. 2009. "Biocompatibility and in vitro antineoplastic drug-loaded trial of titania nanotubes prepared by anodic oxidation of a pure titanium." *Science in China Series B: Chemistry* 52 (12):2161.

Xu, Jingwen, Xuemei Zhou, Zhida Gao, Yan-Yan Song, and Patrik Schmuki. 2016. "Visible-light-triggered drug release from TiO_2 nanotube arrays: A controllable antibacterial platform." *Angewandte Chemie* 128 (2):603–607.

Xu, Wenzhou, Manlin Qi, Xue Li, Xuxu Liu, Lin Wang, Wanqi Yu, Min Liu, A. Lan, Yanmin Zhou, and Yanyan Song. 2019. "TiO_2 nanotubes modified with Au nanoparticles for visible-light enhanced antibacterial and anti-inflammatory capabilities." *Journal of Electroanalytical Chemistry* 842: 66–73.

Yu, Yonglin, Qichun Ran, Xinkun Shen, Hong Zheng, and Kaiyong Cai. 2020. "Enzyme responsive titanium substrates with antibacterial property and osteo/angio-genic differentiation potentials." *Colloids and Surfaces B: Biointerfaces* 185: 110592.

Yuan, Zhang, Suzhou Huang, Shaoxiong Lan, Haizhou Xiong, Bailong Tao, Yao Ding, Yisi Liu, Peng Liu, and Kaiyong Cai. 2018. "Surface engineering of titanium implants with enzyme-triggered antibacterial properties and enhanced osseointegration in vivo." *Journal of Materials Chemistry B* 6 (48):8090–8104.

Zhang, Erlin, Xiaotong Zhao, Jiali Hu, Ruoxian Wang, Shan Fu, and Gaowu Qin. 2021. "Antibacterial metals and alloys for potential biomedical implants." *Bioactive Materials* 6 (8):2569–2612.

Zhang, Xiangyu, Jianfang Li, Xin Wang, Yueyue Wang, Ruiqiang Hang, Xiaobo Huang, Bin Tang, and Paul K. Chu. 2018. "Effects of copper nanoparticles in porous TiO_2 coatings on bacterial resistance and cytocompatibility of osteoblasts and endothelial cells." *Materials Science and Engineering: C* 82: 110–120.

Zhang, Xuejiao, Yong Huang, Bingbing Wang, Xiaotong Chang, Hao Yang, Jinping Lan, Saisai Wang, Haixia Qiao, He Lin, and Shuguang Han. 2020. "A functionalized Sm/Sr doped TiO_2 nanotube array on titanium implant enables exceptional bone-implant integration and also self-antibacterial activity." *Ceramics International* 46 (10):14796–14807.

Zhang, Xuejiao, Xiaolei Zhang, Bingbing Wang, Jinping Lan, Hao Yang, Zhenhui Wang, Xiaotong Chang, Saisai Wang, Xinchao Ma, and Haixia Qiao. 2020. "Synergistic effects of lanthanum and strontium to enhance the osteogenic activity of TiO_2 nanotube biological interface." *Ceramics International* 46 (9):13969–13979.

Zhang, Yanli, Liangjiao Chen, Chundong Liu, Xiaoli Feng, Limin Wei, and Longquan Shao. 2016. "Self-assembly chitosan/gelatin composite coating on icariin-modified TiO_2 nanotubes for the regulation of osteoblast bioactivity." *Materials & Design* 92:471–479.

Zhang, Yanni, Kun Wang, Yang Song, Enping Feng, Kai Dong, Yong Han, and Tingli Lu. 2020. "Ca substitution of Sr in Sr-doped TiO_2 nanotube film on Ti surface for enhanced osteogenic activity." *Applied Surface Science* 528: 147055.

Zhang, Yifan, Karan Gulati, Ze Li, Ping Di, and Yan Liu. 2021. "Dental implant nano-engineering: Advances, limitations and future directions." *Nanomaterials* 11 (10):2489.

Zhao, Lingzhou, Hairong Wang, Kaifu Huo, Xuming Zhang, Wei Wang, Yumei Zhang, Zhifen Wu, and Paul K. Chu. 2013. "The osteogenic activity of strontium loaded titania nanotube arrays on titanium substrates." *Biomaterials* 34 (1):19–29.

Zhou, Juncen, Micael Alonso Frank, Yuyun Yang, Aldo R. Boccaccini, and Sannakaisa Virtanen. 2018. "A novel local drug delivery system: Superhydrophobic titanium oxide nanotube arrays serve as the drug reservoir and ultrasonication functions as the drug release trigger." *Materials Science and Engineering: C* 82: 277–283.

Zong, Mingxiang, Long Bai, Yanlian Liu, Xin Wang, Xiangyu Zhang, Xiaobo Huang, Ruiqiang Hang, and Bin Tang. 2017. "Antibacterial ability and angiogenic activity of Cu-Ti-O nanotube arrays." *Materials Science and Engineering: C* 71:93–99.

Chapter 11

Porous Silicon for Drug Delivery Applications

Ganesh Kokil, Ayad Saeed, Astha Sharma, and Tushar Kumeria

University of New South Wales

CONTENTS

LIST OF ABBREVIATIONS

APTS: 3-Aminopropyltriethoxysilane
CA IX: Carbonic anhydrase IX
Caco-2: Colon epithelial cells
DHC: Dehydrocoupling
DOX: Doxorubicin
Fe_3O_4: Iron oxide
GBM: Glioblastoma multiforme
GOPS: 3-Glycidoxypropyltrimethoxysilane
HF: Hydrofluoric acid

DOI: 10.1201/9781003217114-14

HT29:	Human colorectal adenocarcinoma
KOH:	Potassium hydroxide
MCF-7:	Human breast adenocarcinoma
MDR:	Multidrug-resistant
NPs:	Nanoparticles
pSi:	Porous silicon
Tf:	Transferrin
VEGF:	Vascular endothelial growth factor

11.1 INTRODUCTION

The search for an ideal ubiquitous system that simultaneously diagnoses, achieves targeted drug delivery, and amends the ailment affected organs are primary goals of current nanomedicine-based technologies (Patra et al. 2018; Mitchell et al. 2021). These drug delivery systems utilize nanometer-scale particles as drug carriers with different shapes and geometries, which ideally need to deliver the cargo to the target site in a controlled manner (Mitchell et al. 2021). Most importantly, achieving target selectivity and preventing off-targeted side effects are key objectives of these nanocarriers (Sousa et al. 2019). In contrast, traditional drug delivery systems have inherent shortfalls such as selectivity, biodistribution, and solubility (Edgar and Wang 2017), which can be rectified using properly designed nanocarrier systems.

Moreover, the cutting-edge notion of nanomedicine does not allow to restrict these platforms merely for drug delivery applications but can offer more sophisticated forms with diagnostic setup within these carrier systems (Ingle et al. 2020). These innovative interventions have widened the opportunities to treat, diagnose, and monitor the progress of disease treatment simultaneously using the same nanocarrier platform. Various nanomedicine systems with such capabilities were developed consisting of polymers (Sung and Kim 2020), micelles (Trinh et al. 2017), liposomes (Sercombe et al. 2015), and nanoparticles (Baetke, Lammers, and Kiessling 2015). Mostly these systems are loaded with drugs and imaging agents together to enable therapeutic and diagnosis applications simultaneously. Nevertheless, a few of these nanocarriers due to their physicochemical properties consist of inherent abilities which can be utilized as diagnostic tools without including any supplementary agents. One of these dual-purpose platforms, porous silicon (pSi) is counted as an exceptional material owing to its distinctive physical and chemical properties, which include precise tuning of geometric topographies, surface chemistry, and high porosity (Kumeria et al. 2017).

pSi was first fabricated by the Uhlirs in 1956 at the Bell Laboratories using the electrochemical etching method (Uhlir Jr. 1956). Subsequently, Gösele and Canham demonstrated the quantum confinement effects within pSi structures, which paved the way to extend their applications in optoelectronics (Canham 1990; Lehmann and Gösele 1991). Furthermore, Canham revealed the modular biocompatible and biodegradable characteristics of pSi films based on their degree of porosity and size of pores (micro, meso, and macro) (Li et al. 2003). This research work pioneered the use of pSi in drug delivery applications and facilitated novel prospects to utilize this material in the biomedical field. It was also shown that pSi-based nanoparticles can be utilized for time-gated imaging applications (Gu et al. 2013; Secret et al. 2014; Joo et al. 2015). Due to its potential as a nanocarrier system, some companies started the commercial production of pSi-based nanomedicines for clinical applications. That said, this clinical translation of pSi is not without technical and commercial challenges, which needed extensive clinical trials and a comprehensive long-term investigation. Thus, pSi as a nanocarrier needs systematic development through big pharma company's collaborations and patience.

The pSi demonstrates various favorable properties that make it an ideal candidate as a drug delivery carrier. The fabrication of pSi using electrochemical synthesis allows the tunable pore sizes and volumes, from nanometers to microns. Various convenient methods are available to modify pSi surface chemistries that can be utilized to control the drug loading amount as well as in vivo release profile. Additionally, pSi can be used as a template for organic and biopolymers for composite preparations with a defined nanostructure. Furthermore, the optical properties of pSi photonic structures provide an additional advantage of self-reporting features in in vivo drug delivery monitoring system.

Thus, this chapter focused on the current developments in pSi-based drug delivery systems with an overview on the fabrication, surface chemical properties, and drug delivery applications.

11.2 FABRICATION OF POROUS SILICON (pSi)

The most common method to fabricate porous silicon for biomedical applications is anodic etching (Sailor 2012). Here, the pSi is synthesized by etching crystalline silicon wafers in aqueous hydrofluoric acid (HF) solutions. *Important note: HF is a highly corrosive and toxic acid, and hence any exposure to it should be avoided at all costs.* Generally, the reaction is carried out as a two-electrode electrochemical reaction under galvanostatic control, where the Si wafer acts as the anode, and the platinum wire as the cathode (Figure 11.1), in the presence of fluoride ions. The oxidized Si atoms are removed off the surface as SiF_4 or SiF_6^{2-} (equations 11.1 and 11.2). Additionally, this production technique allows pSi to be formed into a variety of shapes and sizes, including films, microparticles, and nanoparticles.

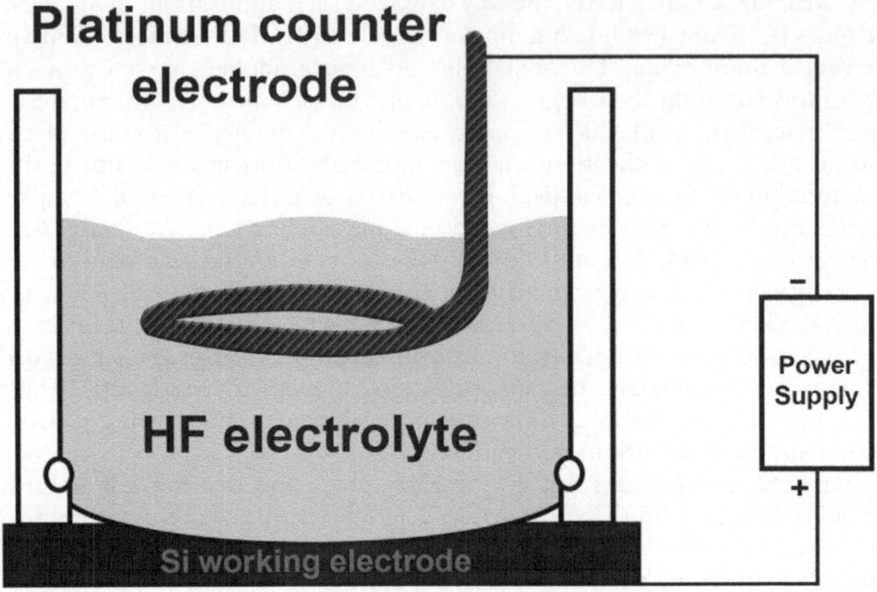

Figure 11.1 Schematic of a two-electrode electrochemical cell used to fabricate pSi. The silicon wafer is the working electrode (anode) where the oxidation reaction is happening, while the platinum electrode is the counter-electrode (cathode) where the reduction reaction occurs.

During the two-electron electrochemical etching process in ethanolic HF (equation 11.1), silicon dissolves selectively in the (100) direction, resulting in pores that are perpendicular to the wafer face (Loni 2014; Uhlir Jr 1956; Unagami 1980).

$$Si + 6F^- + 2H^+ + 2h^+ SiF_6^{2-} + H_2 \tag{11.1}$$

The silicon film can be removed by electropolishing with a simple 4-electron process represented by equation 11.2, which completely dissolves the bulk-to-porous silicon interface without generating pores.

$$Si + 6F^- + 4h^+ SiF_6^{2-} \tag{11.2}$$

These films can be utilized as implants or broken down into micro/nanoparticles for injectable delivery vehicles that could act as a depot for the delivery of specific drugs.

The fabrication conditions have a significant impact on the pore structure of pSi. For instance, in electrochemical etching, parameters such as the type of Si wafer, HF concentration, and current density determine the shape and size of pores (Lehmann, Stengl, and Luigart 2000; Salonen et al. 2008; Salonen and Lehto 2008; Zhang 2003). The pore diameter can be simply modified to meet the desired properties because it can be regulated by several parameters. The size of the pores is influenced by many parameters including the substrate's resistivity, doping type, current density, and etching solution composition (Canham 2014). Higher current densities result in wider and more linear pores and higher porosity, up to the point where the surface is electropolished (Zhang 2003), while using lower current densities the pores are more tortuous, fir tree, or sponge-like.

The synthesis of pSi is based on a top-down method, wherein size-controlled nanoparticles are generated via mechanical size reduction using ultrasonication or milling (A Santos et al. 2011). The particles are subsequently size-selected using filtration (Park et al. 2009) or differential sedimentation in a centrifuge technique (Santos et al. 2010). In an attempt to generate larger quantities of size-controlled pSi NPs, mechanical comminution of a free-standing pSi film was performed. This pSi film was generated with high porosity perforation layers that specifically fracture during the ultrasonic milling proces (Qin et al. 2014).

During the etching process, high-current density pulses are delivered at regular intervals, forming a porous multilayer separated by thin layers of even higher porosity (Qin et al. 2014). The porous film is preferentially cleaved at these high-porosity perforations employing ultrasonic fracturing, resulting in superior size control, and yielded pSi NPs in 160–350 nm range (Qin et al. 2014). pSi for drug delivery applications typically has mesoporous (2–50 nm) sizes (Anglin et al. 2008; Lehto et al. 2013; Liu, Bimbo, et al. 2013; Liu, Mäkilä, et al. 2013; Salonen et al. 2005; Tahvanainen et al. 2012).

11.3 SURFACE CHEMISTRY OF pSi AND THEIR STABILITY THROUGH CHEMICAL MODIFICATION

Biosensing is normally achieved in an aqueous environment, and it is a prerequisite that the sensor used for this application is chemically stable. The major bottleneck of pSi nanostructures is their degradation, initiated immediately after the etching process (Figure 11.2) (Kang et al. 2019). The underlying reason for their degradation is the highly reactive and unstable hydride (Si–Hx, $x=1$, 2, or 3) pores of freshly etched pSi wafer, which is susceptible to oxidation and hydrolysis (Dhanekar and Jain 2013; Sailor 2012; Salonel and Mäkilä 2021). During aging, the pore walls with Si-H bonds are replaced by their respective oxides and are responsible for

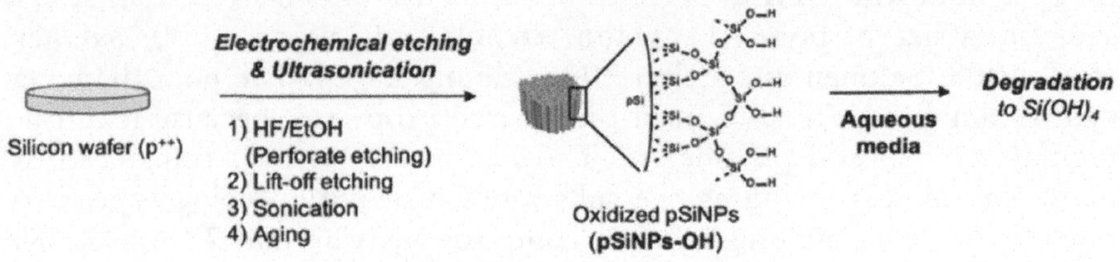

Figure 11.2 Degradation of freshly etched pSi through oxidation reaction (Kang et al. 2019).

amorphous silicon impurity deposition (Canham et al. 1991). These impurities can be challenging to resolve while utilizing the pSi nanostructures for any intended applications.

Surface chemistry plays an important role not only in pSi nanostructure stability but also for biomolecule immobilization and degradation profile. Thus, suitable surface chemical modifications are essential for minimizing the aging and maintaining the integrity of pSi nanostructures. These surface chemical modifications of pSi thin film can be achieved before or after particle size reduction within the dispersion medium or using chemical modifications such as carbonization, hydrosilylation (Si–C), and hydrolytic condensation using organotrialkoxysilane reagents (Si–O–Si) (Figure 11.3). These modifications resulted in hydrophobic or charged surfaces with enhanced stability and therapeutic payload efficiency (Tieu, Dhawan, et al. 2019).

11.4 FORMATION OF SILICON–CARBON BOND

Over the past two decades, various chemical and electrochemical approaches to convert the Si–H_x to Si–C bonds have been reported (Gooding and Ciampi 2011). The silicon–carbon (Si–C) bond formed provides a highly stable coating on pSi surface, thus preventing its degradation. This protective covering can be attributed to the carbon atom's low electronegativity with higher kinetic stability compared to silicon-oxygen (Si–O) bond (Buriak 2002). The methods to convert Si–H_x to Si–C bond are referred to as hydrosilylation and carbonization.

11.4.1 Hydrosilylation

Hydrosilylation (Figure 11.3) involves the reaction of unsaturated organic compounds such as alkenes or alkynes to reactive Si–H_x surface to yield Si–C bond. This process is regarded as the most efficient method to stabilize pSi surfaces (Sweetman et al. 2015). This reaction can be catalyst initiated,

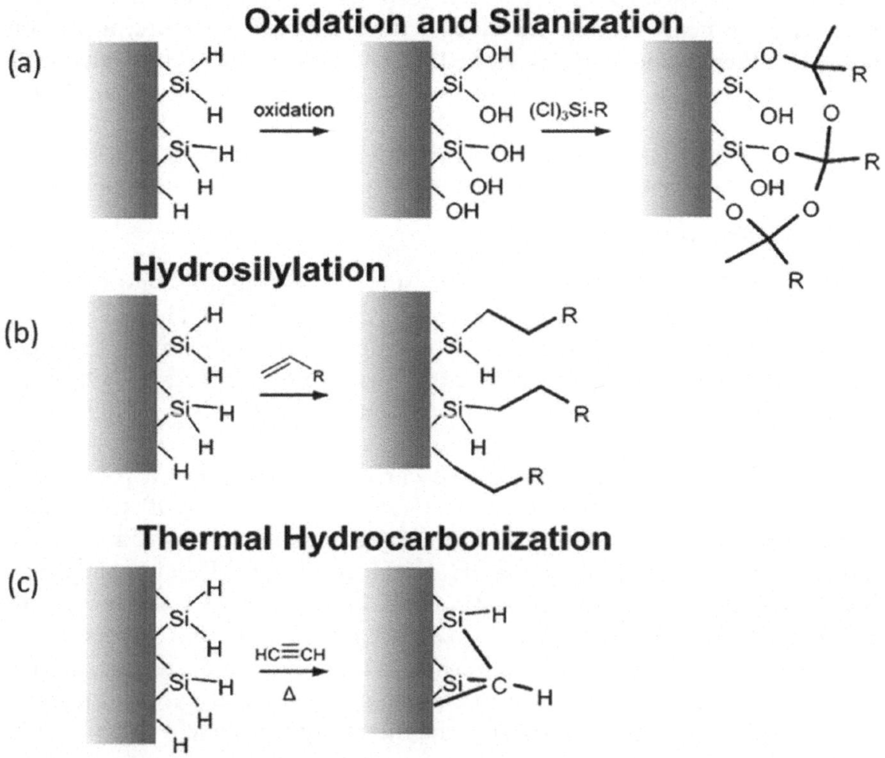

Figure 11.3 A schematic representation showing different strategies to prevent pSi surface degradation (a) oxidation followed by silanization, (b) hydrosilylation, and (c) thermal hydrocarbonization. (Adapted from Park et al. 2019.)

or other factors such as light (Stewart and Buriak 2001), heat (Boukherroub et al. 2002), and electro-grafting (Robins, Stewart, and Buriak 1999) are additional ways to initiate this process. Furthermore, these reactions allow incorporation of a wide range of chemical functional groups onto the pSi surface like thiols (-SH), alcohols (-OH), polyethylene glycols, esters (-COOR), and carboxylic acids (-COOH), which can be further customized into desired modification of interest (Britcher et al. 2008; Schmeltzer et al. 2002). Buriak et al. first reported the hydrosilylation reaction on pSi surface (Buriak et al. 1999). Subsequently, several works have been reported on Si–C bond formation using chemical, thermal, and metal catalyst-based reactions. Of these various reported methods, thermal hydrosilylation is comparatively modest strategy for embedding an extensive variety of functional groups onto pSi surface with 80% or more efficiency proportionate to the available Si–H_x bonds (Hua, Swihart, and Ruckenstein 2005). Consequently, the monolayers produced via thermal hydrosilylation demonstrated stable pSi nanostructure in both physiological and harsh basic environments for the duration of the study. Furthermore, using this method, alkenes and alkynes with different functional groups have been used to attach various biomolecules such as nucleic acids (Lie et al. 2004), antibodies, amino acids (Sam et al. 2010), peptides, enzymes (Kermad et al. 2013), and proteins (Sweetman, Graney, and Voelcker 2007).

11.4.2 Carbonization

Other than hydrosilylation, the formation of Si–C bond for preventing degradation can be achieved using carbonization (Figure 11.3). There are three basic approaches utilizing gaseous, liquid, and solid carbon sources to accomplish satisfactory thermal carbonization of pSi surfaces. Of these, a gas-phase carbon source such as acetylene is frequently used due to its compact, fast diffusing, and powerful physisorbed characteristics (Cheng et al. 1993). Salonen et al. pioneered carbon-stabilization on pSi surface through thermal decomposition of acetylene gas at 600°C–900°C (Salonen et al. 2000). This resulted in a thin protective coating on pSi surface even in harsh acidic (HF) or alkaline (NaOH, KOH) conditions (Delalat, Sheppard, Rasi Ghaemi, et al. 2015; Kim, Zuidema, et al. 2016). Furthermore, this modification was found to be non-toxic in in vitro and in vivo applications (Krueger et al. 2016). Most importantly, carbon-stabilized pSi surfaces retain their distinctive characteristics such as high surface area, adjustable pore morphology, versatile surface chemistry, and provide an appropriate optical platform for sensing.

11.4.3 Dehydrogenative Coupling (DHC)

DHC is the process of creating a bond between two molecules by dihydrogen elimination. This reaction has demonstrated to be effective in molecular chemistry using group 14 elements of the periodic table, where the M–M bond is formed during the reaction between two M–H (e.g., M=Si) species, resulting in the release of hydrogen gas (Melen 2016; Waterman 2013). Thus, DHC reaction has been employed to modify group 14 semiconductor surfaces at both the bulk and nanoscale ranges. Li et al. utilized the DHC reaction catalyzed by zirconocene and titanocene to introduce arylsilanes or alkylsilanes into H-terminated silicon wafers and pSi surfaces (Li and Buriak 2006). Based on prior research, Wilkinson's catalyst chloridotris(-triphenylphosphine)rhodium(I) [$(PPh_3)_3RhCl$] was used to extend DHC to reactions of alkylsilanes with H-terminated SiNPs. Although surface modification was achievable, the method's applicability was limited due to the loss of the material's optical properties (Zhenyu, H., and G.C. 2014). The catalytically DHC chemistry of hydrogen-terminated Si surfaces was originally reported by Buriak, Veinot, and coworkers (Purkait et al. 2014; Li and Buriak 2006). Although it worked effectively, the extremely reactive catalysts caused undesirable oxidative side reactions, and the chemistry was difficult to employ due to limited availability. As an alternative method to hydrosilylation, DHC using a hydridosilane (R-SiH_3) instead of alkene ($RCH=CH_2$) was utilized to minimize the oxidative side reactions of Si–H with trace oxygen and water as shown in Figure 11.4 (Kim, Joo, et al. 2016). In the thermally driven silane dehydrocoupling chemistry, the reaction takes place on the pSi NPs surfaces at mild temperatures (80°C) with no additional catalyst or reactant solvent. The non-catalyzed dehydrogenative coupling of organosilanes to a wide range of substrates, particularly silicon has been successfully reported (Arkles et al. 2012). Dokyoung et al. have found out that this reaction occurs without the need for a catalyst, resulting

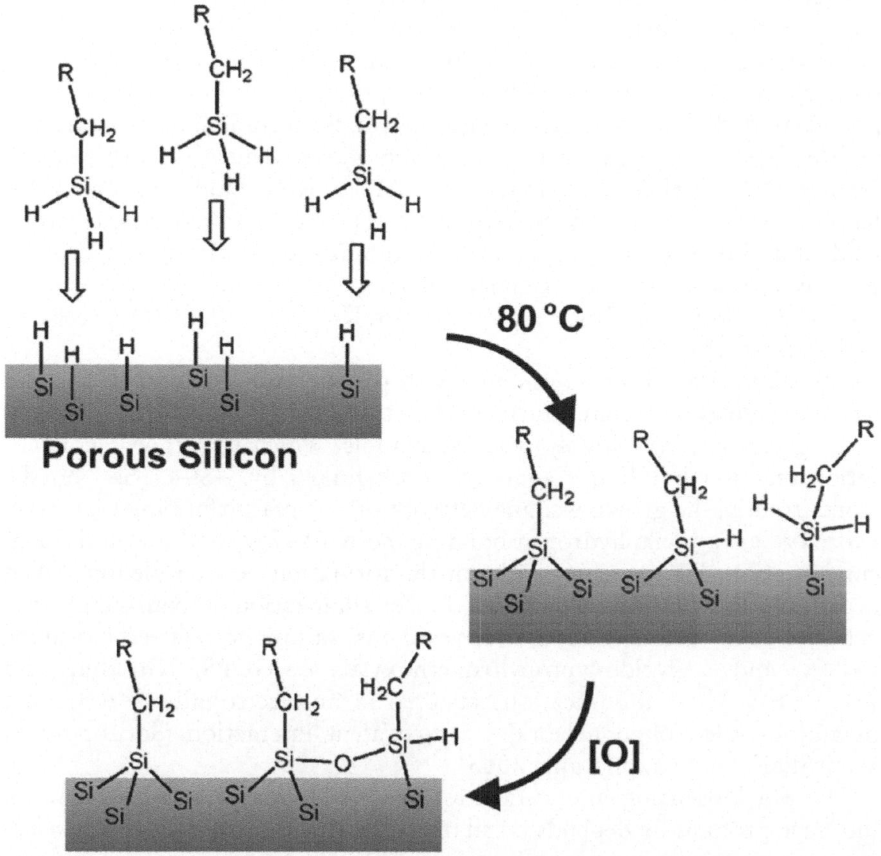

Figure 11.4 Proposed suggested dehydrogenative coupling mechanisms between trihydridosilanes and hydrogenated silicon in the presence of air. (Adapted from Kim, Joo, et al. 2016.)

in long-term functional coatings with minimal oxidation and degradation of the original Si–H surface's electronic quality. Additionally, this coupling reaction was also successfully utilized to graft functional hydridosilanes with terminal groups such as alkene, bromo, and perfluorocarbon, demonstrating the surface-binding molecule is functional group tolerant. Even though the dehydrocoupling reaction can occur on pSi NPs, the hydrophobicity of the resulting nanoparticles hampered further investigation. In another research work, Hyeon and his group introduced this method on pSi NPs and investigated drug release profiles (Oh et al. 2021).

11.4.4 Silanization

Among all surface modifications, silanization is the most common derivatization on silicon-based substrates. Conventionally, it needs incorporation of hydroxide layer through oxidizing the silicon surface. Subsequently, these modifications proceed via silanol-based conjugation with chloro- or alkoxysilane-based compounds. Several chemical compounds with distinctive functional groups can be decorated on pre-oxidized hydroxyl-terminated pSi surface including polyethylene glycol, thiols, and amines (Delalat, Sheppard, Ghaemi, et al. 2015; Kim, Zuidema, et al. 2016; Krueger et al. 2016). Different methods of silanization have been extensively studied and demonstrated that surface stabilization is vital for enhancing pSi low chemical stability (Delalat, Sheppard, Ghaemi, et al. 2015; Kim, Joo, et al. 2016; Kim, Zuidema, et al. 2016; Krueger et al. 2016; Sweetman and Voelcker 2012).

The silanization process initiates with pSi surface oxidation to create a hydroxyl group terminated surfaces. Next, the water-hydrolyzed alkoxysilane species generate highly reactive silanols, which undergoe a condensation reaction building a silane network linked by (–Si–O–Si–) bonds. Concurrently, the growing silane network on the pSi surface interacts with hydroxyl group via hydrogen-bonding network followed by additional condensation. Finally, this results in the formation of a covalently linked organosilane layer (Hermanson 2013). The silanization of oxidized pSi was achieved using various silane derivatives like as 3-aminopropyltriethoxysilane (APTS) and 3-glycidoxypropyltrimethoxysilane (GOPS) (Gooding and Zhu 2014). These modifications resulted in an electrophilic reactive site of amino-ended oligonucleotides for covalent interaction (Sotiropoulou, Vamvakaki, and Chaniotakis 2005).

The pSi biosensing application for the development of biorecognition interface profoundly depends on silane chemistry. Most importantly, selective recognition of species of interest while preventing unwanted interaction with other molecules is one of the key features of such an interface. Sailor et al., in their initial work, explored alkyl silanization surface chemistry in interferometric detection of DNA and protein/DNA for biosensing application (Lin et al. 1997). These modification methods are now widely used for enzymes, DNA, antibodies, and small molecules immobilization on pSi surface for a wide range of biological applications (Ouyang et al. 2005).

11.5 DRUG DELIVERY APPLICATIONS

Drug formulation and the corresponding physicochemical characteristics of a given route of administration play a significant role in therapeutic efficacy and short- or long-term biological effects. The main challenges in drug formulation are poor dissolution/ solubility, poor solid state stability, and poor pharmacokinetic properties of the drug molecules (Kalepu and Nekkanti 2016; Gala, Miller, and Williams III 2020). With the plenty of weekly soluble drug contenders currently under exploration in the drug expansion pipeline, there is a substantial imperative to advance methodologies to control and enhance their in vivo behavior. Thus, enhancement in the current therapeutical strategies is needed to improve the delivery of poorly water-soluble active pharmaceutical ingredients. pSi is one of the materials which can be easily incorporated and utilized as nanomedicine for antimicrobial activity (Kargupta et al. 2014), gene therapy (Kang et al. 2016), targeted chemotherapy (Li et al. 2018), wound healing (Jin et al. 2021), and even combination therapies (Xia et al. 2019). The pSi was used for effective controlled release and localized therapeutic effect, offering increased efficacy with fewer side effects. In addition, the high porous nature of pSi was convenient for surface modifications and can be used for the purpose of diagnostics and therapeutic cargo payload via covalent attachment, physical trapping, or adsorption. The surface can thus be modulated as hydrophilic, hydrophobic, or amphiphilic and can help in determining the amount of drug loading and its released. Hydrophobic molecules such as dexamethasone (Anglin et al. 2004) or hydrophilic molecules such as serum albumin (Tay et al. 2004) can be loaded into these nanostructures. By integrating the drug molecules with the pSi particles, the drug is provided with efficient protection against premature degradation of the drug, while upholding the complete regulation over the drug release. This flexibility is important for the desirable and controlled approach for the biological and therapeutic profiles, such as the bioavailability, pharmacokinetics, and tissue distribution, of drug molecules (Santos et al. 2014). Liu et al. coloaded a hydrophobic drug (IMC) and a hydrophilic peptide (PYY3–36) onto pSi NPs. Sequential loading of these two drugs onto the pSi NPs enhanced the drug release rate and also their amount permeated across Caco-2 (colon epithelial cells) and Caco-2/HT29 (colon epithelial cells/ human colorectal adenocarcinoma) cell monolayers. Conformational analysis specified that the PYY3–36 displayed biological activity after release from the pSi NPs and permeation across the intestinal cell monolayers. Thus, demonstrating the potential for synchronized multi-drug delivery of both hydrophobic and hydrophilic compounds (Liu, Bimbo, et al. 2013). The amount of loaded drug into a pSi microparticle is relatively large due to its large free volume (Thomas, Pacholski, and Sailor 2006). Thus, higher drug doses can be incorporated within well-defined architecture allowing reproducible loading and release of precise quantities (Park et al. 2007).

During the dissolution process, silicic acid is generated and participates in sol–gel reactions. Common ions such as Ca^{2+} and Mg^{2+} usually participate in the silicate precipitation reaction process and act as bioactive material (Kokubo, Kim, and Kawashita 2003; Saravanapavan and Hench 2003; Salinas, Vallet-Regi, and Izquierdo-Barba 2001). Additionally, hybrid materials using organic polymers, or a biopolymer combination, can also serve as effective composites for drug delivery (Soppimath et al. 2001). Due to the combination of two or more chemical entities, they greatly expand the design of the delivery system (Polarz and Antonietti 2002). Templates with micro-mesoporous membranes, zeolites, and crystalline colloidal arrays were mainly useful in electronic, mechanical, and optical structures (Wirtz et al. 2002; C. Hulteen and Martin 1997; Moller and Bein 1998; Xu, Majetich, and Asher 2002). This also assists in tuning the porosity and pore size of the nanostructures (Kordás et al. 2004). This characteristic is advantageous in improving the mechanical stability and controlling the release rate of a drug delivery system. Polymers such as polylactide (Li et al. 2003), polydimethylsiloxane (Sirbuly et al. 2003), polyethylene (Li et al. 2003), polystyrene (Li et al. 2003), polycaprolactone (Mukherjee et al. 2006), zein (a biopolymer derived from maize) (Orosco et al. 2006), and poly(N-isopropylacrylamide) (Segal et al. 2007) were documented to be successfully incorporated in porous Si. Moreover, the incorporation of biocompatible polymers with porous Si also helps in improving the controlled drug release, specificity, and stability in an aqueous environment (Li et al. 2003; Kilian et al. 2007).

Electrochemical etching using aqueous potassium hydroxide (KOH) or HF generates a polymer film with optical characteristics, and the polymer release from the master system relies on the interfacial chemistry and tortuosity of the pore network (Segal et al. 2007; Koshida et al. 1993; Collins et al. 2001). Biocompatible polymer in drug delivery applications mainly uses hydrogels (Caló and Khutoryanskiy 2015). The system is beneficial in ophthalmologic devices, biosensors, bio-membranes, and controlled drug delivery (Annaka and Tanaka 1992). The use of crosslinking polymers assists in volume phase transitions and is sensitive to surrounding factors such as pH and temperature (Aoki et al. 1994).

Different forms of pSi were trialed and tested for various medical applications such as anticancer (Xia et al. 2018), anti-inflammatory (Kalluri et al.

2019), and analgesics (Xu et al. 2022), as well as delivery of proteins and peptides (Navrotsky et al. 2021). Additionally, the system is also useful to fulfill the required dietary supplement (Canham 2014). Construction of porous pSi nanomaterial is also advantageous in the form of films (Canham 2014), chip implants (Tieu, Alba, et al. 2019), composite materials (McMillan and Coffer 2021), and microneedles (Chiappini 2021) with ease of fabrication and administration.

Leigh Canham first demonstrated the restorability and biocompatibility of pSi in the mid-1990s, thus promoting the in vivo use of porous silicon (Li et al. 2003). Since then pSi has been widely explored for applications in drug delivery (Li et al. 2018), self-reporting sensor embedded drug delivery (Wang et al. 2018), and scaffolds (Zuidema et al. 2020; Zuidema et al. 2018), as shown in Figure 11.5. The fundamental properties of pSi such as highly controlled pore size for sustainable drug release (Park et al. 2019), surface modification for targeted drug delivery (Jung, Huh, and Kim 2021), and biodegradability (Hon et al. 2012) make it a potential candidate for drug delivery applications. The pores size of pSi can house large quantities of drug molecules due to their ultrahigh surface area and huge pore volume [9]. For example, Wang et al. developed pSi microparticle-based delivery

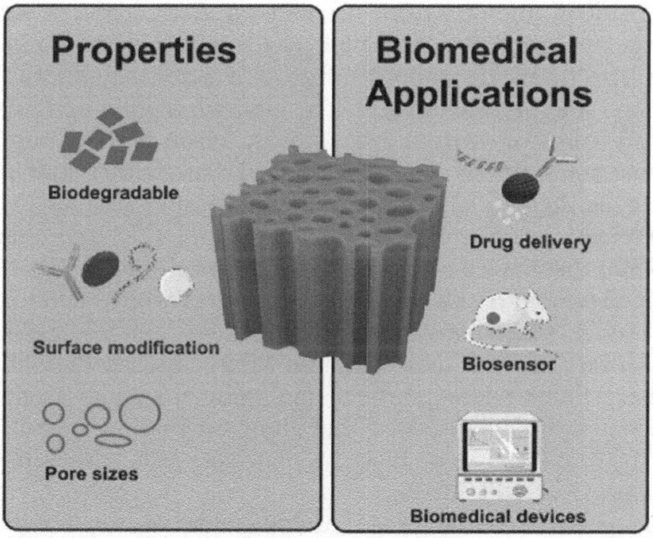

Figure 11.5 Schematic representation of pSi uses in biomedical application. The desirable properties of porous silicon such as biodegradability and surface modification with different groups like antibodies, protein, and tunable pore size make it a perfect candidate for drug delivery agent. Thus, it is widely used for biomedical applications such as drug delivery, biosensors, and biomedical devices.

system. The microparticles contain a core silicon (Si) skeleton surrounded by a SiO_2 shell. Here, two types of pSi were prepared with smaller (10 nm) pores and larger (20 nm) pores. The larger pore material was found to yield a higher mass loading of bovine serum albumin (3 vs 20%) (Wang et al. 2018). Iron oxide (Fe_3O_4) nanoparticles have been documented to be locked into the pores in aqueous ammonia to induce oxidation (Dorvee et al. 2004). The basic pH and nucleophilic nature of ammonia promote the oxidation of freshly etched porous Si in aqueous solutions (Sweryda-Krawiec et al. 1996).

For pSi to be used in medical applications, it is highly important to emphasize the safety and well-being of patients administered for any pSi-based treatment. Therefore, ample work has been focused toward evaluating and establishing the biocompatibility of pSi-based biomaterials. pSi can degrade spontaneously in the physiological environment as silicic acid, which is integrally present in tissues and can be further excreted through urine from the human body (Park et al. 2019). Duan et al. demonstrate a co-delivery platform for synergistic promotion of angiogenesis based on biodegradable, therapeutic, and self-reporting luminescent porous silicon microparticles. The biodegradation of pSi is determined by intrinsic properties such as size, porosity, chemical composition, and pH of the surrounding environment (Salonen and Lehto 2008; Godin et al. 2008). The silicon ions released from the porous silicon microparticles are non-cytotoxic and can significantly stimulate the migration of endothelial cells and fibroblasts. To improve the therapeutic effect, vascular endothelial growth factor (VEGF) was loaded on porous silicon microparticles by electrostatic adsorption and rapid release of VEGF was observed within a few hours, which plays therapeutic roles in promoting angiogenesis (Duan et al. 2021). In another study, Xia et al. developed drug delivery systems to treat multidrug-resistant (MDR) cancer cells. Herein, anticancer drugs (doxorubicin, DOX) and photothermal agents (IR820 dyes) were consecutively integrated into amino-terminated porous silicon nanoparticles via electrostatic attractions, with high loading amount of DOX (13.3%, w/w) and IR820 (18.6%, w/w). The pSi was helpful in the delivery of DOX molecules into MDR cancer cells, while enhancing the intracellular release and accumulation in cellular nuclei. Finally, cytotoxicity assays demonstrated that the combination treatments could offer a synergistic effect to destruct MDR cancer cells with a higher therapeutic efficacy (Xia et al. 2018).

A major barrier to the usage of injectable or implantable porous silicon-based nanostructures as a therapeutic delivery carrier or a diagnostic device is their early degradation and erosion (Tzur-Balter et al. 2015; Shabir et al. 2018). This early degradation of the carrier would lead to the premature release of the cargo. This becomes more fatal when the final aim is to avoid cytotoxic side effects at the targeted site. Thus a long-term stability of the device is required to accomplish the desirable detection limits and sensitivity (Tong et al. 2016). To overcome these challenges, the degradation rate of porous silicon can be enhanced and customized through the modification of the surface chemistry. Liu et al. developed a novel nanohybrid based on porous silicon, gold nanoparticles (Au NPs), and acetylated dextran for liver regeneration and acute-liver-failure (ALF) treatment. This nanohybrid can be used to identify pathological changes in the tissues and selectively deliver drugs to these sites, which have an extremely high potential to ameliorate therapeutic outcomes for patients. It also effectively loads the therapeutic compound (XMU-MP-1) inside, which greatly improves the drug solubility, precise in situ drug delivery, and drug functioning time (Liu et al. 2018).

In the 1990s, with the advancement in silicon microfabrication techniques, silicon microneedle was first fabricated and used for drug delivery (Henry et al. 1998). Brammer et al. first reported the study of porous silicon needles for drug delivery comprised of porous needles having a diameter of 10–40 nm and a length of 1–3 μm. These porous silicon needles provided a sustainable release of penicillin and streptomycin for 42 days (Brammer et al. 2009). In another study, Kim et al. designed bioresorbable, miniaturized porous silicon needles built on a thin, flexible, and water-soluble film with covalently linked drug cargos at doses equivalent to conventional polymeric microneedles. The water-soluble film is provisionally used for the insertion of needles into tissues followed by immediate dissolution within 1 min by the application of saline solution. Subsequently, the needles persisted in tissues without affecting their natural motions. Subsequently, the needle underwent gradual hydrolysis in tissue fluids to degrade into biocompatible byproducts, leading to sustained, long-lasting release of preloaded drug cargos over days at a controlled rate (Kim et al. 2020). Compared to microneedles, nanoneedles offer additional uniform delivery owing to the greater density of nanoneedles per surface area. They also reduce the intrusiveness of the injection confining the treatment to a localized region (Li et al. 2018). Chiappini et al. synthesized porous silicon nanoneedles for intracellular delivery of nucleic acids. These porous silicon nanoneedles (pitch 2 μm and tip diameter 50 nm) displayed easy penetration into the cells for nanoinjection, and their structure was significantly sustained after pressing against skin or muscle. Nanoinjection through porous silicon nanoneedles was accomplished by either cellular activity or application of an external force. Furthermore, nanoinjection did not present significant toxicity and leakage of intracellular material (Chiappini et al. 2015).

The freshly etched porous silicon slowly reacts with the ambient air leading to native oxide growth, thus affecting its structural and optoelectronic properties. Surface modifications can be used to prevent oxide layer growth and for targeted drug delivery by adding functionalities to the porous silicon surface to aid use in particular applications, as summarized in Table 11.1 (Jarvis, Barnes, and Prestidge 2012). Luo et al. systematically developed

Table 11.1 Surface Modification of Porous Silicon and Use in Drug Delivery

Surface Modification Functionalities	*Drugs*	*Result*	*References*
Chitosan, silica xerogel, and a hybrid (chitosan mixed with silica xerogel)	Tamoxifen	Prolonged tamoxifen release	Haidary et al. (2016)
Gold nanoparticles and acetylated dextran	XMU-MP-1	Targeted drug delivery and better drug solubility	Liu et al. (2018)
Undecylenic acid-modified porous silicon functionalized with Fc fragment and coated with chitosan	Glucagon-like peptide-1	Enhanced absorption for oral peptide delivery	Martins et al. (2018)
Transferrin-conjugated porous silicon nanoparticles	Transferrin	Inhibits GBM cells from migrating	Sheykhzadeh et al. (2020)

and evaluated transferrin (Tf) functionalized porous silicon (Tf@pSiNPs) for glioma-targeted drug delivery system. These Tf@pSiNPs nanoparticles presented selective delivery to blood–brain barrier (BBB) forming cells and glioblastoma multiforme (GBM) cells. The anticancer drug doxorubicin (DOX) was effectively loaded and released in a pH-responsive manner, thus enhancing the movement across an in vitro BBB monolayer and presenting cytotoxicity toward GBM cells compared with free DOX. Overall, Tf@ pSiNPs offered a prospective toolbox for targeted therapy to treat GBM (Luo et al. 2019).

Janoniene et al. constructed a nanosystem for precisely targeting cancer cells under hypoxia conditions for cancer therapy. They synthesized a porous silicon-based nanosystem for targeted cancer therapy with VD11–4-2, a novel inhibitor for carbonic anhydrase IX (CA IX) anchored on pSi particles (VD-pSi). The CA IX is mainly expressed on the cancer cell membrane under hypoxia condition, and thus this nanosystem exhibited a strong affinity toward hypoxic human breast adenocarcinoma (MCF-7) cells and a better killing efficiency (Janoniene et al. 2017).

The treatment of multiple diseases frequently necessitates various therapeutics administered simultaneously with uniform biodistribution profiles and pharmacokinetics. In clinical exercise, combination therapy has long been implemented as the primary treatment regimen to lessen drug resistance and enhance therapeutic effectiveness (Santos et al. 2014). Therefore, nanodelivery systems are needed to carry more than one therapeutic compound.

To summarize, porous silicon has been successfully used as a vehicle for the delivery of poorly soluble drugs and protein therapeutics. Pore size and surface modification largely influence drug loading, penetration, and dissolution rate. Surface modification of porous silicon has shown great potential for drug delivery applications. Controlling these interactions allowed specific drug release behaviors to overcome the challenges of therapeutics.

11.6 CONCLUSION

The promising research results for porous silicon structures encourage further exploration for biomedical applications, chiefly in drug delivery and cancer immunotherapy. However, the clinical application of pSi is still in early stages due to the limited understanding of its performance in treating a specific disease, while considering the effects of the surface chemistry, and geometry. This understanding is vital for forecasting the *in vivo* fate of pSi-based materials. It is predicted that the blend of multidiscipline, including chemistry, materials, pharmaceutical science, engineering, biology, and medicine could lead to make exciting innovations in the upcoming future and could fuel the clinical translation of porous silicon.

REFERENCES

Anglin, E. J., L. Cheng, W. R. Freeman, and M. J. Sailor. 2008. Porous silicon in drug delivery devices and materials. *Advanced Drug Delivery Reviews* 60 (11):1266–1277.

Anglin, E. J., M. P. Schwartz, V. P. Ng, L. A. Perelman, and M. J. Sailor. 2004. Engineering the chemistry and nanostructure of porous silicon Fabry-Pérot films for loading and release of a steroid. *Langmuir* 20 (25):11264–11269.

Annaka, M., and T. Tanaka. 1992. Multiple phases of polymer gels. *Nature* 355 (6359):430–432.

Aoki, T., M. Kawashima, H. Katono, et al. 1994. Temperature-responsive interpenetrating polymer networks constructed with poly(acrylic acid) and poly(N, N-dimethylacrylamide). *Macromolecules* 27 (4):947–952.

Arkles, B., Y. Pan, Y. M. Kim, E. Eisenbraun, C. Miller, and A. E.A. Kaloyeros. 2012. Hydridosilane modification of metals: An exploratory study. *Journal of Adhesion Science and Technology* 26 (1–3):41–54.

Baetke, S. C., T. Lammers, and F. Kiessling. 2015. Applications of nanoparticles for diagnosis and therapy of cancer. *The British Journal of Radiology* 88 (1054):20150207.

Boukherroub, R., J. T. C. Wojtyk, D. D. M. Wayner, and D. J. Lockwood. 2002. Thermal hydrosilylation of undecylenic acid with porous silicon. *Journal of the Electrochemical Society* 149 (2):H59.

Brammer, K. S., C. Choi, S. Oh, et al. 2009. Antibiofouling, sustained antibiotic release by Si nanowire templates. *Nano letters* 9 (10):3570–3574.

Britcher, L., T. J. Barnes, H. J. Griesser, and C. A. Prestidge. 2008. PEGylation of porous silicon using click chemistry. *Langmuir* 24 (15):7625–7627.

Buriak, J. M. 2002. Organometallic chemistry on silicon and germanium surfaces. *Chemical Reviews* 102 (5):1271–1308.

Buriak, J. M., M. P. Stewart, T. W. Geders, et al. 1999. Lewis acid mediated hydrosilylation on porous silicon surfaces. *Journal of the American Chemical Society* 121 (49):11491–11502.

Caló, E., and V. V. Khutoryanskiy. 2015. Biomedical applications of hydrogels: A review of patents and commercial products. *European Polymer Journal* 65:252–267.

Canham, L. T. 1990. Silicon quantum wire array fabrication by electrochemical and chemical dissolution of wafers. *Applied Physics Letters* 57 (10):1046–1048.

Canham, L. 2014. Porous silicon and functional foods. In *Handbook of Porous Silicon* Cham: Springer International Publishing.

Canham, L. T., M. R. Houlton, W. Y. Leong, C. Pickering, and J. M. Keen. 1991. Atmospheric impregnation of porous silicon at room temperature. *Journal of Applied Physics* 70 (1):422–431.

Cheng, C. C., P. A. Taylor, R. M. Wallace, et al. 1993. Hydrocarbon surface chemistry on Si (100). *Thin Solid Films* 225 (1–2):196–202.

Chiappini, C. 2021. Porous silicon microneedles and nanoneedles for biomedical applications. doi: 10.1016/B978-0-12-821677-4.00006-9.

Chiappini, C., E. De Rosa, J. O. Martinez, et al. 2015. Biodegradable silicon nanoneedles delivering nucleic acids intracellularly induce localized in vivo neovascularization. *Nature Materials* 14 (5):532–539.

Collins, A., E. Mikeladze, M. Bengtsson, M. Kokaia, T. Laurell, and E. Csöregi. 2001. Interference elimination in glutamate monitoring with chip integrated enzyme microreactors. *Electroanalysis* 13 (6):425–431.

Delalat, B., V. C. Sheppard, S. R. Ghaemi, et al. 2015. Targeted drug delivery using genetically engineered diatom biosilica. *Nature Communications* 6 (1):1–11.

Dhanekar, S., and S. Jain. 2013. Porous silicon biosensor: Current status. *Biosensors and Bioelectronics* 41:54–64.

Dorvee, J. R., A. M. Derfus, S. N. Bhatia, and M. J. Sailor. 2004. Manipulation of liquid droplets using amphiphilic, magnetic one-dimensional photonic crystal chaperones. *Nature Materials* 3 (12):896–899.

Duan, W., Y. Jin, Y. Cui, et al. 2021. A co-delivery platform for synergistic promotion of angiogenesis based on biodegradable, therapeutic and self-reporting luminescent porous silicon microparticles. *Biomaterials* 272: 120772.

Edgar, J. Y. C., and H. Wang. 2017. Introduction for design of nanoparticle based drug delivery systems. *Curr Pharm Des* 23 (14):2108–2112.

Gala, U. H., D. A. Miller, and R. O. Williams III. 2020. Harnessing the therapeutic potential of anticancer drugs through amorphous solid dispersions. *Biochimica et Biophysica Acta (BBA)-Reviews on Cancer* 1873 (1):188319.

Godin, B., J. Gu, R. E. Serda, et al. 2008. Multistage mesoporous silicon-based nanocarriers: biocompatibility with immune cells and controlled degradation in physiological fluids. *Controlled Release Newsletter/Controlled Release Society* 25 (4):9.

Gooding, J. J., and S. Ciampi. 2011. The molecular level modification of surfaces: From self-assembled monolayers to complex molecular assemblies. *Chemical Society Reviews* 40 (5):2704–2718.

Gooding, J. J., and Y. Zhu. 2014. Modifying porous silicon with self-assembled monolayers for biomedical applications. In *Porous Silicon for Biomedical Applications*. Elsevier. doi: 10.1533/9780857097156.1.81.

Gu, L., D. J. Hall, Z. Qin, et al. 2013. In vivo time-gated fluorescence imaging with biodegradable luminescent porous silicon nanoparticles. *Nature Communications* 4 (1):2326.

Haidary, S. M., A. B. Mohammed, E. P. Córcoles, N. K. Ali, and M. R. Ahmad. 2016. Effect of coatings and surface modification on porous silicon nanoparticles for delivery of the anticancer drug tamoxifen. *Microelectronic Engineering* 161: 1–6.

Henry, S., D. V. McAllister, M. G. Allen, and M. R. Prausnitz. 1998. Microfabricated microneedles: A novel approach to transdermal drug delivery. *Journal of Pharmaceutical Sciences* 87 (8):922–925.

Hermanson, G. T. 2013. *Bioconjugate Techniques*. Academic Press, Cambridge, MA.

Hon, N. K., Z. Shaposhnik, E. D. Diebold, F. Tamanoi, and B. Jalali. 2012. Tailoring the biodegradability of porous silicon nanoparticles. *Journal of Biomedical Materials Research Part A* 100 (12):3416–3421.

Hua, F., M. T. Swihart, and E. Ruckenstein. 2005. Efficient surface grafting of luminescent silicon quantum dots by photoinitiated hydrosilylation. *Langmuir* 21 (13):6054–6062.

Hulteen, J. C., and C. R. Martin. 1997. A general template-based method for the preparation of nanomaterials. *Journal of Materials Chemistry* 7 (7):1075–1087.

Ingle, A. P., P. Golińska, A. Yadav, et al. 2020. Nanotechnology. In *Nanobiotechnology in Diagnosis, Drug Delivery, and Treatment*. ISBN: 978-1-119-67177-0.

Janoniene, A., Z. Liu, L. Baranauskiene, et al. 2017. A versatile carbonic anhydrase IX targeting ligand-functionalized porous silicon nanoplatform for dual hypoxia cancer therapy and imaging. *ACS Applied Materials & Interfaces* 9 (16):13976–13987.

Jarvis, K. L., T. J. Barnes, and C. A. Prestidge. 2012. Surface chemistry of porous silicon and implications for drug encapsulation and delivery applications. *Advances in Colloid and Interface Science* 175: 25–38.

Jin, Y., Y. Yang, W. Duan, X. Qu, and J. Wu. 2021. Synergistic and on-demand release of Ag-AMPs loaded on porous silicon nanocarriers for antibacteria and wound healing. *ACS Applied Materials & Interfaces* 13 (14):16127–16141.

Joo, J., X. Liu, V. R. Kotamraju, E. Ruoslahti, Y. Nam, and M. J. Sailor. 2015. Gated luminescence imaging of silicon nanoparticles. *ACS Nano* 9 (6):6233–6241.

Jung, Y., Y. Huh, and D. Kim. 2021. Recent advances in surface engineering of porous silicon nanomaterials for biomedical applications. *Microporous and Mesoporous Materials* 310: 110673.

Kalepu, S., and V. Nekkanti. 2016. Improved delivery of poorly soluble compounds using nanoparticle technology: A review. *Drug Delivery and Translational Research* 6 (3):319–332.

Kalluri, J. R., J. West, G. R. Akkaraju, L. T. Canham, and J. L. Coffer. 2019. Plant-derived tandem drug/mesoporous silicon microcarrier structures for anti-inflammatory therapy. *ACS Omega* 4 (5):8359–8364.

Kang, J., J. Joo, E. J. Kwon, et al. 2016. Self-sealing porous silicon-calcium silicate core–shell nanoparticles for targeted siRNA delivery to the injured brain. *Advanced Materials* 28 (36):7962–7969.

Kang, R. H., S. H. Lee, S. Kang, J. Kang, J. K. Hur, and D. Kim. 2019. Systematic degradation rate analysis of surface-functionalized porous silicon nanoparticles. *Materials (Basel)* 12 (4):580.

Kargupta, R., S. Bok, C. M. Darr, et al. 2014. Coatings and surface modifications imparting antimicrobial activity to orthopedic implants. *Wiley Interdisciplinary Reviews: Nanomedicine and Nanobiotechnology* 6 (5):475–495.

Kermad, A., S. Sam, N. Ghellai, K. Khaldi, and N. Gabouze. 2013. Horseradish peroxidase-modified porous silicon for phenol monitoring. *Materials Science and Engineering: B* 178 (18):1159–1164.

Kilian, K. A., T. Böcking, K. Gaus, M. Gal, and J. J. Gooding. 2007. Peptide-modified optical filters for detecting protease activity. *ACS Nano* 1 (4):355–361.

Kim, D., J. Joo, Y. Pan, et al. 2016. Thermally induced silane dehydrocoupling on silicon nanostructures. *Angewandte Chemie* 128 (22):6533–6537.

Kim, D., J. M. Zuidema, J. Kang, et al. 2016. Facile surface modification of hydroxylated silicon nanostructures using heterocyclic silanes. *Journal of the American Chemical Society* 138 (46):15106–15109.

Kim, H., H. S. Lee, Y. Jeon, et al. 2020. Bioresorbable, miniaturized porous silicon needles on a flexible water-soluble backing for unobtrusive, sustained delivery of chemotherapy. *ACS Nano* 14 (6):7227–7236.

Kokubo, T., H.-M. Kim, and M. Kawashita. 2003. Novel bioactive materials with different mechanical properties. *Biomaterials* 24 (13):2161–2175.

Kordás, K., S. Beke, A. E. Pap, A. Uusimäki, and S. Leppävuori. 2004. Optical properties of porous silicon.: Part II: Fabrication and investigation of multilayer structures. *Optical Materials* 25 (3):257–260.

Koshida, N., H. Koyama, Y. Yamamoto, and G. J. Collins. 1993. Visible electroluminescence from porous silicon diodes with an electropolymerized contact. *Applied Physics Letters* 63 (19):2655–2657.

Krueger, N. A., A. L. Holsteen, S.-K. Kang, et al. 2016. Porous silicon gradient refractive index micro-optics. *Nano Letters* 16 (12):7402–7407.

Kumeria, T., S. J. P. McInnes, S. Maher, and A. Santos. 2017. Porous silicon for drug delivery applications and theranostics: Recent advances, critical review and perspectives. *Expert Opin Drug Deliv* 14 (12):1407–1422.

Lehmann, V., and U. Gösele. 1991. Porous silicon formation: A quantum wire effect. *Applied Physics Letters* 58 (8):856–858.

Lehmann, V., R. Stengl, and A. Luigart. 2000. On the morphology and the electrochemical formation mechanism of mesoporous silicon. *Materials Science and Engineering: B* 69:11–22.

Lehto, V.-P., J. Salonen, H. Santos, and J. Riikonen. 2013. Nanostructured silicon-based materials as a drug delivery system for water-insoluble drugs. *Drug Delivery Strategies for Poorly Water-Soluble Drugs*, 477–508. doi: 10.1002/9781118444726.ch15.

Li, W., Z. Liu, F. Fontana, et al. 2018. Tailoring porous silicon for biomedical applications: From drug delivery to cancer immunotherapy. *Advanced Materials* 30 (24):1703740.

Li, Y. Y., F. Cunin, J. R. Link, et al. 2003. Polymer replicas of photonic porous silicon for sensing and drug delivery applications. *Science* 299 (5615):2045–2047.

Li, Y.-H., and J. M. Buriak. 2006. Dehydrogenative silane coupling on silicon surfaces via early transition metal catalysis. *Inorganic Chemistry* 45 (3):1096–1102.

Lie, L. H., S. N. Patole, A. R. Pike, et al. 2004. Immobilisation and synthesis of DNA on Si (111), nanocrystalline porous silicon and silicon nanoparticles. *Faraday discussions* 125:235–249.

Lin, V. S.-Y., K. Motesharei, K.-P. S. Dancil, M. J. Sailor, and M. Reza Ghadiri. 1997. A porous silicon-based optical interferometric biosensor. *Science* 278 (5339):840–843.

Liu, D., L. M. Bimbo, E. Mäkilä, et al. 2013. Co-delivery of a hydrophobic small molecule and a hydrophilic peptide by porous silicon nanoparticles. *Journal of Controlled Release* 170 (2):268–278.

Liu, D., E. Mäkilä, H. Zhang, et al. 2013. Nanostructured porous silicon-solid lipid nanocomposite: Towards enhanced cytocompatibility and stability, reduced cellular association, and prolonged drug release. *Advanced Functional Materials* 23 (15):1893–1902.

Liu, Z., Y. Li, W. Li, et al. 2018. Multifunctional nanohybrid based on porous silicon nanoparticles, gold nanoparticles, and acetalated dextran for liver regeneration and acute liver failure theranostics. *Advanced Materials* 30 (24):1703393.

Loni, A. 2014. Porous silicon formation by anodization. In: Canham L. (eds.) *Handbook of Porous Silicon*. Springer, Cham.

Luo, M., G. Lewik, J. C. Ratcliffe, et al. 2019. Systematic evaluation of transferrin-modified porous silicon nanoparticles for targeted delivery of doxorubicin to glioblastoma. *ACS Applied Materials & Interfaces* 11 (37):33637–33649.

Martins, J. P., D. Liu, F. Fontana, et al. 2018. Microfluidic nanoassembly of bio-engineered chitosan-modified FcRn-targeted porous silicon nanoparticles@ hypromellose acetate succinate for oral delivery of antidiabetic peptides. *ACS Applied Materials & Interfaces* 10 (51):44354–44367.

McMillan, N. K., and J. L. Coffer. 2021. Chapter 15- Porous silicon and related composites as functional tissue engineering scaffolds. In: H. A. Santos (ed.) *Porous Silicon for Biomedical Applications (Second Edition)*. Woodhead Publishing, Sawston.

Melen, R. L. 2016. Dehydrocoupling routes to element–element bonds catalysed by main group compounds. *Chemical Society Reviews* 45 (4):775–788.

Mitchell, M. J., M. M. Billingsley, R. M. Haley, M. E. Wechsler, N. A. Peppas, and R. Langer. 2021. Engineering precision nanoparticles for drug delivery. *Nature Reviews Drug Discovery* 20 (2):101–124.

Moller, K., and T. Bein. 1998. Inclusion chemistry in periodic mesoporous hosts. *Chemistry of Materials* 10 (10):2950–2963.

Mukherjee, P., M. A. Whitehead, R. A. Senter, D. Fan, J. L. Coffer, and L. T. Canham. 2006. Biorelevant mesoporous silicon / polymer composites: Directed assembly, disassembly, and controlled release. *Biomedical Microdevices* 8 (1):9–15.

Navrotsky, A., R. Hervig, J. Lyons, D.-K. Seo, E. Shock, and A. Voskanyan. 2021. Cooperative formation of porous silica and peptides on the prebiotic Earth. *Proceedings of the National Academy of Sciences* 118 (2):e2021117118.

Oh, J. H., R. H. Kang, J. Kim, E.-K. Bang, and D. Kim. 2021. Thermally induced silane dehydrocoupling on porous silicon nanoparticles for ultra-long-acting drug release. *Nanoscale* 13 (37):15560–15568.

Orosco, M.M., C. Pacholski, G.M. Miskelly, and M.J. Sailor. 2006. Protein-coated porous-silicon photonic crystals for amplified optical detection of protease activity. *Advanced Materials* 18 (11):1393–1396.

Ouyang, H., M. Christophersen, R. Viard, B. L. Miller, and P. M. Fauchet. 2005. Macroporous silicon microcavities for macromolecule detection. *Advanced Functional Materials* 15 (11):1851–1859.

Park, J.-H., L. Gu, G. Von Maltzahn, E. Ruoslahti, S. N. Bhatia, and M. J. Sailor. 2009. Biodegradable luminescent porous silicon nanoparticles for in vivo applications. *Nature Materials* 8 (4):331–336.

Park, J. S., S. O. Meade, E. Segal, and M. J. Sailor. 2007. Porous silicon-based polymer replicas formed by bead patterning. *Physica Status Solidi (a)* 204 (5):1383–1387.

Park, Y., J. Yoo, M.-H. Kang, W. Kwon, and J. Joo. 2019. Photoluminescent and biodegradable porous silicon nanoparticles for biomedical imaging. *Journal of Materials Chemistry B* 7 (41):6271–6292.

Patra, J. K., G. Das, L. F. Fraceto, et al. 2018. Nano based drug delivery systems: Recent developments and future prospects. *Journal of Nanobiotechnology* 16 (1):71.

Polarz, S., and M. Antonietti. 2002. Porous materials via nanocasting procedures: Innovative materials and learning about soft-matter organization. *Chemical Communications* (22):2593–2604.

Purkait, T. K., M. Iqbal, M. H. Wahl, et al. 2014. Borane-catalyzed room-temperature hydrosilylation of alkenes/alkynes on silicon nanocrystal surfaces. *Journal of the American Chemical Society* 136 (52):17914–17917.

Qin, Z., J. Joo, L. Gu, and M. J. Sailor. 2014. Size control of porous silicon nanoparticles by electrochemical perforation etching. *Particle & Particle Systems Characterization* 31 (2):252–256.

Robins, E. G., M. P. Stewart, and J. M. Buriak. 1999. Anodic and cathodic electrografting of alkynes on porous silicon. *Chemical Communications* 24:2479–2480.

Sailor, M. J. 2012. *Porous Silicon in Practice: Preparation, Characterization and Applications*. John Wiley & Sons, Hoboken, NJ.

Salinas, A. J., M. Vallet-Regi, and I. Izquierdo-Barba. 2001. Biomimetic apatite deposition on calcium silicate gel glasses. *Journal of Sol-Gel Science and Technology* 21 (1):13–25.

Salonen, J., L. Laitinen, A. M. Kaukonen, et al. 2005. Mesoporous silicon microparticles for oral drug delivery: Loading and release of five model drugs. *Journal of Controlled Release* 108 (2–3):362–374.

Salonen, J., and V.-P. Lehto. 2008. Fabrication and chemical surface modification of mesoporous silicon for biomedical applications. *Chemical Engineering Journal* 137 (1):162–172.

Salonen, J., V.-P. Lehto, M. Björkqvist, E. Laine, and L. Niinistö. 2000. Studies of thermally-carbonized porous silicon surfaces. *Physica Status Solidi (a)* 182 (1):123–126.

Salonen, J., A. M. Kaukonen, J. Hirvonen, and V.-P. Lehto. 2008. Mesoporous silicon in drug delivery applications. *Journal of Pharmaceutical Sciences* 97 (2):632–653.

Salonen, J. and E. Mäkilä. 2021. Chapter 1 - Thermal stabilization of porous silicon. In: *Porous Silicon for Biomedical Applications* (Second Edition). Woodhead Publishing, Sawston.

Sam, S., J.-N. Chazalviel, A. C. Gouget-Laemmel, et al. 2010. Covalent immobilization of amino acids on the porous silicon surface. *Surface and Interface Analysis* 42 (6-7):515–518.

Santos, H. A., L. M. Bimbo, V.-P. Lehto, A. J. Airaksinen, J. Salonen, and J. Hirvonen. 2011. Multifunctional porous silicon for therapeutic drug delivery and imaging. *Current Drug Discovery Technologies* 8 (3):228–249.

Santos, H. A., E. Mäkilä, A. J. Airaksinen, L. M. Bimbo, and J. Hirvonen. 2014. Porous silicon nanoparticles for nanomedicine: preparation and biomedical applications. *Nanomedicine* 9 (4):535–554.

Santos, H. A., J. Riikonen, J. Salonen, et al. 2010. In vitro cytotoxicity of porous silicon microparticles: effect of the particle concentration, surface chemistry and size. *Acta Biomaterialia* 6 (7):2721–2731.

Saravanapavan, P., and L. L. Hench. 2003. Mesoporous calcium silicate glasses. I. Synthesis. *Journal of Non-Crystalline Solids* 318 (1):1–13.

Schmeltzer, J. M., L. A. Porter, M. P. Stewart, and J. M. Buriak. 2002. Hydride abstraction initiated hydrosilylation of terminal alkenes and alkynes on porous silicon. *Langmuir* 18 (8):2971–2974.

Secret, E., M. Maynadier, A. Gallud, et al. 2014. Two-photon excitation of porphyrin-functionalized porous silicon nanoparticles for photodynamic therapy. *Advanced Materials* 26 (45):7643–7648.

Segal, E., L.A. Perelman, F. Cunin, et al. 2007. Confinement of thermoresponsive hydrogels in nanostructured porous silicon dioxide templates. *Advanced Functional Materials* 17 (7):1153–1162.

Sercombe, L., T. Veerati, F. Moheimani, S. Y. Wu, A. K. Sood, and S. Hua. 2015. Advances and challenges of liposome assisted drug delivery. *Frontiers in Pharmacology* 6: 286.

Shabir, Q., K. Webb, D. K. Nadarassan, et al. 2018. Quantification and reduction of the residual chemical reactivity of passivated biodegradable porous silicon for drug delivery applications. *Silicon* 10 (2):349–359.

Sheykhzadeh, S., M. Luo, B. Peng, et al. 2020. Transferrin-targeted porous silicon nanoparticles reduce glioblastoma cell migration across tight extracellular space. *Scientific Reports* 10 (1):1–16.

Sirbuly, D. J., G. M. Lowman, B. Scott, G. D. Stucky, and S. K. Buratto. 2003. Patterned Microstructures of porous silicon by dry-removal soft lithography. *Advanced Materials* 15 (2):149–152.

Soppimath, K. S., T. M. Aminabhavi, A. R. Kulkarni, and W. E. Rudzinski. 2001. Biodegradable polymeric nanoparticles as drug delivery devices. *Journal of Controlled Release* 70 (1):1–20.

Sotiropoulou, S., V. Vamvakaki, and N. A. Chaniotakis. 2005. Stabilization of enzymes in nanoporous materials for biosensor applications. *Biosensors and Bioelectronics* 20 (8):1674–1679.

Sousa, D., D. Ferreira, J. L. Rodrigues, and L. R. Rodrigues. 2019. Chapter 14-Nanotechnology in targeted drug delivery and therapeutics. In: S. S. Mohapatra, S. Ranjan, N. Dasgupta, R. K. Mishra, and S. Thomas (eds.) *Applications of Targeted Nano Drugs and Delivery Systems*. Elsevier, Amsterdam.

Stewart, M. P., and J. M. Buriak. 2001. Exciton-mediated hydrosilylation on photoluminescent nanocrystalline silicon. *Journal of the American Chemical Society* 123 (32):7821–7830.

Sung, Y. K., and S. W. Kim. 2020. Recent advances in polymeric drug delivery systems. *Biomaterials Research* 24 (1):12.

Sweetman, M. J., S. D. Graney, and N. H. Voelcker. 2007. Interfacing porous silicon with biomolecules. Paper read at BioMEMS and Nanotechnology III. doi: 10.1117/12.759211.

Sweetman, M. J., S. J. P. McInnes, R. B. Vasani, T. Guinan, A. Blencowe, and N. H. Voelcker. 2015. Rapid, metal-free hydrosilanisation chemistry for porous silicon surface modification. *Chemical Communications* 51 (53):10640–10643.

Sweetman, M. J., and N. H. Voelcker. 2012. Chemically patterned porous silicon photonic crystals towards internally referenced organic vapour sensors. *RSC Advances* 2 (11):4620–4622.

Sweryda-Krawiec, B., R. R. Chandler-Henderson, J. L. Coffer, Y. G. Rho, and R. F. Pinizzotto. 1996. A comparison of porous silicon and silicon nanocrystallite photoluminescence quenching with amines. *The Journal of Physical Chemistry* 100 (32):13776–13780.

Tahvanainen, M., T. Rotko, E. Mäkilä, et al. 2012. Tablet preformulations of indomethacin-loaded mesoporous silicon microparticles. *International Journal of Pharmaceutics* 422 (1–2):125–131.

Tay, L., N. L. Rowell, D. Poitras, J. W. Fraser, D. J. Lockwood, and R. Boukherroub. 2004. Bovine serum albumin adsorption on passivated porous silicon layers. *Canadian Journal of Chemistry* 82 (10):1545–1553.

Thomas, J. C., C. Pacholski, and M. J. Sailor. 2006. Delivery of nanogram payloads using magnetic porous silicon microcarriers. *Lab on a Chip* 6 (6):782–787.

Tieu, T., M. Alba, R. Elnathan, A. Cifuentes-Rius, and N. H. Voelcker. 2019. Advances in porous silicon–based nanomaterials for diagnostic and therapeutic applications. *Advanced Therapeutics* 2 (1):1800095.

Tieu, T., S. Dhawan, V. Haridas, et al. 2019. Maximizing RNA loading for gene silencing using porous silicon nanoparticles. *ACS Applied Materials & Interfaces* 11 (26):22993–23005.

Tong, W. Y., M. J. Sweetman, E. R. Marzouk, C. Fraser, T. Kuchel, and N. H. Voelcker. 2016. Towards a subcutaneous optical biosensor based on thermally hydrocarbonised porous silicon. *Biomaterials* 74:217–230.

Trinh, H. M., M. Joseph, K. Cholkar, R. Mitra, and A. K. Mitra. 2017. Chapter 3-Nanomicelles in diagnosis and drug delivery*. In: A. K. Mitra, K. Cholkar, and A. Mandal (eds.) *Emerging Nanotechnologies for Diagnostics, Drug Delivery and Medical Devices*. Boston, MA: Elsevier.

Tzur-Balter, A., Z. Shatsberg, M. Beckerman, E. Segal, and N. Artzi. 2015. Mechanism of erosion of nanostructured porous silicon drug carriers in neoplastic tissues. *Nature Communications* 6 (1):1–8.

Uhlir Jr., A. 1956. Electrolytic shaping of germanium and silicon. *Bell System Technical Journal* 35 (2):333–347.

Unagami, T. 1980. Formation mechanism of porous silicon layer by anodization in HF solution. *Journal of the Electrochemical Society* 127 (2):476.

Wang, J., T. Kumeria, M. T. Bezem, J. Wang, and M. J. Sailor. 2018. Self-reporting photoluminescent porous silicon microparticles for drug delivery. *ACS Applied Materials & Interfaces* 10 (4):3200–3209.

Waterman, R. 2013. Mechanisms of metal-catalyzed dehydrocoupling reactions. *Chemical Society Reviews* 42 (13):5629–5641.

Wirtz, M., M. Parker, Y. Kobayashi, and C. R. Martin. 2002. Template-synthesized nanotubes for chemical separations and analysis. *Chemistry* 8 (16):3572–3578.
Xia, B., Q. Zhang, J. Shi, J. Li, Z. Chen, and B. Wang. 2018. Co-loading of photothermal agents and anticancer drugs into porous silicon nanoparticles with enhanced chemo-photothermal therapeutic efficacy to kill multidrug-resistant cancer cells. *Colloids Surf B Biointerfaces* 164:291–298.
Xia, B., W. Zhang, H. Tong, J. Li, Z. Chen, and J. Shi. 2019. Multifunctional chitosan/porous silicon@ Au nanocomposite hydrogels for long-term and repeatedly localized combinatorial therapy of cancer via a single injection. *ACS Biomaterials Science & Engineering* 5 (4):1857–1867.
Xu, W., Z. Zhao, J. Falconer, et al. 2022. Sustained release ketamine-loaded porous silicon-PLGA microparticles prepared by an optimized supercritical CO(2) process. *Drug Delivery and Translational Research* 12 (3):676–694.
Xu, X., S. A. Majetich, and S. A. Asher. 2002. Mesoscopic monodisperse ferromagnetic colloids enable magnetically controlled photonic crystals. *Journal of the American Chemical Society* 124 (46):13864–13868.
Zhang, X. G. 2003. Morphology and formation mechanisms of porous silicon. *Journal of the Electrochemical Society* 151 (1):C69.
Zhenyu, Y., M. H. Wahl, and J. G. C. Veinot. 2014. Size-independent organosilane functionalization of silicon nanocrystals using Wilkinson's catalyst. *Canadian Journal of Chemistry* 92 (10):951–957.
Zuidema, J. M., A. Bertucci, J. Kang, M. J. Sailor, and F. Ricci. 2020. Hybrid polymer/porous silicon nanofibers for loading and sustained release of synthetic DNA-based responsive devices. *Nanoscale* 12 (4):2333–2339.
Zuidema, J. M., T. Kumeria, D. Kim, et al. 2018. Oriented nanofibrous polymer scaffolds containing protein-loaded porous silicon generated by spray nebulization. *Advanced Materials* 30 (12):1706785.

Chapter 12

Surface Modified Graphene Oxide (GO) for Chemotherapeutic Drug Delivery

Manoj Kumar Singh and Pratap Singh
Central University of Haryana

Nahid Tyagi
Central University of Haryana and Jamia Millia Islamia

Manika Khanuja
Centre of Nanoscience and Nanotechnology, Jamia Millia Islamia

CONTENTS

DOI: 10.1201/9781003217114-15

12.1 INTRODUCTION

The term cancer refers to a category of diseases characterized by abnormal cell proliferation and protruding growth. The extension of cancer cells in the human body has led to an increase in mortality rate and morbidity throughout the globe. More than ten million cases of cancer occurred each year globally. It is estimated by the World Health Organization (WHO)-, that ~13.1 million cancer-associated demised may be materialized by 2030. However, ground-breaking efforts of the scientific community toward medical sciences and better understanding of tumor biology with bio-safety and biocompatibility reduce mortality rate upto 5%. For inhibiting or killing tumor cells'- toxicities to normal cells, multi-drug resistance, low aqueous solubility, non-specific cytotoxicity, and various side effects have made conventional chemotherapy a terrible idea for cancer treatment. For this reason, determining the optimal dosage range of therapeutic agents requires the development of extremely efficient therapeutic treatment systems that can conquer biological restrictions, especially identify cancerous tissue from healthy tissue, and act prudently to the heterogeneous and typical tumor micro-environment [1–4]. The scientific community suggested the advanced NDD system focused on carbon and its allotropes, metals, polymers, and metal oxides. Out of all, graphene-based nanomaterials and associated therapeutic methods have exposed incredible capacity in cancer treatment due to their biocompatibility, simple modification, high surface area, and nontoxic nature [5,6]. Because of some restraints on using pristine graphene and graphene derivatives including time- and dose-dependent cytotoxicity, researchers developed numerous functionalizations and modifications schemes of graphene oxide (GO) via various organic and inorganic materials including polymers, antibodies, and metal nanocomposites to mitigate this limitation. These materials not only settled down this problem but also develop and enhance various stunning properties of graphene and its derivatives in nano-drug delivery systems.

It is our goal in the current chapter to provide an update and overview on recent advancements in the field of chemotherapeutic drug delivery systems focused on nanomaterials and their composites. The first section concludes with the central idea of the NDD system and its necessities in anti-cancer treatment. Section 12.2 is dedicated to the fundamental information of carbon, graphene, and graphene oxide and their structures associated with their properties.

The synthesis part will be discussed in the third section. Section 12.4 gives a brief idea of surface modification of nanomaterials (graphene, GO) related to metal nanocomposites, antibody nanocomposites, and polymer nanocomposites. Various characterization techniques are covered in the next section. In Section 12.6, the participation of GO in the gene delivery system and chemotherapeutic drug delivery system has been discussed. Section 12.7 is dedicated to biocompatibility (the easy going to the biological environment) and harmfulness of the human cells to the GO nanocomposites.

12.2 FUNDAMENTAL OF CARBON AND ITS ALLOTROPES

Carbon is likely derived from the Latin word carbon, which can signify "coal" or "coke" and advertised as ${}^{12}_{6}C$ (12 amu of average atomic mass) in group 14 (VIa) of the periodic table [7]. Carbon is the fourth most plentiful element in the solar system and is essential to all kinds of life on Earth. The electronic configuration of carbon is $1s^2\ 2s^2\ 2p^2$ where, four electrons are coupled through the π bonding, establishes four bonds and no electrons are left unpaired. Consequently, the diamagnetic behavior has been observed due to the minimal possibility of retaining unpaired electrons. It is possible for carbon atoms to form a variety of bonds with one another. Carbon exists hybridization (processes of intermixing s and p orbitals) of sp: 1-single and 1-triple bond associated with a line arrangement, sp^2: 1-double and 2-single bonds associated with the trigonal arrangement, and sp^3: 4 single bonds associated with tetrahedral arrangement [8,9], as shown in Figure 12.1.

The chemical elements have the ability to exist in two or more distinct forms identified as allotropes. On the basis of dimensionality, nanostructures/carbon allotropes can be organized into four manners as three-dimensional (graphite, diamond), two-dimensional (graphene), one-dimensional (CNT, nanoribbons, nanohorns), and zero-dimensional (fullerenes, quantum dots) structures [10,11]. Various types of allotropes are depicted in Figure 12.2. Among them, graphene (single layer of graphite), CNT, and buckminsterfullerene are used the most for versatile applications. The most thermodynamically stable form of carbon is graphite at ordinary temperatures and pressures while all allotropes have in the solid form [12]. The vast properties of carbonaceous materials have been widely studied because of their variety, advantageous characteristics, and active uses, including chemical, biomedical, and energy storage regions. Finally, we will discuss potential approaches for improving the performance of nano-drug efficiency that have yet to be explored.

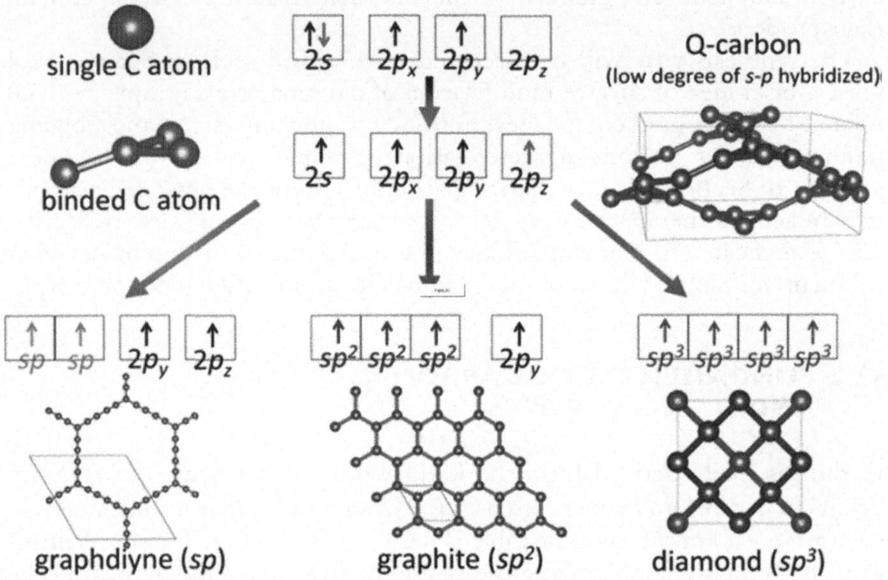

Figure 12.1 Scheme of different types of hybridization in carbon and its allotropes. (Reprint from "ACS Applied Material Interfaces", Lian R., 2020, with permission).

12.2.1 Graphene

In 2004 Novoselov et al. synthesized graphene in their renowned paper "Electric field effect in atomically thin carbon films, honored with the Nobel Prize (2004), and explored a new area of research for the scientific community [13,14]. A single layer of graphite tagged as graphene adopts a hexagonal honeycomb lattice structure with sp^2 hybridization, as displayed in Figure 12.3. Graphene is connected with two triangular Bravais lattices superimposed on each other. For semiconducting nature with zero gap, there is a cone-like arrangement of electronic bands touching one other known as the Dirac point, as shown in Figure 12.4. It is composed of sp^2 hybridized bonds between carbon atoms, while an outside the plane p orbital supplies the delocalization network of the electron. Graphene has been shown to have a wide range of attributes such as very large specific surface area-(~2,630 m^2/g^1), breaking strength (~30 GPa), superior charge carrier mobility (~200,000 cm^2/Vs to ~500,000 cm^2/Vs), mechanical stiffness (1,060 GPa), electrical conductivity ~10^4 Ω^{-1}/cm, thermal conductivity/ ~3×10^3 W/m/K, 300 K, Young's modulus ~1.1 TPa, transparency ~97.7% including visible spectrum and many more [15–18]. Graphene has been publicized a great potential in the zone of medical and drug delivery system due to high surface area that provides the different functionalization

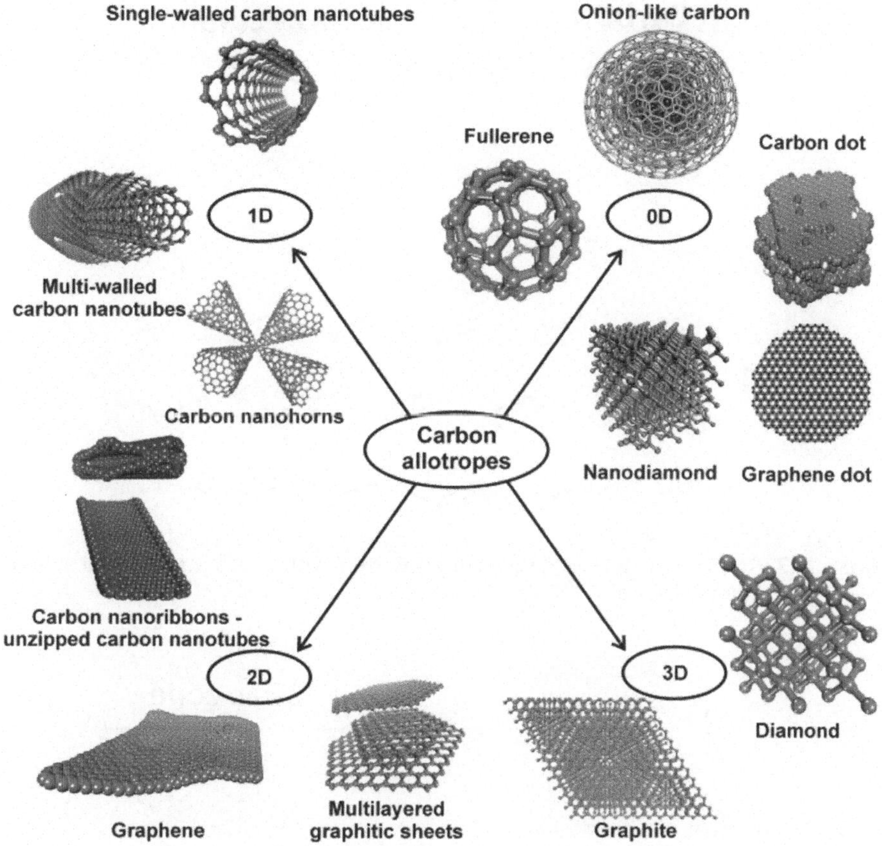

Figure 12.2 Scheme of different types of hybridization in carbon and its allotropes. (Reprintfrom"ACSAppliedMaterialInterfaces",LianR.,2020,withpermission).

scheme with flexible cargo burdening. The solubility inside environments (aqueous) and successive interaction through lipids (in cell membranes) have been promoted by the hydrophilic and hydrophobic consolidation graphene (surface). Physical characteristics of graphene may be impacted by interact antagonistically with biological systems and capacity to interact adversely with biological systems, which is important for biomedical uses. The non-covalent interaction among the carbon rings through π-π stacking is the consequence of the pinion of graphene and aromatic molecules [19]. Furthermore, the enormous surface zone of the two-dimensional shape allows for a single flake of graphene an array of various aromatic groups can be applied to bio-compatible products. For graphene in its purest form, π-π stacking and hydrophobic interactions are important and deliver the main source of drug-binding [20].

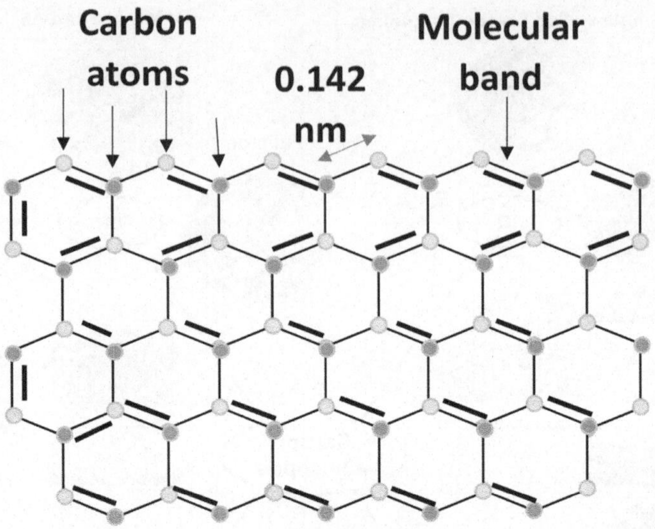

Figure 12.3 Atomic structure of Graphene single layer with 6 carbons arranged in honeycomb lattice.

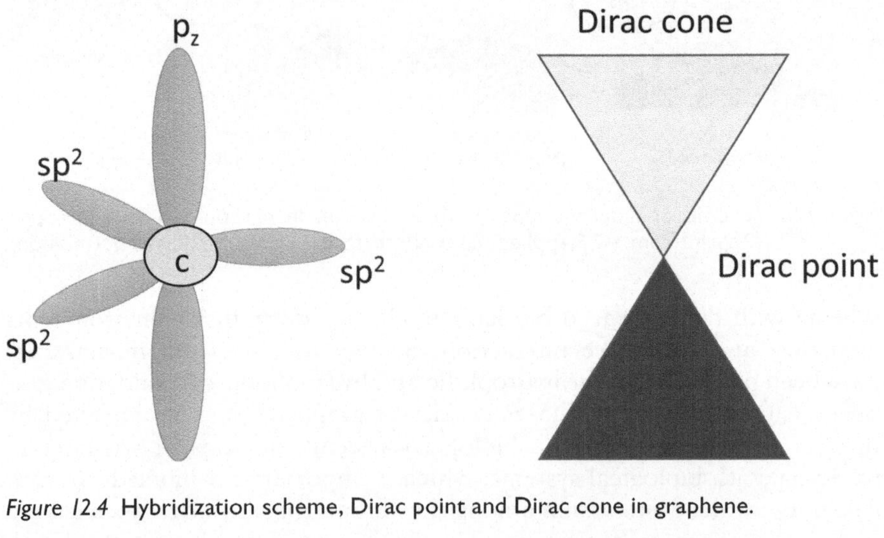

Figure 12.4 Hybridization scheme, Dirac point and Dirac cone in graphene.

Besides these the phenomenon of steric interference has occurred on the graphene-surface due to the exploitation, and it changes the geometry of flake (graphene). It is necessary to eliminate non-polar solvent's leftover molecules while transferring the molecule from the solvent's flakes into the water. Conclusively, on the flake surface, both surfactants and remaining solvent molecules (non-polar) are adsorbed and combine with toxicities in the synthesis [21]. Therefore, biological applications have been limited in their use of pristine graphene, and the use of different graphene forms has been favored in the research. In this account, nanomaterials such as GO and reduced-graphene oxide (rGO) have the most promise in biological areas because of their large surface, tunable physicochemical, flexible, loading properties, excellent biocompatibility, and ease of accessibility.

12.2.2 Graphene Oxide (GO)

The fundamental strof GO characterized like single graphene sheet improved through several sorts of functional groups such as; epoxy (-O-), hydroxyl (–OH), carboxyl (–COOH), and oxygen, epoxide groups are present on GO's surface [22], as shown in Figure 12.5. The hydrophilicity and solubility of several water-insoluble medicines are attributed to such GO's oxide groups. To promote surface interactions, GO possesses aromatic (sp^2), with aliphatic (sp^3) zones, due to the epoxy and hydroxyl groups are located on the graphene oxide sheet's basal plane, whereas some of its edge locations are tethered to carbonyl and carboxyl groups [23,24]. There is a straightforward modification of functional groups such that they are compatible with bioactive chemicals due to the medication loading or delivery effectiveness may be enhanced [25].

Besides, hyaluronic acid (HA) is a molecule that may be applied to transport chemotherapeutics to specific locations. A few cell surface proteins (receptors), associated with HA and, CD44 (surface adhesion receptor), enhance tissue integrity and facilitate cell attachment. Consequently,

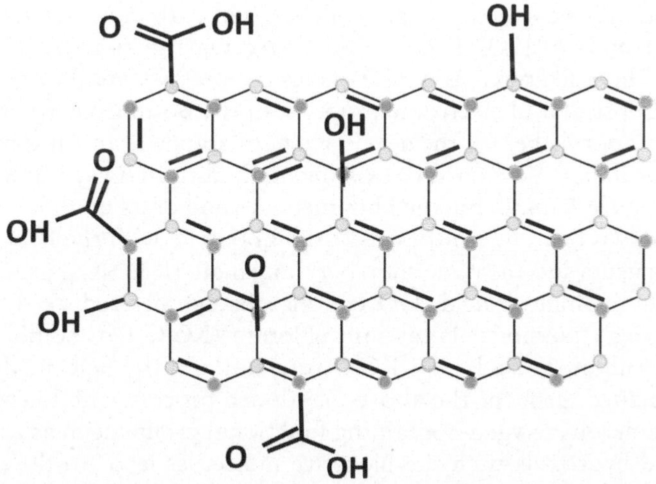

Figure 12.5 Single layer structure of graphene oxide having -O- and -OH groups

target-specific drug delivery chemotherapeutic agents have improved by GO-HA arrangement [26, 27]. It is observed that adding water-insoluble SN38 to GO and polyethylene glycol (PEG) conjugates resulted in increased solubility and antineoplastic effectiveness of medications/drugs [28]. Similarly, the PEG functionalization, GO's biocompatibility, tumor tissue distribution, and photodynamic anticancer activity were improved upon. Another significant aspect of GO's characteristics and functions, in this sequence of functional groups, is the GO's size. Size-dependent biological activities may be obtained by producing GO in a variety of sizes using various methods and utilities like:- submicron-sized GO/390.2±51.4 nm and nano-sized GO/NGO; 65.5±16.3 nm, but the micro-sized GO/ 1,089.9±135.3 nm could increase the rate of cell death while generating no visible putrefaction [29,30]. Biotechnological applications promise to benefit from GO's superior surface functionalization capabilities, aqueous processability, and amphiphilicity, among other things.Nnanocomposites of GO with nobel metals, metals and polymers shows a great potential application such as;- gene delivery, phototherapy, biosensing, bio-imaging, antibacterial action, drug, and more in the region of biomedical and NDD systems. For this purpose, controllable, environmentally approachable, and toxicity free synthesis are required for nanomaterials and GO.

12.3 SYNTHESIS AND SURFACE MODIFICATION OF GO

GO consisting of 2D planer structure is an oxidized and more hydrophilic product derived from graphene. Due to the attachments of diverse oxygen atoms on graphene sheets, some sp^2 hybridized carbon atoms get replaced into sp^3 carbons of GO. These oxygen carrying functionalities such as – OH, -COOH, and epoxides of GO makes it more hydrophilic and provides intensified optical and electronic properties [31]. Bottom-up and top-down are the two approaches for the development of graphene and graphene oxide via graphite flakes. Schematic of existing methods for GO synthesis is represented in Figure 12.6. Using the Hummers method or its modified form graphene oxide GO can be synthesized from graphene with the help of strong oxidizing agents such as potassium permanganate ($KMNO_4$) acidified with concentrated sulphuric acid. GO can also be synthesized via Brodie's or Staudenmaier's methods. Potassium chlorate ($KClO_3$) in combination of nitric and sulphuric acids and $KClO_3$ in fuming nitric acid medium used as an oxidizing agent for the above-mentioned processes [32]. The interactions of numerous oxygen-containing functional groups such as carboxylic, epoxy, and hydroxyls with the bioactive molecules leads to the change in the surface chemistry of GO. Hydrophobicity, zero band gap, sharp edgess and poor solubility in the majority of solvents of the graphene demands

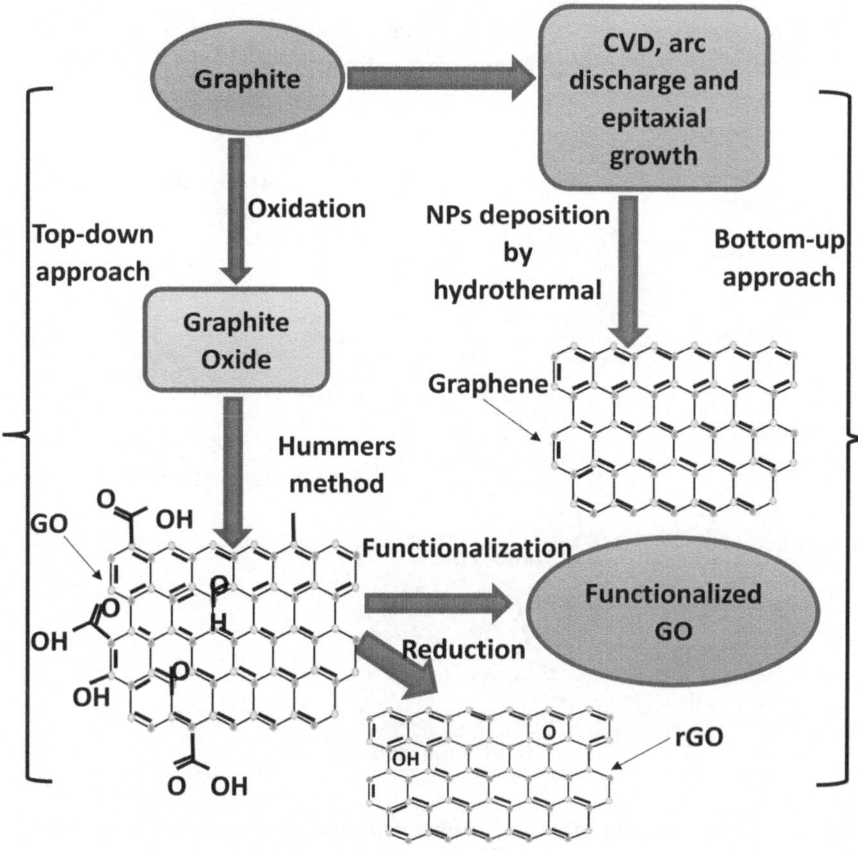

Figure 12.6 Schematics for the synthesis of graphene and graphene oxide via both approaches.

functionalization of graphene for its large array of applications [33,34]. And after doing proper modification or functionalization of GO, its water solubility and cellular internalization can be increased while toxicity can be reduced [35]. Sun et al. (2008) developed techniques for the functionalization of GO, which makes it compatible for biological use. "Smart tumor responsive" properties can also be generated through the functionalization of GO in addition to pH and temperature [36]. Applications of GO and modified GO in drug delivery or cancer therapy have become an imminent tool, in the medical field as shown in Figure 12.7.

In the field of drug delivery system (DDS), covalent and non-covalent functionalization of GO by the researcher's community has become a golden era in medical science. The modification of GO through covalent bonds involved two mechanisms: The first one is covalent bonding between free

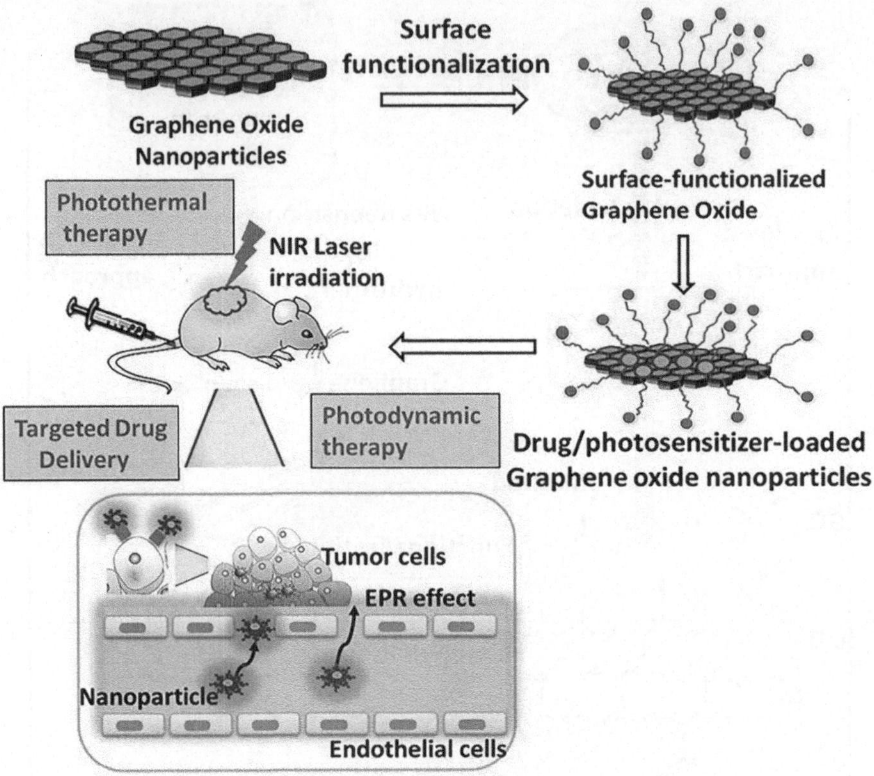

Figure 12.7 Surface functionalized GO loaded with drugs and photosensitizer using in Drug delivery system (DDS) in photodynamic therapy via NIR radiations. (Reprint from "MDPA", H Sharma, 2020, with permission).

radicals and carbon-carbon bonds or between dineophiles, and the second is covalent bonding between oxygen functionalities of GO and organic functional groups. In the former mechanism, covalent bond is formed between the sp^2-hybridized carbon atoms of graphene with free radicals obtained by the calcinations of diazonium salts. In addition, with free radicals, dieneophiles also interact with the sp^2 carbon atoms of graphene. To make graphene more soluble in solvents and to circumvent stacking, non-covalent functionalization is indispensable with the diverse organic molecules. This non-covalent functionalization of graphene offers π-π stacking and Van der wall interactions between graphene and functionalized molecules [35,37].

On the other hand, non-covalent functionalizations via π-π stacking offer a new roadmap for the attachment of functional groups without the distortion of electronic map of graphene [38,39]. Bai et al. used non-covalent modification of graphene by using nanoplatelets of graphene and sulfonated polyaniline to coerce it water soluble. Yang et al. fabricated a highly conductive and long-lasting graphene based material via non-covalent functionalization of graphene [40]. Dai et al. functionalized GO by using six arm PEG to tailor the surface properties of GO for making it biocompatible, more stable in various biological solvents and these modified nano GO used for insoluble anticancer drug SN38 via π-π stacking [28].

12.4 FUNCTIONALIZATION SCHEMES

As discussed the various advantages of the functionalization of GO nanoparticles over the pristine nanoparticles of GO,- we have a variety of schemes for synthesizing functionalized GO including the decoration of diverse types of antibodies, polymers, and metal nanoparticles on the surface of GO,-for inhibiting or killing the tumor cells. A detailed study on the application of functionalized GO has been discussed in this section. Different types of GO synthesis are portrayed in Figure 12.8.

12.4.1 GO associated with Antibody Nanocomposites

Besides having various advantages of nanoparticles in drug delivery including size in nano range, high surface to volume ratio, and targeting drug delivery in a controlled fashion, some limitations of these miraculous particles can never be avoided [41,42]. To overcome the limitations of pristine

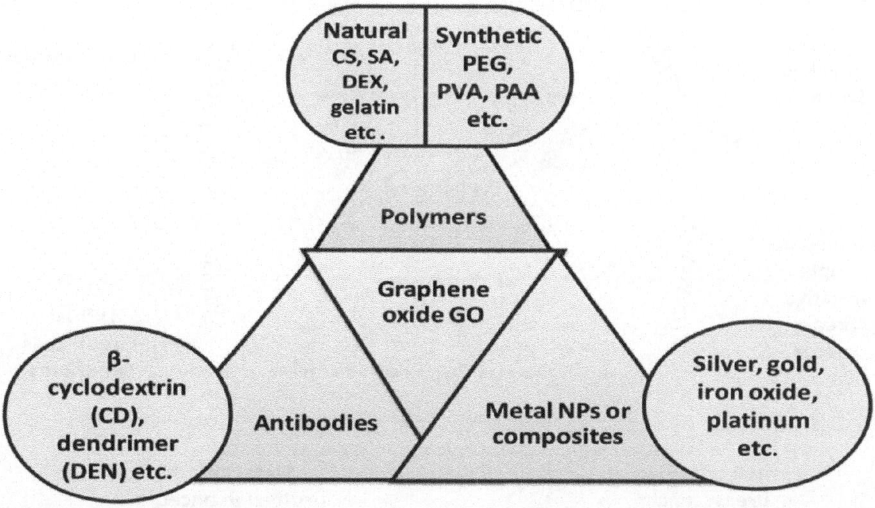

Figure 12.8 Materials used for the surface Functionalization of GO with their examples.

graphene synthesis nanoparticles such as the mechanism of induction via multiple drug resistance and diffusion of drugs into the tumor in an inefficient ways, antibodies decoration on the surface of NPs are the best option in this cancer crisis era worldwide [43]. Antibodies or antibody fragments can be decorated on the surface of GO NPs via covalent bonding or adsorptions. Prior activation of the NPs is a must for the covalent binding. For improving therapeutic index and targeted or controlled drug delivery therapies, antibody-drug conjugates (ADCs) are the best systems for targeted drug delivery.

By the United States Food and Drug Administration (FDA), a total of eight ADCs have been approved up to now shown in Figure 12.9. The potential of antibody-conjugated nanoparticles (ACNPs) and antibody-associated nanocomposites (ADCs) resides in both nanotechnology and antibody conjugation. ACNPs have many advantages over ADCs together with the delivery of drugs in a targeted or controlled manner, preserving drugs' chemical shapes, less toxic, and also neglect unpredicted metabolization [44]. Graphene and its derivatives such as GO are serving as the superior nanoparticles for antibody conjugation in cancer therapies. Recently, hybrid nanocomposites of GO coated with the antibodies β-cyclodextrin (CD), dendrimer (DEN), and poly amido amide were used for the delivery of chemotherapeutic drugs doxorubicin (DOX), photosensitizer (protoporphyrin

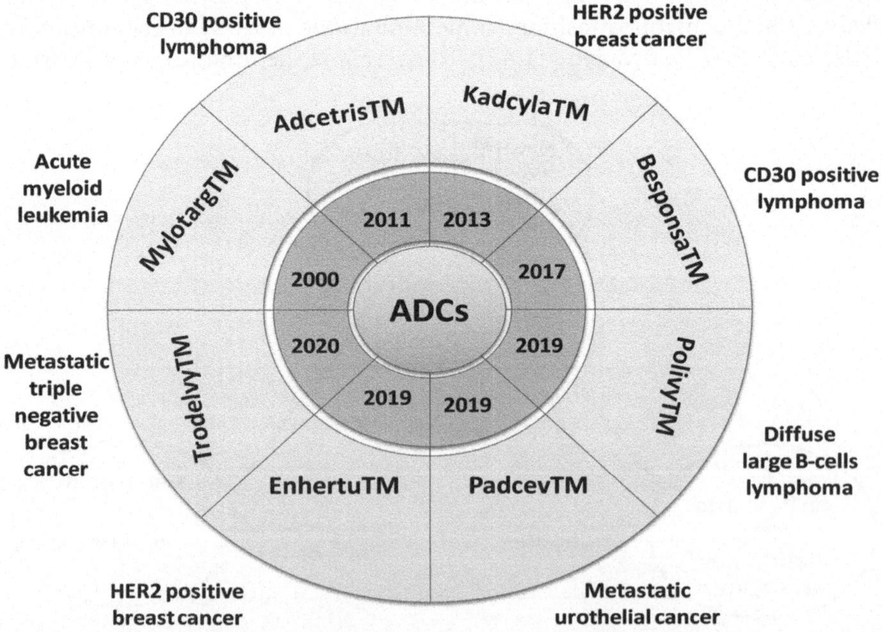

Figure 12.9 Eight types of antibody drug conjugates (ADCs) approved by FDA.

IX (PpIX)), and camptothecin (CPT). Furthermore, the order of the capacity for the drugs loading by using these hybrid nanocomposites of GO was camptothecin>protoporphyrin IX>doxorubicin, but cytotoxicity was enhanced [45]. Graphene quantum dots modified with polyethylene glycol (PEG) and loaded with the platinum used to restrict the hypoxia-mediated chemoresistance oral squamous cells carcinoma (OSCC). These quantum dots show a very fabulous inhibitory effect for the growth of tumor cells with minimal systematic drugs toxicity [46]. Another group used a merger of chemotherapy and photothermal therapies by using magnetic GO modified with PEG and cetuximab against CT-26 murine colorectal cells [47]. Cetuximab, which is an epidermal growth receptor factor (EGRF) monoclonal type antibody used for the active targeting of the drugs because EGFR is highly expressible on the surface of tumor of colorectal cancer cells. By this study, it is also showed that the drug releases more effectively at lower pH (~5.5) than at higher value of pH (~7.4) and then effectively targets EGRF CT-26 murine colorectal cancer cells. Liu et al. used chitosan (CS)-modified GO carried by the conjugation of HA and loaded with the anti-cancer drug SNX-2112 for inhibiting or killing the A549 cancerous cells. These nanocomposites show a very lesser cytotoxicity for the normal human bronchial epithelial cells [48]. GO with galactosylated CS and loaded with DOX has also been used by another group of researchers for the treatment of cancerous cells. This is much better in vivo anti-tumor effect than former, demonstrated on the basis of tumor weight and volume [49]. All these demonstrations of GO associated with antibody are really motivational and may also lead to change the face of tumor treatment and management worldwide.

12.4.2 GO associated with Metal Nanoparticle Composites

Metal-based nanoparticles and compounds have great potential in the therapeutic domain from date back to ancient times. Assyrians, Egyptians, and Chinese used these metal-based composites for various types of disease treatments such as mercury sulfides (Cinnabar) for the treatment of ailments. Recently, metal-based nanocomposites or complexes for the decoration of GO surface and widely applied them for the treatment of cancer and other incurable diseases. Some recent studies show that GO-metal composites have a good anticancer effect without loading any chemotherapeutic agents. In 2015, for the treatment of ovarian cancer (A2780) cells, Gurunathan et al. synthesized GO/rGO-AgNPs composites decorated with *Tilia amurensis* plant extract without any external anti-cancerous agents [50].

Functionalized GO with metal NPs has promising applications in energy, catalysis, and biomedical fields. Such as in a recently reported work by

Yang et al., GO with associated iron oxide (GO-IO NPs) nanoparticles was used as a drug carrier agent for tumor tissues [51]. In 2011, Ma et al. used GO-IO NPs and functionalized them with the branched-chain polyethylene glycol (GO-IO-PEG) NPs loaded with DOX for in vitro photothermal therapy (PTT) and highly magnetically targeted drug delivery to destroy cancerous cells guided by magnetic fields. These nanocomposites have a fabulous stability in all types of physiological solutions. Besides this in vivo for the imaging of MR mice tumor, these nanocomposites are also used. It is reported that these GO-IO-PEG nanocomposites show a promising platform for cancer imaging and therapy [52]. DOX-loaded GO@Ag nanocomposites were synthesized by another group for the inhibition or death of cancerous cells in chemo-PTT therapy and X-rays imaging [53]. It is also reported that the highest tumor growth inhibition capability of these nanocomposites was 83.9% under NIR irradiations. In a recently reported work, GO nanosheets were decorated with magnetic iron nanoparticles and then functionalized them with CS or sodium alginate for the delivery of DOX in killing of cancerous cells via PTT therapy, and it is also noted that the better release of DOX takes place at a lower value of pH [54]. Thapa et al. synthesized GO-AgNPs nanocomposites loaded with methotrexate (MTX) for the folate receptor tumor-targeted therapy [55]. Kang et al. decorated gold nanoparticles on GO (GO-AuNPs) and investigated its potential in PTT for inhibiting or killing tumor tissues. GO-AuNPs sheets are also stuffed into tumor-tropic mesenchymal stem cells (MSCs) for the intensified efficiency of PTT [56].

12.4.3 GO associated with Polymer Nanocomposites

To overcome the aggregation of GO in presence of salt and serum components in the form of physiological buffer and dose-dependent cytotoxicity, functionalization of GO using polymers including PEG, CS, polyacrylic acid (PAA), polyvinyl alcohol (PVA), and others is the best strategy [52,57–59].

For the drug delivery applications in chemotherapy and other tumor treatment therapies, GO surface modified with CS has become a fabulous functionalization scheme because of its hydrophilic, non-toxic, biocompatible, and biodegradable nature. The solubility of GO can also be enhanced with the addition of CS on its surface. CS polymer is an amino polysaccharides and belongs to the family of acetyl glucosamine and glucosamine [48,60–61]. Because of its mucoadhesive and nontoxic nature, it enhances the strength, stability, and biocompatibility of GO-CS nanocomposites. Fabrication of GO-CS nanocomposites resides on the amide coupling between COOH and amine group of GO and CS,respectively and surface charge/particle size aslo changed through this coupling as a function of pH. Rana et al. synthesize GO-CS functionalized nanocomposites for controlled release of in vitro drugs ibuprofen (IBU) and 5-fluorouracil

(5-FU). These drugs are bonded on the surface of GO-CS via physisorption. Cytotoxicity of 5-FU loaded on GO-CS functionalized nanocomposites was evaluated in CEM human lymphoblastic leukemia and human breast cancer cells Michigan cancer foundation-7 (MCF-7) [62]. Lei et al. synthesized GO-CS nanocomposites modified with sodium alginate (SA) via electrostatic self-assembly. Anti-cancer medicine DOX was loaded on the surface of these nanocomposites by using electrostatic interactions and π-π stacking [63]. Zho et al. fabricated another drug delivery-based system by using GO-CS nanocomposites for the delivery of DOX to HepG2 tumor cells. For killing the PC-3 prostate cancer cell line, Harsha et al. fabricate GO-CS nanocomposites loaded with DOX with a drug-loading capacity of about 65% and releasing capacity of 50% in 48 hours [64]. Xie et al. designed dextran (Dex) loaded GO-CS functionalized composites for the controlled release of Dex in MCF-7 cancer cells. Functionalization of Dex and CS was carried out by a non-covalent self-assembly technique. The author also reported the role of these GO-CS/Dex nanocomposites in killing or inhibiting the HepG2 cancer cell lines [65].

PEG is another "stealth" type of polymer; it enhances the circulating time of NPs in the bloodstream and also protects therapeutic drugs from degradation. PEG has many applications in biomedical and pharmaceutical domains. Because of its safety and biocompatibility, it is registered as "Generally Regarded as Safe" (GRAS) by FDA [66]. Sun et al. designed GO-PEG nanocomposites and reported their diverse applications in the biomedical field. They attached B-specific antibody Rituxan on the surface of GO-PEG nanocomposites for the selective targeting of cancerous cells. Further combination of GO-PEG/Rituxan was used in vitro drugs delivery of doxorubicin to CEM-NKT cells and Raji cell lines [67]. Another group of researchers designed nanocomposites of GO with iron oxide (GO-IO) and functionalized them with PEG for the treatment of cancer. Then these composites were used in the delivery of DOX. And DOX was loaded on the surface of GO-IO-PEG via π–π stacking interactions between the DOX and GO. GO-IO-PEG-DOX composites were also tested for the delivery of drugs to murine breast cancer 4T1 cells [46]. Xu et al. designed GO functionalized with PEG and reported their way of carrier for the paclitexal (PTX) an anti-cancer drug. Synthesis steps for these GO-PEG-PTX nanocomposites are shown in figure 12.10. Drug-loading capacity of these nanocarriers was reported as 11.2% by weight. It is also demonstrated in this work that GO-PEG-PTX composites have a much significant cytotoxicity to A549 and MCF-7 cells as compared to nude PTX [68].

Through hydrolysis and polymerization of vinyl acetate, another water-soluble polymer polyvinyl alcohol (PVA) was synthesized by the researchers. Because of low propensity for adhesion of proteins, biocompatibility, and non-toxic behavior, PVA is highly used in biomedical applications [69]. Aqueous stability and biocompatibility of GO can be

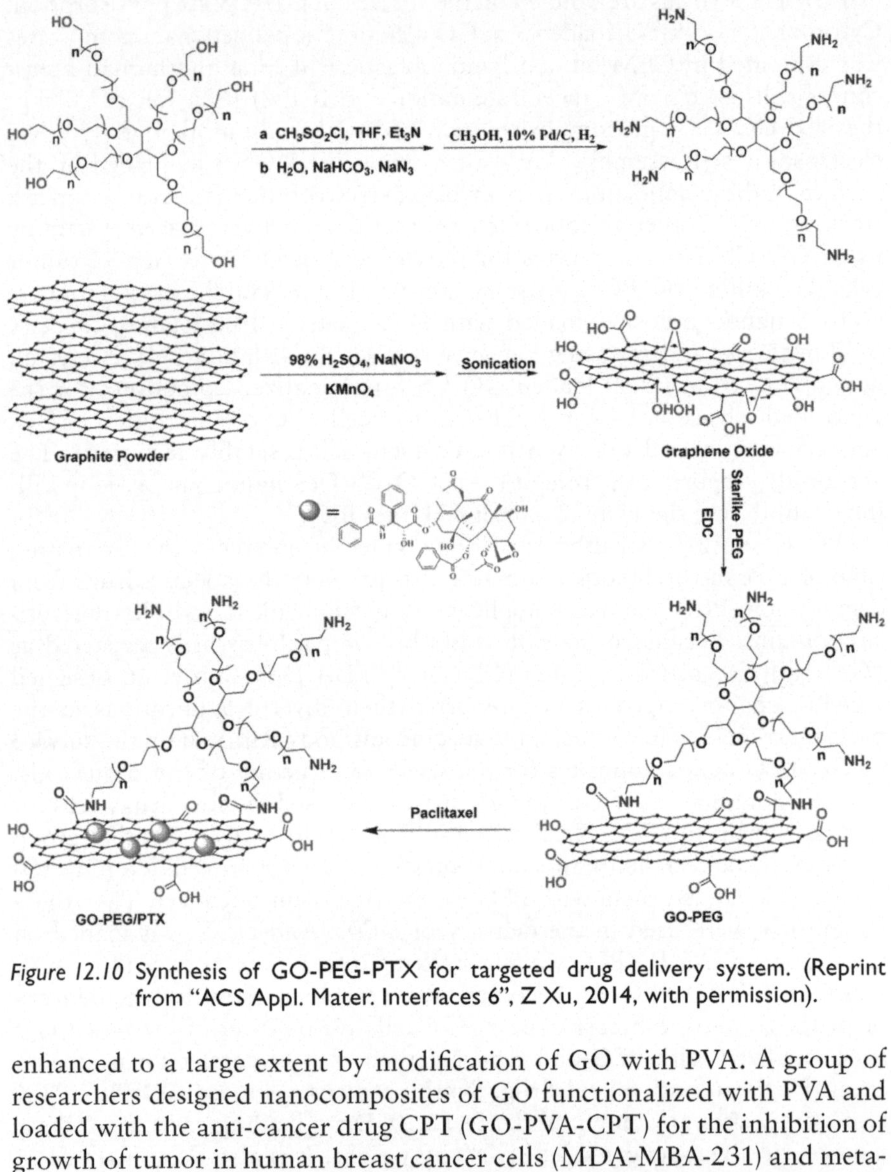

Figure 12.10 Synthesis of GO-PEG-PTX for targeted drug delivery system. (Reprint from "ACS Appl. Mater. Interfaces 6", Z Xu, 2014, with permission).

enhanced to a large extent by modification of GO with PVA. A group of researchers designed nanocomposites of GO functionalized with PVA and loaded with the anti-cancer drug CPT (GO-PVA-CPT) for the inhibition of growth of tumor in human breast cancer cells (MDA-MBA-231) and metastatic skin tumor cell lines (A-5RT3). These composites cause greater than 50% inhibition of tumor cells. GO-PVA-CPT composites show superior strength and potential towards nano-drugs carriers in chemotherapeutic treatment [70].

HA polymer consists of very good stability and aqueous solubility, and is cost effective, due to it's natural occurrence. It is also a biocompatible, non-immunogenic, and biodegradable polysaccharidespolymer [71]. Various research groups have reported diverse drug delivery applications of HA acids. Song et al. synthesized GO modified with HA as a nanocarriers for the carriage of DOX in vitro H22 hepatic cancer cells. Loading of DOX on the surface of GO-HA occurs via π–π stacking and H-bonding interactions. It is also reported by the author that GO-HA-DOX composites show greater cytotoxicity toward HepG2 cancer cells as compared to free DOX or GO-DOX composites. Inhibition towards growth of tumor cells in mice occurs in a dose-dependent manner, and the most effective dose was 6 mg/kg. Jung et al. also designed GO-HA nanocarriers for the targeted delivery of epirubicin. The drug epirubicin was decorated on the surface of GO-HA through π–π stacking interactions [72]. Recently, Pramanik et al. reported various uses of HA-modified GO in vitro drug delivery for methodical tumor therapies [73].

The author used two anti cancer drugs, DOX and PTX, simultaneously for the selective targeting of MDA-MB-231 cancer cells.

PAAis a polymer of acrylic acid and monomers that comes under the category of synthetic polymers. It is less toxic, biocompatible, mucoadhesive, and pH-sensitive polymer. Lu et al. designed GO-PAA composites and explored their potential in specific targeted delivery for 1,3-bis(2-chloroet hyl)-1-nitrosourea (BCNU) brain tumor therapy. PAA was attached to the surface of GO via free radical polymerization reactions. Surface modification by PAA improves various qualities of GO including solubility, thermal stability, and cell-penetrating capability [74]. AFM studies of GO and functionalized GO-PAA shows that both haves same lateral width dimensions. The thickness of PAA-modified GO ranges from 0.9 to 1.9 nm with no contaminates on the surface of GO-PAA. These nanocomposites showed superior dispersibility and did not agglomerate in an aqueous solution even after several months of aging [74,75].

12.5 CHARACTERIZATION TECHNIQUES

12.5.1 UV-Vis Spectroscopy

UV/Vis/NIR spectroscopy was utilized to determine how gefitinib (GEF) and quercetin (QSR) are loaded on top of the nanocarrier delivery system. This was done by first comparing the UV/Vis picture of the medication and GO-PVP in order to determine the loading capacity of the system. H. Tiwari et al. observed that carbon-carbon aromatic double bonds (C=C) at 225 nm in graphene oxide while GO-PVP, a new peak was observed at 275 and 225 nm peak has vanished. Quercetin and gefitinib showed as peaks in the UV/Vis peaks of the dual-drug-loaded scheme at wavelengths of 380and 331 nm, respectively [76]. Furthermore, the optical characteristics of PEG-GO are determined by UV/Vis/NIR spectrophotometer (PerkinElmer LAMBDA 1050, USA). The UV/Vis/NIR spectrum is depicted in Figure 12.11.

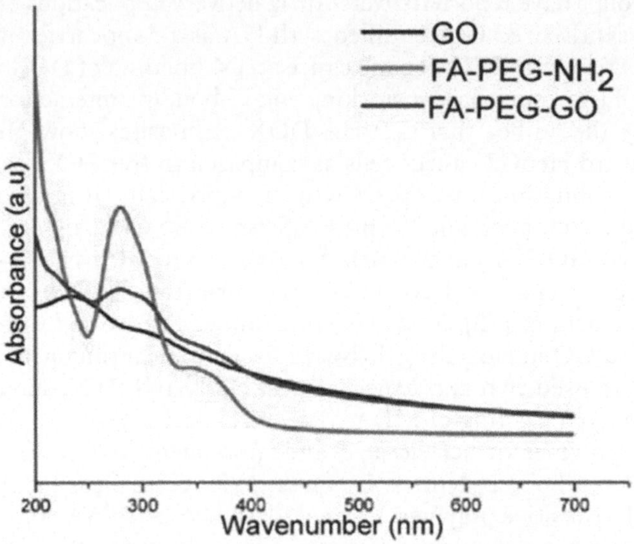

Figure 12.11 GO, FA-PEG-NH2 and FAPEG-GO spectra using UV/Vis/Nir spectroscopy (Reprint from "ACS Biomater. Science Engineering", A Basu, 2018, with permission).

GO's UV-Visible spectrum showed that it has two prominent spectra humps: the 232 nm peak and the 310 nm while there was a peak swing from 232 to 275 nm that could be observed in the spectra of FA-PEG-GO [77]. It was an additional wide-ranging absorbance peak in the range of 340–380nm, which was most likely due to a mixture of FA's second absorbance peak at 370 nm, together with GO's displaced shoulder. These results give the existence of drug loading on the GO.

12.5.2 Fourier Transform Infrared Spectroscopy (FTIR)

Fourier transform infrared spectroscopy will be used to elucidate the structure of the compound and hence, compound identification, i.e., types of the samples. Other than this, FTIR has applications in determining the trace gases in human breath and determining blood chemistries by using surface techniques. It was determined that GO-PVP was effectively connected to the sheet of GO using FTIR spectrum comparisons. The bands observed at the intensities:- 3,406 cm^{-1}/OH, 1,730 cm^{-1}/C-O, 1,623 cm^{-1}/C-C, 1,222 cm^{-1}/C-O, and 1,054 cm^{-1}/C-O-C [78]. Besides these, an intense band at 1,639/cm was caused by GO and FA-PEG joining to create an amide bond between them, as depicted in Figure 12.12. On the other hand, comparing GO and GO-PVP in FTIR spectroscopy

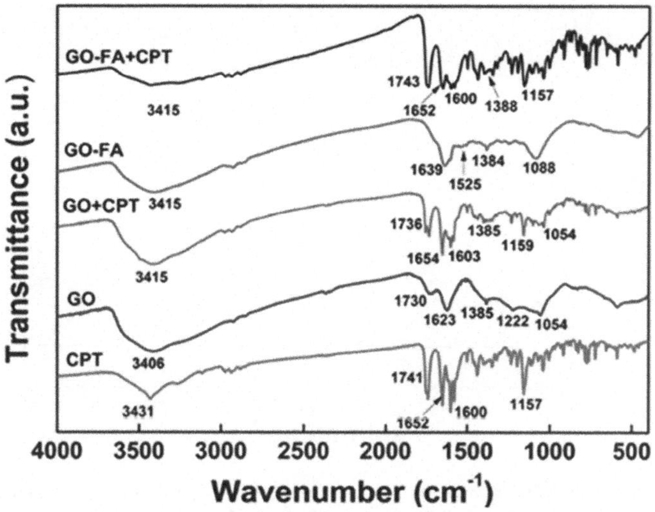

Figure 12.12 FTIR spectra of GO-FA+CPT camptothecin with different bond group including nano-carrier load. (Reprint from "ACS Appl. Nano Mater", M Sous, 2018, with permission).

confirmed that the polymer was successfully attached to the sheet of Go. The spectrum shows the peaks:- 3,435 cm^{-1}/ hydroxyl groups, 1,732 cm^{-1}/ carbonyls of –COOH, 1,635 cm^{-1}/ C-C skeletal, 1,412 cm^{-1}/ carboxy C-O, 1,222 cm^{-1}/ epoxy C-O-C, and 1,048 cm^{-1}/ alkoxy stretching [76].

12.5.3 Raman Spectroscopy

Raman (Indian scientist) cultivates an informative tool focusing on the trace of vibrational characteristics of the molecules and honored with Noble (1930) for it. Specific phase cognate with the vibrational band has been used by the Raman spectroscopy to identify the surface defects. Furthermore, this spectroscopy is widely used to identify the orientation of crystal and phase character of the sample. Raman spectroscopy is also an effective instrument to recognize the composition of the metal (sample). In this sequence, Raman spectroscopy is the key device to investigate the nano-materials and their composites. As a non-destructive method of characterizing graphene and its derivatives, Raman spectroscopy is a decent choice. In order to allow combination chemotherapy in one system, PEGylated nano-graphene oxide (pGO) is loaded with both doxorubicin (DOX) and cisplatin (Pt) clearly presented in Figure 12.13.

After the modification technique, the intensity curve visualized as Pt (black), pGO (blue), and pGO-Pt (red), G and D bonds of graphene could be found at 1,580and 1,340 cm^{-1}, suggested it did not cause any significant

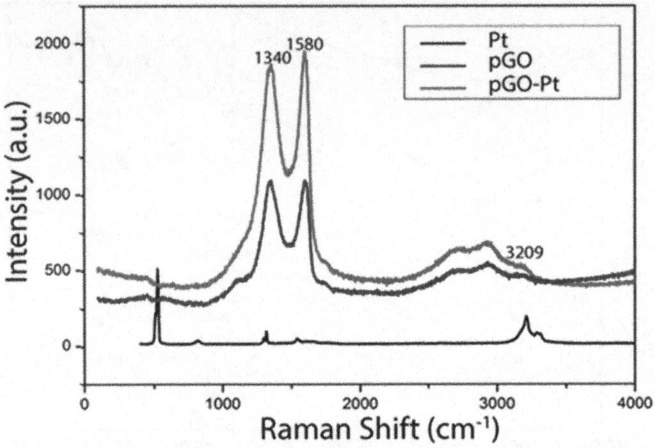

Figure 12.13 pGO, pGO-Pt, and Pt Raman spectrum.Reprinted with permission from [73]. Copyright (2020) Nature. (Reprint from "Scientific report", A Pawlak, 2020, with permission).

structural damage. Raman spectra is displayed in Figure 12.13. With of difference 3,209 cm^{-1}, pGO-Pt followed the same trend as pGO showed that Pt was linked to pGO without altering the fundamental structure [79].

12.5.4 Thermo Gravimetric Analysis (TGA)

TGA is a qualitative technique that is used for monitoring the mass of the sample from 1 mg to several gm as a furnace ramps temperature up to 1,600°C under the stable gas flow atmosphere. TGA instruments vary from the temperature range of 60°C –1,600°C under ambient conditions. The chemical and physical characteristics of the materials are calculated with respect to time or temperature. Under 100°C, mass of graphene is lost owing to π-stacking latticeevaporation of water molecules. TGA analysis is used to investigate the thermal stability of pristine and functionalized graphene. The TGA curves of GO and polydopamine functionalized graphene oxide (GO-PDA) samples reveal multi-stage of weight loss, as shown in Figure 12.14. The derivative curve is specified by the heat degradation of unstable oxygenic functional groups such as carboxyl, epoxy, and hydroxyl, which leads to a significant weight reduction of the GO and GO-PDA sample. As seen by the curves, the largest weight loss of GO and GO-PDA arose at temperatures of 243°C and 263°C, respectively [80,81]. It confirms that GO-PDA is more thermally stable than pure GO at this stage, due to the partial GO reduction and the substitution of some oxygen-containing functional groups with amine groups, which retard thermal degradation.

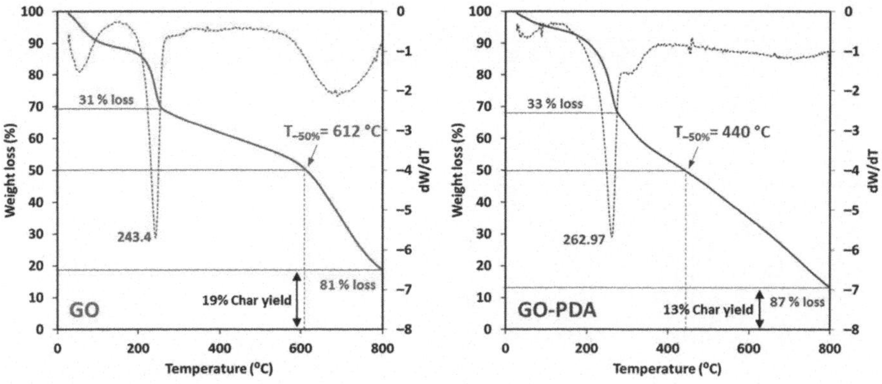

Figure 12.14 TGA analysis of CS, sGO, CMC. (Thermally decomposition). (Reprint from "ACS Appl. Bio Mater", Y Low., 2021, with permission).

12.5.5 Atomic Force Microscopy (AFM)

The family of scanning probe microscopy (SPM) is the key feature to characterize low-dimensional materials, specially focused on multidimensional information in atomic and nanoscale with controlled fashion. The thickness and the height profile of nanomaterials have been measured very accurately. AFM operation can be categorized into three modes;- contact mode, non-contact mode, and tapping mode. The contact potential difference (CPD) and work function energy scanning tunneling microscopy (STM), atomic force microscopy (AFM), shear force microscopy (SFM), scanning probe lithography (SPL), scanning probe microscopy (SPM) required to move a single electron from the highest filled energy level to the vacuum energy level) are vital factors to deal with KPFM (Kelvin probe force microscopy). The CPD (V_{CPD}), the difference between the tip work function (φ Tip) and the surface material work function (φ Sample), is described by the equation:

$$V_{CPD} = (\varphi\,\text{Tip} - \varphi\,\text{Sample}) / q \tag{12.1}$$

Where;- q (1.6×10^{-19}C) is the charge of the electron. It has the ability to measure the thickness and lateral size of the graphene and atomically sized nanocomposites. According to AFM analysis (Figure 12.15), the size range of GO particles is 1–1.5 μm while the height profile indicates the diameter of about 1–1.2 nm [82].

12.5.6 X-ray Photoelectron Spectroscopy (XPS)

In 1960, an ideal, surface-sensitive, quantitative, and valuable instrument has been advanced by K. Siegbahn (Nobel for Physics in 1981) and his

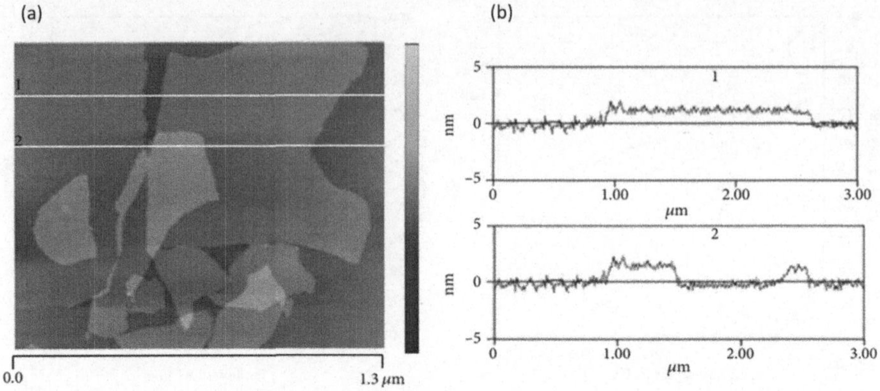

Figure 12.15 GO imaging including height profile by AFM. (reprint from "Hindawi BioMed Research International", A Rhazouani, 2021, with permission).

colleague, who focused on the idea of electron ejection from the surface of the sample. The XPS spectra is based on the interaction of highly energetic X-ray with the sample and coetaneous analyzing the number of electrons and kinetic energy ejects from the sample surface. Therefore, XPS is applicable for the measurement of empirical formula, chemical state, elemental composition, and electronic state of the sample surface. When it comes to graphene oxide with chitosan functionalized on its surface, the XPS technique has been used to confirm the presence of surface composition. ChrGO's oxygen and nitrogen levels were higher than GO's, while its carbon content was lower than GO's. The bump of the ChrGO spectra is present at the 533 eV/ O1s, 399 eV/ N1s, and 284 eV/ C1s. Besides that, the separated peaks related to the ChrGO bond are: 284.7 eV/C-C, 286.4 eV/C-O, 288.2 eV/C=C, and 289 eV/O=C-O, respectively (Figure 12.16) [83]. In the ChrGO spectrum, the presence of an amide peak indicates that CS has been functionalized.

12.5.7 Scanning Electron Microscopy (SEM)

In the account of electron microscopy, SEM stands for the accurate and realistic information provider tool for the nanomaterials by the highly energetic electron scanning method. This scanning method exists the interaction between the sample and electrons and produces super-fine surface imaging. Therefore, SEM apparently measures the compositional and morphological map of the material. In addition, the crystalline structure, surface rift, and surface impurity details have been wildly analyzed by the scanning technique in high vacuum or natural environmental conditions. As shown in the SEM in Figure 12.17, NGO have a schistose-like structure.

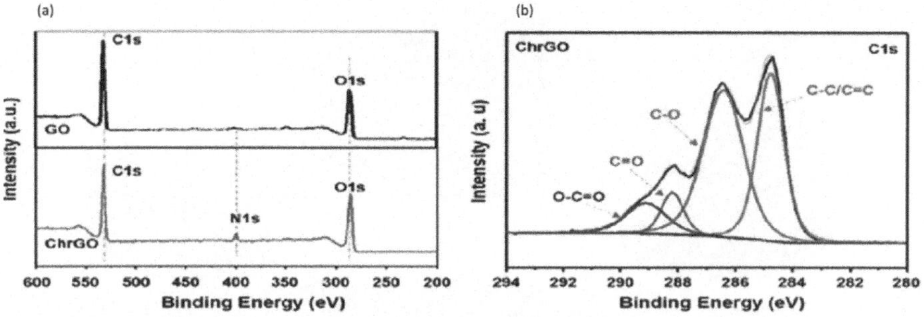

Figure 12.16 The XPS spectra of functionalized GO (ChrGO). (Reprint from "ACS Appl. Bio Mater", Y Low., 2021, with permission).

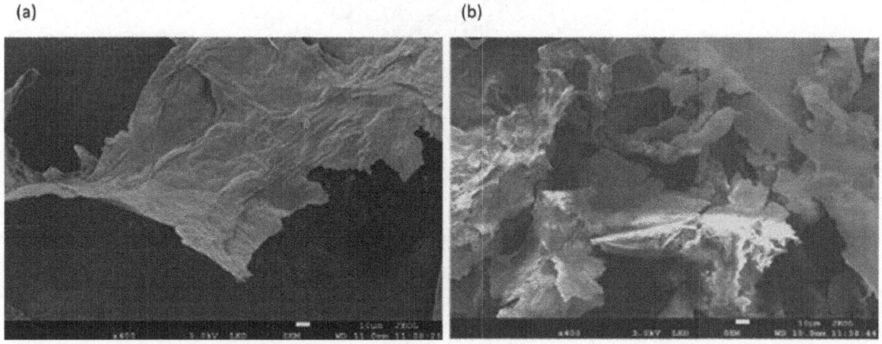

Figure 12.17 (a), (b) SEM imaging of NGO and, DOX@NGO-PEG-HN. (Reprint from "Scientific Report", R. Li., 2021, with permission).

SEM image shows that,- DOX@NGO-PEG-HN(TSPLNIHNGQKL)-1 has pronounced more creases and curls with the comparison of NGO. Due to the π–π stacking bond between the aromatic DOX ring and graphene oxide plates makes the structure almost porous. It is observed that after the treatment of PEG and HN-1, the internal spacing between the layers of GO has been enlarged [48]

12.6 GO NANOCOMPOSITES IN THERAPEUTICAL DOMAIN

Having unique intrinsic physical as well as chemical properties of GO such as large surface region, good nanocarriers, reactive oxygen-containing sites on its basal planes, and effective biocompatibility, graphene and its derived products (GO) have plenty of applications in the therapeutic domain.

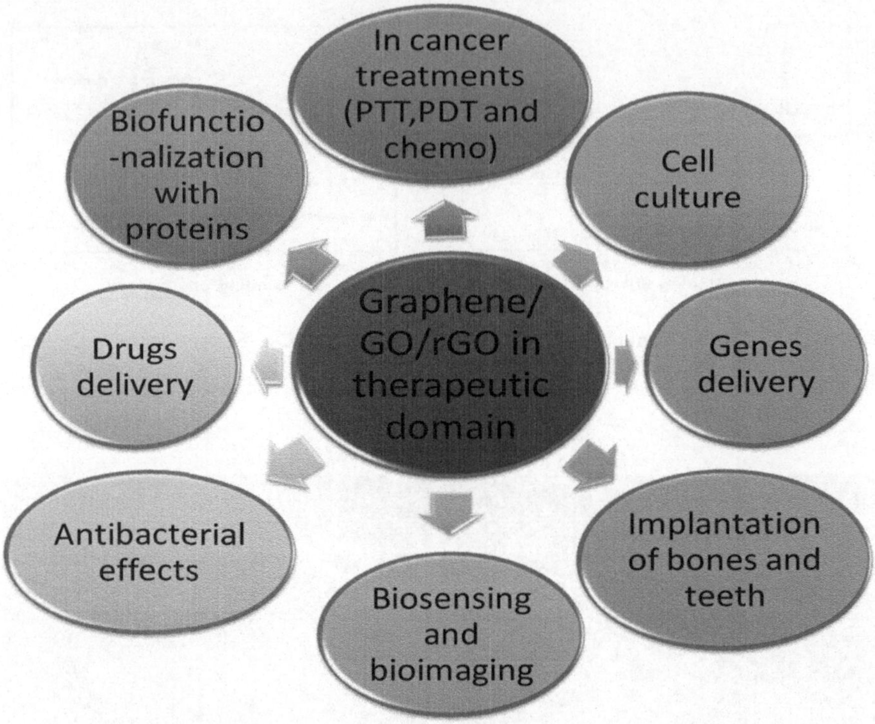

Figure 12.18 Depicting various biomedical applications of graphene family under the domain of drug delivery system.

Because of their promising properties, GO has a variety of applications in biomedical applications such as cancer treatment, bioimaging, antibacterial effects, drug delivery, gene delivery, and more. Various areas of applications of graphene and its derivatives GO/rGO are clearly portrayed in Figure 12.18.

12.6.1 GO in the Direction of Chemotherapeutic Drug Delivery System

Normal clinical chemotherapeutic drugs produce toxic effects and various side effects on the normal cells and also have low cellular uptake. To abolish these limitations in clinical applications of chemotherapeutic drugs, nano-drug delivery system grabs the attention of researcher's community [1–3]. GO offers outstanding properties in this regard, such as high drug-loading capacity, pH responsive, greater surface area, and bio-safety [4–6]. Hence intensive investigations are underway for determining nano-carrier capacity of GO for the delivery of chemotherapeutic drugs in cancer therapy [33]. It is demonstrated by the scientific community on the basis of various studies that GO is a novel approach for performing on-demand chemotherapy coupled with PTT and PDT. Besides having as an effective drug carrier, GO also shows inhibitory actions on the tumor and cancerous tissues and hence stops their growth [59].

Diverse types of anticancer drugs like DOX, SN 38, and methotrexate can be loaded and delivered by using GO as a nano-carrier [84]. Moreover, in 2008 Yang et al. demonstrated that the highest loading capacity of nano-graphene oxide (NGO) for DOX was reported nearly 200% [85]. Because the loading of NGO by using hydrophobic drugs affects its stability in an aqueous medium and also reduces biocompatibility, some modifications are required for attaining fabulous strength of GO in the drug delivery system [86,87]. And hence, for improving stability and biocompatibility of GO, functionalization techniques are the best options, by which we can generate superb biomaterials having various biomedical applications, especially in the drug delivery system [48]. Various functionalization schemes including polymers, antibodie, and metal nanocomposites have been discussed already. Zhou et al. reported that the PEG-functionalized GO works as a promising nanocarrier as well as also resists breast cancer cells' metastasis by selectively down-regulated PGC-1α through the inhibition of OXPHOS [88]. In a recent study, Taun et al. combined photothermal therapy with dual chemotherapies by using two anti-cancer drugs. For this, they- synthesized GO loaded with dual anti-cancer drugs doxorubicin and irinotecan (GO-DI) which was stabilized with poloxamer 188 for heat generation and drugs delivery for killing the cancerous tissues via NIR irradiations. Schematic for the anticnacer activity of GO-DI nanocomposites is represented in Figure 12.19. This combined chemo-photothermal therapy not only improves therapeutic efficacy but also shows superb efficiency to overcome drug resistance [89].

12.6.2 GO in the Gene Delivery System

Gene delivery is a process of introducing external DNA into the cells, for curing various genetically transmitted diseases and complex genetic disorders. On the basis of ethics and safety, scope of gene delivery is controversial, bone marrow and bloods required for gene therapeutic strategies should be remains within the domain of legal grounds. Recently, scientists have investigated various non-viral gene carriers out of which GO emerged as a promising gene carrier for gene delivery because of having fabulous properties including bio-safety, good biocompatibility, large surface area, negative charges, and better adsorption efficiency [90]. In 2019, Di Santo et al. investigated gene therapy as an ideal strategy for the treatments of diverse tumor tissues [91]. A vector is required for gene therapy, which

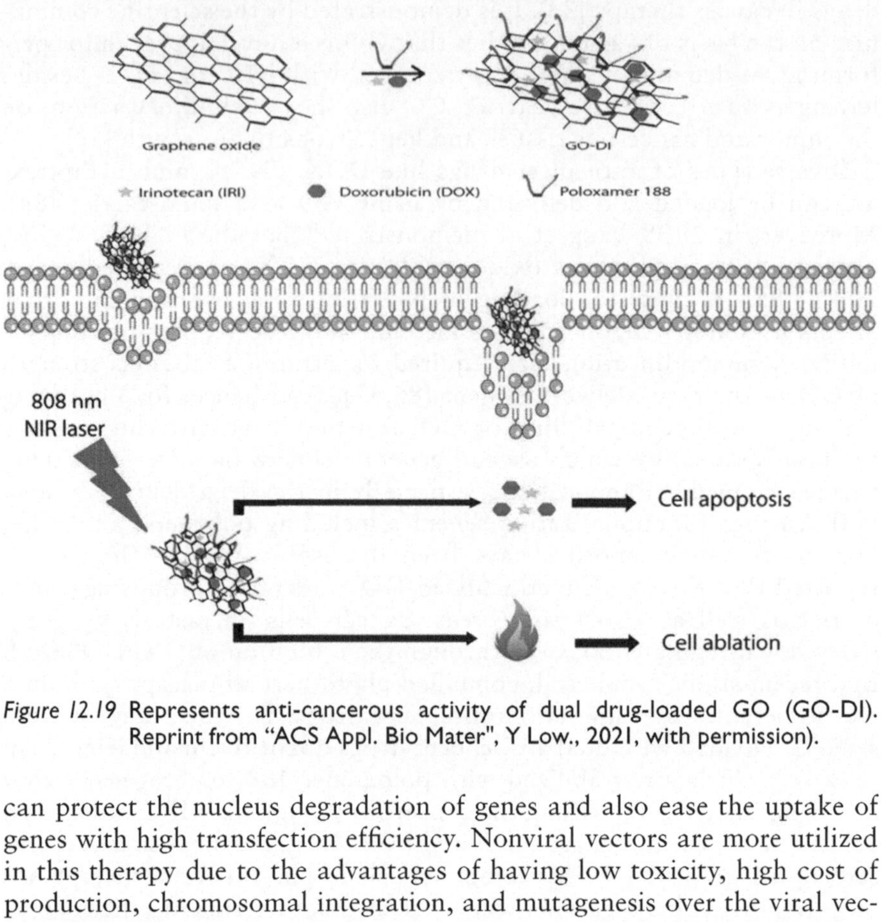

Figure 12.19 Represents anti-cancerous activity of dual drug-loaded GO (GO-DI). Reprint from "ACS Appl. Bio Mater", Y Low., 2021, with permission).

can protect the nucleus degradation of genes and also ease the uptake of genes with high transfection efficiency. Nonviral vectors are more utilized in this therapy due to the advantages of having low toxicity, high cost of production, chromosomal integration, and mutagenesis over the viral vectors [92,93].

Nowadays, functionalized GO has become a superior tool for the gene delivery system. GO sheets functionalized with PEI were used for the cellular gene delivery via electrostatic or covalent interaction for plasmid DNA (pDNA) stacking [94]. In a study by Lu et al., it is demonstrated that nude GO can load single-stranded DNA (ssDNA) via π–π stacking,- but difficult to load double-stranded DNA (dsDNA). Recently, researchers group fabricated nano GO functionalized with PEG and PEI (NGO-PEG-PEI) loaded with pDNA and ssRNA and,- gene carriers active in the NIR region for the efficient delivery of genes and to get a better transfection effect. It is also demonstrated that the expression and silence of genes can be regulated by controlling NIR irradiations [95,96]. In 2018, Du et al. synthesized GO functionalized with PEI, PEG, and FA for the inhibition of growth of the ovarian cancer cells through the delivery of ssRNA [97]. Chain et al. synthesized a novel gene delivery system using GO-PEI nanocomposites for carrying reporter plasmids. In green fluorescent protein (pGFP)-expressing plasmids and luciferase-expressing (pGL-3) plasmids, genetic materials were delivered by using GO-PEI composites on the nucleus of HeLa cells. By using fluorescence microscopy, the delivery of this genetic material was confirmed [98].

Recently, nuclear localization signals (NLSs) have become the most effective tools for providing direct entry of any external substances into the cells via semi-permeable membrane. Most utilized and effective NLS is PV7 peptide (PKKKRKV). To fabricate a nuclear-localized gene delivery system, Ren et al. synthesized GO-PEI composites modified with PV7 peptides [99]. Besides, all of these many latest studies demonstrated that the GO works as a promising tool in gene delivery therapy. But more analysis and studies about the biocompatibility and bio-safety of GO are required to prepare a formulation for the real-life applications of gene delivery in clinical and practical biomedical approaches.

12.7 BIOCOMPATIBILITY AND NOXIOUSNESS OF GO NANOCOMPOSITES

After doing an exhaustive investigation by using cells and animal models, biocompatibility and toxicity of graphene and graphene oxide GO are specified:-, subsequently, clinical and practical applications of GO can be easily elaborated. By rising solubility and dispersibility of graphene, its biocompatibility can be increased [100]. Because of having various carboxyl, hydroxyl, and epoxy groups on the basal plane of GO, it is more hydrophilic and hence more biocompatible than pristine graphene. Biocompatibility of GO can be enhanced to a greater extent by surface functionalization with various hydrophilic agents. Functionalization of GO using polymer PEG not only enhances its biocompatibility and in vivo pharmacokinetics for targeting tumor tissues but also reduces non-specific bindings [28]. Various reports demonstrated that the functionalized GO nano-carriers reduce the risk of cytotoxicity over the major organs such as hearts, liver, spleen, and kidney or on mice even after the treatment of approximately 30 days [101]. But it is also investigated that GO shows dose and time-dependent cytotoxicity. A dose less than 20 μg/Ml, is safe for human fibroblast cells, but greater than 50 μg/mL quantity of GO shows cytotoxic effects such as reducing cell adhesion, inducing cell apoptosis, and entering into mitochondria, lysosomes, cell nucleus, and endoplasm. Long-term stays of GO in kidneys also have various adverse effects on it and also become a very challenging task to clean it from the kidney [57]. GO and its nanocomposites also have antibacterial activity, but besides this, GO shows noxious and cytotoxic effects on prokaryotic cells [102].

12.8 CONCLUSION AND FUTURE SCOPE

Over the past few decades, graphene and its family especially GO have become significant and promising materials for biomedical applications. As we have already discussed in this chapter, GO has emerged as an encouraging and hopeful material in this cancer crisis era. However, functionalization of GO is also a majestic exploration by the scientific community to mitigate some basic limitations of GO such as dose and time-dependent cytotoxicity and some issues related to bio-safety. Functionalization of GO with metal nanoparticles also enhances its efficiency in PTT and PDT therapies. Hence, surface functionalized GO has become a fabulous material as a nano-carrier in chemotherapeutic drug delivery, gene delivery, and also for the loading of various anti-cancerous drugs such as DOX, Dex, methotrexate, and many more. Various biological issues for the normal cells and human bodies have been discussed in the above section. However, next-generation cancer therapies and drug delivery systems in clinical trials are completely based on bio-safety, active targeting, stimuli-response, and multifunctional materials and nanocomposites. As aforementioned functionalized GO reduces this current challenge to a greater extent and also looks forward to providing new and biocompatible clinical options for fighting this cancer crisis era and other lethal diseases. It is also expected that more intensive researches in this direction may open a new window for biomedical sciences for the upcoming period and beyond.

REFERENCES

1. Uthappa, U. T., G. Sriram, Varsha Brahmkhatri et al. "Xerogel modified diatomaceous earth microparticles for controlled drug release studies." *New Journal of Chemistry* 42, no. 14 (2018): 11964–11971.
2. Uthappa, U. T., Varsha Brahmkhatri, G. Sriram, Ho-Young Jung et al. "Nature engineered diatom biosilica as drug delivery systems." *Journal of Controlled Release* 281 (2018): 70–83.
3. Uthappa, U. T., Mahaveer D. Kurkuri, and Madhuprasad Kigga. "Nanotechnology advances for the development of various drug carriers." In: Prasad, R., Kumar, V., Kumar, M., Choudhary, D. (eds.) *Nanobiotechnology in Bioformulations*, Springer, Cham, 2019: 187–224.
4. Uthappa, U. T., Madhuprasad Kigga, G. Sriram et al. "Facile green synthetic approach of bio inspired polydopamine coated diatoms as a drug vehicle for controlled drug release and active catalyst for dye degradation." *Microporous and Mesoporous Materials* 288 (2019): 109572.
5. Uthappa, U. T., G. Sriram, O. R. Arvind et al. "Engineering MIL-100 (Fe) on 3D porous natural diatoms as a versatile high performing platform for controlled isoniazid drug release, Fenton's catalysis for malachite green dye degradation and environmental adsorbents for Pb^{2+} removal and dyes." *Applied Surface Science* 528 (2020): 146974.

6. Uthappa, U. T., O. R. Arvind, G. Sriram et al. "Nanodiamonds and their surface modification strategies for drug delivery applications." *Journal of Drug Delivery Science and Technology* 60 (2020): 101993.
7. Loos, Marcio. "Allotropes of carbon and carbon nanotubes." In: *Carbon Nanotube Reinforced Composites* (2015): 73–101. doi: 10.1016/B978-1-4557-3195-4.00003-5.
8. Tucek, J., Piotr Błonski, Juri Ugolotti et al. "Emerging chemical strategies for imprinting magnetism in graphene and related 2D materials for spintronic and biomedical applications." *Chemical Society Reviews* 47, no. 11 (2018): 3899–3990.
9. Lian, Ruqian, Jianrui Feng, Xin Chen et al. "Q-Carbon: A new carbon allotrope with a low degree of s–p orbital hybridization and its nucleation lithiation process in lithium-ion batteries." *ACS Applied Materials & Interfaces* 12, no. 1 (2019): 619–626.
10. Titirici, Maria-Magdalena, Robin J. White et al. "Sustainable carbon materials." *Chemical Society Reviews* 44, no. 1 (2015): 250–290.
11. Deng, Junjiao, Yi You, Veena Sahajwalla, and Rakesh K. Joshi. "Transforming waste into carbon-based nanomaterials." *Carbon* 96 (2016): 105–115.
12. Georgakilas, Vasilios, Jason A. Perman, Jiri Tucek, and Radek Zboril. "Classification, chemistry, and applications of fullerenes, carbon dots, nanotubes, graphene, nanodiamonds, and combined superstructures." *Chemical Reviews* 115 (2015): 4744–4822.
13. Novoselov Kostya, S., Andre K. Geim, Sergei V. Morozov et al. "Electric field effect in atomically thin carbon films." *Science* 306, no. 5696 (2004): 666–669.
14 Geim Andre K., and Novoselov Konstantin S. "The rise of graphene." 6,ournals, pp. 11-19. 2010.
15. Smith, Andrew T., Anna Marie LaChance et al. "Synthesis, properties, and applications of graphene oxide/reduced graphene oxide and their nanocomposites." *Nano Materials Science* 1, no. 1 (2019): 31–47.
16. Das, Sonali, Deepak Pandey, Jayan Thoma and Tania Roy. "The role of graphene and other 2D materials in solar photovoltaics." *Advanced Materials* 31, no. 1 (2019): 1802722.
17. Cao, Mu, Ding-Bang Xiong, Li Yang et al. "Ultrahigh electrical conductivity of graphene embedded in metals." *Advanced Functional Materials* 29, no. 17 (2019): 1806792.
18. Li, Li-Xiang, and Feng Li. "The effect of carbonyl, carboxyl and hydroxyl groups on the capacitance of carbon nanotubes." *New Carbon Materials* 26, no. 3 (2011): 224–228.
19. Yang, Huihui, David H. Bremner, Lei Tao et al. "Carboxymethyl chitosan-mediated synthesis of hyaluronic acid-targeted graphene oxide for cancer drug delivery." *Carbohydrate Polymers* 135 (2016): 72–78.
20. Loh, Kian Ping, Qiaoliang Bao, Priscilla Kailian Ang et al. "The chemistry of graphene." *Journal of Materials Chemistry* 20, no. 12 (2010): 2277–2289.
21. Ali-Boucetta, Hanene, Dimitrios Bitounis, Rahul Raveendran-Nair et al. "Purified graphene oxide dispersions lack in vitro cytotoxicity and in vivo pathogenicity." *Advanced Healthcare Materials* 2, no. 3 (2013): 433–441.

22. McCallion, Catriona, John Burthem, Karen Rees-Unwin et al. "Graphene in therapeutics delivery: Problems, solutions and future opportunities." *European Journal of Pharmaceutics and Biopharmaceutics* 104 (2016): 235–250.
23. Huang, Xiao, Xiaoying Qi, Freddy Boey, and Hua Zhang. "Graphene-based composites." *Chemical Society Reviews* 41, no. 2 (2012): 666–686.
24. Georgakilas, Vasilios, Jitendra N. Tiwari, K. Christian Kemp et al. "Noncovalent functionalization of graphene and graphene oxide for energy materials, biosensing, catalytic, and biomedical applications." *Chemical Reviews* 116, no. 9 (2016): 5464–5519.
25. Spinato, Cinzia, Cecilia Menard-Moyon, and Alberto Bianco. "Chemical functionalization of graphene for biomedical applications." In: Georgakilas, V. (ed.) *Functionalization of Graphene* (2014): 95–138. Wiley-VCH Verlag GmbH & Co. KGaA, Weinheim.
26. Song, Erqun, Weiye Han, Cheng Li, et al. "Hyaluronic acid-decorated graphene oxide nanohybrids as nanocarriers for targeted and pH-responsive anticancer drug delivery." *ACS Applied Materials & Interfaces* 6, no. 15 (2014): 11882–11890.
27. Wu, Huixia, Haili Shi, Yapei Wang, et al. "Hyaluronic acid conjugated graphene oxide for targeted drug delivery." *Carbon* 69 (2014): 379–389.
28. Liu, Zhuang, Joshua T. Robinson, Xiaoming Sun, and Hongjie Dai. "PEGylated nanographene oxide for delivery of water-insoluble cancer drugs." *Journal of the American Chemical Society* 130, no. 33 (2008): 10876–10877.
29. Lim, Mi-Hee, In Cheul Jeung, Jinyoung Jeong et al. "Graphene oxide induces apoptotic cell death in endothelial cells by activating autophagy via calcium-dependent phosphorylation of c-Jun N-terminal kinases." *Acta Biomaterialia* 46 (2016): 191–203.
30. Kang, Ee-Seul, Inbeom Song, Da-Seul Kim et al. "Size-dependent effects of graphene oxide on the osteogenesis of human adipose-derived mesenchymal stem cells." *Colloids and Surfaces B: Biointerfaces* 169 (2018): 20–29.
31. Sharma, Horrick, and Somrita Mondal. "Functionalized graphene oxide for chemotherapeutic drug delivery and cancer treatment: A promising material in nanomedicine." *International Journal of Molecular Sciences* 21, no. 17 (2020): 6280–6322.
32. Poh, Hwee Ling, Filip Sanek, Adriano Ambrosi et al. "Graphenes prepared by Staudenmaier, Hofmann and Hummers methods with consequent thermal exfoliation exhibit very different electrochemical properties." *Nanoscale* 4, no. 11 (2012): 3515–3522.
33. Liu, Cui-Cui, Jing-Jing Zhao, Rui Zhang et al. "Multifunctionalization of graphene and graphene oxide for controlled release and targeted delivery of anticancer drugs." *American Journal of Translational Research* 9, no. 12 (2017): 5197–5219.
34. Loh, Kian Ping, Qiaoliang Bao, Priscilla Kailian Ang, and Jiaxiang Yang. "The chemistry of graphene." *Journal of Materials Chemistry* 20, no. 12 (2010): 2277–2289.
35. Jonoush, Zahra A., Masoumeh Farahani, et al. "Surface modification of graphene and its derivatives for drug delivery systems." *Mini-Reviews in Organic Chemistry* 18, no. 1 (2021): 78–92.

36. Shim, Gayong, Mi-Gyeong Kim, Joo Yeon Park, and Yu-Kyoung Oh. "Graphene-based nanosheets for delivery of chemotherapeutics and biological drugs." *Advanced Drug Delivery Reviews* 105 (2016): 205–227.
37. Jain, Vijay Prakash, Shivani Chaudhary, Deepa Sharma et al. "Advanced functionalized nanographene oxide as a biomedical agent for drug delivery and anticancerous therapy: A review." *European Polymer Journal* 142 (2021): 110124.
38. Vinters, Harry V., Gérard Debrun, John C.E. Kaufmann, and Charles G. Drake. "Pathology of arteriovenous malformations embolized with isobutyl-2-cyanoacrylate (bucrylate): Report of two cases." *Journal of Neurosurgery* 55, no. 5 (1981): 819–825.
39. Salice, Patrizio, Emiliano Rossi, et al. "Chemistry of carbon nanotubes in flow." *Journal of Flow Chemistry* 4, no. 2 (2014): 79–85.
40. Yang, Huafeng, Qixian Zhang, et al. "Stable, conductive supramolecular composite of graphene sheets with conjugated polyelectrolyte." *Langmuir* 26, no. 9 (2010): 6708–6712.
41. Malaspina, David C., Gabriel Longo, and Igal Szleifer. "Behavior of ligand binding assays with crowded surfaces: Molecular model of antigen capture by antibody-conjugated nanoparticles." *PLoS One* 12, no. 9 (2017): 1–21.
42. Duncan, Ruth, and Rogerio Gaspar. "Nanomedicine (s) under the microscope." *Molecular Pharmaceutics* 8, no. 6 (2011): 2101–2141.
43. Ocana, Alberto, Eitan Amir, and Atanasio Pandiella. "HER2 heterogeneity and resistance to anti-HER2 antibody-drug conjugates." *Breast Cancer Research* 22, no. 1 (2020): 1–3.
44. Juan, Alberto, Francisco J. Cimas et al. "Antibody conjugation of nanoparticles as therapeutics for breast cancer treatment." *International Journal of Molecular Sciences* 21, no. 17 (2020): 6018, 1–21.
45. Siriviriyanun, Ampornphan, Ya-Ju Tsai, et al. "Cyclodextrin-and dendrimer-conjugated graphene oxide as a nanocarrier for the delivery of selected chemotherapeutic and photosensitizing agents." *Materials Science and Engineering: C* 89 (2018): 307–315.
46. Wei, Zheng, Xiteng Yin, Yu Cai, et al. "Antitumor effect of a Pt-loaded nanocomposite based on graphene quantum dots combats hypoxia-induced chemoresistance of oral squamous cell carcinoma." *International Journal of Nanomedicine* 13 (2018): 1505–1524.
47. Lu, Yu-Jen, Pin-Yi Lin, et al. "Magnetic graphene oxide for dual targeted delivery of doxorubicin and photothermal therapy." *Nanomaterials* 8, no. 4 (2018): 193.
48. Li, Ran, Yimei Wang, Jie Du, Xiangyu Wang et al. "Graphene oxide loaded with tumor-targeted peptide and anti-cancer drugs for cancer target therapy." *Scientific Reports* 11, no. 1 (2021): 1–10.
49. Wang, Chen, Zhiqiang Zhang, et al. "Design and evaluation of galactosylated chitosan/graphene oxide nanoparticles as a drug delivery system." *Journal of Colloid and Interface Science* 516 (2018): 332–341.
50. Gurunathan, Sangiliyandi, Jae Woong Han et al. "Reduced graphene oxide–silver nanoparticle nanocomposite: A potential anticancer nanotherapy." *International Journal of Nanomedicine* 10 (2015): 6257–6276.
51. Yang, Xiaoying, Xiaoyan Zhang, et al. "Superparamagnetic graphene oxide–Fe_3O_4 nanoparticles hybrid for controlled targeted drug carriers." *Journal of Materials Chemistry* 19, no. 18 (2009): 2710–2714.

52. Ma, Xinxing, Huiquan Tao et al. "A functionalized graphene oxide-iron oxide nanocomposite for magnetically targeted drug delivery, photothermal therapy, and magnetic resonance imaging." *Nano Research* 5, no. 3 (2012): 199–212.
53. Shi, Jinjin, Lei Wang, Jing Zhang, Rou Ma, et al. "A tumor-targeting near-infrared laser-triggered drug delivery system based on GO@ Ag nanoparticles for chemo-photothermal therapy and X-ray imaging." *Biomaterials* 35, no. 22 (2014): 5847–5861.
54. Xie, Meng, Feng Zhang, et al. "Layer-by-layer modification of magnetic graphene oxide by chitosan and sodium alginate with enhanced dispersibility for targeted drug delivery and photothermal therapy." *Colloids and Surfaces B: Biointerfaces* 176 (2019): 462–470.
55. Thapa, Raj Kumar, Jae Hee Kim et al. "Silver nanoparticle-embedded graphene oxide-methotrexate for targeted cancer treatment." *Colloids and Surfaces B: Biointerfaces* 153 (2017): 95–103.
56. Kang, Seokyung, Junghee Lee, et al. "Gold nanoparticle/graphene oxide hybrid sheets attached on mesenchymal stem cells for effective photothermal cancer therapy." *Chemistry of Materials* 29, no. 8 (2017): 3461–3476.
57. Wang, Kan, Jing Ruan, Hua Song et al. "Biocompatibility of graphene oxide." *Nanoscale Research Letters* 6 (2011) 1–8.
58. Muxika A., Etxabide A., Uranga J., Guerrero P., and Caba K D L.. "Chitosan as a bioactive polymer: Processing, properties and applications." *International Journal of Biological Macromolecules* 105 (2017): 1358–1368.
59. Loutfy, Samah A., Taher A. Salaheldin, et al "Synthesis, characterization and cytotoxic evaluation of graphene oxide nanosheets: in vitro liver cancer model." *Asian Pacific Journal of Cancer Prevention: APJCP* 18, no. 4 (2017): 955–961.
60. Liu, Baoqing, Chengchuan Che, et al. "Fabrication and antitumor mechanism of a nanoparticle drug delivery system: Graphene oxide/chitosan oligosaccharide/γ-polyglutamic acid composites for anticancer drug delivery." *ChemistrySelect* 4, no. 43 (2019): 12491–12502.
61. Sohrabi, Shohreh, Azadeh Haeri et al. "Chitosan gel-embedded moxifloxacin niosomes: An efficient antimicrobial hybrid system for burn infection." *International Journal of Biological Macromolecules* 85 (2016): 625–633.
62. Rana, Vijay Kumar, Myeon-Cheon Choi et al. "Synthesis and drug-delivery behavior of chitosan-functionalized graphene oxide hybrid nanosheets." *Macromolecular Materials and Engineering* 296, no. 2 (2011): 131–140.
63. Lei, Hailin, Meng Xie, Yongwei Zhao et al. "Chitosan/sodium alginate modificated graphene oxide-based nanocomposite as a carrier for drug delivery." *Ceramics International* 42, no. 15 (2016): 17798–17805.
64. SreeHarsha, Nagaraja, Rahul Maheshwari et al. "Graphene-based hybrid nanoparticle of doxorubicin for cancer chemotherapy." *International Journal of Nanomedicine* 14 (2019): 7419–7429.
65. Xie, Meng, Hailin Lei et al. "Non-covalent modification of graphene oxide nanocomposites with chitosan/dextran and its application in drug delivery." *RSC Advances* 6, no. 11 (2016): 9328–9337.

66. Suk, Jung Soo, Qingguo Xu et al. "PEGylation as a strategy for improving nanoparticle-based drug and gene delivery." *Advanced Drug Delivery Reviews* 99 (2016): 28–51.
67. Sun, Xiaoming, Zhuang Liu, et al. "Nano-graphene oxide for cellular imaging and drug delivery." *Nano Research* 1, no. 3 (2008): 203–212.
68. Xu, Zhiyuan, Song Wang, Yongjun Li et al. "Covalent functionalization of graphene oxide with biocompatible poly (ethylene glycol) for delivery of paclitaxel." *ACS Applied Materials & Interfaces* 6, no. 19 (2014): 17268–17276.
69. Aslam, Muhammad, Mazhar Ali Kalyar, and Zulfiqar Ali Raza. "Polyvinyl alcohol: A review of research status and use of polyvinyl alcohol based nanocomposites." *Polymer Engineering & Science* 58, no. 12 (2018): 2119–2132.
70. Sahoo, Nanda Gopal, Hongqian Bao et al. "Functionalized carbon nanomaterials as nanocarriers for loading and delivery of a poorly water-soluble anticancer drug: A comparative study." *Chemical Communications* 47, no. 18 (2011): 5235–5237.
71. Lee, So Yun, Moon Sung Kang et al. "Hyaluronic acid-based theranostic nanomedicines for targeted cancer therapy." *Cancers* 12, no. 4 (2020): 940.
72. Jung, Ho Sang, Min-Young Lee, et al. "Nano graphene oxide–hyaluronic acid conjugate for target specific cancer drug delivery." *RSC Advances* 4, no. 27 (2014): 14197–14200.
73. Pramanik, Nilkamal, Santhalakshmi Ranganathan et al. "A composite of hyaluronic acid-modified graphene oxide and iron oxide nanoparticles for targeted drug delivery and magnetothermal therapy." *ACS Omega* 4, no. 5 (2019): 9284–9293.
74. Lu, Yu-Jen, Hung-Wei Yang et al. "Improving thermal stability and efficacy of BCNU in treating glioma cells using PAA-functionalized graphene oxide." *International Journal of Nanomedicine* 7 (2012): 1737–1747.
75. Chen, Yunping, Yuanyuan Qi, and Bin Liu. "Polyacrylic acid functionalized nanographene as a nanocarrier for loading and controlled release of doxorubicin hydrochloride." *Journal of Nanomaterials* 2013 (2013) 1–8.
76. Tiwari, Himani, Neha Karki et al. "Functionalized graphene oxide as a nanocarrier for dual drug delivery applications: The synergistic effect of quercetin and gefitinib against ovarian cancer cells." *Colloids and Surfaces B: Biointerfaces* 178 (2019): 452–459.
77. Basu, Arijita, Priyanka Upadhyay, Avijit Ghosh et al. "Folic-acid-adorned PEGylated graphene oxide interferes with the cell migration of triple negative breast cancer cell line, MDAMB-231 by targeting miR-21/PTEN axis through NFκB." *ACS Biomaterials Science & Engineering* 5, no. 1 (2018): 373–389.
78. Sousa, Marcelo, Luis Augusto Visani de Luna, Leandro Carneiro Fonseca, et al. "Folic-acid-functionalized graphene oxide nanocarrier: synthetic approaches, characterization, drug delivery study, and antitumor screening." *ACS Applied Nano Materials* 1, no. 2 (2018): 922–932.
79. Pei, Xibo, Zhou Zhu, Zhoujie Gan et al. "PEGylated nano-graphene oxide as a nanocarrier for delivering mixed anticancer drugs to improve anticancer activity." *Scientific Reports* 10, no. 1 (2020): 1–15.

80. Alkhouzaam, Abedalkader, Hazim Qiblawey, and Majeda Khraisheh "Polydopamine functionalized graphene oxide as membrane nanofiller: Spectral and structural studies." *Membranes* 11, no. 2 (2021): 86, 1–17.
81. Pawlak A., and Mucha M . "Thermogravimetric and FTIR studies of chitosan blends." *Thermochimica Acta* 396, no. 1–2 (2003): 153–166.
82. Rhazouani, Asmaa, Halima Gamrani, Mounir El Achaby et al. "Synthesis and toxicity of graphene oxide nanoparticles: A literature review of in vitro and in vivo studies." *BioMed Research International* 2021 (2021): 5518999.
83. Shu, Mengjun, Feng Gao, Min Zeng et al. "Microwave-assisted chitosan-functionalized graphene oxide as controlled intracellular drug delivery nanosystem for synergistic antitumour activity." *Nanoscale Research Letters* 16, no. 1 (2021): 1–12.
84. Dasari Shareena, Thabitha P., Danielle McShan et al. "A review on graphene-based nanomaterials in biomedical applications and risks in environment and health." *Nano-micro Letters* 10, no. 3 (2018): 1–34.
85. Yang, Xiaoying, Xiaoyan Zhang, Zunfeng Liu et al. "High-efficiency loading and controlled release of doxorubicin hydrochloride on graphene oxide." *The Journal of Physical Chemistry C* 112, no. 45 (2008): 17554–17558.
86. Cheon, Yeong Ah, Jun Hyuk Bae, and Bong Geun Chung. "Reduced graphene oxide nanosheet for chemo-photothermal therapy." *Langmuir* 32, no. 11 (2016): 2731–2736.
87. Yu, Jing, Yanmin Ju, Lingyun Zhao et al. "Multistimuli-regulated photochemothermal cancer therapy remotely controlled via Fe_5C_2 nanoparticles." *ACS Nano* 10, no. 1 (2016): 159–169.
88. Zhou, Teng, Bo Zhang, Peng Wei, Yipeng Du, Hejiang Zhou, Meifang Yu, Liang Yan et al. "Energy metabolism analysis reveals the mechanism of inhibition of breast cancer cell metastasis by PEG-modified graphene oxide nanosheets." *Biomaterials* 35, no. 37 (2014): 9833–9843.
89. Tran, Tuan Hiep, Hanh Thuy Nguyen, Tung Thanh Pham et al. "Development of a graphene oxide nanocarrier for dual-drug chemo-phototherapy to overcome drug resistance in cancer." *ACS Applied Materials & Interfaces* 7, no. 51 (2015): 28647–28655.
90. Priyadarsini, Subhashree, Swaraj Mohanty, Sumit Mukherjee, Srirupa Basu, and Monalisa Mishra. "Graphene and graphene oxide as nanomaterials for medicine and biology application." *Journal of Nanostructure in Chemistry* 8, no. 2 (2018): 123–137.
91. Di Santo, Riccardo, Erica Quagliarini, Sara Palchetti et al. "Microfluidic-generated lipid-graphene oxide nanoparticles for gene delivery." *Applied Physics Letters* 114, no. 23 (2019): 233701.
92. Kim, Hyunwoo, and Won Jong Kim. "Photothermally controlled gene delivery by reduced graphene oxide–polyethylenimine nanocomposite." *Small* 10, no. 1 (2014): 117–126.
93. Kim, Hyunwoo, Ran Namgung, Kaushik Singha, Il-Kwon Oh, and Won Jong Kim. "Graphene oxide–polyethylenimine nanoconstruct as a gene delivery vector and bioimaging tool." *Bioconjugate Chemistry* 22, no. 12 (2011): 2558–2567.

94. Liu, Lijun, Qingming Ma, Jie Cao, Yang Gao et al. "Recent progress of graphene oxide-based multifunctional nanomaterials for cancer treatment." *Cancer Nanotechnology* 12, no. 1 (2021): 1–31.
95. Liu, Jingquan, Liang Cui, and Dusan Losic. "Graphene and graphene oxide as new nanocarriers for drug delivery applications." *Acta Biomaterialia* 9, no. 12 (2013): 9243–9257.
96. Wu, Liping, Jinshan Xie, Tan Li, Zihao Mai et al. "Gene delivery ability of polyethylenimine and polyethylene glycol dual-functionalized nanographene oxide in 11 different cell lines." *Royal Society Open Science* 4, no. 10 (2017): 170822.
97. Du, Shibin, Yunfei Wang, Junping Ao et al. "Targeted delivery of sirna to ovarian cancer cells using functionalized graphene oxide." *Nano Life* 8, no. 1 (2018): 1850001.
98. Chen, Biao, Min Liu, Liming Zhang et al. "Polyethylenimine-functionaliz ed graphene oxide as an efficient gene delivery vector." *Journal of Materials Chemistry* 21, no. 21 (2011): 7736–7741.
99. Ren, Tianbin, Lan Li, Xiaojun Cai et al. "Engineered polyethylenimine/graphene oxide nanocomposite for nuclear localized gene delivery." *Polymer Chemistry* 3, no. 9 (2012): 2561–2569.
100. Dreyer, Daniel R, Sungjin Park, Christopher W. Bielawski, and Rodney S. Ruoff. "The chemistry of graphene oxide Chem." *Society Reviews* 39 (2010): 228–240.
101. Sun, Xia, Junpeng Shi, Xiaoyan Fu and Yi Yang, and Hongwu Zhang. "Long-term in vivo biodistribution and toxicity study of functionalized near-infrared persistent luminescence nanoparticles." *Scientific Reports* 8, no. 1 (2018): 1–11.
102. Kumar, Parveen, Peipei Huo, Rongzhao Zhang, and Bo Liu. "Antibacterial properties of graphene-based nanomaterials." *Nanomaterials* 9, no. 5 (2019): 737, 1–32.

Chapter 13

Fullerene Derivatives for Drug Delivery Applications

Pranita Rananaware and Varsha P. Brahmkhatri
Jain (Deemed-to-be University)

CONTENTS

13.1 INTRODUCTION

The fullerene C60 was found in 1985 by Kroto, Curl, and Smalley. They discovered the third allotropic form of carbon belonging to diamond and graphite (Castro et al. 2017). They were awarded a Nobel Prize in 1996 for Chemistry for this seminal discovery (Kroto et al. 1985). C60 is the most abundant and is symbolic of the fullerene family. Fullerene molecules were made entirely of carbon, in the form of a hollow sphere and ellipsoid or tube. Spherical fullerenes can be called buckyballs (Ajie et al. 1990). Allotrope was named fullerene referred to the architect's name (Yadav 2018). The possible forms of fullerenes are not only C60, C70, and fullenerol, but there are various forms that can be designed with hexagons and pentagons. The structures can contain a number of hexagons, but every structure of fullerenes must have only 12 pentagons. Pentagons are essential to form a closed network. Figure 13.1 represents many possible fullerenes such as C28, C32, C44, C50, C58, C70, C76, C84, C240, C540, C960, and many more, out of all the commonly used fullerenes are

DOI: 10.1201/9781003217114-16

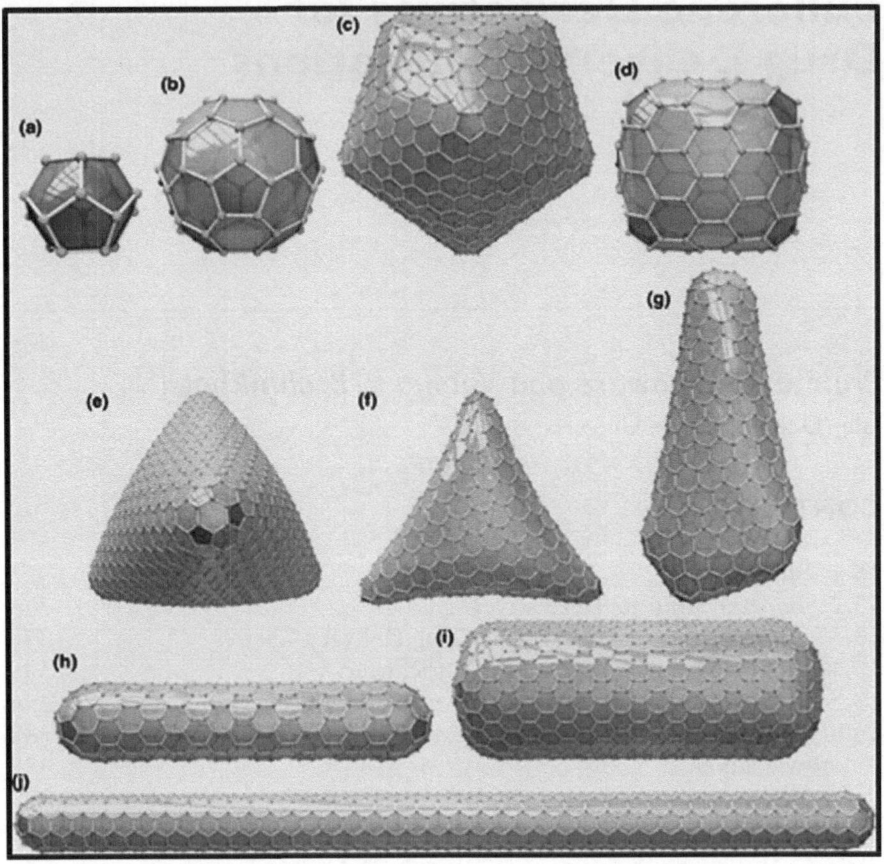

Figure 13.1 (a) C20, (b) C60, (c) C960; (d) barrel-shaped C140; (e) trigonal pyramidally shaped C1140; (f) trihedrally shaped C440-D3; (g) nano-cone C524; (h) cylindrically shaped (tubes) C360, (i) C1152, and (j) C840. (Reprinted with permission from Schwerdtfeger, Wirz, and Avery 2015. Copyright 2016, Nanoscale.)

C60 and C70. C60 molecule has high symmetry, which is one of the main properties (Schwerdtfeger, Wirz, and Avery 2015). The structure of C60 fullerene surface contains 12 pentagons and 20 hexagons. In its 60 carbon atoms, the van der Waals diameter of the C60 molecule is 1 nm in its 60 carbon atom, which resembles the length of a C_8H_{18} molecule (Jensen, Wilson, and Schuster 1996).

In 1990, the functionalized fullerene was first synthesized in the macroscopic amount (Krätschmer et al. 1990). Fullerenes are functionalized to achieve better solubility and improved physical and chemical properties, allowing them to be explored in different fields (Wudl 1992). Fullerenes are the recognized allotropes of carbon that can be dissolved in solvents at room temperature. The bioactive compounds that implement affinity to particular nucleic acids, proteins, and cell receptors such as peptides (Vance et al. 2016) and saccharides (Muñoz et al. 2016) can be functionalization with fullerenes. The functionalization with polar or ionic groups like hydroxyl (Semenov et al. 2016), carbonyl (Kataoka et al. 2016), or quaternary ammonium salts (Castro et al. 2016) and finally encapsulation with macromolecules (Ikeda et al. 2017) are some of the most common approaches to synthesize water-soluble fullerene derivatives for biomedical applications (Castro et al. 2017; Vance et al. 2016). These applications were feasible because of the specific factors present in this carbon allotrope, including its three-dimensional structure, chemical reactivity, and solubility (Moussa 2018).

Buckminsterfullerenes (C60) is a shortened icosahedron that contains 60 carbon atoms with C5–C5 single bonds forming pentagons and C5–C6 double bonds forming hexagons. The width of a fullerene molecule is 0.7 nm (Kroto et al. 1985). Fullerene-based nanomaterials are considered well in chemistry, physics, and biology because of their excellent rigidity, high symmetry structure, and stability. In the last 25 years, the reports on fullerenes have increased exceptionally and exhibit more efficacy in terms of applications (Moussa 2018). Moreover, C60 has less solubility in aqueous solvents, limiting its biomedical applications. Currently, numerous reports have been coming up toward variation of biocompatible fullerenes and water-soluble fullerene, which benefit further and expand the studies of C60-based fullerenes (Ma and Liang 2010). The method of improving the solubility of fullerene to form its complex with surfactants like polyethylene glycol (PEG), cyclodextrin, etc. The fullerene surface was modified with multi-polar groups to produce a water-soluble compound, including hydroxylated fullerenes, amination of fullerenes, carboxy fullerenes (malonic acid substituted fullerenes), and endohedral metallofullerenes. The modification of fullerene was widely used not only to keep the spherical structure and physical properties intact but also to retain some chemical and biological activities. These fullerene nanoparticles were accumulated with different surfaces, sizes, and morphological properties. It has been shown that they find varied applications in biomedicine, including radiotracers (Okumura et al. 2002) and magnetic resonance imaging (MRI) contrast agents for metallo fullerenols (Shevtsov et al. 2014).

The functionalization and surface modification of fullerene and its derivatives are shown in Figure 13.2. In this chapter, we have discussed the fullerenes as important drug delivery carriers for various drugs, genes, and DNA and RNA biomolecules, and their therapeutic potential in targeted therapies will be enlightened.

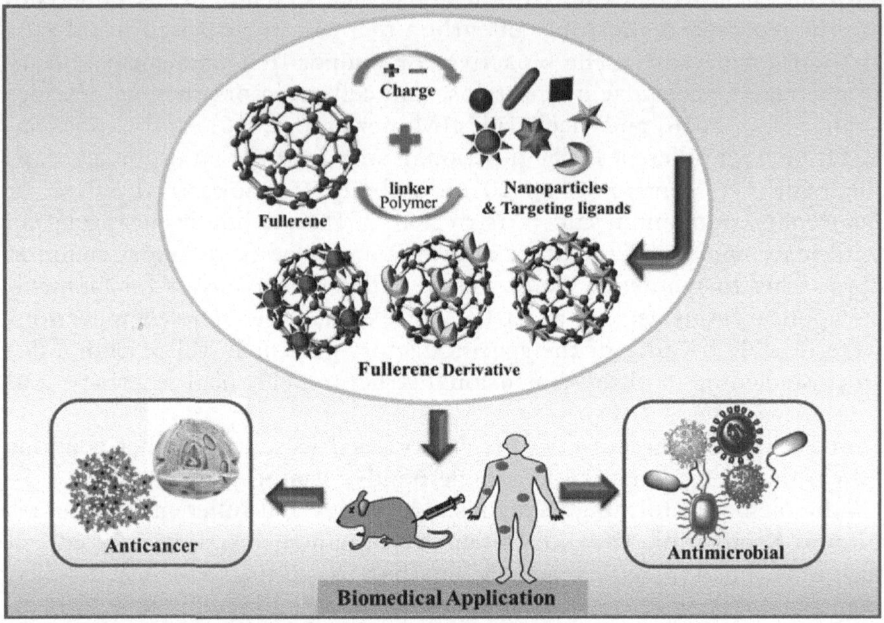

Figure 13.2 Fullerene derivative for biomedical application.

13.2 FULLERENE AND ITS DERIVATIVES

There are numerous synthesis methods for the preparation of fullerene C60 nanotubes (FNTs), like solution evaporation (Wang et al. 2006), template technique (Liu et al. 2002), surfactant-assisted method (Ji et al. 2007), and liquid-liquid interfacial precipitation method (LLIP) (Minato, Miyazawa, and Suga 2005). While discriminating with another synthesis method, the LLIP method is effortless and commercially viable for the direct development of FNTs at room temperature and without necessary catalysts or surface-active agents (Qu et al. 2011).

In the classic LLIP process, pyridine was used as a suitable solvent and isopropyl alcohol (IPA) was used as a precipitation agent (Li et al. 2010). Moreover, in preparing FNTs, pyridine exhibits a highly toxic and irritant smell, which is unsuitable for mass or industrial manufacture. N-methyl-2-pyrrolidone (NMP) is replaced by pyridine as the better solvent to prepare FNTs, giving good solubility for C60 at a meager price. FNFs were prepared in NMP/IPA system with several morphologies for the earliest. The different morphologies of FNFs in the NMP/IPA system were established by scanning electron microscopy (Qu et al. 2011).

Another functionalization strategy of fullerene with silver carbonate was investigated, wherein the reaction of fullerene with (Z)-N-aryl benzamidines provided unique C60-fused imidazoline products with high yields. Substrates with both electron-donating and electron-withdrawing groups acting on aromatic rings could be working. Fulleroimidazolines should be further functionalized for giving regioisomeric derivatives with 1,2,3,4-configuration or nitroxide products, which can be difficult to synthesize by available methods (He et al. 2013).

The functionalization of C60 by various functional groups can lead to different biomedical applications, as shown in Figure 13.3. Many of the functionalized fullerenes were reported with a good yield to excellent yields resulting in several functional and distinctive fullerene-based materials. Moreover, the application of these derivatives has not been studied completely. Though various methods have been developed to synthesize the flexible structures, the construction of definite nanostructures according

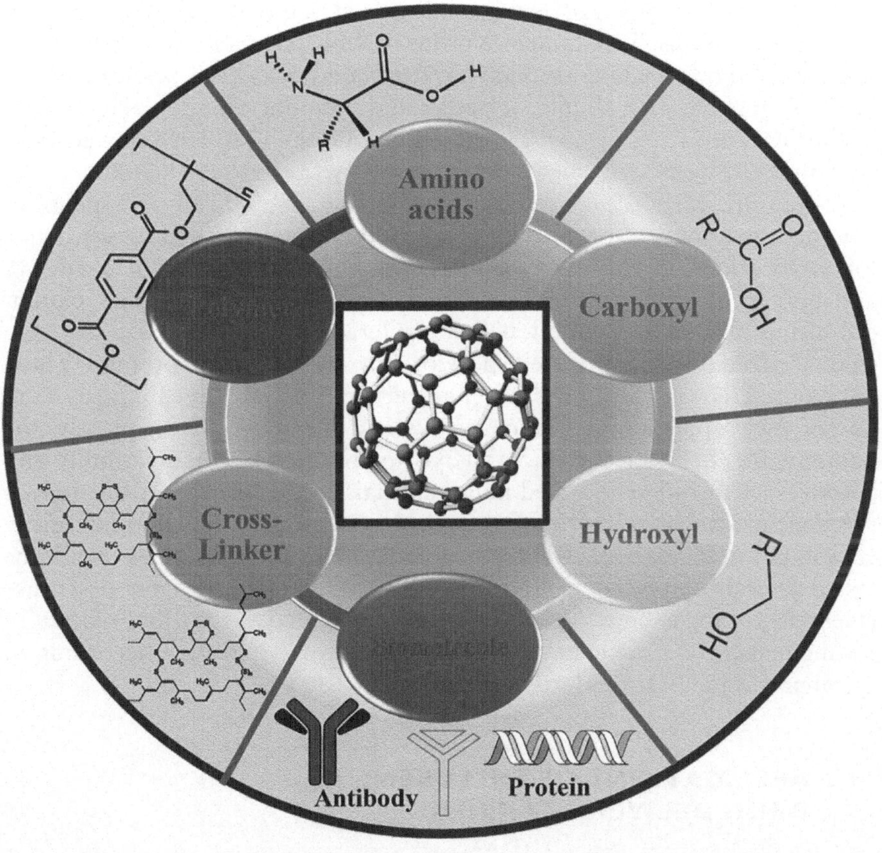

Figure 13.3 Various functional groups for fullerene functionalization toward the biomedical application.

to the requirement of functional fullerene materials and biologically useful molecules is still a challenge (Yan et al. 2015).

The chemical oxidation of fullerene C60 into a highly oxidized analog (oxC60) using Staudenmaier's procedure was reported (Zygouri et al. 2020). This simple oxidation protocol is broadly used in the chemical oxidation of graphite. This oxidation leads to the formation of a highly soluble fullerene's derivative (known as "fullerene oxide" comparable to graphene oxide) by forming oxygen-carrying functional polar groups on the surface of C60 while holding its spherical structure. Apart from its simplicity, the main advantage of this method compared with other derivatives for soluble C60 products is the invention of epoxy groups on the surface of the fullerene. In this synthetic approach, hydrophilic C60 molecules were created with epoxy elements in higher yields at a low cost. Additionally, these groups are allowed for further functionalization and thus for inventing the new hydrophilic fullerene product without any requirement of higher temperatures and complicated synthetic reactions. Epoxy groups are readily modified via ring-opening reactions under different conditions. For example, a primary aliphatic amine (octadecylamine) was achieved by attaching through covalent bonding. This is achieved by the method representing a simple, versatile, and reproducible approach for controlling the derivatives of various well-defined and stable fullerene products by exploiting the well-established carbon chemistry (Zygouri et al. 2020).

The unique carbon cage structure which can give numerous opportunities for functionalization provides the nanomaterials with great efficiency for applications in the medical field. Analyzing the physical, chemical, and biological properties of fullerenes and their derivatives, they exhibit promising results. The functionalized fullerene-based nanomaterials were characterized by using infrared spectroscopy and by aquaphotomics. These nanomaterials were also used for engineering a new skin cream formula in one of their applications like cosmetics and medicine. Consequently, the nano-cream effects on the skin and existing results of biocompatibility and cytotoxicity of fullerene-based nanomaterials can confirm that fullerene is not toxic in low concentrations when functionalized. Investigation of fullerenes to get new materials for cosmetic and medical applications should be tested as there can be some effects on sensitive tissue like eye tissue. Future research will focus on various types of acute systemic, irritation, sensitivity testing, subchronic toxicity, and *in vitro* genotoxicity testing according to the appropriate ISO standards (Zygouri et al. 2020).

13.3 APPLICATIONS OF FULLERENE AS DRUG DELIVERY CARRIER

Fullerene molecules are self-possessed of carbon in the form of a hollow sphere, ellipsoid, or tube. Fullerenes in the form of a cylindrical structure

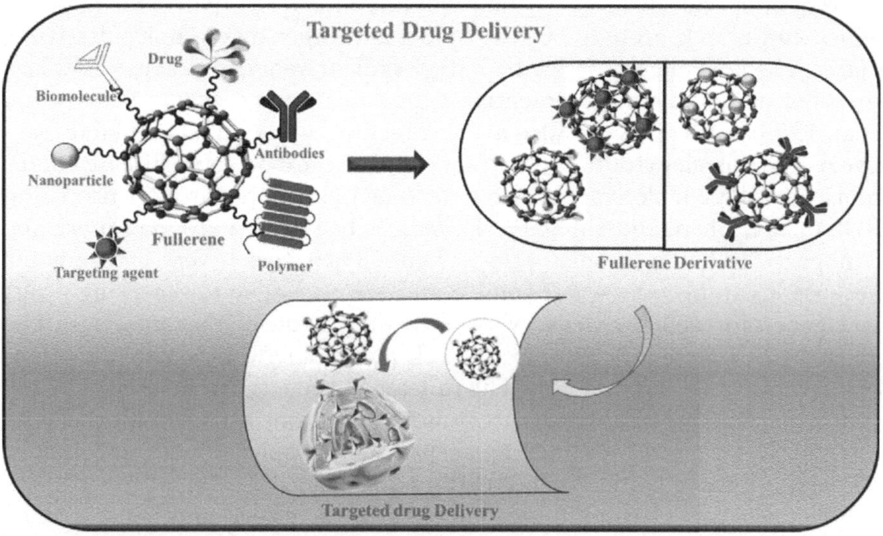

Figure 13.4 Fullerene as a targeted drug delivery agent.

are called carbon nanotubes (CNTs) or buckytubes and fullerenes in the spherical shape are known as buckyballs. The special carbon cage structure coupled with immense scope for derivatization makes them an efficient therapeutic agent for biomedical applications (Uthappa, Kurkuri, and Kigga 2019). Fullerene has great potential as a targeted drug delivery agent, as shown in Figure 13.4. The fullerenes can be used in organic photovoltaic (OPV), medical purposes, portable power, biopharmaceuticals, and as antioxidants (Bhakta and Barthunia 2020).

The conjugation of fullerene-based biomolecules has become a preliminary strategy in ov0ercoming the intrinsic hydrophobic obstacles wrecked by fullerenes to use such molecules for biological purposes. The applications of fullerenes in various physicochemical and pharmacological fields are active. They are found to be flexible and lightweight but are stronger than steel. They have good resistance to heat while transferring better than any other material. These characteristics apply to different applications like super-strong cables and biomedical devices for drug delivery and tips for scanning probe microscopes, medical diagnostic, and therapeutic applications. In most of the studies, it is observed that C60-fullerenes are not cytotoxic to human and animal cells in vitro, and the acute toxicity against animal tissues is low for in vivo conditions (Bhakta and Barthunia 2020).

Fullerene-based materials have been reported as anti-HIV agents by rapidly fitting in the active site of the viral protease. The fullerenes of anionic and cationic types prevent the duplication of HIV-RT and hepatitis C virus (Mashino et al. 2005). Fullerenes have neuroprotective activity in response to oxygen species such as O_2 (Superoxide) and OH (Hydroxyl) radicals, which can attack proteins, DNA, lipids, and other macromolecules without ingesting. Fullerenes can be called radical sponges because they are reported as world's most potential radical scavenging agents (Tokuyama et al. 1993). Fullerenes can also act as a medical antioxidant. Cellular reactive oxygen species (ROS) production can cause apoptosis in disease conditions. So fullerene derivatives can defend against apoptosis by neutralizing ROS (Yang, Chen, and Shi 2019). Fullerenes belong to a group of inorganic nanoparticles having a small size (~ 1 nm). Their core is very hydrophobic because it can become water soluble and are accessible for carrying drugs and genes for cellular delivery by attaching hydrophobic moieties. The products of fullerenes can cross the cell membrane to bind the mitochondria (Azzam and Domb 2004). The fullerene products can be used as X-ray contrast agents. C60 fullerenes are found to be a contrast agent for the MRI method. It is a good MR imaging agent when complexed with gadolinium (Ghiassi, Olmstead, and Balch 2014).

Fullerenes can trap toxic heavy metals in their cage and hence can be used as radiotracers *in vivo* (Shinohara 2000). The fullerenes were established to have efficient antimicrobial activity due to their intercalation with biological membranes. The various strains of fungi and bacteria like *B. subtilis*, *C. albicans*, *M. avium*, and *E. coli* display positive results (Mashino et al. 1999). It acts as a preservative in antiaging cosmetics, and to prevent oxidation, it is formulated with zinc oxide (Hirlekar et al. 2009). Due to its capacity to fluorescence with some biomolecules, protein-captured nanotubes can be used as implantable biosensors. For the study of cells and biological systems, they have been used as nanosized robots and motors (Lacerda et al. 2006).

In the past few years, the important aspects of the carbon molecules are claimed to develop a new exciting scientific field (Zhao et al. 2017). This progress recommends the idea of fullerene applications as an extensive choice in the areas such as diagnostics, pharmaceuticals, environmental, and energy industries along with medical and dental fields with complex resin and coating materials for dental implants, bonding systems, and dental restorations (Zhao et al. 2017). These developments lead to a wide range of efficient commercial applications, including anticancer drug delivery systems using photodynamic therapy, HIV drugs, and cosmetics to slow down human skin aging. In the detection, fullerene products become constant immune effector cells for avoiding or obstructing the release of proinflammatory molecules, making them potential candidates for various diseases like arthritis, asthma, and multiple sclerosis. Gadolinium contains endohedral fullerenes, as MRI contrast agents for diagnosing numerous diseases. Therefore, a new group of fullerenes-based theranostics is developed, which can combine therapeutic and diagnostic capabilities for detecting and killing cancer cells (Bhakta and Barthunia 2020).

13.4 APPLICATION OF FULLERENE FOR ANTICANCER

Developments in nanotechnology and nanomaterials can attain the objective of early diagnosis and early therapy of cancer in the forthcoming decades (Chen et al. 2012). Over the past few years, fullerene and its by-products have been reflected as the most inspiring nanomaterials because of its exclusive properties that accelerate various medicinal applications. The drugs can be delivered through a small therapeutic molecule to the cancer cells. It has been described how fullerene and its derivatives have been reported for cancer therapy and diagnosis. It will be emphasized that fullerene derivatives are used as antitumor drugs.

Fullerene and its products as antitumor agents is a new commencement that has appeared in recent years (Chen, Mao, and Liu 2012). In many tumor analysis studies, fullerene and its by-products were more efficient in overcoming tumor growth than predictable antitumor chemicals (Chen et al. 2005). The mechanism for antitumor activity of fullerene and its derivatives included anti-angiogenesis (Meng et al. 2010), oxidative stress regulation, effective immunomodulator, and autophagy inducement (Chen et al. 2012).

Fullerene C60 and its products have been well established for their efficiency as drug carriers for local cancer chemotherapy. The coupling of C60 derivatives with the high clinical active anticancer drugs has been measured as a demonstrative strategy to impart C60-specific properties for enhanced preparation (Chen, Mao, and Liu 2012). Wilson and coworkers created a C60-paclitaxel conjugate as a slow-release drug for aerosol liposome transfer of paclitaxel for lung cancer therapy. The outcomes endorsed that the conjugate was similar to free paclitaxel in antitumor influence in vitro and held assurances for enriched therapeutic efficacy of paclitaxel in vivo. The in vitro therapeutic efficacy of the paclitaxel-embedded fullerene was suppressed toward the MCF-7 breast cancer cell growth compared with Abraxane, a commercially available, nanoparticle-albumin-bound formulation of paclitaxel. The results demonstrated that the paclitaxel-embedded buck exhibits similar efficacy to Abraxane in cell viability studies. Moreover, empty bucks were not cytotoxic (Partha et al. 2008). Doxorubicin (DOX) is also a highly effective drug used for cancer chemotherapy and can be used as self-labeled fluorescent probes in bioimaging and other mechanistic investigations on drug delivery. To upgrade the side effects of DOX drug delivery, improving the cellular uptake and selective targeting of cancer cells conjugation with fullerenes may be beneficial (Liu et al. 2010). Hydrophilic covalent conjugates of fullerene and DOX were synthesized for the anti-neoplastic activities of DOX. By comparing fullerenol-DOX antitumor efficacy to the free drug, conjugate exhibited better performance without any systemic toxicity of free DOX in vitro (Lu, Haque, et al. 2009).

Photodynamic therapy (PDT) is usually used for severe disease treatment through visible light irradiating photosensitizing agents or photosensitizers to activate ROS to kill cells. ROS is an aggressive chemical species that can rapidly react with any nearby biomolecules, and cells, including normal and abnormal cells, can be killed by apoptosis or necrosis (Dolmans, Fukumura, and Jain 2003). Recent reports on targeting photosensitizers on the tumor by linking antibodies or antibody fragments suggest that when injecting them into the bloodstream, the photosensitizers were absorbed specifically by cancer cells. However, they are still in pre-clinical trials (Lu, Hu, et al. 2009). Another interesting fullerene analog, C60-PEG, was investigated for antitumor activity. It was found that the C60-PEG conjugates with methyl-terminated PEG, with the highest molecular weight, exhibit the longest half-life period in the blood circulation and the highest tumor accumulation with a maximum suppression of the tumor growth (Lu, Hu, et al. 2009).

A fullerene-based tumor-targeted multifunctional magnetic nanocomposite (C60-IONP-PEG-FA) showed negligible toxicity both in vitro and in vivo. Nanoparticles were found to be powerful tumor diagnostic agents as well as a strong photosensitizer for photothermal ablation of the tumor, as shown in Figure 13.5a. The C60-IONP nanocomposite is synthesized via decorating iron oxide nanoparticles (IONP) onto fullerene (C60) and then functionalized by polyethene glycol (PEG2000), giving C60-IONP-PEG with excellent stability in physiological solutions. Finally, folic acid (FA), a widely used tumor-targeting molecule, was linked to C60-IONP-PEG to obtain an active tumor-targeting effect on MCF-7 cells and malignant tumors in mice models. C60-IONP-PEG-FA is the very effective photosensitizer and powerful agent for photothermal ablation of tumor and depicts minimum toxicity as shown in Figure 13.5c and d. It served as a powerful tumor diagnostic MRI contrast agent, and furthermore, for better enhancement, PDT is combined with radio frequency (RF) thermal therapy (RTT) during the treatment in both in vitro and in vivo. Moreover, the versatile nanoplatform can selectively kill cancer cells which can be highly localized in regions via excellent active tumor-targeting and magnetic-targeted abilities. The multifunctional C60-IONP-PEG-FA nanoplatform had great potential for cancer theragnostic applications (Shi et al. 2014).

A recently reported, water-soluble nano-conjugate of fullerene-glycine derivative with the FDA-approved drug gemcitabine (nanoC60GEM) (Nalepa et al. 2020). The physiochemical characteristics of the fullerene nanomaterial confirm that two gemcitabine units are attached to the fullerene scaffold via the formation of amide bonds, as shown in Figure 13.5 D. The nanoC60GEM showed that the cytotoxicity effect was concentration dependent in PAN02 cells, as depicted in Figure 13.5e. However, it offers mild phototoxic effects due to the protein corona formation on the surface of the fullerene scaffold and the low quantum yields of the singlet oxygen

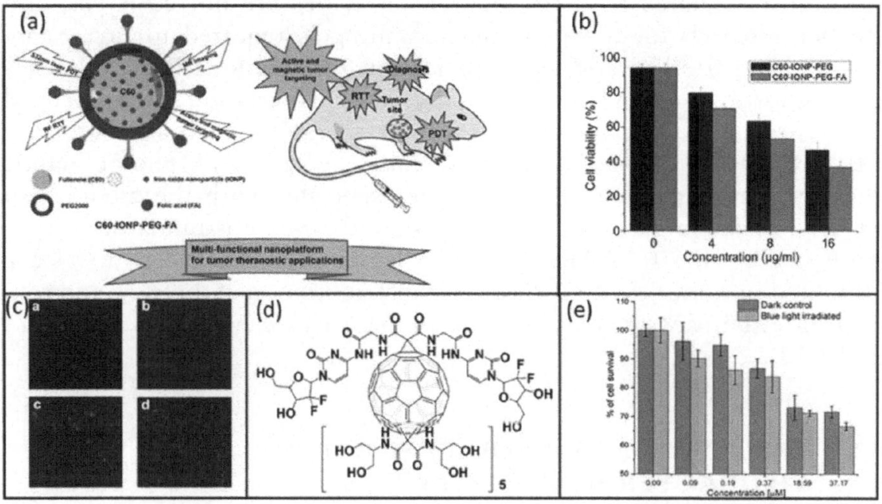

Figure 13.5 (a) Schematic representation of C60eIONPePEGeFA and its biofunctions. (b) Viabilities of MCF-7 cells. (c) Fluorescence images of stained cells treated with C60eIONPePEGeFA. (Reprinted with permission from Shi et al. 2014. Copyright 2014, Biomaterials.) (d) Chemical structure of nanoC60-GEM. (e) Phototoxicity effect on the PAN02 cancer cell line of nanoC60GEM. (Reprinted with permission from Nalepa et al. 2020. Copyright 2020, Cancer Nanotechnology.)

generation. Further in biological studies, 3D spheroids and murine models were used to evaluate the efficacy of therapy using nanoC60GEM. The results acquired from biological assays on pancreatic cancer cell lines show the enhanced cytotoxic effects of nanoC60GEM by generating ROS after blue LED irradiation on fullerene nanomaterial (Nalepa et al. 2020).

Figure 13.5 (a) Schematic representation of C60eIONPePEGeFA and its biofunctions. (b) Viabilities of MCF-7 cells. (c) Fluorescence images of stained cells treated with C60eIONPePEGeFA. (Reprinted with permission from Shi et al. 2014. Copyright 2014, Biomaterials.) (d) Chemical structure of nanoC60-GEM. (e) Phototoxicity effect on the PAN02 cancer cell line of nanoC60GEM. (Reprinted with permission from Nalepa et al. 2020. Copyright 2020, Cancer Nanotechnology.)

Fullerene has a unique chemical structure that possesses interesting photophysical properties, making it a potentially strong candidate for photodynamic therapy in biological systems (Arbogast et al. 1991). The physicochemical properties of fullerenes and functionalized fullerenes encourage developing tumor theranostics for potential applications in tumor imaging and therapy (Chen et al. 2012).

The interesting properties of fullerenes can bring new insights for anti-tumor therapeutics, including gene therapy. However, the underlying mechanisms related to their apparent activities are not clear yet, and further research for a better understanding is required to investigate the biocompatibility and safe application of functionalized fullerenes as diagnostic tools and therapeutic agents. Furthermore, functionalized fullerenes show their potential in tumor therapies, such as photothermal treatment, chemotherapeutics, radiotherapy, and photodynamic therapy. The antitumor effects can be associated with the modulation of anti-angiogenesis, oxidative stress, and immunostimulatory activity (Chen et al. 2012). The diverse varieties of fullerene derivatives are exploited in tumor theranostics; their distribution, metabolism, and toxicity in organisms are the concern among researchers as mentioned in Table 13.1.

13.5 APPLICATIONS OF FULLERENE FOR ANTIBACTERIAL ACTIVITY

Fullerene derivative possesses antibacterial activity against both Gram negative (*E. coli*) and positive bacteria (*S. aureus*). The antibacterial activities are dependent on time and concentration. In the first hour of incubation, most of the bacteria are inactivated, and when there is an increase in material concentration, the rate of cell death also increases (Chen, Ma, et al. 2016). Due to direct physical contact, bacterial cytotoxicity can be attributed to membrane stress and causes cell death, as shown in Figure 13.6. The suppression of energy metabolism (Shvedova et al. 2012), direct physical contact (Lyon et al. 2008), respiratory chain inhibition, and photosensitizing effects (Sharma, Chiang, and Hamblin 2011) of fullerene derivatives are considered to be responsible for the observed antibacterial action. The ability of fullerenes is discovered to interact with biological membranes and to evaluate their antimicrobials applications. For example, Deryabin et al. revealed that the important correlations between these physicochemical characters and contacts of fullerene products with bacterial cell surface are involved in bioenergetics violation and toxic effects (Deryabin et al. 2015).

An amphiphilic photosensitizing agent based on a tricationic fullerene C60 ($DMC60^{3+}$) was efficiently synthesized from the non-charged analog MMC60. The fullerenes exhibit a strong UV absorption, with a broad range of less intense absorption up to 710 nm. Both compounds showed low fluorescence emission and were able to photosensitize ROS production. Photodecomposition of L-tryptophan was sensitized by fullerenes which indicated the involvement of the type II pathway. $DMC60^{3+}$ is an effective agent that produces the photodynamic inactivation (PDI) of *S. aureus*, *C. albicans*, and *E. coli*. Mechanistic insight shows that the photodynamic action was sensitized by DMC60 3+ mediated by photo processes in

Table 13.1 Fullerene Derivatives and Their Applications in Cancer

Material	*Functionalization (Drug)*	*Application*	*Reference*
Fullerene (C60)	Doxorubicin	Targeted breast cancer therapy	Kepinska, Kizek, and Milnerowicz (2018)
Fullerene-nanodiamond	–	Photosensitized water treatment and photodynamic cancer therapy	Lee et al. (2021)
$Gd@C_{82}(OH)_2$ fullerene derivatives	Gadolinium	Cancer therapy	Meng et al. (2013)
Aminofullerenes (Monoamino C60 and Hexakisamino C60)	N1-Tritylethane-1,2-Diamine and N1,N3-Bis(2 (triethylamine)-ethyl)malonamide	Photodynamic Treatment of non-melanoma skin cancers	Serda et al. (2020)
Glycofullerene JK39	D-glucosamine	Prostate cancer model for siRNA delivery	Korzuch et al. (2021)
Glycofullerene (called Sweet-C60)	–	Drug delivery vehicle in treating pancreatic cancer	Barańska et al. (2021)
Fullerene (Cs-$C60Ar_6$, $C60Ar_5X$ (X=Cl, H) and Cs-$C60Ar_4$)	–	Lung cancer cell inhibitors	Voronov, Troshin, and Hsu
Aminated fullerene (C60-EDA)	Ethylenediamine	A promising candidate for cancer Metastasis-targeting drugs	Zhou et al. (2020)
Fullerene (C60)	Pluronic F127-chitosan nanoparticles (PCNPs)	Targeted heating via fullerene for enhanced cancer treatment by microwave hyperthermia	Sun et al. (2016)
Fullerenes	Doxorubicin and magnetic gold nanoparticles	Target interaction with mutated gene BRCA2 in breast cancer	Skaličková et al. (2017)
Fullerene	Antenna nanoparticles (DA NPS)	Photosensitizer design for enhanced cancer phototheranostics	Shi et al. (2019)

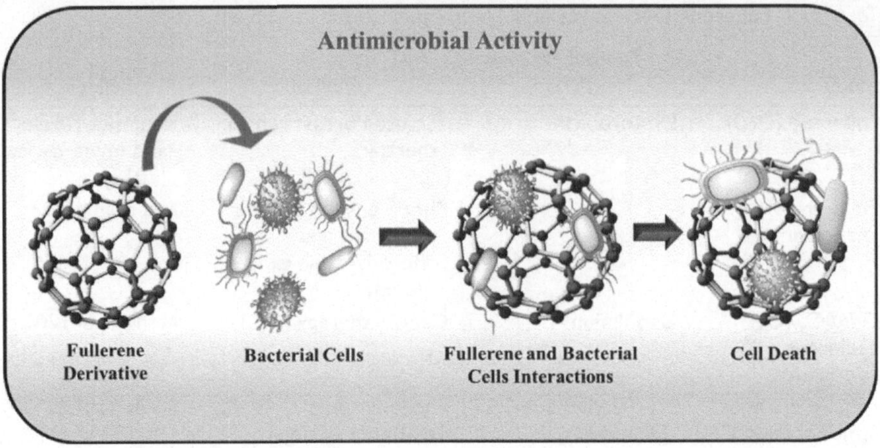

Figure 13.6 Fullerene derivatives for antimicrobial activity.

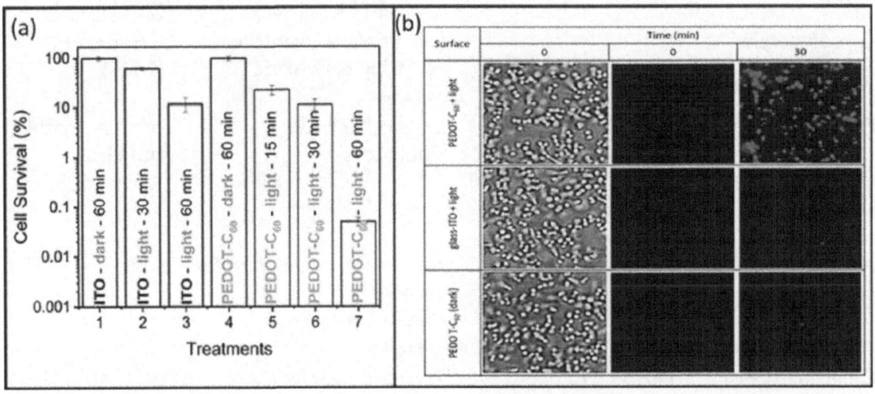

Figure 13.7 (a) Survival of *S. aureus* biofilm on ITO electrode and on PEDOT-C60 and (b) Bright-field (first column) and fluorescence microscopy (second and third columns) images of *S. aureus*. (Reprinted with permission from Reynoso et al. 2021, Copyright 2021, RSC Advances.)

bacteria, while a majority of the type II pathway was found in *C. albicans*. In potassium iodide, a potentiation of PDI was observed due to the formation of reactive iodine species. Therefore, the amphiphilic $DMC60^{3+}$ can be used as an effective potential broad-spectrum antimicrobial photosensitizer (Agazzi et al. 2021).

A photostable and photodynamic antimicrobial surface was successfully obtained and applied to photoinactivation microorganisms. This proposition

Table 13.2 Fullerene Derivatives Exploit the Antimicrobial Activity

Material	*Functionalization*	*Application*	*Reference*
Fullerene (C_{60})	Methoxyethyleneglycol	Antimicrobial (Gram-positive and Gram-negative bacterial cells) photodynamic inactivation	Thota et al. (2012)
Fullerene (C_{60})	N-Fmoc-L-glutamic acid alpha-tert-butyl ester	Antimicrobial activity against *S. aureus* and *E. coli*	Pellarini et al. (2001)
Fullerene (C_{60})	Cyclen	Antimicrobial activity against *S. aureus* and *E. coli* by electrostatic attraction	Chen, Liu, et al. (2016)
Fullerene (C_{60})	-	Increase in membrane permeability	Grinholc et al. (2015)
Fullerene (C_{70})	Ag-NP and polystyrene-(PS-P4VP)	Multifunctional antimicrobial agent C_{70} and Ag-NPs, synergistically target bacterial cells that increase photo-generated ROS	Moor, Osuji, and Kim (2016)
Fullerene (C_{60})	-	Bacterial phospholipids and membrane phase behavior of *Pseudomonas putida* (Gram negative) and *Bacillus subtilis* (Gram positive)	Fang et al. (2007)
Fullerene (C_{60})	C_{60}-OH, C_{60}-COOH, C_{60}-NH_2	Fullerenes cause more membrane stress than perturbation to energy metabolism	Tang et al. (2007)
Fullerene (C_{60})	C(60)-bis (N,N-dimethylpyrrolidinium iodide)	Fullerene derivatives effectively inhibited bacteria cell growth	Mashino et al. (2003)
Fullerenopyrrolidine	Glycopeptide antibiotic derivative teicoplanin ψ-aglycone	Antibacterial activity against enterococci resistant to teicoplanin	Tollas et al. (2012)
Fullerene (C_{70})	Monoadduct and bisadduct	Antimicrobial and photodynamic therapy (with decacationic monoadducts and bisadducts)	Tollas et al. (2012)
Fullerene (C_{60})	Decaquaternary chain and deca-tertiary-amino groups	Antimicrobial photodynamic inactivation mediated by a cationic fullerene	Zhang et al. (2015)

was based on synthesizing a fullerene derivative (EDOT-C60), where fullerene is covalently linked with 3,4-ethylene dioxythiophene (EDOT) through a 1,3-dipolar cycloaddition reaction. This dual-functional monomer bears an EDOT center connected with an alkyl chain to a fullerene moiety. EDOT acts as an electropolymerizable unit that allows film formation over conducting substrates, while fullerene performs the photodynamic antimicrobial activity. Moreover, photodynamic properties of PEDOT-C60 were compared with fullerene and showed that electrodeposited films were able to produce singlet molecular oxygen (type II) and superoxide radical anion (type I). The photodynamic action sensitized by PEDOT-C60 was observed in vitro against *S. aureus*, as shown in Figure 13.7a. Fullerenes with antimicrobial photodynamic effects are promising for photoinactivation microorganisms and obtaining photostable self-sterilizing surfaces, as shown in Figure 13.7b. Fullerene derivatives, such as amino fullerenes and Fullerenopyrrolidine, were activated against Gram-positive and Gram-negative bacteria, as shown in Table 13.2 (Reynoso et al. 2021).

13.6 CONCLUSION AND FUTURE PERSPECTIVES

The unique properties of fullerenes make them a potential candidate for applications in biomedicine. It is well established that the different functionalized fullerenes with -NH_2, -OH, -COOH, polymer, peptide, and drug modifications enhance their wider scope in various fields. These functionalized fullerene and fullerene vesicles promote their efficiency in drug delivery. The biological applications of fullerene derivatives in cancer therapy with low toxicity can selectively kill the cancer cells in highly localized regions and in antimicrobial activity, and the target-specific drug delivery can be achieved. Despite increasing interest in the development of fullerene derivatives with vast functionalities, getting low-cost fullerene adducts is still a challenge. This chapter highlights the tremendous activities regarding the functionalization of fullerene and its biomedical applications with improved properties. Moreover, further concerns remain after these remarkable improvements, such as enhancement of properties in fullerene by its derivatization and to get low toxicology impact on long-term exposure in biomedical applications.

ACKNOWLEDGMENTS

We are thankful to Jain (Deemed-to-be University), Bangalore, India, for providing facilities. VB also acknowledges TARE-SERB File No. TAR/2018/000547.

REFERENCES

Agazzi, M. L., J. E. Durantini, E. D. Quiroga, M. Gabriela Alvarez, and E. N. Durantini. 2021. A novel tricationic fullerene C 60 as broad-spectrum antimicrobial photosensitizer: Mechanisms of action and potentiation with potassium iodide. *Photochemical & Photobiological Sciences* 20 (3):327–341.

Ajie, H., M. M. Alvarez, S. J. Anz, et al. 1990. Characterization of the soluble all-carbon molecules C60 and C70. *Journal of Physical Chemistry* 94 (24):8630–8633.

Arbogast, J. W., A. P. Darmanyan, C. S. Foote, et al. 1991. Photophysical properties of sixty atom carbon molecule (C60). *The Journal of Physical Chemistry* 95 (1):11–12.

Azzam, T., and A. J. Domb. 2004. Current developments in gene transfection agents. *Current Drug Delivery* 1 (2):165–193.

Barańska, E., O. Wiecheć-Cudak, M. Rak, and A. Bienia. 2021. Interactions of a water-soluble glycofullerene with glucose transporter 1. *Analysis of the Cellular Effects on a Pancreatic Tumor Model* 11 (2): 513.

Bhakta, P., and B. Barthunia. 2020. Fullerene and its applications: A review. *Journal of Indian Academy of Oral Medicine and Radiology* 32 (2):159.

Castro, E., A. H. Garcia, G. Zavala, and L. Echegoyen. 2017. Fullerenes in biology and medicine. *Journal of Materials Chemistry B* 5 (32):6523–6535.

Castro, E., Z. S. Martinez, C.-S. Seong, et al. 2016. Characterization of new cationic N, N-Dimethyl [70] fulleropyrrolidinium iodide derivatives as potent HIV-1 maturation inhibitors. *Journal of Medicinal Chemistry* 59 (24):10963–10973.

Chen, C., G. Xing, J. Wang, et al. 2005. Multihydroxylated [Gd@C82(OH)22] n nanoparticles: Antineoplastic activity of high efficiency and low toxicity. *Nano Lett* 5 (10):2050–2057.

Chen, Q., G. F. Liu, H. Wei, and X. L. Xie. 2016. Antibacterial activity of cationic cyclen-functionalized fullerene derivatives: Membrane stress. *Digest Journal of Nanomaterials and Biostructures* 11:753–761.

Chen, Q., Z. Ma, G. Liu, H. Wei, and X. Xie. 2016. Antibacterial activity of cationic cyclen-functionalized fullerene derivatives: Membrane stress. *Digest Journal of Nanomaterials and Biostructures* 11:753–761.

Chen, Z., L. Ma, Y. Liu, and C. Chen. 2012. Applications of functionalized fullerenes in tumor theranostics. *Theranostics* 2 (3):238–250.

Chen, Z., R. Mao, and Y. Liu. 2012. Fullerenes for cancer diagnosis and therapy: Preparation, biological and clinical perspectives. *Current Drug Metabolism* 13 (8):1035–1045.

Deryabin, D. G., L. V. Efremova, A. S. Vasilchenko, et al. 2015. A zeta potential value determines the aggregate's size of penta-substituted [60] fullerene derivatives in aqueous suspension whereas positive charge is required for toxicity against bacterial cells. *Journal of Nanobiotechnology* 13:50.

Dolmans, D. E., D. Fukumura, and R. K. Jain. 2003. Photodynamic therapy for cancer. *Nature Reviews Cancer* 3 (5):380–387.

Fang, J., D. Y. Lyon, M. R. Wiesner, J. Dong, and P. J. Alvarez. 2007. Effect of a fullerene water suspension on bacterial phospholipids and membrane phase behavior. *Environ Sci Technol* 41 (7):2636–2642.

Ghiassi, K. B., M. M. Olmstead, and A. L. Balch. 2014. Gadolinium-containing endohedral fullerenes: Structures and function as magnetic resonance imaging (MRI) agents. *Dalton Transactions* 43 (20):7346–7358.

Grinholc, M., J. Nakonieczna, G. Fila, et al. 2015. Antimicrobial photodynamic therapy with fulleropyrrolidine: Photoinactivation mechanism of Staphylococcus aureus, in vitro and in vivo studies. *Appl Microbiol Biotechnol* 99 (9):4031–4043.

He, C.-L., R. Liu, D.-D. Li, S.-E. Zhu, and G.-W. Wang. 2013. Synthesis and functionalization of [60] fullerene-fused imidazolines. *Organic Letters* 15 (7):1532–1535.

Hirlekar, R., M. Yamagar, H. Garse, M. Vij, and V. Kadam. 2009. Carbon nanotubes and its applications: A review. *Asian Journal of Pharmaceutical and Clinical Research* 2 (4):17–27.

Ikeda, A., S. Satake, T. Mae, et al. 2017. Photodynamic Activities of porphyrin derivative–cyclodextrin complexes by photoirradiation. *ACS Medicinal Chemistry Letters* 8 (5):555–559.

Jensen, A. W., S. R. Wilson, and D. I. Schuster. 1996. Biological applications of fullerenes. *Bioorganic & Medicinal Chemistry* 4 (6):767–779.

Ji, H.-X., J.-S. Hu, Q.-X. Tang, et al. 2007. Controllable preparation of submicrometer single-crystal C60 rods and tubes trough concentration depletion at the surfaces of seeds. *The Journal of Physical Chemistry C* 111 (28):10498–10502.

Kataoka, H., T. Ohe, K. Takahashi, S. Nakamura, and T. Mashino. 2016. Novel fullerene derivatives as dual inhibitors of Hepatitis C virus NS5B polymerase and NS3/4A protease. *Bioorganic & Medicinal Chemistry Letters* 26 (19):4565–4567.

Kepinska, M., R. Kizek, and H. Milnerowicz. 2018. Fullerene as a doxorubicin nanotransporter for targeted breast cancer therapy: Capillary electrophoresis analysis. *Electrophoresis* 39 (18):2370–2379.

Korzuch, J., M. Rak, K. Balin, et al. 2021. Towards water-soluble [60] fullerenes for the delivery of siRNA in a prostate cancer model. *Scientific Reports* 11 (1):10565.

Krätschmer, W., L. D. Lamb, K. H. D. R. Fostiropoulos, and D. R. Huffman. 1990. Solid C 60: A new form of carbon. *Nature* 347 (6291):354–358.

Kroto, H. W., J. R. Heath, S. C. O'Brien, R. F. Curl, and R. E. Smalley. 1985. C 60: Buckminsterfullerene. *Nature* 318 (6042):162–163.

Lacerda, L., A. Bianco, M. Prato, and K. Kostarelos. 2006. Carbon nanotubes as nanomedicines: From toxicology to pharmacology. *Advanced Drug Delivery Reviews* 58 (14):1460–1470.

Lee, H., J. S. Lee, K. J. Moor, et al. 2021. Hand-ground fullerene-nanodiamond composite for photosensitized water treatment and photodynamic cancer therapy. *Journal of Colloid and Interface Science* 587:101–109.

Li, G., P. Liu, Z. Han, et al. 2010. A novel approach to fabrication of fullerene C60 nanotubes: Using C60–pyridine colloid as a precursor. *Materials Letters* 64 (3):483–485.

Liu, H., Y. Li, L. Jiang, et al. 2002. Imaging as-grown [60] fullerene nanotubes by template technique. *Journal of the American Chemical Society* 124 (45):13370–13371.

Liu, J. H., L. Cao, P. G. Luo, et al. 2010. Fullerene-conjugated doxorubicin in cells. *ACS Applied Materials & Interfaces* 2 (5):1384–1389.

Lu, F., S. A. Haque, S. T. Yang, et al. 2009. Aqueous compatible fullerene-doxorubicin conjugates. *The Journal of Physical Chemistry C Nanomater Interfaces* 113 (41):17768.

Lu, F., Z. Hu, J. Sinard, A. Garen, and R. A. Adelman. 2009. Factor VII-verteporfin for targeted photodynamic therapy in a rat model of choroidal neovascularization. *Investigative Ophthalmology & Visual Science* 50 (8):3890–3896.

Lyon, D. Y., L. Brunet, G. W. Hinkal, M. R. Wiesner, and P. J. Alvarez. 2008. Antibacterial activity of fullerene water suspensions (nC60) is not due to ROS-mediated damage. *Nano Letters* 8 (5):1539–1543.

Ma, H. L., and X.-J. Liang. 2010. Fullerenes as unique nanopharmaceuticals for disease treatment. *Science China Chemistry* 53 (11):2233–2240.

Mashino, T., D. Nishikawa, K. Takahashi, et al. 2003. Antibacterial and antiproliferative activity of cationic fullerene derivatives. *Bioorganic & Medicinal Chemistry Letters* 13 (24):4395–4397.

Mashino, T., K. Okuda, T. Hirota, M. Hirobe, T. Nagano, and M. Mochizuki. 1999. Inhibition of *E. coli* growth by fullerene derivatives and inhibition mechanism. *Bioorganic & Medicinal Chemistry Letters* 9 (20):2959–2962.

Mashino, T., K. Shimotohno, N. Ikegami, et al. 2005. Human immunodeficiency virus-reverse transcriptase inhibition and hepatitis C virus RNA-dependent RNA polymerase inhibition activities of fullerene derivatives. *Bioorganic & Medicinal Chemistry Letters* 15 (4):1107–1109.

Meng, H., G. Xing, B. Sun, et al. 2010. Potent angiogenesis inhibition by the particulate form of fullerene derivatives. *ACS Nano* 4 (5):2773–2783.

Meng, J., X. Liang, X. Chen, and Y. Zhao. 2013. Biological characterizations of [Gd@ $C8_2$ $(OH)_{22}$] n nanoparticles as fullerene derivatives for cancer therapy. *Integrative Biology* 5 (1):43–47.

Minato, J., K. Miyazawa, and T. Suga. 2005. Morphology of C60 nanotubes fabricated by the liquid–liquid interfacial precipitation method. *Science and Technology of Advanced Materials* 6 (3–4):272.

Moor, K. J., C. O. Osuji, and J. H. Kim. 2016. Dual-functionality fullerene and silver nanoparticle antimicrobial composites via block copolymer templates. *ACS Applied Materials & Interfaces* 8 (49):33583–33591.

Moussa, F. 2018. [60] Fullerene and derivatives for biomedical applications. *Nanobiomaterials*, pp. 113–136. doi: 10.1016/B978-0-08-100716-7.00005-2.

Muñoz, A., D. Sigwalt, B. M. Illescas, et al. 2016. Synthesis of giant globular multivalent glycofullerenes as potent inhibitors in a model of Ebola virus infection. *Nature Chemistry* 8 (1):50–57.

Nalepa, P., R. Gawecki, G. Szewczyk, et al. 2020. A [60] fullerene nanoconjugate with gemcitabine: Synthesis, biophysical properties and biological evaluation for treating pancreatic cancer. *Cancer Nanotechnology* 11 (1):1–21.

Okumura, M., M. Mikawa, T. Yokawa, Y. Kanazawa, H. Kato, and H. Shinohara. 2002. Evaluation of water-soluble metallofullerenes as MRI contrast agents. *Academic Radiology* 9 (2):S495–S497.

Partha, R., L. R. Mitchell, J. L. Lyon, P. P. Joshi, and J. L. Conyers. 2008. Buckysomes: Fullerene-based nanocarriers for hydrophobic molecule delivery. *ACS Nano* 2 (9):1950–1958.

Pellarini, F., D. Pantarotto, T. Da Ros, A. Giangaspero, A. Tossi, and M. Prato. 2001. A novel [60] fullerene amino acid for use in solid-phase peptide synthesis. *Organic Letters* 3 (12):1845–1848.

Qu, Y., W. Yu, S. Liang, S. Li, J. Zhao, and G. Piao. 2011. Structure and morphology characteristics of fullerene C60 nanotubes fabricated with n-methyl-2-pyrrolidone as a good solvent. *Journal of Nanomaterials* 2011. doi: 10.1155/2011/706293.

Reynoso, E., A. M. Durantini, C. A. Solis, et al. 2021. Photoactive antimicrobial coating based on a PEDOT-fullerene C 60 polymeric dyad. *RSC Advances* 11 (38):23519–23532.

Schwerdtfeger, P., L. N. Wirz, and J. Avery. 2015. The topology of fullerenes. *Wiley Interdisciplinary Reviews: Computational Molecular Science* 5 (1):96–145.

Semenov, K. N., N. A. Charykov, V. N. Postnov, et al. 2016. Fullerenols: Physicochemical properties and applications. *Progress in Solid State Chemistry* 44 (2):59–74.

Serda, M., G. Szewczyk, O. Krzysztyńska-Kuleta, et al. 2020. Developing [60] fullerene nanomaterials for better photodynamic treatment of non-melanoma skin cancers. *ACS Biomaterials Science & Engineering* 6 (10):5930–5940.

Sharma, S. K., L. Y. Chiang, and M. R. Hamblin. 2011. Photodynamic therapy with fullerenes in vivo: Reality or a dream? *Nanomedicine (Lond)* 6 (10):1813–1825.

Shevtsov, M. A., B. P. Nikolaev, Y. Y. Marchenko, et al. 2014. Magnetic resonance imaging of rat C6 glioma model enhanced by using water-soluble gadolinium fullerene. *Applied Magnetic Resonance* 45 (4):303–314.

Shi, H., R. Gu, W. Xu, et al. 2019. Near-infrared light-harvesting fullerene-based nanoparticles for promoted synergetic tumor phototheranostics. *ACS Applied Materials & Interfaces* 11 (48):44970–44977.

Shi, J., L. Wang, J. Gao, et al. 2014. A fullerene-based multi-functional nanoplatform for cancer theranostic applications. *Biomaterials* 35 (22):5771–5784.

Shinohara, H. 2000. Endohedral metallofullerenes. *Reports on Progress in Physics* 63 (6):843.

Shvedova, A. A., A. Pietroiusti, B. Fadeel, and V. E. Kagan. 2012. Mechanisms of carbon nanotube-induced toxicity: Focus on oxidative stress. *Toxicology and Applied Pharmacology* 261 (2):121–133.

Skaličková, S., M. Löfelmann, M. Gargulák, et al. 2017. Fullerene Doxorubicin Nanotransporter for Target Interaction with mutated gene BRCA2. *Klinická onkologie: casopis Ceské a Slovenské onkologické spolecnosti* 30 (Supplementum1):177–179.

Sun, M., A. Kiourti, H. Wang, et al. 2016. Enhanced microwave hyperthermia of cancer cells with fullerene. *Molecular Pharmaceutics* 13 (7):2184–2192.

Tang, Y. J., J. M. Ashcroft, D. Chen, et al. 2007. Charge-associated effects of fullerene derivatives on microbial structural integrity and central metabolism. *Nano Letters* 7 (3):754–760.

Thota, S., M. Wang, S. Jeon, S. Maragani, M. R. Hamblin, and L. Y. Chiang. 2012. Synthesis and characterization of positively charged pentacationic [60] fullerene monoadducts for antimicrobial photodynamic inactivation. *Molecules* 17 (5):5225–5243.

Tokuyama, H., S. Yamago, E. Nakamura, T. Shiraki, and Y. Sugiura. 1993. Photoinduced biochemical activity of fullerene carboxylic acid. *Journal of the American Chemical Society* 115 (17):7918–7919.

Tollas, S., I. Bereczki, A. Sipos, et al. 2012. Nano-sized clusters of a teicoplanin ψ-aglycon-fullerene conjugate. Synthesis, antibacterial activity and aggregation studies. *European Journal of Medicinal Chemistry* 54:943–948.

Uthappa, U. T., M. D. Kurkuri, and M. Kigga. 2019. Nanotechnology advances for the development of various drug carriers. In Prasad, R., Kumar, V., Kumar, M., Choudhary, D. (eds.) *Nanobiotechnology in Bioformulations*. Springer, Cham.

Vance, S. J., V. Desai, B. O. Smith, M. W. Kennedy, and A. Cooper. 2016. Aqueous solubilization of C60 fullerene by natural protein surfactants, latherin and ranaspumin-2. *Biophysical Chemistry* 214: 27–32.

Voronov, II, P. A. Troshin, and S. H. Hsu. 2020. Fullerene derivatives as lung cancer cell inhibitors: investigation of potential descriptors using QSAR approaches. *International Journal of Nanomedicine* 15:2485..

Wang, L., B. Liu, D. Liu, et al. 2006. Synthesis of thin, rectangular C60 nanorods using m-xylene as a shape controller. *Advanced Materials* 18 (14):1883–1888.

Wudl, F. 1992. The chemical properties of buckminsterfullerene (C60) and the birth and infancy of fulleroids. *Accounts of Chemical Research* 25 (3):157–161.

Yadav, J. 2018. Fullerene: Properties, synthesis and application. *Research & Reviews: Journal of Physics* 6 (3):1–6.

Yan, W., S. M. Seifermann, P. Pierrat, and S. Braese. 2015. Synthesis of highly functionalized C 60 fullerene derivatives and their applications in material and life sciences. *Organic & Biomolecular Chemistry* 13 (1):25–54.

Yang, B., Y. Chen, and J. Shi. 2019. Reactive oxygen species (ROS)-based nanomedicine. *Chemical Reviews* 119 (8):4881–4985.

Zhang, Y., T. Dai, M. Wang, D. Vecchio, L. Y. Chiang, and M. R. Hamblin. 2015. Potentiation of antimicrobial photodynamic inactivation mediated by a cationic fullerene by added iodide: In vitro and in vivo studies. *Nanomedicine (Lond)* 10 (4):603–614.

Zhao, Q., Y. Lin, N. Han, et al. 2017. Mesoporous carbon nanomaterials in drug delivery and biomedical application. *Drug Delivery* 24 (sup1):94–107.

Zhou, W., J. Huo, Y. Yang, X. Zhang, S. Li, and C. Zhao. 2020. Aminated fullerene abrogates cancer cell migration by directly targeting myosin heavy chain 9. *ACS Appl Mater Interfaces* 12 (51):56862–56873.

Zygouri, P., K. Spyrou, E. Mitsari, et al. 2020. A facile approach to hydrophilic oxidized fullerenes and their derivatives as cytotoxic agents and supports for nanobiocatalytic systems. *Scientific Reports* 10 (1):1–13.

Chapter 14

Applications of Carbon Nanotubes in Drug Delivery

Zhenxu Yang, Yogambha Ramaswamy, and Gurvinder Singh
The University of Sydney

CONTENTS

DOI: 10.1201/9781003217114-17

14.1 INTRODUCTION

Carbon nanotubes (CNTs) are one-dimensional (1D) cylindrical nanomaterials (NMs) with a diameter in the nanometer range (Iijima and Ichihashi 1993). Based on their structural characteristics, CNTs can be classified into two main types: (i) single-walled CNTs formed by rolling a single layer of graphite sheet into a cylindrical tube (Bougrine et al. 1999) and (ii) multi-walled CNTs comprised from multiple layers of concentric cylinders with the space of about 0.34 nm between the adjacent layers (Iijima 1991). In the twenty-first century, CNTs have been considered the most promising NMs because of their optical (Zhao, Chen, and Xie 2006), electrical (Bandaru 2007), mechanical (Spitalsky et al. 2010), and thermal properties (Dresselhaus et al. 2004; Popov 2004). These properties can be tailored by varying the diameter, length of CNTs, wall nature, and chirality (Zhang and Zheng 2010; Gavrel et al. 2014). Over the last few decades, the applications of CNTs have been explored in a range of disciplines, from bioengineering to materials science, energy, environment, construction, and nanoelectronics (Bati et al. 2019; Saliev 2019). The most versatile physicochemical characteristics of CNTs that make them suitable for biomedical applications are high surface area, ultra-light weightiness, chemical inertness, and enhanced antibacterial and antifungal properties (Gupta, Gupta, and Sharma 2019; Prajapati et al. 2022; Wang, Zhou, and Chen 2017). Also, CNTs offer rich surface chemistry to bind various biological entities, such as pharmaceutical drugs, imaging agents, target molecules, and functionalized polymers via covalent and noncovalent strategies (Aboofazeli 2010; Chen and Mitra 2019; Assali et al. 2018). These properties have enabled the rational design of multifunctional CNTs for different biomedical applications, including diagnostic, biosensors, cellular therapy, and targeted drug delivery. Furthermore, CNTs have been used as a scaffolding material for supporting the growth of bone cells (Pei et al. 2019), cardiomyocytes (Gorain et al. 2018), and neurons (Cellot et al. 2009) and promoting stem cell differentiation into specific lineages, for example, human mesenchymal stem cells into bone cells (Mooney et al. 2008).

In principle, CNTs can be considered a nanocontainer because the tips of CNTs are open (Gupta, Gupta, and Sharma 2019). As a result, CNTs possess a high surface area due to the accessibility to the inner and outer surfaces of CNTs. Different biomolecules or drug molecules can be incorporated into the internal as well as outer space of CNTs via surface functionalization strategies, and they have high drug-loading capacity, hence CNTs are considered promising nanocarriers for drug delivery (Bianco,

Kostarelos, and Prato 2005). Traditional drug delivery approaches contain numerous limitations, such as poor water solubility, low selectivity or targeting, low therapeutic indices, and the induction of drug resistance (Patra et al. 2018; Tiwari et al. 2012; Edgar and Wang 2017). The therapeutic efficacy of the treatment can be improved by delivering the drugs with high selectivity and specificity to diseased tissues. To achieve the targeted therapy for disease treatment, it is essential to develop intelligent drug delivery systems that offer improved efficiency and viability. An ideal vehicle for target drug delivery systems should meet three requirements: (i) target effects; (ii) strong adsorptive effects to ensure the transport of drugs to the disease sites; (iii) control release of drugs to the disease sites by relevant mechanisms, such as chemical reaction (pH change, hydrolysis, and enzymatic), stimuli responsive (temperature, magnetic field, and light), and diffusion; and (iv) minimal side effects and reduced toxicity. The transporting capabilities of CNTs combined with relevant surface modifications and their unique physicochemical properties show a great potential to meet these four requirements.

CNTs possess several intriguing features that make them attractive nanovehicles for controlled and targeted drug delivery. Firstly, the unique needle-like morphology of CNTs enables them to passively cross the cell membranes and enter the cell via energy-dependent endocytosis, independent of cell types and surface functionality. The size of CNTs can influence their cell penetration mechanism (Lacerda et al. 2012). Secondly, like other nanovehicles (liposomes and spherical nanoparticles), CNTs also experience the enhanced permeability and retention (EPR) effect, facilitating the increased accumulation of CNTs in diseased tissues due to the large pore size of vasculatures in abnormal tissues as compared to healthy tissues (Iyer et al. 2006). Third, intravenous administration of nanosized CNTs can circulate in the bloodstream for a longer time. However, the size of CNTs should be optimal to avoid their excretion by the kidney (small size below 5 nm) or detection and trapped by the reticuloendothelial system (large size above 200 nm). Fourth, a high surface area of CNTs enables them to carry multiple moieties, such as nanoparticles, drugs, and other biomolecules. These multiple moieties can be attached to the exterior or interior space of CNTs. For example, the diagnostic capability of CNTs can be enhanced by incorporating nanoparticle-based optical or magnetic probes in the interior space of CNTs for imaging purposes. This offers an exciting opportunity to develop targeted CNTs-based nanotheranostics (combining diagnosis and treatment capabilities) agents for simultaneous diagnosis, transport, and targeted drug delivery. In addition, CNTs-based nanotheranostics agents can help in tracking the administrated nanovehicles to assess in real-time spatial distribution to measure their biodistribution profile, monitoring the drug release, and evaluating the therapeutic efficacy of the treatment. CNTs hold great potential for future drug discovery based on the intracellular targets that have been hard to reach. Therefore, CNTs have extensively been used to efficiently deliver numerous therapeutic agents with reduced toxicity from small molecules, such as chemotherapeutic drugs (Liu et al. 2008), anti-inflammatory (Luo et al. 2011), antimicrobial (Benincasa et al. 2011) to more complex biological moieties, including small interference ribonucleic acids (siRNA) (Podesta et al. 2009), antibodies (McDevitt et al. 2007), and peptide-based vaccines (Pantarotto et al. 2003).

14.1.1 Chemical Properties of CNTs

To begin the discussion of CNTs, it is essential to first review the knowledge of carbon as an element. Carbon is an element that has an atomic number 6, an electronic configuration of $1s^2 2s^2 2p^2$ (Blackman 2016), and an electronegativity of 2.55 (Allen 1989), which offers great versatility in chemical reactions. Carbon is one of the most abundant elements in the universe (Fischer et al. 2020). In our body, carbon acts as the backbone of our DNA, cells, and our flesh (Rikhvanov and Baranovskaya 2013). It has a variety of allotropes, having the same elemental composition but in different forms, such as crystallinity ("Allotropy" 2021). Diamond, graphite, fullerenes, graphene, and carbon nanotubes (Tanaka 2014). What makes them different from other carbon allotropes? To answer this, the concept of hybridization is introduced.

Carbon has four valence electrons sitting in 2s and 2p orbitals (Blackman 2016; Sattler 2016). During a bonding formation process, as in the case of methane, these orbitals will re-arrange via a process called hybridization to create four degenerated single bonds or four sigma bonds and can be termed sp^3 hybridization. (Penotti et al. 1988; Blackman 2016). Diamond is considered one of the hardest materials with sp^3 hybridization found naturally on earth (Delhaes 2000). Unlike methane (CH_4), diamond is interconnected with itself rather than other heterogeneous atoms, such as hydrogen in methane (Delhaes 2000; Dresselhaus 2001). There are three sigma bonds and a pi-bond for each carbon center (Hay, Hunt, and Goddard III 1972; Xu and Dunning 2020). In this case, the carbon has a hybridization of sp^2. In the case of graphite, the carbon has a hybridization state of sp^2 (Morris 2013). As shown in Figure 14.1, graphite has a planar structure where different layers are only held by weak van der Waals' forces (Charlier, Gonze, and Michenaud 1994; Meyyappan 2004). It has been found that by pealing graphite layer by layer (Novoselov et al. 2004), a new kind of material, graphene, could be produced. Since there is no structural change between graphene (a single layer of graphite) and graphite, graphene is also sp^2 hybridization (Morris 2013).

Hybridization can aid the classification of carbon compounds (Tanaka 2014). As shown in Figure 14.2, the degree of hybridization, sp^n (where n=0, 1, 2, 3), in relation to the [H]/[C] atomic ratio can be plotted and used to

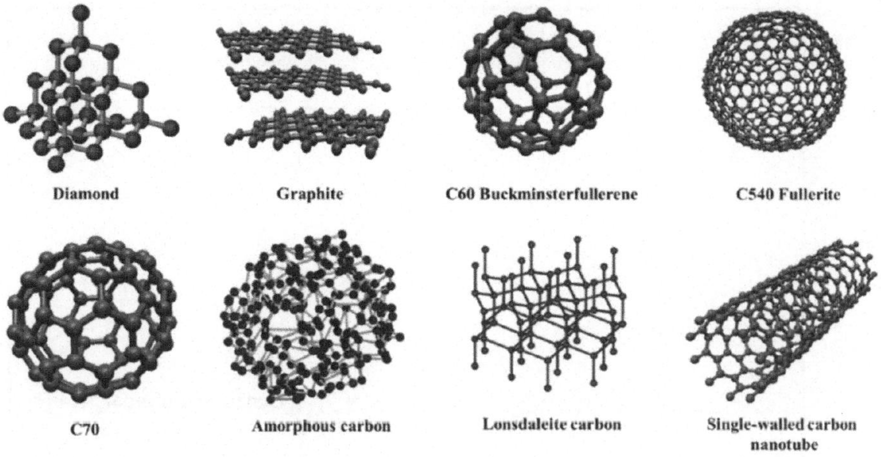

Figure 14.1 Illustration of eight carbon allotropes and their structure.

classify the carbon compounds. Since neither diamond, graphite, nor graphene has hydrogen attached, all of them are plotted against the x-axis where $y=0$. It can be noticed that carbon nanotube and fullerene are situated between $n=2$ and $n=3$. The intermediate degree of hybridization is one of the features of carbon (Ebbesen and Takada 1995). The formation of CNTs can be imagined as rolling a sheet of graphene to form a tube structure and capped with half fullerene at two ends (Kushwaha et al. 2013), as shown in Figure 14.1. As the curvature forms, the degree of hybridization of CNTs must increase from sp^2 of the graphene to a closer state of sp^3 (like a diamond) (Tanaka 2014). To be precise, the degree of hybridization for CNTs can be denoted as $sp^{2+\delta}$, where δ depends on the degree of curvature of the bend in CNTs, as suggested in Figure 14.2.

14.1.2 Classification of CNTs

The carbon-carbon bond distance of CNTs is roughly 1.4Å (Robertson, Brenner, and Mintmire 1992), and CNTs can be further categorized into two main groups based on the number of graphene sheets existent in nanotubes (Tomanek 2008): single-walled carbon nanotube (SWCNT) and multiwalled carbon nanotube (MWCNT). SWCNTs are CNTs consisting of a single graphene sheet layer, whereas MWCNTs are multiple graphene sheets (Anzar et al. 2020). Although the discovery of MWCNTs was recognized in 1959 by Roger Bacon (Bacon 1960; Tanaka 2014), it was fully characterized and designated with the appropriate terminology by Iijima in 1991 and was produced using the arc-discharge evaporation method (Iijima 1991). This discovery further led to the development of SWCNT (1 nm in

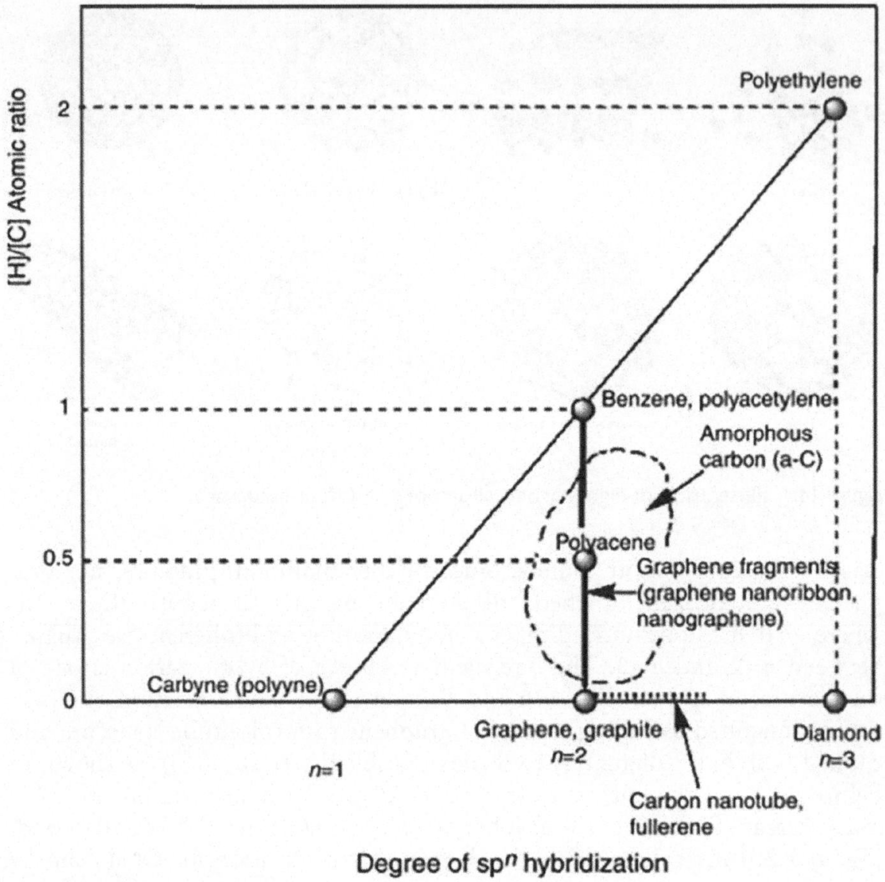

Figure 14.2 Domain map of carbon material family illustrating the classification of carbon materials based on the degree of sp^n hybridization (Tanaka 2014). (Copyright © 2014 Elsevier Ltd. All rights reserved.)

diameter) by Iijima in 1993 (Iijima and Ichihashi 1993) and was found in a soot-like deposit in the carbon-arc chamber.

MWCNT as the name suggests has several layers of CNTs (Figure 14.3d). These CNTs arrange themselves concentrically layer by layer. The inter-layer distance of MWCNTs was measured to be approximately 0.34 nm on an average (Kharissova and Kharisov 2014). SWCNTs are found to have limited length due to the tendency to collapse, and the SWCNT diameter was found to be between 0.6 and 2.0 nm (Wang et al. 2000). In MWCNT, the innermost tube was found to be as small as 0.4 nm in diameter and the outermost tube to be as large as hundreds of nm. However, a typical MWCNT would find its innermost diameter larger than 2 nm and outer-most diameter less than 100 nm (Meyyappan 2004).

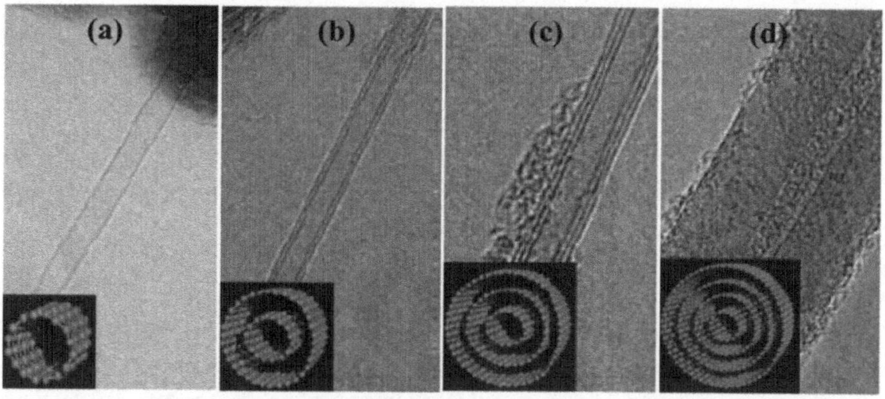

Figure 14.3 High-resolution transmission electron microscopy (HRTEM) images of (a) single-walled, (b) double-walled, (c) triple-walled, and (d) multiwalled CNTs. Insets are the corresponding models of these CNTs (Endo 2007).

As discussed above, SWCNT could be visualized as a hollow tube that is rolled from a single graphene sheet (Iijima and Ichihashi 1993). The properties of SWCNT are fundamentally linked to the direction of rolling or its chirality (Iijima and Ichihashi 1993; Anzar et al. 2020), and hence CNTs can also be classified on the basis of chirality.

A vector representation of the graphene sheet can be described as:

$$C_h = n\,\hat{a}_1 + m\,\hat{a}_2$$

where $\hat{a}_1$ and $\hat{a}_2$ are the two unit vectors in terms of the graphene lattice vectors. C_h is defined as the chiral vector that consists of integer (n, m). The diameter of the SWCNT d_t can be obtained from the chiral vector via the following equation:

$$d_t = \frac{|C_h|}{\pi} = \frac{a}{\pi}\sqrt{n^2 + m^2 + nm}$$

where $a = |\hat{a}_1| = |\hat{a}_2|$ is lattice constant. From the vector representation, two main groups of SWCNT could be described, achiral and chiral SWCNT. The chirality is defined based on the symmetry of the SWCNT. In C_h, if $n = m$, the SWCNT is commonly referred to as armchair tubes. If $m = 0$, the tubes are referred to as zigzag tubes. Both are referred to as achiral since axes of symmetry exist in the center of the tubes. In contrast, chiral SWCNT has no center of symmetry where $n \neq m$ as shown in Figure 14.4b. It has been understood that the direction in which the SWCNT joins itself can drastically affect physical properties like electrical conductivity. When $n = m$, metallic armchair SWCNT can be found (metallic SWCNTs); when

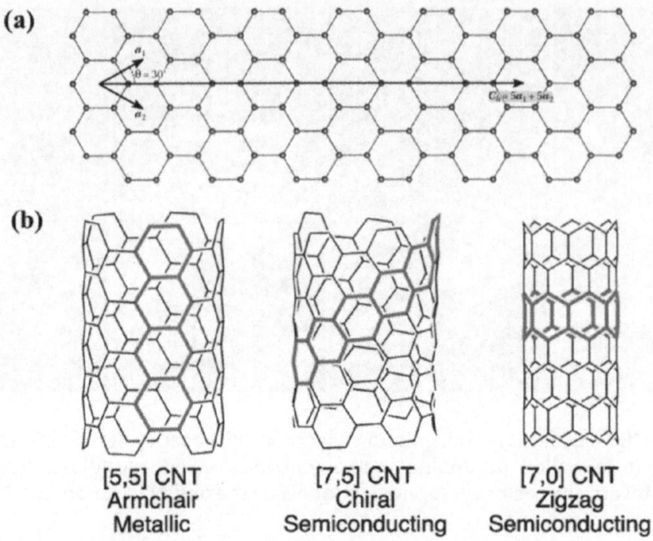

Figure 14.4 (a) The graphene lattice making up a section of the (5,5) single-walled carbon nanotube with graphene lattice vectors (a_1, a_2), the chiral vector Ch and chiral angle θ marked. $C_h = 5a_1 + 5a_2$ (Proctor et al. 2017). (b) Representation of CNT [5,5] armchair, [7,5] chiral, and [7,0] zigzag conformation (Sisto et al. 2016). (Copyright © 2020, CRC Press.)

$m = 0$, semiconducting zigzag SWCNTs can be found (semiconducting SWCNTs). When $n \neq m$, two situations will occur. If $|n - m| = 3q$ where q is an integer, the SWCNT is predicted to be metallic; if $|n - m| \neq 3q$, the SWNT is predicted to be semiconducting.

14.1.3 General Properties of CNTs

Since the discovery of CNTs, researchers have been fascinated by their excellent properties, such as high tensile strength and high electrical and heat conductivity due to their unique bonding formation or perfect structural characteristics (Dresselhaus 2001; Tomanek 2008). The tensile strength of CNTs is 100 times greater than steel, which is the highest among the existing materials. They also display elasticity under axial compressive forces and strength depending on the chirality of CNTs. For example, CNTs of small diameter and near-armchair configurations show the highest tensile strengths. Their excellent intrinsic stability and structural flexibility are important for their applications for drug delivery as they can penetrate or perforate cell membranes as needles (Fabbro et al. 2012). Depending on the rolling configuration of graphite/graphene sheets or the chirality, CNTs can behave as conducting or semiconducting materials.

The electrical conductivity in CNTs arises from the presence of delocalized electrons in their ring structure. The emergence of a high density of surface electrons in conducting (or metallic) CNTs facilitates the biomolecular binding and wrapping of the tubes with peptides or proteins to design delivery nanovehicles. Semiconducting CNTs show fluorescence emission in the near-infra red (NIR) region of the electromagnetic spectrum because CNTs can absorb light in the NIR region in which components of cells and tissues, such as water and protein, have negligible absorption. This property can be exploited to reveal the tumor location and spatial distribution of CNTs within the tissue. Therefore, CNTs exhibit both electrical and optical properties.

Another unique physical property of CNTs is their exceptionally high thermal conductivity. They conduct heat by the vibration of covalent bonds holding carbon atoms together, followed by heat transmission via the vibration throughout the nanotube. This property of CNTs can be employed to develop standalone novel imaging probes or hybrid probes by combining them with specific compounds for tissue imaging. Also, CNTs can absorb and convert electromagnetic radiation (specifically NIR absorption) into heat and sonic energy (Moon, Lee, and Choi 2009), which have been exploited for developing CNTs-based photothermal and photoacoustic therapies to treat cancerous diseases (Zhou et al. 2012). They can also retain energy and resist thermal ablation. Additionally, semiconducting CNTs can be used to improve and control drug release by NIR laser (Ghosh et al. 2009).

14.2 SYNTHESIS

Several synthetic strategies have been developed for the large-scale production of CNTs. However, in this chapter, the most common methods for synthesizing CNTs will be discussed. Table 14.1 lists the advantages and disadvantages of the three discussed synthesis methods (Dresselhaus 2001; Anzar et al. 2020; Ferreira et al. 2019; Karimi, Solati, Amiri, et al. 2015).

Table 14.1 Advantages and Disadvantages of Three Commonly Adopted Carbon Nanotube Synthesis Methods (Ferreira et al. 2019)

Method	*Advantages*	*Disadvantages*
Electric arc discharge	High degree of structural perfection	Carbon impurities and short CNTs
Laser vaporization	High degree of structural perfection and high purity	High cost, low yield
Chemical vapor deposition	Large-scale production, good alignment, and control over diameter and shell number	Higher defect density

14.2.1 Electric Arc-Discharge Method

In 1991, Iijima used the arc-discharge evaporation method to discover MWCNTs, as shown in Figure 14.5a. This method was similar to the synthesis of fullerene (Iijima 1991; Iijima and Ichihashi 1993). A typical system consists of two graphite electrodes surrounded by inert gas connected to the external power supply. A direct current (DC) at nominal conditions of 100 A and 20 V is applied across a pair of graphite electrodes located close to each other in the presence of inert gas (helium gas or argon gas at about 500 torr) (Ishigami et al. 2000). As a result, the arc produced between the graphite electrodes would bring the temperature up to 6000°C which is high enough to sublime the carbon from the graphite electrode (i.e., the transition of carbon from the solid state to the gaseous state) [36]. A plasma is formed by ejected electrons from the high-energy sublimed carbon atoms.

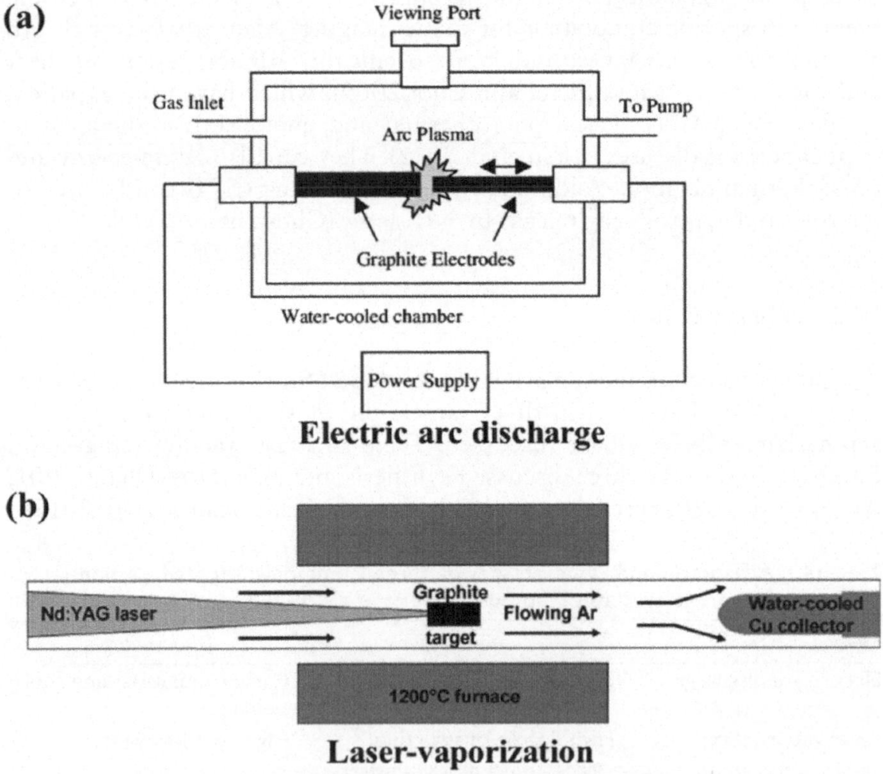

Figure 14.5 Schematic representations of (a) an arc discharge. (Reprinted by permission from Kingston and Simard (2003). Copyright 2013, Taylor & Francis.) and (b) laser vaporization apparatus. (Permission from Guo et al. (1995). Copyright 1995, Elsevier B.V.)

And these ejected electrons impact the anode with high velocity to produce vaporized carbon and subsequent carbon ions. These carbon ions and carbon vapor would move to a colder zone within the chamber, allowing the deposition of CNTs on the cathode, which has a lower temperature than the anode. The MWCNTs can be found in the soot (Iijima 1991). A slightly modified approach of arc discharge was explored for producing SWCNTs. In a modified approach, an anodic electrode is decorated with a metal catalyst, for instance Fe, Co, Mo, and Ni (Dresselhaus 2001; Tomanek 2008). In general, the synthesis of SWCNTs requires the use of catalysts (metal or a metal mixture), while catalytic precursor is not necessary for the production of MWCNTs.

A low-cost electric arc-discharge method has the capability to produce large quantities of CNTs. However, this method has poor control over the growth and unknown growth mechanism, leading to the increased concentration of reaction by-products (e.g., fullerene, amorphous carbon, graphitic nanoparticles) (Lu et al. 2012). Several parameters, such as the dispersion and concentration of carbon vapor inside the inert gas, the temperature of the reactor, the composition of catalysts, and the presence of hydrogen, strongly influence the diameter of CNTs (inner and outer) as well as the type of predominant nanotubes (MWCNTs or SWCNTs) (Kingston and Simard 2003). For example, the fabrication and purity of MWCNTs depend on the gas pressure inside the chamber. MWCNTs of large diameters are formed in the presence of high gas pressure, whereas a low gas pressure inside the chamber leads to thin and long MWCNTs. The type of gas can also influence the morphology of CNTs. For example, the incorporation of hydrogen into the methane and helium in the chamber results in the formation of long and good-quality MWCNTs in high yield.

14.2.2 Laser Ablation Method

In 1995, Guo et al. (1995) unexpectedly discovered the growth of MWNT in the soot during the synthesis of fullerene. In a laser vaporization oven apparatus at high temperature (800°C–1,500°C) (Figure 14.5b), intense Nd:YAG (neodymium-doped yttrium aluminum garnet) laser beam is focused on the graphite target surface under 500 torr in the presence of inert gas, such as argon. A low-temperature collector plate made of copper is used for the deposition of the soot produced by the laser ablation. This technique can also produce high-quality SWCNTs by employing bimetal mixtures of Co with Ni as the catalyst. With the improvement of the original method proposed by Rinzler et al. (1998), laser vaporization synthesis of SWNTs became the "standard method," where the resulting soot was found to contain 60%–90% SWNT. Laser ablation can produce CNTs in small quantity with high purity and in large quantity with high impurity (Maser et al. 2001). Several parameters such as gas flow rate, carrier gas type, catalyst, the substrate for nucleation, and time can significantly affect the structure and growth of the CNTs. For instance, the composition of the target materials plays an important role in the synthesis of CNTs. When a pure graphite target is used, carbon nano-onions (concentric buckyballs) and fullerenes are the dominant products as compared to the CNTs. In the laser ablation process, SWCNTs of high purity and yield are formed by doping the graphite targets with Ni or Co. Additionally, the reaction temperature can also control the quantity and quality of CNTs. A lower reaction temperature causes low-quality CNTs, whereas a high temperature (1,200°C) enables high-quality CNTs. However, the technique is expensive due to laser cost and energy.

14.2.3 Chemical Vapor Deposition (CVD)

The electric arc-discharge and laser vaporization processes enable the high-quality synthesis of CNTs; however, these approaches are not suitable for economical large-scale production of CNTs. To overcome these limitations of these processes, a more controlled synthesis and continuous operation based on CVD have been developed for the production of SWCNTs and MWCNTs (Figure 14.6a). CVD was explored for the production of

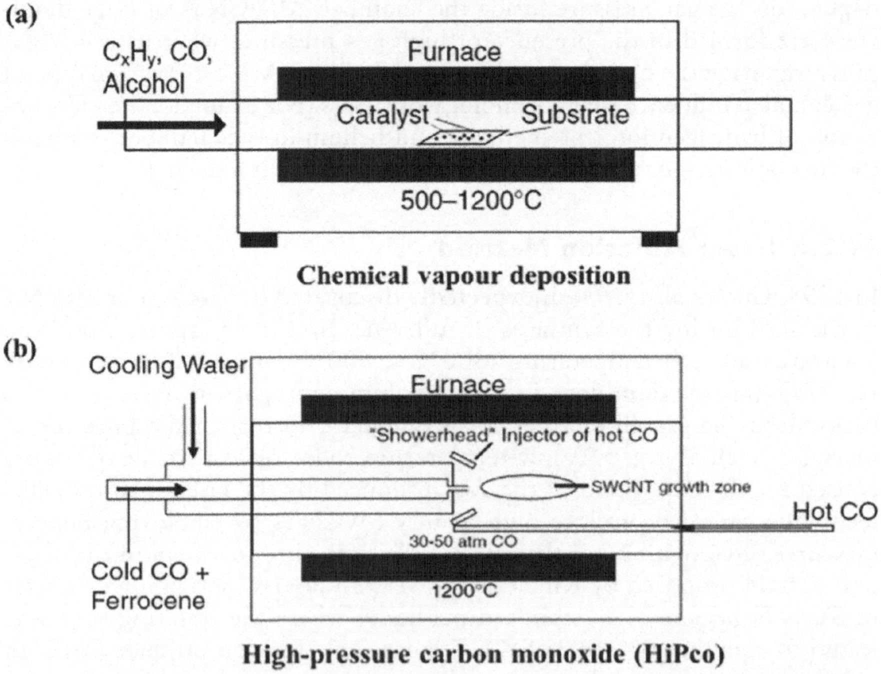

Figure 14.6 Schematics of (a) a CVD furnace and (b) HiPco furnace (O'Connell 2006). (Copyright 2006, CRC Press.)

carbon fibers and filaments for many years, and in 1993, Endo et al. used this method for the production of MWCNTs (Endo et al. 1993). CVD process involves the catalytic decomposition of volatile or gaseous precursors in the presence of metallic nanoparticles. These metallic nanoparticles act as a nucleation site for the growth of CNTs. Carbon monoxide (CO), methane (CH_4), ethanol, ethylene, and acetylene are commonly used as the sources of carbon in this method. CNTs can be produced by heating a gaseous hydrocarbon source, such as ethanol, at 600°C–1,000°C in the presence of a metal catalyst (Ni, Fe, Co, etc.) (Dresselhaus 2001). CNTs fabrication by CVD is a two-step process: (i) deposition of catalyst on the solid substrate by thermal annealing and nucleation; and (ii) the growth of CNTs at the sites of the metal catalysts. Catalytic nanoparticles stay either at the tip of the growing CNTs or at the base, depending on the adhesion strength between the substrate and catalytic nanoparticles. Later, these catalytic nanoparticles can be removed from CNTs by acid treatment. The length of CNTs depends on the reaction time, and nanotubes up to 60 mm in length can be produced by this method. Moreover, the size of CNTs can be tailored by changing the size of the catalytic nanoparticles.

CVD process offers several advantages, including the large-scale production of CNTs with high yield (Anzar et al. 2020), controlled growth of CNTs on a solid substrate, and low production costs in terms of low-energy consumption and low production of waste by-products (more economical). By adjusting the geometry of the reaction chamber, CVD can even produce vertically aligned CNTs as high-performance field emitters. The yield of CNTs from CVD is generally higher than that produced from the arc-discharge method. Despite several advantages, CNTs produced by the CVD process are often not pure, thus adding the additional purification step to get rid of contaminants using thermal annealing and chemical treatment. In CVD, the overall cost of SWCNTs production is much higher than MWCNTs.

14.2.4 High-Pressure Carbon Monoxide (HiPco) Synthesis

To increase the mass scaling ratio of CVD process, a modified technique, HiPco synthetic technique based on the decomposition of carbon monoxide (CO) in the presence of metal carbonyl was developed at Rice University by Nikolaev and Smalley et al. (Figure 14.6b). SWCNTs were produced by mixing high-pressure CO gas (10–100 atm) and a catalytic precursor iron carbonyl or metallocene in the reaction chamber (Nikolaev et al. 1999; Chiang et al. 2001). The decomposition of iron pentacarbonyl results in the synthesis of iron nanoparticles that act as catalytic sites for nucleation and growth of CNTs from the transformation of CO to carbon. HiPco synthesis method allows the continuous production of SWCNTs, and the produced

SWCNTs are of high quality and narrow diameter (from 0.7 to 1.4 nm), becoming the de facto standard for SWCNTs production.

14.3 PURIFICATION AND MODIFICATION OF CNTs

CNTs produced by arc discharge, laser ablation, and CVD methods often contain a large quantity of impurities, including carbonaceous by-products (amorphous carbon, fullerenes, amorphous and graphitic nanoparticles) and catalytic metal nanoparticles (Chiang et al. 2001; Hou, Liu, and Cheng 2008). While the carbonaceous impurities can be minimized by adjusting the experimental parameters during the synthesis of CNTs, the presence of metal impurities cannot be avoided as-synthesized CNTs are highly aggregated and hydrophobic due to strong van der Waals' interactions. The presence of impurities and aggregated hydrophobic nanotubes can increase the potential toxicity of CNTs as well as induce innate immune responses, which could defeat the purpose of using CNTs as drug delivery nanovehicles (Yuan et al. 2019). Therefore, the purification and modification strategies are required to remove impurities and introduce hydrophilicity (for improving solubility in water) in the CNTs structure for using them in biomedical applications.

The purification strategies can broadly be categorized into two approaches: physical and chemical and a multistep strategies are commonly employed to remove the impurities generated during the production of CNTs (Liu, Gao, et al. 2007), thus improving their solubility in water. A typical process involves three steps of purification: two oxidative processes (either liquid- or gas-phase oxidation) and a combination of physical separation methods, including centrifugation, filtration, and sonication. The gas-phase oxidation process involves using oxidative gases, such as dry or moist O_2, O_2-air mixture, NH_3, H_2, and CO_2 at a constant temperature ranging from 250°C to 1,000°C to remove catalytic nanoparticles and amorphous carbon from crude CNTs product (Nish et al. 2007; Mercier et al. 2013; Sheng et al. 2011). The main limitation of this treatment is that both the impurities and CNTs get oxidized. In liquid-phase oxidation, strong acids, such as HCl, HNO_3 H_2SO_4, and H_2O_2, are used to remove the impurities (both the carbonaceous and metal) (Bougrine et al. 1999). Also, the treatment of pristine CNTs with strong acids can introduce different hydrophilic functional groups in CNTs, thus making functional CNTs dispersible in the aqueous phase. The surface functionality depends on the type of acid used for the purification of CNTs (Figure 14.7). This is the most common procedure used in the industrial scale. Since the chemical nature of carbonaceous impurities is very identical to CNTs, a final step of purification is required, and it involves the separation of impurities based on their physical differences by several methods, including ultra-sonication (Liu, Gao, et al. 2007),

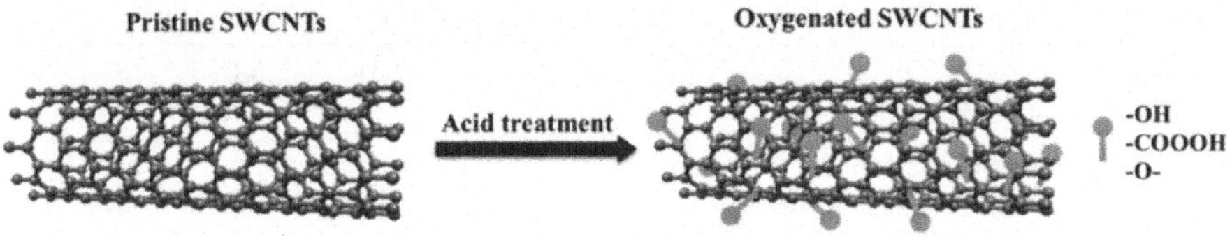

Figure 14.7 Schematic illustration of oxygenated SWCNTs.

microfiltration (Chiang et al. 2001), and size exclusion chromatography (Flavel et al. 2014).

In addition, acid treatments of CNTs will also result in the creation of structural defects with the formation of certain functional groups, which is unavoidable in such a corrosive acid environment. These functional groups change the chemical properties of CNTs entirely, by converting them from hydrophobic to hydrophilic (Figure 14.7) (Zhang, Zhang, and Zhang 2011). Unmodified CNTs have poor solubilities due to their strong van der Waals' interaction among the CNTs [50, 51], which could also be termed agglomeration. The creation of oxidative functional groups would repel the CNTs in close proximity in terms of increasing the solubility of CNTs. The existence of carboxylic groups would also form hydrogen bonds with surrounding aqueous media, increasing the solubility of the modified CNTs. Table 14.2 shows examples of acid modification methods and their applicability in drug delivery for CNTs. Also, the hollow structure of CNTs is a perfect host for drug storage (Bianco, Kostarelos, and Prato 2005). To open the tips of CNTs, a mixture of strong acids is used. Commonly, H_2SO_4/HNO_3 is used, and the tips of CNTs would be opened with newly generated oxidative functional groups, such as carboxylic acid (-COOH) and hydroxyl (-OH).

14.4 FUNCTIONALIZATION STRATEGIES FOR CNTs

In terms of using CNTs for drug delivery applications, maintaining the solubility of CNTs in biological media is one of the key hurdles because pristine CNTs are hardly dispersible in the aqueous phase and tend to aggregate due to strong hydrophobic interactions. These large size of aggregated CNTs are not suitable for drug delivery applications due to low blood circulation time, inefficient cellular uptake, clearance by macrophages, and toxicity. Therefore, surface functionalization is required to improve the efficacy of using CNTs as drug delivery vehicles in biological environments for appropriate and proper absorption of drug molecules, selective transport to the target site, longer blood circulation time, half-clearance time, biocompatibility, and reduced toxicity arising from the use of CNTs. In the next

Table 14.2 Compiled Data for Drug Load of Oxidized CNTs

Type of CNTs	*Modification Method*	*Drug/Loading System*	*System and Release Control*	*References*
MWCNTs	Acid oxidation (3:1 = H_2SO_4:HNO_3) to produce carboxylic acid groups	Aspirin	Suspension in alcohol solution	Yusof et al. (2009)
MWCNTs	Nitric acid treatment to produce carbonyl groups	Epirubicin hydrochloride (EPI)	Supramolecular complexes via	Chen et al. (2011)
MWCNTs	Carboxylated CNTs	Doxorubicin (DOX)	pH responsive, where low pH benefits the desorption	Wang et al. (2012)
SWCNTs	Carboxylated CNTs	Small interfering RNA (siRNA)	Combined with tumor marker (i.e. p53 siRNA, TNF-	Neagoe et al. (2012)
CNTs	Wet-chemical treatment with nitric acid for hollow tube production	Carboplatin	Encapsulation of drugs within the hollow tubes	Hampel et al. (2008)
CNTs	Cell-homing indole-load with EphB4-binding peptide	Peptide labeling	Near-infrared (NIR) irradiation for controlled release	Su et al. (2011)
MWCNTs	Acid sonication to open two ends of MWCNTs and sealed using polypyrrole (PPy) via electropolymerization	Dexamethasone (Dex)	Using electrical stimulation to achieve controlled release of drugs	Luo et al. (2011)
SWCNTs	None	Combretastatin A4 (CA4)	5–15 nm SWCNTs covalently filled with CA4	Assali et al. (2018)
MWCNTs	Acid oxidation (3:1 = H_2SO_4: HNO_3) to obtain carboxylated MWCNTs	N-desmethyl-tamoxifen-tosyl-tetraethylene glycol and quercetin	pH responsive	Kumar et al. (2018)

section, two strategies based on noncovalent and covalent interactions for attaching inorganic, organic, or biological entities to CNTs are discussed (Figure 14.8).

14.4.1 Physical or Noncovalent Functionalization

In noncovalent functionalization, a wide range of molecules are attached to the primary structure of CNTs by physical interactions. This attachment

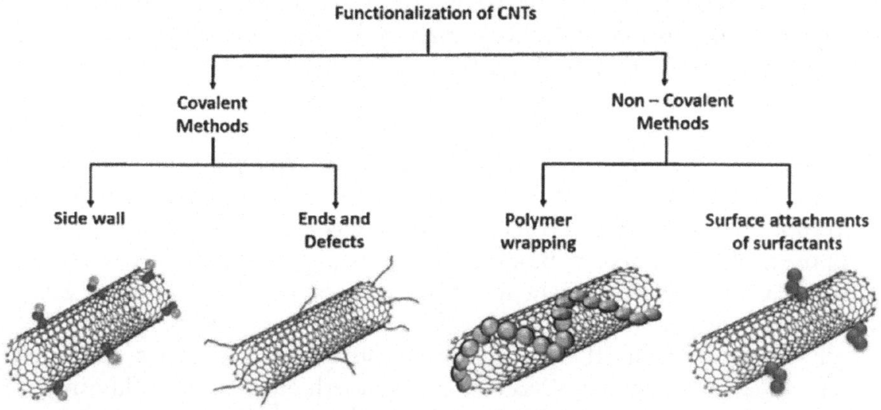

Figure 14.8 Various surface functionalization strategies for CNTs. (Reprinted by permission from Karimi, Solati, Amiri, et al. (2015). Copyright 2018, Elsevier B.V.)

or functionalization is facilitated by various forces acting between the molecules and the surface of CNTs, including electrostatic, hydrogen bond, van der Waals, and π-π stacking interactions. Electrostatic interactions mainly occur when two oppositely charged species come together, for example, the interaction between the negatively charged CNTs (acid purified) and cationic polyelectrolyte (polyethylene imine (PEI)) surfactant leading to surfactant wrapped CNTs (Yang et al. 2020). Hydrogen bonding interaction plays a key role in the adsorption of various organic molecules or chemicals to the surface of acid-purified CNTs. The presence of surface groups, such as carboxylic acid (-COOH), hydroxyl (-OH), amine ($-NH_2$) on CNTs, acts as hydrogen bonding doners (Liu, Sun, et al. 2007; Sobhani et al. 2011). Organic or drug molecules can be adsorbed to the surface of CNTs via π-π stacking interactions. For instance, the formation of supramolecular complexes between doxorubicin and CNTs via π-π stacking interactions occurs as both have many π electrons (Ali-Boucetta et al. 2008). This strategy involves the use of ultrasonic, centrifugation, and filtration processes to achieve the physical attachment of various molecules to CNTs. In the case of noncovalent functionalization, a single-step straightforward, non-destructive, and inexpensive strategy is used, and the functionalization does not cause damage to the side walls of CNTs, thus preserving the original electronic structure and properties of CNTs.

To obtain the stable dispersion of CNTs for drug delivery applications, three types of molecules are utilized: surfactants, biomolecules (nucleic acids and peptides), and polymeric molecules. These molecules are easily available at low cost, and several surfactant molecules (anionic, cationic, and nonionic) are found to be efficient in improving the solubility of CNTs in water. The stability of CNTs dispersion in water is highly dependent on the appropriate selection of surfactant molecules. For example, the use of Triton X-100 (nonionic) and sodium dodecyl sulfonate (anionic) creates an aqueous suspension of CNTs with a concentration of below<0. 1 mg/mL and stability up to 1 week (Islam et al. 2003). The use of cationic surfactant (sodium dodecyl benzene sulfonate) produces a stable suspension of CNTs (more than a month) at a concentration of 10 mg/mL. However, these surfactants cannot be used for drug delivery applications because of their toxicity profile. Therefore, a research effort has been made to develop biocompatible surfactant molecules. Pluronic is a biocompatible surfactant composed of a series of triblock nonionic copolymers, and its brush-like architecture provides a repellent surface to proteins (Granite et al. 2011). These molecules are commonly used for creating stable dispersion of CNTs which originate from their amphiphilic structure and steric hindrance effects. 1,2-Distearoyl-sn-glycero-3-phosphoethanol-amine-N-[amino(polyethylene glycol)-2000] (DSPE-PEG2000) surfactant molecules have been used to functionalize CNTs (Choudhary and Northrop 2012; Wang et al. 2013). These surfactant molecules offer advantages over others, such as being biocompatible, enhance the blood circulation of CNTs, and serve as a linker molecule for attaching targeting moieties to CNTs.

Biomolecules, which are biocompatible in biological environments, have a high affinity with the graphitic network of CNTs. They can strongly adsorb on the exterior surface of CNTs via van der Waals interaction, π-interactions, and electrostatic and hydrophobic interactions. For instance, DNA molecules are utilized for CNT dispersion via π-π interaction between a double-stranded DNA sequence and CNT's surface, adding great versatility to the noncovalent functionalization strategy (Chou et al. 2005). Here, the electrostatic repulsion of the negatively charged phosphate backbone of the DNA gives a stable dispersion of CNTs, which can be obtained by sonication of DNA molecules with pristine CNTs (here pristine CNTs refers to CNTs with any surface modification). It is known that the physicochemical properties of polymers can influence their ability to disperse CNTs as well as also affect the properties of CNTs. One such example can be the use of polypyrrole (PPy) that is a promising conductive polymeric molecule, and the wrapping of this polymer around CNTs provides good stability to CNTs suspension and enhances the electrical conductivity of CNTs (Karadas and Ozkan 2014). These large molecular weight and long-chain polymeric molecules can wrap around CNTs surface via electrostatic and van der Waals interactions to form a coating around CNTs. Therefore, incorporating polymeric molecules of different physical characteristics into CNTs can be used to construct hybrid NMs with improved physical properties for biomedical applications.

14.4.2 Covalent Functionalization

Covalent functionalization of CNTs involves the permanent and irreversible attachment of chemical moieties to the tubular structure of CNTs by forming covalent bonds, which share at least one pair of electrons between the introduced chemical moieties and CNTs. The purpose of a covalent bond is to increase the dispersibility of CNTs and their attachments with various biologically active moieties used for drug delivery. Owing to the hydrophobic and chemical inertness of as-synthesized CNTs, the covalent attachment of functional groups on the surface of CNTs is a difficult task. Therefore, this strategy requires the modification of CNTs via grafting of oxygenated species (carboxylic group, alcohol, ester, and ketone groups) onto the surface using aggressive acid treatment or plasma etching (Figure 14.7). Later, a direct or indirect functionalization strategy using carboxylic moieties on the surface of CNTs can be employed for covalent functionalization. The advantages of the covalent functionalization are counterbalanced by partial or complete disruption of the π-conjugated backbones of the CNTs, thus severely influencing the electronic, optical, and mechanical properties. Moreover, covalent bonding affinity to CNTs is higher and can resist any desorption of attached molecules compared with noncovalent bonding.

The covalent functionalization of CNTs can be adapted by two methods: (i) utilizing the structural defects along the sidewalls and the tips of the CNTs, and (ii) the formation of direct bond along the entire CNTs (Hirsch and Vostrowsky 2005). A first strategy based on the structural defects can be a useful platform for initiating the covalent functionalization of CNTs. These structural defects can be introduced during the synthesis and purification steps, such as introducing the five- and seven-membered rings in the structure of CNTs instead of the usual two six-membered rings. This leads to the change in the hybridization of carbons from sp^2 to sp^3. The treatment of CNTs with strong acids under harsh conditions (heating and sonication) causes damage to the backbone of the CNTs with the insertion of different functional groups, such as carboxyl, carbonyl, and hydroxyl groups. Also, these defects can potentially induce an increased local strain, resulting in higher chemical reactivity of neighboring carbon atoms. These highly reactive sites, such as the amide groups on CNTs, can be used for the purpose of additional functionalization of CNTs with biologically active molecules, such as protein, enzymes, antibodies, targeting ligands, and drug molecules. Carboxylic acid functionalization is a common strategy to bind the amine site of biomolecules with CNTs via amidation reaction (Zardini et al. 2012). In these reactions, numerous cross-linking agents, such as carbo-di-imides, oxalyl chloride, thionyl, or esters, are employed to the carboxylic acids in the amidation reaction. Apart from targeting the defect site for functionalization, it can also be achieved by the direct covalent method attachment that is based on the generation of highly reactive species to the surface of CNTs via cycloadditions (Kumar, Rana, and Cho 2011), fluorination (Tasis et al. 2006), electrophilic (Hauke and Hirsch 2010) or nucleophilic (Sgobba, Ehli, and Guldi 2012). These reactive species also attack the sp^2 structure of CNTs and change the hybridization from sp^2 to sp^3. The fluorinated CNTs have C-F bonds that are weaker than those in alkyl fluorides, thus providing substitution sites for additional functionalization, such as replacing fluorine atoms with amino, carboxyl, hydroxyl, and alkyl groups (Stevens et al. 2003).

14.5 APPLICATION OF CNTs IN DRUG DELIVERY

14.5.1 Considerations of CNTs as Drug Delivery System

Drug delivery systems (DDSs) are considered vehicles designed for transporting and releasing a drug to certain tissue or organ (Uthappa, Kurkuri, and Kigga 2019). These systems enhance the therapeutic efficacy of conventional medicines by overcoming limitations associated with traditional drug delivery systems (Uthappa, Sriram, et al. 2020), such as toxicity of cargo (Bhat et al. 2021), aggregation (Uthappa, Brahmkhatri, et al. 2018), lack of selectivity (Kurkuri and Aminabhavi 2004), drug degradation (Uthappa, Arvind, et al. 2020), and poor biodistribution (Uthappa, Sriram, et al. 2018; Uthappa et al. 2019). Two essential properties of CNTs encourage their use as DDSs: (i) large surface area that allows loading of multiple biologically active moieties; and (ii) ability to penetrate different types of cells and undergo endocytosis. CNTs-based DDSs increase the biological activity of drug molecules via controlling the release rates, protect the drug from degradation, decrease the quantity of the drug, and consequently, reduce the undesirable effects of the drug and toxicity. To use CNTs for targeted drug delivery, CNTs need to be uptook by cells. Three main routes for CNT delivery are known, including endocytosis, phagocytosis, and direct translocation through the plasma membrane (Raffa et al. 2010). In the endocytosis mechanism, CNTs are internalized inside endosome vesicles before entering the lysosomes localized in the perinuclear compartment. Endocytosis is an energy-dependent process, predominantly receptor-mediated for both SWCNTs and MWCNTs. For example, SWCNTs/doxorubicin complexes can be accumulated in the lysosomal compartment of endothelial cells after endocytosis (Wang et al. 2010; Kang et al. 2012). While SWCNTs remained entrapped into lysosomes, drug molecules (doxorubicin) detached in the acidic environment of lysosomes, diffused into the cytoplasm, and reached the nucleus to induce cell damage.

CNTs of a size less than 1 µm in length possess needle-like morphology, and they can penetrate the cell membrane more efficiently than large-sized CNTs without energy consumption (i.e., passive diffusion of CNTs) (Shi et al. 2011). The internalization of the CNTs can happen due to passive diffusion, and this can be split into three steps: (i) landing of functionalized CNTs to the membrane surface; (ii) penetration of the lipid head groups;

and (iii) sliding through the lipid tails. Phagocytosis, which is identical to endocytosis, is a cellular process of ingesting and eliminating large-sized particles of diameter (>0.5 μm). CNTs of extremely large size (i.e., a bundle of CNTs) are taken up by cells via the phagocytosis process. CNTs of extremely large lengths are impractical for drug delivery applications because phagocytosis of large size CNTs can lead to granuloma formation (Hirano, Kanno, and Furuyama 2008). Despite the significant efforts dedicated to understanding the internalization mechanism of CNTs, there is no single best strategy for delivery of CNTs into cells because each strategy can be affected by several factors, such as the length of nanotubes, type of surface coating, surface charge, the preparation method of CNTs, and their degree of aggregation in the biological medium. Also, the type of functionalization strategy (covalent vs noncovalent) and cell type can influence the cellular uptake mechanism of CNTs. In the following section, we will discuss the main parameters that should be considered for designing CNTs-based drug delivery vehicles.

14.5.1.1 Size and Structure

For developing efficient DDSs, the size of CNTs plays a vital role in various delivery steps, such as drug loading, transporting, and targeting. CNTs of smaller size possess a high surface area and the ability to bind a wide variety of therapeutics, such as drugs, siRNA, DNA, enzymes, and antibodies. To reach the target site, drug molecules attached to the outer or interior space of CNTs with similar sizes can be transported via the blood or the lymphatic system. For this, the size of CNTs should be optimized for long blood circulation time, which decreases with the increase in the size of CNTs. In addition, SWCNTs have also been shown to cross the blood–brain barrier (BBB) while preventing the release of drug molecules into healthy tissues (Beg et al. 2011).

For delivering and releasing drug molecules to tissue cells, CNTs should be uptaken by cells. The size of CNTs is one of the most significant parameters that can influence cellular uptake. In the literature, it has been shown the highest uptake of CNTs of length ~320 nm. However, the cellular uptake decreases with increase in the length of CNTs above >660 nmand decrease in the length of CNTs below <130 (Sciortino et al. 2017; Jin et al. 2017). In another work, it has been shown that the cellular uptake mechanism depends on the length of CNTs. CNTs with a length larger than 400 nm undergo cellular internalization through endocytosis, whereas smaller CNTs enter by penetrating the cellular membrane (Antonelli et al. 2010). Therefore, the length of CNTs should be optimized to achieve high cellular uptake, which is also an essential consideration for formulating an efficient drug delivery vehicle. Apart from the size of CNTs, the cellular uptake of CNTs depends on their structure (SWCNTs vs MWCNTs). For example, when MWCNTs and SWCNTs of similar sizes are compared, MWCNTs are uptook by endocytosis, and SWCNTs undergo cell penetration through the membrane. Also, MWCNTs of large size showed better results acting as drug vehicles to reach the target under the same conditions than smaller SWCNTs (Kushwaha et al. 2013).

14.5.1.2 Surface-Decorated Molecules

The surface functionalization of CNTs can improve the therapeutic efficacy of drugs because surface properties can control the stability of CNTs in a biological medium and cellular uptake of CNTs. Furthermore, CNTs can transport the drug molecules attached to their surface or into the matrix. After the internalization of CNTs-based delivery vehicles, the cellular microenvironment destructs the binding of drug molecules and releases the therapeutic drug content inside the cells. If the targeting molecules are not attached to CNTs, drug molecules can release before entering the cells, thus affecting the healthy tissues and cells. For designing an optimal drug delivery vehicle, decorating surfaces with appropriate biologically active molecules or polymeric molecules are essential for preventing aggregation, stability, efficient targeting, and pharmacological effects of the drug. Since CNTs are hydrophobic, they are likely to be cleared due to their high binding affinity to blood components (Kou et al. 2013). Introducing hydrophilicity to CNTs by functionalizing with biocompatible surfactants or polymers will prevent their clearance and increase their blood circulation time. For example, polyethylene glycol (PEG) is a relatively inert and hydrophilic molecule (Li and Huang 2010). When PEG molecules are attached to the surface of CNTs via surface functionalization strategies, PEG coating stabilizes the dispersion of CNTs in a biological medium. PEG coating also prevents the adsorption of plasma proteins (opsonization) on CNTs. Therefore, the surface coating can prevent the substantial loss of drug molecules from CNTs during circulation. PEG-coated CNTs can be referred to as "stealth" CNTs because they cannot be detected by the reticuloendothelial system (RES) without opsonization. Additionally, surface functionalization can help in preventing the toxicity associated with the use of drug molecules. For example, the functionalization of MWCNTs with poly(dopamine) improves their dispersibility in the biological medium, thus reducing the formation of inflammatory factors and cytokines (Sun et al. 2017). The loading of doxorubicin drug molecules to CNTs causes lower toxic effects in organs than free drug molecules (Perepelytsina et al. 2018).

Cellular uptake and intracellular localization of CNTs depend on the type of surface charge (positive or negative) and its charge density. It has been shown that charged NMs are taken up better than their uncharged counterparts (Thorek and Tsourkas 2008). When the surface charge is present on the surface, it is likely that positively charged CNTs are generally better uptook than negatively charged CNTs because of the electrostatic attraction between the negatively charged cell membrane and positively charged CNTs (Hassan et al. 2016). For instance, Budhathoko-Uprety et al. have shown that cellular uptake of amine-CNTs was higher than carboxyl-CNTs (Budhathoki-Uprety et al. 2017). It has been demonstrated that the reduction in the negative surface charge can lead to better cellular uptake both in vitro and in vivo. Therefore, one can design an efficient drug delivery vehicle by considering the surface charge of CNTs.

14.5.1.3 Agglomeration Tendency

CNTs have a strong tendency to agglomerate due to the π-π interaction between tubes. The formation of bundles from unmodified CNTs is unavoidable. The degree of agglomeration and aggregation can impact cellular internalization and increase cytotoxicity as a drug delivery vector. For example, the accumulation of aggregated SWCNTs (2–5 μm in length and 1.2 in diameter) in the liver can cause inflammation and oxidative stress (Principi et al. 2016). An efficient surface coating around CNTs is crucial to obtain the stable dispersion of CNTs in a sufficient degree for drug delivery applications. However, it is unlikely to achieve a complete dispersion of CNTs in the aqueous phase due to the lack of efficient surface coating molecules. Song et al. used oxidized MWCNTs (200–700 nm in length and 10–20 nm in diameter) to investigate the influence of agglomerated MWCNTs concentration on cellular uptake and cytotoxicity (Song et al. 2016). When the concentration of larger agglomerates of MWCNTs was decreased, a high cellular uptake with no obvious cytotoxicity was noticed. As the concentration of agglomerated MWCNTs increased, the toxicity level was elevated. From these experiments, it can be concluded that agglomeration can assist the endocytosis of MWCNTs owing to their effective interaction of agglomerates with cells. Therefore, a high cellular uptake and low cytotoxicity of agglomerated CNTs can facilitate drug delivery by controlling the concentration of agglomerated CNTs.

14.5.1.4 Cell Type

Since different cell types have different rates of cellular uptake due to their different biological functions, this can alter the internalization mechanism of CNTs. Summers et al. investigated the cellular internalization of CNTs in various cell lines, including human lung cancer cells (Calu-6 and A549), human breast cells (MCF-7), and mouse macrophage cells (J774) (Summers et al. 2017). Among different cell lines, the J774 cell line showed the highest cellular uptake of CNTs after 24 hours. Calu-6 and MCF-7 did not reveal any significant differences (30% less cellular uptake than J774), whereas A549 showed 40% less cellular uptake than J774. A high cellular uptake of macrophage cells (J774) is facilitated by phagocytosis process, taking a large amount of large-sized CNTs (>500 nm). However, other cells primarily use the endocytosis process for cellular uptake for CNTs of size <200 nm. These phagocytic cells can be employed as carriers of CNTs into tumor cells for cancer therapy.

14.5.1.5 Drug Loading and Release Mechanism

Drug loading and release profile from nanovehicle also play an essential role in developing efficient CNTs-based DDSs. The controlled release of drug molecules helps to keep the drug concentration within the therapeutic range and avoid toxic effects arising from uncontrolled release. The drug-loading efficiency depends on the specific drug type. Three drug-loading strategies have been established: (i) physical adsorption equilibrium, (ii) solvent evaporation, and (iii) melting (Debnath and Srivastava 2021). In the physical adsorption method, the drug molecules penetrate drug vehicles and distribute until the equilibrium is reached. After adsorption, drug-loaded CNTs can be separated from the solution by centrifugation. In a solvent evaporation technique, the evaporation of the solvent is required after the adsorption of drug molecules to CNTs. In this method, the drug molecules are evenly distributed through the drug vehicle. The melting method is not suitable for drug loading due to low drug-loading efficiency (Mozafari 2020). The drug release from nanovehicles is influenced by several parameters, such as the composition of surface molecules attached to CNTs (drug, targeting, and polymer), physiochemical interaction of surface molecules with the surrounding biological environment, materials type, and morphology of nanovehicles. The drug release can also be classified into three mechanisms: (i) diffusion-controlled release, (ii) solvent-controlled release, and (iii) stimuli-sensitive release (Figure 14.9) (Lee and Yeo 2015). In diffusion-controlled drug release, the release is driven by the concentration gradient across the membrane (outer surface) of nanovehicles. This system shows high initial drug release, followed by a decreasing release rate along with increasing the diffusion distance for drug molecules located at nanovehicles. In a solvent-controlled release, the drug molecules are released by flowing the water from outside of the drug vehicles (a region of low drug concentration) to the drug-loaded core (a region of high drug concentration). This mechanism is also known as osmosis-controlled release. Drug release from stimuli-responsive nanovehicles is controlled by either internal or external stimuli, e.g., pH, light, temperature, or magnetic field. In stimuli-responsive release, the drug molecules are incorporated into CNTs through stimuli-sensitive molecules, rather than the release vehicles from stimuli.

Among various mechanisms, pH-responsive controlled release is the most common strategy that has been exploited in the design of CNTs-based

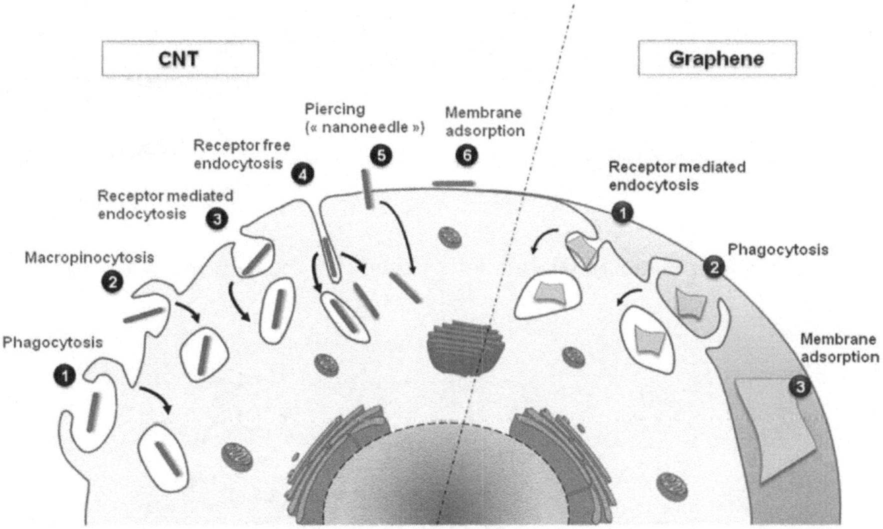

Figure 14.9 Illustration of CNT and graphene cellular uptake pathways (Bussy, Ali-Boucetta, and Kostarelos 2013). (Copyright © 2013, American Chemical Society.)

drug delivery vehicles. The microenvironment of tumor tissues is generally recognized as acidic, which deviates from the slightly basic healthy tissue environment (Warburg, Wind, and Negelein 1927; Griffiths 1991). Such a trait was exploited to the full extent by the intelligent design of the drug delivery systems. Since the pH change would work as a triggering mechanism, the CNTs could be designed to release the drug once it enters the microenvironment of cancerous cells. In 2018, Ünlü et al. demonstrated the possibility of unfunctionalized short SWNTs (1–1.3 µm in length) loaded with DOX as an agent for cancer therapy (Unlu et al. 2018). It was reported that SWCNTs would have a higher load and better stability than DOX/SWCNTs at basic conditions. Upon endocytosis by cancer cells, the acidic extracellular medium triggers the release of DOX and subsequent cell apoptosis. Kumar et al. also utilized the characteristic acidic microenvironment of cancer cells where carboxylated MWCNTs were conjugated with N-dimethyl-tamoxifen-tetraethylene-glycol-quercetin or N-TAM-TEG-MWCNTs-QT conjugate (referred to as N-TAM-conjugate from now on) (Kumar et al. 2018). The N-TAM-conjugate was successfully observed to release two drugs over time: fast release of QT to inhibit the activity of P-glycoproteins (multidrug resistance or MDR proteins) and CYP3A4 (microsomal enzymes) (Persidis 2000); higher accumulation and sustained release of TAM (estrogen receptor modulator to treat breast cancer) in the acidic microenvironment of tumor tissues. Such a technique offers a new strategy to approach MDR-cancer cells treatment,

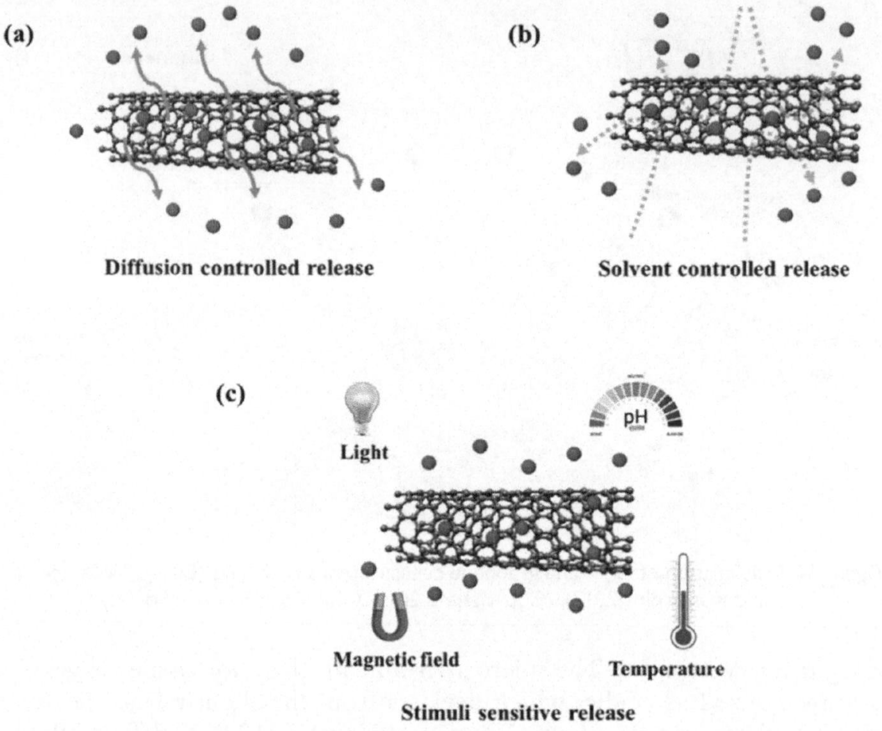

Figure 14.10 Various mechanisms of drug release from CNTs.

potentially providing benefits of enhanced efficacy and dose reduction in cancer chemotherapy.

14.5.2 Applications of CNTs

14.5.2.1 Drug Delivery Vector

Doxorubicin (DOX) is commonly used as a chemotherapeutic medication to treat patients suffering from cancer, including the brain, ovarian, breast, bladder, cervical, lung, mesothelioma, and testicular. However, it has disadvantages, such as irreversible side effects, poor selectivity after intravenous administration, low ability to cross through cellular membranes, and irreversible toxicity (Pugazhendhi et al. 2018). CNTs can transport DOX molecules to target tissue cells with reduced toxicity and minimal side effects because their unique physicochemical properties such as large surface area, excellent chemical stability, and ability to pass through the cell membrane and BBB (Shityakov et al. 2015). For example, Heister et al. developed a smart DDS based on oxidized SWCNTs functionalized with a monoclonal antibody together with DOX and fluorescein molecules (Heister et al. 2009). The results showed the binding of DOX molecules to the antigen target sites after the recognition of the carcinoembryonic antigen and the tumor markers by the antibody. The released DOX molecules were able to reach the nucleus while SWCNTs remained in the cytoplasm. The designed DOX-SWCNTs complexes allowed the successful targeted delivery of the anticancer drug (DOX) to cancer cells along with the visualization of the cellular uptake of SWCNTs using fluorescence probe molecules. In another work, Dai et al. developed a DDS consisting of SWCNTs, phospholipids (PL)-PEG chain, a cyclic tripeptide (arginine-glycine-aspartic acid, RGD), and DOX (Liu et al. 2009). In this design, PL-PEG molecules were attached to SWCNTs via noncovalent interaction between the PL chain and SWCNTs, PEG pointing to aqueous solutions, where DOX molecules were adsorbed to the side walls of SWCNTs. The coverage of PL-PEG and DOX molecules on the surface area of SWCNTs were 10% and 75%, respectively. RGD molecules (targeting moieties) act as recognition elements for integrin receptors, which are upregulated in a range of cancerous tumors. These DDSs have shown the efficient, targeted delivery of DOX molecules with less toxicity than free DOX molecules. The release of DOX molecules was triggered by a change in pH from basic to acidic. The hydrophobic DOX molecules strongly bind to SWCNTs due to poor solubility in the solution of pH more than 7. As the acidity of the solution increases (or pH of the solution decreases), the amine groups in DOX molecules protonate at low pH values, which enhances the hydrophilicity of DOX molecules, thus the solubility of DOX. Since the extracellular or physiological environment is weakly basic and the intracellular environment is acidic, the important strategy based on pH can be used to regulate drug loading or release of drug molecules from SWCNTs. For instance, Uttekar et al. designed nanocarriers consisting of MWCNTs conjugated with a combination of folic acid (FA: targeting agent for cancerous tumor) and ethylene diamine (EDA) for delivery of DOX molecules to MCF-7 breast cancer cells (Uttekar et al. 2019). In vitro results showed more than 60% release of drug molecules from FA-EDA-MWCNTs-DOX at pH in the acidic range after 48 hours compared to the drug release with the pH in the basic range. DOX molecules can also be encapsulated in polyethylenimine (PEI)-modified MWCNTs covalently conjugated with a fluorescent protein and hyaluronic acid (HA) for targeted delivery to cancer cells overexpressing CD-44 receptors (Cao et al. 2015). The results showed the increased release rate of DOX from DDSs under acidic conditions, pH 5.8 within tumor cell microenvironment, compared to the physiological environment (pH 7.4).

Paclitaxel (PTX) is another anticancer drug, which is insoluble and tends to accumulate in the physiological environment. The attachment of these drug molecules to CNTs by covalent and noncovalent functionalization strategies provides an alternative platform for cancer therapy. The drug loading and its release can also be controlled by pH. For example, HA-chitosan-CNTs-PTX based on a smart DDS has been developed to release drugs to lung cancer tumor cells having an acidic microenvironment (Yu et al. 2016). Karnati et al. have developed a novel drug delivery platform by co-loading two drug molecules (PTX and DOX) on the chitosan-functionalized SWCNTs (Karnati and Wang 2018). Molecular dynamic simulation results showed that both PTX and DOX molecules strongly bind with the pristine SWCNTs with the same binding strength. However, incorporating these drug molecules on chitosan-coated SWCNTs results in decreased binding of DOX and PTX with the sidewalls of the SWCNTs. The protonation of chitosan and drug molecules in the acidic environment weakens the interaction between PTX/DOX and SWCNTs, thus triggering the release of drug molecules in the acidic environment. Gemcitabine (GEM) is another type of anticancer agent, primarily used for non-small cell lung and pancreatic cancers. The use of GEM in a clinical setting is very limited because of its short plasma half-life (17 minutes) and rapid metabolism. These limitations require the frequent administration of a high dose of GEM drugs which can cause severe side effects. To improve the delivery of GEM drugs, SWCNTs were employed to construct DDSs by conjugating PEG and drug molecules to SWCNTs (Razzazan et al. 2016). The release of GEM from PEG-SWCNTs-GEM was high at a low pH of 5.0 as compared to a pH of 7.4. In vitro and in vivo results from the human lung and pancreatic carcinoma cell lines and B6 nude mice showed increased antinuclear activity and decreased tumor cell growth compared to free GEM.

14.5.2.2 CNTs for Therapeutic Brain Delivery

The delivery of therapeutic drugs to the brain is hindered by the presence of the BBB, which is composed of endothelial cells, astrocytes, and other types of support cells (Pardridge 2012). The role of BBB is to protect the brain from circulating toxins or pathogens in the blood, supply nutrients to brain tissues, and filter harmful compounds from the brain back to the bloodstream. Therefore, the therapeutic treatment of brain disorders and gliomas remains a challenge. To cross the BBB, the size of the particle should be below 100 nm (Ohta et al. 2020). CNTs of smaller size functionalized with target moieties have the capacity to cross the BBB by receptor-mediated transcytosis (energy-dependent pathways) and passive penetration (an energy-independent mechanism) (Kafa et al. 2015). In addition to their intrinsic ability to cross the BBB, the high surface area makes them suitable for loading and delivering brain therapeutics. Moreover, the specific targeting to the brain is crucial for increasing the accumulation of delivery vehicles to the brain and reducing systemic side effects. Two different pathways have been explored for brain delivery: (i) intracranial administration and (ii) systemic administration.

In intracranial administration, therapeutic drugs are locally administrated to bypass the BBB. This approach can be helpful in treating brain disorders, such as tumors and stroke, where a surgical procedure is often required. Zhao et al. used functionalized SWCNTs conjugated with CpG oligonucleotides to treat glioma-bearing mice (Zhao et al. 2011). The results from the animal model showed the increased uptake of SWCNTs-CpG by tumor cells after a single intracranial injection compared to free CpG. This led to a strong antitumoral response, decreased tumor size, and increased animal survival time. Since CNTs have the ability to absorb NIR light and convert it to heat, they can be used as a therapeutic agent for photothermal therapy. Santos et al. employed functionalized CNTs to develop photothermal mediated brain tumor therapy (Santos et al. 2014). A combination of intracranial injection of SWCNTs and NIR exposure to mice-bearing glioblastoma multiforme (GBM) tumor showed significant suppression of tumor growth compared to individual therapeutic treatment (SWCNTs or NIR exposure). Also, this combined therapeutic treatment inhibited tumor occurrence for up to 80 days. The intracranial administration of drugs can be applied in clinical settings; however, its applications are restricted by the invasiveness of the technique and patient compliance. Researchers have introduced systemic administration of drug molecules to the brain by crossing the BBB. The results from preclinical studies involving intravenous (IV) injection of CNTs evidenced the penetration of CNTs to the tissues beyond the BBB. For instance, Kafa et al. developed angiopep-2 (ANG)-targeted chemically functionalized MWCNTs to cross the BBB in vivo model (Kafa et al. 2016). The conjugation of ANG ligand to MWCNTs enhanced BBB of MWCNTs-ANG compared to non-targeted MWCNTs. In vivo results revealed higher uptake of MWCNTs-ANG in glioma brain than to non-targeted MWCNTs at 24 hours post-injection. Therefore, the improved brain targeting with ANG allows the future clinical applications of functionalized MWCNTs-ANG to deliver active therapeutic agents for glioma therapy.

14.5.2.3 Gene Delivery Vector

In 2003, the world's first commercially available gene therapy, Gendicine, to treat head and neck squamous cell carcinoma was approved by China's regulatory agency (Daley 2019). Fourteen years later in 2017, FDA approved United States' first gene therapy, Kymriah (tisagenlecleucel) to treat acute lymphoblastic leukemia (Braendstrup, Levine, and Ruella 2020). Ever since, the proven benefits of gene therapy have accelerated the pace of approval of gene therapy. To date ("Allotropy" 2021), more than 20 gene-based medicines have been approved by drug regulatory agencies in various countries (Ma et al. 2020). One of the most used delivery vectors for gene therapy is adenoviruses. Adenoviruses are modified to insert their therapeutic genes into infected cells, restoring the cells to a healthy state. Similarly, other viral vectors such as adeno-associated viruses, retrovirus, lentivirus, and RNA viruses can also achieve high transfection efficiencies (Karimi, Solati, Ghasemi, et al. 2015). Unfortunately, viral vectors have concerns about potentially inducing cancers and limited genetic payload. Notably, the immune response of the viral vector still hinders its uniform efficacy (Shirley et al. 2020). The death of Jesse Gelsinger in 1999 halted the development of gene therapy (Sibbald 2001). Researchers are finding an alternative to reduce vector immunogenicity.

One approach is to use nonviral delivery vectors, such as CNTs. The advantages of nonviral vectors are relatively safe, chemically controllable, enhanced biocompatibility, and unrestricted gene sizes (Karimi, Solati, Ghasemi, et al. 2015). However, nonviral vectors also face limitations, such as incapability of transversing nuclear membrane, low transfection efficiencies, and poor transgene expression (Wang, Upponi, and Torchilin 2012). Despite these limitations, CNTs have attracted much attention for the delivery of genetic materials. CNTs are highly tunable and versatile. By modifying the surface chemistry of CNTs, they can become biocompatible and nonimmunogenic and achieve specific targeting (Mohammadi et al. 2020). Various reports on delivering plasmid DNA (pDNA), small interfering RNA (siRNA), and micro-RNA (miRNA) have been published (Kushwaha et al. 2013; Neagoe et al. 2012; Singh et al. 2005). CNTs have abundant π-electrons, which stabilize the nucleic acids due to π-π stacking interactions (Goujun and Fayun 2017). Nucleic acid-loaded CNTs show excellent stability outside the target tissues and cells, achieve high loading of genetic cargos, and protect nucleic acids against enzymatic degradation (Jampilek and Kralova 2021). In a study, the delivery of miRNA to endothelial cells to regulate cell proliferation and in vitro angiogenesis has been demonstrated by employing functionalized CNTs, such as polyethylenimine and polyamidoamine (Masotti et al. 2016).

14.5.2.4 Photothermal and Photodynamic Therapy

Photothermal therapy (PTT) has emerged as a promising noninvasive therapeutic technique due to the targeted killing of cells using heat energy, particularly cancer research. CNTs have exceptional optical absorbance in visible and NIR regions, which could release a significant amount of heat and enhance the thermal ablation of cells during NIR laser irradiation and radiofrequency irradiation. Since biological tissues show a deep-tissue penetration with very low absorption of NIR wavelengths from 700 to 1,100 nm, CNTs with NIR absorption can be promising candidates for PTT. In PTT, CNTs absorb photon energy and convert rapidly into heat to increase the local temperature for killing tumor cells. PPT and commercially available chemotherapy can be combined to improve the therapeutic efficacy of cancer treatment. In a study, PEG-wrapped MWCNTs were targeted to cancerous mice having melanoma tumor (Sobhani et al. 2017). When NIR (λ=808 nm, P=2 W) laser light was exposed to mice for 10 minutes, the average size of the tumor in mice decreased sharply because of the hyperthermia effect induced by PTT. PEG-coated CNTs can be used as PTT agents for eradicating solid tumors. PPT can also be combined with chemotherapy to obtain enhanced antitumor efficacy by delivering drugs and converting NIR into heat. For example, Dong et al. formulated chitosan-functionalized MWCNTs encapsulated with DOX drug molecules (Dong et al. 2017). These DDSs have shown enhanced antitumor efficacy through the synergistic function of chemotherapy (sustain release of DOX) and photothermal ablation (inducing hypothermia under NIR irradiation).

Besides PTT, photodynamic therapy (PDT) is also another emerging therapeutic technology. PDT utilizes light of a particular wavelength to activate photosensitizers (PS) to destroy the cancerous tumor. In PDT, the excitation of PS molecules by a specific light produces reactive oxygen species (ROS), leading to cell necrosis or apoptosis. A limitation of this PDT is that the majority of used PS molecules are hydrophobic. This can be overcome by incorporating PS molecules into CNTs for significantly enhanced efficacy and tumor selectivity in cells. For instance, the synthesis of SWCNTs coupled with hyaluronic acid (targeting agent) and chlorin e6 (PS molecules) has been reported (Sundaram and Abrahamse 2020). Chlorin e6 is a naturally derived chlorophyll with crucial advantages. These include low toxicity, fast and selective accumulation in the target tissue, strong absorption wavelength at 650–670 nm, high singlet oxygen quantum yield, and no side effects. These nanocomposite systems displayed PDT-enhanced apoptosis of cancer cells at laser irradiation of 10 J/cm^2. Instead of using PS molecules, SWCNTs can also be used as PS because of their metallic and semiconducting properties (Wang et al. 2014). In recent years, attempts have been made in the development of multimodal therapeutic agents by combining two or more therapeutic functionalities (Zhang et al. 2018). Carbon quantum dots and iron oxide nanoparticles were conjugated to PEG functionalized SWCNTs, followed by loading of DOX molecules. When PDT was applied, 30% of the cancer cell remained alive at the highest dose. When therapeutic treatments were combined at the same dose (combination of PTT, PDT, and chemotherapy), more than 95% of cancer cells were killed. Additionally, this multimodal therapeutic technique can also be combined with magnetic resonance imaging (MRI) to monitor the efficacy of therapeutic treatment.

14.6 CONCLUSION AND FUTURE OF NANOTHERAPEUTICS

Safety is still one of the primary concerns for nanotherapeutics (Faunce 2007; Wolfram et al. 2015). The lack of standard protocols for evaluating nanotherapeutics hinders the clinical translations of benchtop science. Without a doubt, since the discovery of CNTs in 1991, researchers have made tremendous progress in this field (Heidarian, Khazaei, and Saien 2021; Jampilek and Kralova 2021). With the accelerating growth of nanotherapeutics in research, it is expected that next-generation precision and high-efficient nanotherapeutics will be made available in the next few decades. The market growth of commercializing nanotherapeutics is rapidly growing worldwide with North America and Europe dominating the global market (Nance 2019; Matteucci et al. 2018). There is also an increasing number of approved nanotherapeutics in clinical trials (Dri et al. 2021; Mitchell et al. 2021).

As much as the future prospect of CNTs is promising, it is impossible to overlook the lack of international regulatory guidelines on the safety of NMs. The commercialization of NMs relies on regulatory guidelines. Without a comprehensive and clear policy in place, the development of NMs-based DDS will see slow growth in clinical trials. The pharmacological and toxicological profiles must be thoroughly investigated before their translation to clinical use (Zhang, Zhang, and Zhang 2011; Seyhan 2019). As the field of nanomedicine is rapidly expanding, the regulatory bodies would hopefully respond to guide the clinical practices of NMs-based DDS. We can remain hopeful for the standardization of clinical assessment of the safety of nanotherapeutics. The increasing number of approved nanotherapeutics will fuel the research and generate more and more discussion in this field. The future of nanotherapeutics is bright, and so are CNTs as DDS.

REFERENCES

Aboofazeli, R. 2010. "Carbon nanotubes: A promising approach for drug delivery." *Iranian Journal of Pharmaceutical Research: IJPR* 9 (1):1–3.

Ali-Boucetta, H., K. T. Al-Jamal, D. McCarthy, M. Prato, A. Bianco, and K. Kostarelos. 2008. "Multiwalled carbon nanotube–doxorubicin supramolecular complexes for cancer therapeutics." *Chemical Communications* (4):459–461. doi: 10.1039/B712350G.

Allen, L. C. 1989. "Electronegativity is the average one-electron energy of the valence-shell electrons in ground-state free atoms." *Journal of the American Chemical Society* 111 (25):9003–9014. doi: 10.1021/ja00207a003.

"Allotropy." 2021. Accessed 17 September. https://www.britannica.com/science/allotropy.

Antonelli, A., S. Serafini, M. Menotta, C. Sfara, F. Pierigé, L. Giorgi, G. Ambrosi, L. Rossi, and M. Magnani. 2010. "Improved cellular uptake of functionalized single-walled carbon nanotubes." *Nanotechnology* 21 (42):425101. doi: 10.1088/0957-4484/21/42/425101.

Anzar, N., R. Hasan, M. Tyagi, N. Yadav, and J. Narang. 2020. "Carbon nanotube - A review on Synthesis, Properties and plethora of applications in the field of biomedical science." *Sensors International* 1. doi: 10.1016/j.sintl.2020.100003.

Assali, M., A. N. Zaid, N. Kittana, D. Hamad, and J. Amer. 2018. "Covalent functionalization of SWCNT with combretastatin A4 for cancer therapy." *Nanotechnology* 29 (24):245101. doi: 10.1088/1361-6528/aab9f2.

Bacon, R. 1960. "Growth, structure, and properties of graphite whiskers." *Journal of Applied Physics* 31 (2):283–290. doi: 10.1063/1.1735559.

Bandaru, P. R. 2007. "Electrical properties and applications of carbon nanotube structures." *Journal of Nanoscience and Nanotechnology* 7 (4–5):1239–1267. doi: 10.1166/jnn.2007.307.

Bati, A. S. R., L. P. Yu, M. Batmunkh, and J. G. Shapter. 2019. "Recent advances in applications of sorted single-walled carbon nanotubes." *Advanced Functional Materials* 29 (30). doi: 10.1002/adfm.201902273.

Beg, S., M. Rizwan, A. M. Sheikh, M. Saquib Hasnain, K. Anwer, and K. Kohli. 2011. "Advancement in carbon nanotubes: Basics, biomedical applications and toxicity." *Journal of Pharmacy and Pharmacology* 63 (2):141–163. doi: 10.1111/j.2042-7158.2010.01167.x.

Benincasa, M., S. Pacor, W. Wu, M. Prato, A. Bianco, and R. Gennaro. 2011. "Antifungal activity of amphotericin B conjugated to carbon nanotubes." *ACS Nano* 5 (1):199–208. doi: 10.1021/nn1023522.

Bhat, S., U. T. Uthappa, T. Altalhi, H. Y. Jung, and M. D. Kurkuri. 2021. "Functionalized porous hydroxyapatite scaffolds for tissue engineering applications: A focused review." *ACS Biomaterials Science & Engineering*. doi: 10.1021/acsbiomaterials.1c00438.

Bianco, A., K. Kostarelos, and M. Prato. 2005. "Applications of carbon nanotubes in drug delivery." *Current Opinion in Chemical Biology* 9 (6):674–679. doi: 10.1016/j.cbpa.2005.10.005.

Blackman, A. G. 2016. *Chemistry*. Milton: Wiley. Edited by Steve Bottle, Siegbert Schmid, Mauro Mocerino and Uta Wille.

Bougrine, A., A. Naji, J. Ghanbaja, and D. Billaud. 1999. "Purification and structural characterization of single-walled carbon nanotubes." *Synthetic Metals* 103 (1–3):2480–2481.

Braendstrup, P., B. L. Levine, and M. Ruella. 2020. "The long road to the first FDA-approved gene therapy: Chimeric antigen receptor T cells targeting CD19." *Cytotherapy* 22 (2):57–69. doi: 10.1016/j.jcyt.2019.12.004.

Budhathoki-Uprety, J., J. D. Harvey, E. Isaac, R. M. Williams, T. V. Galassi, R. E. Langenbacher, and D. A. Heller. 2017. "Polymer cloaking modulates the carbon nanotube protein corona and delivery into cancer cells." *Journal of Materials Chemistry B* 5 (32):6637–6644. doi: 10.1039/C7TB00695K.

Bussy, C., H. Ali-Boucetta, and K. Kostarelos. 2013. "Safety considerations for graphene: Lessons learnt from carbon nanotubes." *Accounts of Chemical Research* 46 (3):692–701. doi: 10.1021/ar300199e.

Cao, X., L. Tao, S. Wen, W. Hou, and X. Shi. 2015. "Hyaluronic acid-modified multiwalled carbon nanotubes for targeted delivery of doxorubicin into cancer cells." *Carbohydrate Research* 405:70–77 doi: 10.1016/j.carres.2014.06.030.

Cellot, G., E. Cilia, S. Cipollone, V. Rancic, A. Sucapane, S. Giordani, L. Gambazzi, H. Markram, M. Grandolfo, D. Scaini, F. Gelain, L. Casalis, M. Prato, M. Giugliano, and L. Ballerini. 2009. "Carbon nanotubes might improve neuronal performance by favouring electrical shortcuts." *Nature Nanotechnology* 4 (2):126–133. doi: 10.1038/nnano.2008.374.

Charlier, J. C., X. Gonze, and J. P. Michenaud. 1994. "Graphite interplanar bonding: Electronic delocalization and van der waals interaction." *Europhysics Letters (EPL)* 28 (6):403–408. doi: 10.1209/0295-5075/28/6/005.

Chen, K., and S. Mitra. 2019. "Incorporation of functionalized carbon nanotubes into hydrophobic drug crystals for enhancing aqueous dissolution." *Colloids and surfaces. B, Biointerfaces* 173:386–391. doi: 10.1016/j.colsurfb.2018.09.080.

Chen, Z., D. Pierre, H. He, S. Tan, C. Pham-Huy, H. Hong, and J. Huang. 2011. "Adsorption behavior of epirubicin hydrochloride on carboxylated carbon nanotubes." *International Journal of Pharmaceutics* 405 (1–2):153–161. doi: 10.1016/j.ijpharm.2010.11.034.

Chiang, I. W., B. E. Brinson, A. Y. Huang, P. A. Willis, M. J. Bronikowski, J. L. Margrave, R. E. Smalley, and R. H. Hauge. 2001. "Purification and characterization of single-wall carbon nanotubes (SWNTs) obtained from the gas-phase decomposition of CO (HiPco Process)." *The Journal of Physical Chemistry B* 105 (35):8297–8301. doi: 10.1021/jp0114891.

Chou, S. G., F. Plentz, J. Jiang, R. Saito, D. Nezich, H. B. Ribeiro, A. Jorio, M. A. Pimenta, Ge G. Samsonidze, A. P. Santos, M. Zheng, G. B. Onoa, E. D. Semke, G. Dresselhaus, and M. S. Dresselhaus. 2005. "Phonon-assisted excitonic recombination channels observed in DNA-wrapped carbon nanotubes using photoluminescence spectroscopy." *Physical Review Letters* 94 (12):127402. doi: 10.1103/PhysRevLett.94.127402.

Choudhary, U., and B. H. Northrop. 2012. "Rotaxanes and biofunctionalized pseudorotaxanes via thiol-maleimide click chemistry." *Organic Letters* 14 (8):2082–2085. doi: 10.1021/ol300614z.

Daley, J. 2019. "Gene therapy arrives." *Nature* 576 (7785):S12–S13. doi: 10.1038/d41586-019-03716-9.

Debnath, S. K., and R. Srivastava. 2021. "Drug delivery with carbon-based nanomaterials as versatile nanocarriers: Progress and prospects." *Frontiers in Nanotechnology* 3 (15). doi: 10.3389/fnano.2021.644564.

Delhaes, P. 2001. *Graphite and Precursors*. 1st edition, CRC Press. doi: 10.1201/9781482296921.

Dong, X., Z. Sun, X. Wang, and X. Leng. 2017. "An innovative MWCNTs/DOX/TC nanosystem for chemo-photothermal combination therapy of cancer." *Nanomedicine: Nanotechnology, Biology and Medicine* 13 (7):2271–2280. doi: 10.1016/j.nano.2017.07.002.

Dresselhaus, M. S. 2001. *Carbon Nanotubes: Synthesis, Structure, Properties, and Applications*. Springer.

Dresselhaus, M. S., G. Dresselhaus, J. C. Charlier, and E. Hernandez. 2004. "Electronic, thermal and mechanical properties of carbon nanotubes." *Philosophical Transactions of the Royal Society a-Mathematical Physical and Engineering Sciences* 362 (1823):2065–2098. doi: 10.1098/rsta.2004.1430.

Dri, D. A., C. Marianecci, M. Carafa, E. Gaucci, and D. Gramaglia. 2021. "Surfactants, nanomedicines and nanocarriers: A critical evaluation on clinical trials." *Pharmaceutics* 13 (3):381.

Ebbesen, T. W., and T. Takada. 1995. "Topological and SP3 defect structures in nanotubes." *Carbon* 33 (7):973–978. doi: 10.1016/0008-6223(95)00025*9.

Edgar, Y. C. J., and H. Wang. 2017. "Introduction For Design Of Nanoparticle Based Drug Delivery Systems." *Current Pharmaceutical Design* 23 (14):2108–2112. doi: 10.2174/1381612822666161025154003.

Endo, M., Hayashi, T., Kim, Y. A., Muramatsu, H. Development and application of carbon nanotubes, Jap. J. Appl. Phys., 45, 4883–4892 (2006).

Endo, M., K. Takeuchi, S. Igarashi, K. Kobori, M. Shiraishi, and H.W. Kroto. 1993. "The production and structure of pyrolytic carbon nanotubes (PCNTs)." *Journal of Physics and Chemistry of Solids* 54 (12):1841–1848. doi: 10.1016/0022-3697(93)90297-5.

Fabbro, C., H. Ali-Boucetta, T. D. Ros, K. Kostarelos, A. Bianco, and M. Prato. 2012. "Targeting carbon nanotubes against cancer." *Chemical Communications* 48 (33):3911–3926. doi: 10.1039/C2CC17995D.

Faunce, T. A. 2007. "Nanotherapeutics: New challenges for safety and cost-effectiveness regulation in Australia." *Medical Journal of Australia* 186 (4):189–191. doi: 10.5694/j.1326-5377.2007.tb00860.x.

Ferreira, F. V., W. Franceschi, B. R.C. Menezes, A. F. Biagioni, A. R. Coutinho, and L. S. Cividanes. 2019. Synthesis, characterization, and applications of carbon nanotubes. In Srinivasarao Yaragalla, Raghvendra Mishra, Sabu Thomas, Nandakumar Kalarikkal, and Hanna J. Maria (eds.) *Carbon-Based Nanofillers and Their Rubber Nanocomposites*. Elsevier, Amsterdam.

Fischer, R. A., E. Cottrell, E. Hauri, K. K. M. Lee, and M. Le Voyer. 2020. "The carbon content of Earth and its core." *Proceedings of the National Academy of Sciences* 117 (16):8743. doi: 10.1073/pnas.1919930117.

Flavel, B. S., K. E. Moore, M. Pfohl, M. M. Kappes, and F. Hennrich. 2014. "Separation of single-walled carbon nanotubes with a gel permeation chromatography system." *ACS Nano* 8 (2):1817–1826. doi: 10.1021/nn4062116.

Gavrel, G., B. Jousselme, A. Filoramo, and S. Campidelli. 2014. "Supramolecular chemistry of carbon nanotubes." In M. Marcaccio and F. Paolucci (eds.) *Making and Exploiting Fullerenes, Graphene, and Carbon Nanotubes*, 95–126. Springer, Berlin.

Ghosh, S., S. Dutta, E. Gomes, D. Carroll, R. D'Agostino, J. Olson, M. Guthold, and W. H. Gmeiner. 2009. "Increased heating efficiency and selective thermal ablation of malignant tissue with DNA-encased multiwalled carbon nanotubes." *ACS Nano* 3 (9):2667–2673. doi: 10.1021/nn900368b.

Gorain, B., H. Choudhury, M. Pandey, P. Kesharwani, M. M. Abeer, R. K. Tekade, and Z. Hussain. 2018. "Carbon nanotube scaffolds as emerging nanoplatform for myocardial tissue regeneration: A review of recent developments and therapeutic implications." *Biomedicine & Pharmacotherapy* 104:496–508 doi: 10.1016/j.biopha.2018.05.066.

Goujun, Z., and Z. Fayun. 2017. "Conformation and electronic structure of DNA in carbon nanotubes: A molecular dynamics and first-principles study." *Micro & Nano Letters* 12 (7):490–493. doi: 10.1049/mnl.2017.0030.

Granite, M., A. Radulescu, W. Pyckhout-Hintzen, and Y. Cohen. 2011. "Interactions between block copolymers and single-walled carbon nanotubes in aqueous solutions: A small-angle neutron scattering study." *Langmuir* 27 (2):751–759. doi: 10.1021/la103096n.

Griffiths, J. R. 1991. "Are cancer cells acidic?" *British Journal of Cancer* 64 (3):425–427. doi: 10.1038/bjc.1991.326.

Guo, T., P. Nikolaev, A. Thess, D. T. Colbert, and R. E. Smalley. 1995. "Catalytic growth of single-walled manotubes by laser vaporization." *Chemical Physics Letters* 243 (1–2):49–54. doi: 10.1016/0009-2614(95)00825-o.

Gupta, N., S. M. Gupta, and S. K. Sharma. 2019. "Carbon nanotubes: Synthesis, properties and engineering applications." *Carbon Letters* 29 (5):419–447. doi: 10.1007/s42823-019-00068-2.

Hampel, S., D. Kunze, D. Haase, K. Kramer, M. Rauschenbach, M. Ritschel, A. Leonhardt, J. Thomas, S. Oswald, V. Hoffmann, and B. Buchner. 2008. "Carbon nanotubes filled with a chemotherapeutic agent: A nanocarrier mediates inhibition of tumor cell growth." *Nanomedicine (Lond)* 3 (2):175–182. doi: 10.2217/17435889.3.2.175.

Hassan, H. A. F. M., L. Smyth, N. Rubio, K. Ratnasothy, J. T. W. Wang, S. S. Bansal, H. D. Summers, S. S. Diebold, G. Lombardi, and K. T. Al-Jamal. 2016. "Carbon nanotubes' surface chemistry determines their potency as vaccine nanocarriers in vitro and in vivo." *Journal of Controlled Release: Official Journal of the Controlled Release Society* 225:205–216. doi: 10.1016/j.jconrel.2016.01.030.

Hauke, F., and A. Hirsch. 2010. Covalent functionalization of carbon nanotubes. In: Guldi, D.M., Martín, N. (eds.) *Carbon Nanotubes and Related Structures*. Wiley-VCH, Weinheim.

Hay, P. J., W. J. Hunt, and W. A. Goddard III. 1972. "Generalized valence bond description of simple alkanes, ethylene, and acetylene." *Journal of the American Chemical Society* 94 (24):8293–8301.

Heidarian, M., A. Khazaei, and J. Saien. 2021. "Grafting drugs to functionalized single-wall carbon nanotubes as a potential method for drug delivery." *Physical Chemistry Research* 9 (1):57–68. doi: 10.22036/pcr.2020.232018.1775.

Heister, Elena, Vera Neves, Carmen Tîlmaciu, Kamil Lipert, Vanesa Sanz Beltrán, Helen M. Coley, S. Ravi P. Silva, and Johnjoe McFadden. 2009. "Triple functionalisation of single-walled carbon nanotubes with doxorubicin, a monoclonal antibody, and a fluorescent marker for targeted cancer therapy." *Carbon* 47 (9):2152–2160. doi: 10.1016/j.carbon.2009.03.057.

Hirano, Seishiro, Sanae Kanno, and Akiko Furuyama. 2008. "Multi-walled carbon nanotubes injure the plasma membrane of macrophages." *Toxicology and Applied Pharmacology* 232 (2):244–251. doi: 10.1016/j.taap.2008.06.016.

Hirsch, Andreas, and Otto Vostrowsky. 2005. "Functionalization of carbon nanotubes." In: Schlüter, A. Dieter (ed.) *Functional Molecular Nanostructures*, 193–237. Springer, Berlin.

Hou, Peng-Xiang, Chang Liu, and Hui-Ming Cheng. 2008. "Purification of carbon nanotubes." *Carbon* 46 (15):2003–2025. doi: 10.1016/j.carbon.2008.09.009.

Iijima, Sumio. 1991. "Helical microtubules of graphitic carbon." *Nature* 354 (6348):56–58. doi: 10.1038/354056a0.

Iijima, Sumio, and Toshinari Ichihashi. 1993. "Single-shell carbon nanotubes of 1-nm diameter." *Nature* 363 (6430):603–605. doi: 10.1038/363603a0.

Ishigami, M., John Cumings, A. Zettl, and S. Chen. 2000. "A simple method for the continuous production of carbon nanotubes." *Chemical Physics Letters* 319 (5):457–459. doi: 10.1016/S0009-2614(00)00151-2.

Islam, M. F., E. Rojas, D. M. Bergey, A. T. Johnson, and A. G. Yodh. 2003. "High weight fraction surfactant solubilization of single-wall carbon nanotubes in water." *Nano Letters* 3 (2):269–273. doi: 10.1021/nl025924u.

Iyer, Arun K., Greish Khaled, Jun Fang, and Hiroshi Maeda. 2006. "Exploiting the enhanced permeability and retention effect for tumor targeting." *Drug Discovery Today* 11 (17):812–818. doi: 10.1016/j.drudis.2006.07.005.

Jampilek, J., and K. Kralova. 2021. "Advances in drug delivery nanosystems using graphene-based materials and carbon nanotubes." *Materials (Basel)* 14 (5). doi: 10.3390/ma14051059.

Jin, Sumin, Piyumi Wijesekara, Patrick D. Boyer, Kris Noel Dahl, and Mohammad F. Islam. 2017. "Length-dependent intracellular bundling of single-walled carbon nanotubes influences retention." *Journal of Materials Chemistry B* 5 (32):6657–6665. doi: 10.1039/C7TB00735C.

Kafa, Houmam, Julie Tzu-Wen Wang, Noelia Rubio, Rebecca Klippstein, Pedro M. Costa, Hatem A.F.M. Hassan, Jane K. Sosabowski, Sukhvinder S. Bansal, Jane E. Preston, and N. Joan Abbott. 2016. "Translocation of LRP1 targeted carbon nanotubes of different diameters across the blood–brain barrier in vitro and in vivo." *Journal of Controlled Release* 225: 217–229.

Kafa, Houmam, Julie Tzu-Wen Wang, Noelia Rubio, Kerrie Venner, Glenn Anderson, Elzbieta Pach, Belén Ballesteros, Jane E. Preston, N. Joan Abbott, and Khuloud T. Al-Jamal. 2015. "The interaction of carbon nanotubes with an in vitro blood-brain barrier model and mouse brain in vivo." *Biomaterials* 53:437–452 doi: 10.1016/j.biomaterials.2015.02.083.

Kang, Bin, Jun Li, Shuquan Chang, Mingzhu Dai, Chao Ren, Yaodong Dai, and Da Chen. 2012. "Subcellular tracking of drug release from carbon nanotube vehicles in living cells." *Small* 8 (5):777–782. doi: 10.1002/smll.201101714.

Karadas, Nurgul, and Sibel A. Ozkan. 2014. "Electrochemical preparation of sodium dodecylsulfate doped over-oxidized polypyrrole/multi-walled carbon nanotube composite on glassy carbon electrode and its application on sensitive and selective determination of anticancer drug: Pemetrexed." *Talanta* 119:248–254 doi: 10.1016/j.talanta.2013.10.065.

Karimi, M., N. Solati, M. Amiri, H. Mirshekari, E. Mohamed, M. Taheri, M. Hashemkhani, A. Saeidi, M. A. Estiar, P. Kiani, A. Ghasemi, S. M. Basri, A. R. Aref, and M. R. Hamblin. 2015. "Carbon nanotubes part I: Preparation of a novel and versatile drug-delivery vehicle." *Expert Opin Drug Deliv* 12 (7):1071–1087. doi: 10.1517/17425247.2015.1003806.

Karimi, M., N. Solati, A. Ghasemi, M. A. Estiar, M. Hashemkhani, P. Kiani, E. Mohamed, A. Saeidi, M. Taheri, P. Avci, A. R. Aref, M. Amiri, F. Baniasadi, and M. R. Hamblin. 2015. "Carbon nanotubes part II: A remarkable carrier for drug and gene delivery." *Expert Opinion on Drug Delivery* 12 (7):1089–1105. doi: 10.1517/17425247.2015.1004309.

Karnati, K. R., and Y. Wang. 2018. "Understanding the co-loading and releasing of doxorubicin and paclitaxel using chitosan functionalized single-walled carbon nanotubes by molecular dynamics simulations." *Physical Chemistry Chemical Physics* 20 (14):9389–9400. doi: 10.1039/C8CP00124C.

Kharissova, O. V., and B. I. Kharisov. 2014. "Variations of interlayer spacing in carbon nanotubes." *RSC Advances* 4 (58):30807–30815. doi: 10.1039/C4RA04201H.

Kingston, C. T., and B. Simard. 2003. "Fabrication of carbon nanotubes." *Analytical Letters* 36 (15):3119–3145. doi: 10.1081/al-120026564.

Kou, L., J. Sun, Y. Zhai, and Z. He. 2013. "The endocytosis and intracellular fate of nanomedicines: Implication for rational design." *Asian Journal of Pharmaceutical Sciences* 8 (1):1–10. doi: 10.1016/j.ajps.2013.07.001.

Kumar, I., S. Rana, and J. W. Cho. 2011. "Cycloaddition reactions: A controlled approach for carbon nanotube functionalization." *Chemistry – A European Journal* 17 (40):11092–11101. doi: 10.1002/chem.201101260.

Kumar, M., G. Sharma, C. Misra, R. Kumar, B. Singh, O. P. Katare, and K. Raza. 2018. "N-desmethyl tamoxifen and quercetin-loaded multiwalled CNTs: A synergistic approach to overcome MDR in cancer cells." *Materials Science and Engineering: C Materials for Biological Applications* 89:274–282. doi: 10.1016/j.msec.2018.03.033.

Kurkuri, M. D., and T. M. Aminabhavi. 2004. "Poly(vinyl alcohol) and poly(-acrylic acid) sequential interpenetrating network pH-sensitive microspheres for the delivery of diclofenac sodium to the intestine." *Journal of Controlled Release* 96 (1):9–20. doi: 10.1016/j.jconrel.2003.12.025.

Kushwaha, S. K. S., S. Ghoshal, A. K. Rai, and S. Singh. 2013. "Carbon nanotubes as a novel drug delivery system for anticancer therapy: A review." *Brazilian Journal of Pharmaceutical Sciences* 49 (4):629–643. doi: 10.1590/s1984-82502013000400002.

Lacerda, L., J. Russier, G. Pastorin, M. A. Herrero, E. Venturelli, H. Dumortier, K.T. Al-Jamal, M. Prato, K. Kostarelos, and A. Bianco. 2012. "Translocation mechanisms of chemically functionalised carbon nanotubes across plasma membranes." *Biomaterials* 33 (11):3334–3343. doi: 10.1016/j.biomaterials.2012.01.024.

Lee, J. H., and Y. Yeo. 2015. "Controlled drug release from pharmaceutical nanocarriers." *Chemical Engineering Science* 125:75–84. doi: 10.1016/j.ces.2014.08.046.

Li, S.-D., and L. Huang. 2010. "Stealth nanoparticles: High density but sheddable PEG is a key for tumor targeting." *Journal of Controlled Release* 145 (3):178–181. doi: 10.1016/j.jconrel.2010.03.016.

Liu, Y., L. Gao, J. Sun, S. Zheng, L. Jiang, Y. Wang, H. Kajiura, Y. Li, and K. Noda. 2007. "A multi-step strategy for cutting and purification of single-walled carbon nanotubes." *Carbon* 45 (10):1972–1978.

Liu, Z., K. Chen, C. Davis, S. Sherlock, Q. Cao, X. Chen, and H. Dai. 2008. "Drug delivery with carbon nanotubes for in vivo cancer treatment." *Cancer Research* 68 (16):6652. doi: 10.1158/0008-5472.CAN-08-1468.

Liu, Z., A. C. Fan, K. Rakhra, S. Sherlock, A. Goodwin, X. Chen, Q. Yang, D. W. Felsher, and H. Dai. 2009. "Supramolecular stacking of doxorubicin on carbon nanotubes for in vivo cancer therapy." *Angewandte Chemie International Edition* 48 (41):7668–7672.

Liu, Z., X. Sun, N. Nakayama-Ratchford, and H. Dai. 2007. "Supramolecular chemistry on water-soluble carbon nanotubes for drug loading and delivery." *ACS Nano* 1 (1):50–56. doi: 10.1021/nn700040t.

Lu, W., M. Zu, J.-H. Byun, B.-S. Kim, and T.-W. Chou. 2012. "State of the art of carbon nanotube fibers: Opportunities and challenges." *Advanced Materials* 24 (14):1805–1833. doi: 10.1002/adma.201104672.

Luo, X., C. Matranga, S. Tan, N. Alba, and X. T. Cui. 2011. "Carbon nanotube nanoreservior for controlled release of anti-inflammatory dexamethasone." *Biomaterials* 32 (26):6316–6323. doi: 10.1016/j.biomaterials.2011.05.020.

Ma, C.-C., Z.-L. Wang, T. Xu, Z.-Y. He, and Y.-Q. Wei. 2020. "The approved gene therapy drugs worldwide: From 1998 to 2019." *Biotechnology Advances* 40:107502. doi: 10.1016/j.biotechadv.2019.107502.

Maser, W. K., A. M. Benito, E. Muñoz, G. Marta de Val, M. Teresa Martínez, Á. Larrea, and G. F. de la Fuente. 2001. "Production of carbon nanotubes by CO_2-laser evaporation of various carbonaceous feedstock materials." *Nanotechnology* 12 (2):147.

Masotti, A., M. R. Miller, A. Celluzzi, L. Rose, F. Micciulla, P. W. F. Hadoke, S. Bellucci, and A. Caporali. 2016. "Regulation of angiogenesis through the efficient delivery of microRNAs into endothelial cells using polyamine-coated carbon nanotubes." *Nanomedicine: Nanotechnology, Biology, and Medicine* 12 (6):1511–1522. doi: 10.1016/j.nano.2016.02.017.

Matteucci, F., R. Giannantonio, F. Calabi, A. Agostiano, G. Gigli, and M. Rossi. 2018. "Deployment and exploitation of nanotechnology nanomaterials and nanomedicine." *AIP Conference Proceedings* 1990 (1):020001. doi: 10.1063/1.5047755.

McDevitt, M. R., D. Chattopadhyay, B. J. Kappel, J. S. Jaggi, S. R. Schiffman, C. Antczak, Jon T. Njardarson, R. Brentjens, and D. A. Scheinberg. 2007. "Tumor targeting with antibody-functionalized, radiolabeled carbon nanotubes." *Journal of Nuclear Medicine* 48 (7):1180. doi: 10.2967/jnumed.106.039131.

Mercier, G., C. Hérold, J.-F. Marêché, S. Cahen, J. Gleize, J. Ghanbaja, G. Lamura, C. Bellouard, and B. Vigolo. 2013. "Selective removal of metal impurities from single walled carbon nanotube samples." *New Journal of Chemistry* 37 (3):790–795. doi: 10.1039/C2NJ41057E.

Meyyappan, M. 2004. *Carbon Nanotubes: Science and Applications.* 1st ed: CRC Press.

Mitchell, M. J., M. M. Billingsley, R. M. Haley, M. E. Wechsler, N. A. Peppas, and R. Langer. 2021. "Engineering precision nanoparticles for drug delivery." *Nature Reviews Drug Discovery* 20 (2):101–124. doi: 10.1038/s41573-020-0090-8.

Mohammadi, E., M. Zeinali, M. Mohammadi-Sardoo, M. Iranpour, B. Behnam, and A. Mandegary. 2020. "The effects of functionalization of carbon nanotubes on toxicological parameters in mice." *Human & Experimental Toxicology* 39 (9):1147–1167. doi: 10.1177/0960327119899988.

Moon, H. K., S. H. Lee, and H. C. Choi. 2009. "In vivo near-infrared mediated tumor destruction by photothermal effect of carbon nanotubes." *ACS Nano* 3 (11):3707–3713. doi: 10.1021/nn900904h.

Mooney, E., P. Dockery, U. Greiser, M. Murphy, and V. Barron. 2008. "Carbon nanotubes and mesenchymal stem cells: Biocompatibility, proliferation and differentiation." *Nano Letters* 8 (8):2137–2143. doi: 10.1021/nl073300o.

Morris, J. E. 2013. *Graphene, Carbon Nanotubes, and Nanostructures: Techniques and Applications*. CRC Press.

Mozafari, M. 2020. *Nanoengineered Biomaterials for Advanced Drug Delivery*. Elsevier, Amsterdam. Edited by S. Pattnaik, Y. Surendra, J. V. Rao, and K. Swain.

Nance, E. 2019. "Careers in nanomedicine and drug delivery." *Advanced Drug Delivery Reviews* 144:180–189. doi: 10.1016/j.addr.2019.06.009.

Neagoe, I. B., C. Braicu, C. Matea, C. Bele, G. Florin, K. Gabriel, C. Veronica, and A. Irimie. 2012. "Efficient siRNA delivery system using carboxilated single-wall carbon nanotubes in cancer treatment." *Journal of Biomedical Nanotechnology* 8 (4):567–574. doi: 10.1166/jbn.2012.1411.

Nikolaev, P., M. J. Bronikowski, R. Kelley Bradley, F. Rohmund, D. T. Colbert, K. A. Smith, and R. E. Smalley. 1999. "Gas-phase catalytic growth of single-walled carbon nanotubes from carbon monoxide." *Chemical Physics Letters* 313 (1–2):91–97. doi: 10.1016/s0009-2614(99)01029-5.

Nish, A., J.-Y. Hwang, J. Doig, and R. J. Nicholas. 2007. "Highly selective dispersion of single-walled carbon nanotubes using aromatic polymers." *Nature Nanotechnology* 2 (10):640–646. doi: 10.1038/nnano.2007.290.

Novoselov, K. S., A. K. Geim, S. V. Morozov, D. Jiang, Y. Zhang, S. V. Dubonos, I. V. Grigorieva, and A. A. Firsov. 2004. "Electric field effect in atomically thin carbon films." *Science* 306 (5696):666–669. doi: 10.1126/science.1102896.

O'Connell, M. J. 2006. *Carbon Nanotubes: Properties and Applications*. 1st ed: CRC Press, Taylor & Francis Group.

Ohta, S., E. Kikuchi, A. Ishijima, T. Azuma, I. Sakuma, and T. Ito. 2020. "Investigating the optimum size of nanoparticles for their delivery into the brain assisted by focused ultrasound-induced blood–brain barrier opening." *Scientific Reports* 10 (1):18220. doi: 10.1038/s41598-020-75253-9.

Pantarotto, D., C. D. Partidos, R. Graff, J. Hoebeke, J.-P. Briand, M. Prato, and A. Bianco. 2003. "Synthesis, structural characterization, and immunological properties of carbon nanotubes functionalized with peptides." *Journal of the American Chemical Society* 125 (20):6160–6164. doi: 10.1021/ja034342r.

Pardridge, W. M. 2012. "Drug transport across the blood–brain barrier." *Journal of Cerebral Blood Flow & Metabolism* 32 (11):1959–1972. doi: 10.1038/jcbfm.2012.126.

Patra, J. K., G. Das, L. F. Fraceto, E. V. Ramos Campos, M. del Pilar Rodriguez-Torres, L. S. Acosta-Torres, L. A. Diaz-Torres, R. Grillo, M. Kumara Swamy, S. Sharma, S. Habtemariam, and H.-S. Shin. 2018. "Nano based drug delivery systems: Recent developments and future prospects." *Journal of Nanobiotechnology* 16 (1):71. doi: 10.1186/s12951-018-0392-8.

Pei, B., W. Wang, N. Dunne, and X. Li. 2019. "Applications of carbon nanotubes in bone tissue regeneration and engineering: Superiority, concerns, current advancements, and prospects." *Nanomaterials (Basel, Switzerland)* 9 (10):1501. doi: 10.3390/nano9101501.

Penotti, F., J. Gerratt, D. L. Cooper, and M. Raimondi. 1988. "The ab initio spin-coupled description of methane: Hybridization without preconceptions." *Journal of Molecular Structure: THEOCHEM* 169:421–436. doi: 10.1016/0166-1280(88)80274-4.

Perepelytsina, O. M., A. P. Ugnivenko, A. V. Dobrydnev, O. N. Bakalinska, A. I. Marynin, and M. V. Sydorenko. 2018. "Influence of carbon nanotubes and its derivatives on tumor cells in vitro and biochemical parameters, cellular blood composition in vivo." *Nanoscale Research Letters* 13 (1):286. doi: 10.1186/s11671-018-2689-9.

Persidis, A. 2000. "Cancer multidrug resistance." *Nature Biotechnology* 18 (S10): IT18-IT20. doi: 10.1038/80051.

Podesta, J. E., K. T. Al-Jamal, M. Antonia Herrero, B. Tian, H. Ali-Boucetta, V. Hegde, A. Bianco, M. Prato, and K. Kostarelos. 2009. "Antitumor activity and prolonged survival by carbon-nanotube-mediated therapeutic siRNA silencing in a human lung xenograft model." *Small* 5 (10):1176–1185. doi: 10.1002/smll.200801572.

Popov, V. N. 2004. "Carbon nanotubes: Properties and application." *Materials Science & Engineering R-Reports* 43 (3):61–102. doi: 10.1016/j.mser.2003.10.001.

Prajapati, S. K., A. Malaiya, P. Kesharwani, D. Soni, and A. Jain. 2022. "Biomedical applications and toxicities of carbon nanotubes." *Drug and Chemical Toxicology* 45 (1):435–450. doi: 10.1080/01480545.2019.1709492.

Principi, E., R. Girardello, A. Bruno, I. Manni, E. Gini, A. Pagani, A. Grimaldi, F. Ivaldi, T. Congiu, and D. De Stefano. 2016. "Systemic distribution of single-walled carbon nanotubes in a novel model: Alteration of biochemical parameters, metabolic functions, liver accumulation, and inflammation in vivo." *International Journal of Nanomedicine* 11:4299.

Proctor, John E., Daniel Melendrez Armada, and Aravind Vijayaraghavan. 2017. *An Introduction to Graphene and Carbon Nanotubes*. 1st ed. CRC Press, Boca Raton, FL.

Pugazhendhi, A., T. N. J. I. Edison, B. K. Velmurugan, J. A. Jacob, and I. Karuppusamy. 2018. "Toxicity of Doxorubicin (Dox) to different experimental organ systems." *Life Sciences* 200:26–30. doi: 10.1016/j.lfs.2018.03.023.

Raffa, V., G. Ciofani, O. Vittorio, C. Riggio, and A. Cuschieri. 2010. "Physicochemical properties affecting cellular uptake of carbon nanotubes." *Nanomedicine* 5 (1):89–97. doi: 10.2217/nnm.09.95.

Razzazan, A., F. Atyabi, B. Kazemi, and R. Dinarvand. 2016. "In vivo drug delivery of gemcitabine with PEGylated single-walled carbon nanotubes." *Materials Science and Engineering: C* 62:614–625. doi: 10.1016/j.msec.2016.01.076.

Rikhvanov, L. P., and N. V. Baranovskaya. 2013. "Element composition of human body." *International Conference on Frontiers of Environment, Energy and Bioscience (ICFEEB 2013)*.

Rinzler, A. G., J. Liu, H. Dai, P. Nikolaev, C. B. Huffman, F. J. Rodríguez-Macías, P. J. Boul, A. H. Lu, D. Heymann, D. T. Colbert, R. S. Lee, J. E. Fischer, A. M. Rao, P. C. Eklund, and R. E. Smalley. 1998. "Large-scale purification of single-wall carbon nanotubes: Process, product, and characterization." *Applied Physics A: Materials Science & Processing* 67 (1):29–37. doi: 10.1007/s003390050734.

Robertson, D. H., D. W. Brenner, and J. W. Mintmire. 1992. "Energetics of nanoscale graphitic tubules." *Physical Review B* 45 (21):12592–12595. doi: 10.1103/PhysRevB.45.12592.

Saliev, T. 2019. "The advances in biomedical applications of carbon nanotubes." *C-Journal of Carbon Research* 5 (2). doi: 10.3390/c5020029.

Santos, T., X. Fang, M.-T. Chen, W. Wang, R. Ferreira, N. Jhaveri, M. Gundersen, C. Zhou, P. Pagnini, F. M. Hofman, and T. C. Chen. 2014. "Sequential administration of carbon nanotubes and near-infrared radiation for the treatment of gliomas." *Frontiers in Oncology* 4 (180). doi: 10.3389/fonc.2014.00180.

Sattler, K. D. 2016. *Carbon Nanomaterials Sourcebook: Graphene, Fullerenes, Nanotubes, and Nanodiamonds, Volume I*. CRC Press.

Sciortino, N., S. Fedeli, P. Paoli, A. Brandi, P. Chiarugi, M. Severi, and S. Cicchi. 2017. "Multiwalled carbon nanotubes for drug delivery: Efficiency related to length and incubation time." *International Journal of Pharmaceutics* 521 (1):69–72. doi: 10.1016/j.ijpharm.2017.02.023.

Seyhan, A. A. 2019. "Lost in translation: The valley of death across preclinical and clinical divide – identification of problems and overcoming obstacles." *Translational Medicine Communications* 4 (1):18. doi: 10.1186/s41231-019-0050-7.

Sgobba, V., C. Ehli, and D. M. Guldi. 2012. "Chapter 15 Covalent approaches towards multifunctional carbon-nanotube materials." In *Fullerenes: Principles and Applications*, 549–612. The Royal Society of Chemistry. doi: 10.1039/9781849732956-00549.

Sheng, L., L. Shi, K. An, L. Yu, Y. Ando, and X. Zhao. 2011. "Effective and efficient purification of single-wall carbon nanotubes based on hydrogen treatment." *Chemical Physics Letters* 502 (1–3):101–106.

Shi, X., A. von dem Bussche, R. H. Hurt, A. B. Kane, and H. Gao. 2011. "Cell entry of one-dimensional nanomaterials occurs by tip recognition and rotation." *Nature Nanotechnology* 6 (11):714–719. doi: 10.1038/nnano.2011.151.

Shirley, J. L., Y. P. de Jong, C. Terhorst, and R. W. Herzog. 2020. "Immune responses to viral gene therapy vectors." *Molecular Therapy* 28 (3):709–722. doi: 10.1016/j.ymthe.2020.01.001.

Shityakov, S., E. Salvador, G. Pastorin, and C. Förster. 2015. "Blood-brain barrier transport studies, aggregation, and molecular dynamics simulation of multiwalled carbon nanotube functionalized with fluorescein isothiocyanate." *International Journal of Nanomedicine* 10:1703–1713. doi: 10.2147/IJN.S68429.

Sibbald, B. 2001. "Death but one unintended consequence of gene-therapy trial." *CMAJ: Canadian Medical Association Journal=journal de l'Association medicale canadienne* 164 (11):1612–1612.

Singh, R., D. Pantarotto, D. McCarthy, O. Chaloin, J. Hoebeke, C. D. Partidos, J. P. Briand, M. Prato, A. Bianco, and K. Kostarelos. 2005. "Binding and condensation of plasmid DNA onto functionalized carbon nanotubes: Toward the construction of nanotube-based gene delivery vectors." *Journal of the American Chemical Society* 127 (12):4388–4396. doi: 10.1021/ja0441561.

Sisto, T. J., L. N. Zakharov, B. M. White, and R. Jasti. 2016. "Towards pi-extended cycloparaphenylenes as seeds for CNT growth: Investigating strain relieving ring-openings and rearrangements." *Chemical Science* 7 (6):3681–3688. doi: 10.1039/C5SC04218F.

Sobhani, Z., R. Dinarvand, F. Atyabi, M. Ghahremani, and M. Adeli. 2011. "Increased paclitaxel cytotoxicity against cancer cell lines using a novel functionalized carbon nanotube." *International Journal of Nanomedicine* 6:705–719. doi: 10.2147/IJN.S17336.

Sobhani, Z., M. A. Behnam, F. Emami, A. Dehghanian, and I. Jamhiri. 2017. "Photothermal therapy of melanoma tumor using multiwalled carbon nanotubes." *International Journal of Nanomedicine* 12: 4509.

Song, Z.-M., L. Wang, N. Chen, A. Cao, Y. Liu, and H. Wang. 2016. "Biological effects of agglomerated multi-walled carbon nanotubes." *Colloids and Surfaces B: Biointerfaces* 142:65–73. doi: 10.1016/j.colsurfb.2016.02.032.

Spitalsky, Z., D. Tasis, K. Papagelis, and C. Galiotis. 2010. "Carbon nanotube-polymer composites: Chemistry, processing, mechanical and electrical properties." *Progress in Polymer Science* 35 (3):357–401. doi: 10.1016/j.progpolymsci.2009.09.003.

Stevens, J. L., A. Y. Huang, H. Peng, I. W. Chiang, V. N. Khabashesku, and J. L. Margrave. 2003. "Sidewall amino-functionalization of single-walled carbon nanotubes through fluorination and subsequent reactions with terminal diamines." *Nano Letters* 3 (3):331–336. doi: 10.1021/nl025944w.

Su, Z., S. Zhu, A. D. Donkor, C. Tzoganakis, and J. F. Honek. 2011. "Controllable delivery of small-molecule compounds to targeted cells utilizing carbon nanotubes." *Journal of the American Chemical Society* 133 (18):6874–6877. doi: 10.1021/ja1084282.

Summers, H. D., P. Rees, J. T. W. Wang, and K. T. Al-Jamal. 2017. "Spatially-resolved profiling of carbon nanotube uptake across cell lines." *Nanoscale* 9 (20):6800–6807. doi: 10.1039/C7NR01561E.

Sun, X., H. Shao, K. Xiang, Y. Yan, X. Yu, D. Li, W. Wu, L. Zhou, K.-F. So, Y. Ren, S. Ramakrishna, A. Li, and L. He. 2017. "Poly(dopamine)-modified carbon nanotube multilayered film and its effects on macrophages." *Carbon* 113:176–191. doi: 10.1016/j.carbon.2016.11.040.

Sundaram, P., and H. Abrahamse. 2020. "Effective photodynamic therapy for colon cancer cells using chlorin e6 coated hyaluronic acid-based carbon nanotubes." *International Journal of Molecular Sciences* 21 (13):4745. doi: 10.3390/ijms21134745.

Tanaka, K. 2014. *Carbon Nanotubes and Graphene*. 2nd ed: Elsevier.

Tasis, D., N. Tagmatarchis, A. Bianco, and M. Prato. 2006. "Chemistry of carbon nanotubes." *Chemical Reviews* 106 (3):1105–1136. doi: 10.1021/cr050569o.

Thorek, D. L. J., and A. Tsourkas. 2008. "Size, charge and concentration dependent uptake of iron oxide particles by non-phagocytic cells." *Biomaterials* 29 (26):3583–3590. doi: 10.1016/j.biomaterials.2008.05.015.

Tiwari, G., R. Tiwari, B. Sriwastawa, L. Bhati, S. Pandey, P. Pandey, and S. K. Bannerjee. 2012. "Drug delivery systems: An updated review." *International Journal of Pharmaceutical Investigation* 2 (1):2–11. doi: 10.4103/2230-973X.96920.

Tomanek, D. 2008. *Carbon Nanotubes: Advanced Topics in the Synthesis, Structure, Properties and Applications, Topics in Applied Physics*. Springer-Verlag, Berlin Heidelberg.

Unlu, A., M. Meran, B. Dinc, N. Karatepe, M. Bektas, and F. S. Guner. 2018. "Cytotoxicity of doxrubicin loaded single-walled carbon nanotubes." *Molecular Biology Reports* 45 (4):523–531. doi: 10.1007/s11033-018-4189-5.

Uthappa, U. T., O. R. Arvind, G. Sriram, D. Losic, J. H. Young, M. Kigga, and M. D. Kurkuri. 2020. "Nanodiamonds and their surface modification strategies for drug delivery applications." *Journal of Drug Delivery Science and Technology* 60. doi: 10.1016/j.jddst.2020.101993.

Uthappa, U. T., V. Brahmkhatri, G. Sriram, H. Y. Jung, J. Yu, N. Kurkuri, T. M. Aminabhavi, T. Altalhi, G. M. Neelgund, and M. D. Kurkuri. 2018. "Nature engineered diatom biosilica as drug delivery systems." *Journal of Controlled Release* 281:70–83. doi: 10.1016/j.jconrel.2018.05.013.

Uthappa, U. T., M. Kigga, G. Sriram, K. V. Ajeya, H.-Y. Jung, G. M. Neelgund, and M. D. Kurkuri. 2019. "Facile green synthetic approach of bio inspired polydopamine coated diatoms as a drug vehicle for controlled drug release and active catalyst for dye degradation." *Microporous and Mesoporous Materials* 288. doi: 10.1016/j.micromeso.2019.109572.

Uthappa, U. T., M. D. Kurkuri, and M. Kigga. 2019. "Nanotechnology advances for the development of various drug carriers." In: Prasad, R., Kumar, V., Kumar, M., Choudhary, D. (eds.) *Nanobiotechnology in Bioformulations*, 187–224. Springer, Cham.

Uthappa, U. T., G. Sriram, O. R. Arvind, S. Kumar, J. H. Young, G. M. Neelgund, D. Losic, and M. D. Kurkuri. 2020. "Engineering MIL-100(Fe) on 3D porous natural diatoms as a versatile high performing platform for controlled isoniazid drug release, Fenton's catalysis for malachite green dye degradation and environmental adsorbents for Pb^{2+} removal and dyes." *Applied Surface Science* 528. doi: 10.1016/j.apsusc.2020.146974.

Uthappa, U. T., G. Sriram, V. Brahmkhatri, M. Kigga, H.-Y. Jung, T. Altalhi, G. M. Neelgund, and M. D. Kurkuri. 2018. "Xerogel modified diatomaceous earth microparticles for controlled drug release studies." *New Journal of Chemistry* 42 (14):11964–11971. doi: 10.1039/c8nj01238e.

Uttekar, P. S., S. H. Lakade, V. K. Beldar, and M. T. Harde. 2019. "Facile synthesis of multi-walled carbon nanotube via folic acid grafted nanoparticle for precise delivery of doxorubicin." *IET Nanobiotechnology* 13 (7):688–696. doi: 10.1049/iet-nbt.2018.5421.

Wang, L., J. Shi, R. Liu, Y. Liu, J. Zhang, X. Yu, J. Gao, C. Zhang, and Z. Zhang. 2014. "Photodynamic effect of functionalized single-walled carbon nanotubes: A potential sensitizer for photodynamic therapy." *Nanoscale* 6 (9):4642–4651. doi: 10.1039/C3NR06835H.

Wang, L., J. Shi, H. Zhang, H. Li, Y. Gao, Z. Wang, H. Wang, L. Li, C. Zhang, C. Chen, Z. Zhang, and Y. Zhang. 2013. "Synergistic anticancer effect of RNAi and photothermal therapy mediated by functionalized single-walled carbon nanotubes." *Biomaterials* 34 (1):262–274. doi: 10.1016/j.biomaterials.2012.09.037.

Wang, M., S. Yu, C. Wang, and J. Kong. 2010. "Tracking the endocytic pathway of recombinant protein toxin delivered by multiwalled carbon nanotubes." *ACS Nano* 4 (11):6483–6490. doi: 10.1021/nn101445y.

Wang, N., Z. K. Tang, G. D. Li, and J. S. Chen. 2000. "Single-walled 4 Å carbon nanotube arrays." *Nature* 408 (6808):50–51. doi: 10.1038/35040702.
Wang, T., J. R. Upponi, and V. P. Torchilin. 2012. "Design of multifunctional non-viral gene vectors to overcome physiological barriers: Dilemmas and strategies." *International Journal of Pharmaceutics* 427 (1):3–20. doi: 10.1016/j.ijpharm.2011.07.013.
Wang, X., Z. Zhou, and F. Chen. 2017. "Surface modification of carbon nanotubes with an enhanced antifungal activity for the control of plant fungal pathogen." *Materials (Basel, Switzerland)* 10 (12):1375. doi: 10.3390/ma10121375.
Wang, Y., S. T. Yang, Y. Wang, Y. Liu, and H. Wang. 2012. "Adsorption and desorption of doxorubicin on oxidized carbon nanotubes." *Colloids Surf B Biointerfaces* 97:62–69. doi: 10.1016/j.colsurfb.2012.04.013.
Warburg, O., F. Wind, and E. Negelein 1927. "The metabolism of tumors in the body." *Journal of General Physiology* 8 (6):519–530. doi: 10.1085/jgp.8.6.519.
Wolfram, J., M. Zhu, Y. Yang, J. Shen, E. Gentile, D. Paolino, M. Fresta, G. Nie, C. Chen, H. Shen, M. Ferrari, and Y. Zhao. 2015. "Safety of nanoparticles in medicine." *Current Drug Targets* 16 (14):1671–1681. doi: 10.2174/1389450115666140804124808.
Xu, L. T., and T. H. Dunning, Jr. 2020. "Orbital hybridization in modern valence bond wave functions: Methane, ethylene, and acetylene." *Journal of Physical Chemistry A* 124 (1):204–214. doi: 10.1021/acs.jpca.9b11054.
Yang, S., Z. Wang, Y. Ping, Y. Miao, Y. Xiao, L. Qu, L. Zhang, Y. Hu, and J. Wang. 2020. "PEG/PEI-functionalized single-walled carbon nanotubes as delivery carriers for doxorubicin: Synthesis, characterization, and in vitro evaluation." *Beilstein Journal of Nanotechnology* 11:1728–1741. doi: 10.3762/bjnano.11.155.
Yu, B., L. Tan, R. Zheng, H. Tan, and L. Zheng. 2016. "Targeted delivery and controlled release of Paclitaxel for the treatment of lung cancer using single-walled carbon nanotubes." *Materials Science and Engineering: C* 68:579–584. doi: 10.1016/j.msec.2016.06.025.
Yuan, X., X. Zhang, L. Sun, Y. Wei, and X. Wei. 2019. "Cellular toxicity and immunological effects of carbon-based nanomaterials." *Particle and Fibre Toxicology* 16 (1):18. doi: 10.1186/s12989-019-0299-z.
Yusof, A. M., N. A. Buang, L. S. Yean, M. L. Ibrahim, M. Rusop, and T. Soga. 2009. "The use of multi-walled carbon nanotubes as possible carrier in drug delivery system for aspirin." In: *AIP Conference Proceedings*.
Zardini, H. Z., A. Amiri, M. Shanbedi, M. Maghrebi, and M. Baniadam. 2012. "Enhanced antibacterial activity of amino acids-functionalized multi walled carbon nanotubes by a simple method." *Colloids and Surfaces B: Biointerfaces* 92:196–202. doi: 10.1016/j.colsurfb.2011.11.045.
Zhang, M., W. Wang, Y. Cui, X. Chu, B. Sun, N. Zhou, and J. Shen. 2018. "Magnetofluorescent Fe_3O_4/carbon quantum dots coated single-walled carbon nanotubes as dual-modal targeted imaging and chemo/photodynamic/photothermal triple-modal therapeutic agents." *Chemical Engineering Journal* 338:526–538. doi: 10.1016/j.cej.2018.01.081.
Zhang, W., Z. Zhang, and Y. Zhang. 2011. "The application of carbon nanotubes in target drug delivery systems for cancer therapies." *Nanoscale Research Letters* 6:555. doi: 10.1186/1556-276X-6-555.

Zhang, Y. N., and L. X. Zheng. 2010. "Towards chirality-pure carbon nanotubes." *Nanoscale* 2 (10):1919–1929. doi: 10.1039/c0nr00222d.

Zhao, D., D. Alizadeh, L. Zhang, W. Liu, O. Farrukh, E. Manuel, D. J. Diamond, and B. Badie. 2011. "Carbon nanotubes enhance CpG uptake and potentiate antiglioma immunity." *Clinical Cancer Research* 17 (4):771. doi: 10.1158/1078-0432.CCR-10-2444.

Zhao, J. J., X. S. Chen, and J. R. H. Xie. 2006. "Optical properties and photonic devices of doped carbon nanotubes." *Analytica Chimica Acta* 568 (1-2):161–170. doi: 10.1016/j.aca.2006.02.006.

Zhou, F., S. Wu, Y. Yuan, W. R. Chen, and D. Xing. 2012. "Mitochondria-targeting photoacoustic therapy using single-walled carbon nanotubes." *Small* 8 (10):1543–1550. doi: 10.1002/smll.201101892.

Index